HUMAN MOTOR CONTROL

SECOND EDITION

HUMAN MOTOR CONTROL

SECOND EDITION

DAVID A. ROSENBAUM
Pennsylvania State University
University Park, PA

ELSEVIER

AMSTERDAM • BOSTON • HEIDELBERG • LONDON
NEW YORK • OXFORD • PARIS • SAN DIEGO
SAN FRANCISCO • SINGAPORE • SYDNEY • TOKYO
Academic Press is an imprint of Elsevier

30 Corporate Drive, Suite 400, Burlington, MA 01803, USA
525 B Street, Suite 1900, San Diego, California 92101-4495, USA
84 Theobald's Road, London WC1X 8RR, UK

Library of Congress Cataloging-in-Publication Data
Application submitted

British Library Cataloguing-in-Publication Data
A catalogue record for this book is available from the British Library.

ISBN: 978-0-12-374226-1

For information on all Academic Press publications
visit our Web site at www.elsevierdirect.com

Printed and bound by CPI Group (UK) Ltd, Croydon, CR0 4YY
Transferred to digital print 2012

Contents

Acknowledgments   xiii
Preface   xv

I

PRELIMINARIES

1. Introduction

Understanding Human Motor Control   2
Levels of Analysis   4
Fields Contributing to Research on Human Motor Control   6
  Physics   6
  Engineering   6
  Statistics   7
  Behavioral Science, Cognitive Science, and Human Factors   7
  Physiology, Neuroscience, Medicine, and Allied Fields   7
Organization of the Book   7
Summary   9

2. Core Problems

The Degrees of Freedom Problem   12
  Whose Problem Is the Degrees of Freedom Problem?   13
  Why the Term "Degrees of Freedom"?   14
  Synergies   14
  Relying on Mechanics   18
  Efficiency   18
The Sequencing and Timing Problem   20
  Speech Errors   20
  Coarticulation   22
  Timing   23
The Perceptual-Motor Integration Problem   25
  Feedback   25
  Feedforward   26
  Movement Enhances Perception   28
  Movement Informs Perception   29
  Mirror Neurons   31
The Learning Problem   32
  Learning by Doing   33
  Learning by Practicing Deliberately   34
  Learning Through Specificity of Practice   35
  Learning Through Neural Plasticity   37

Summary   39
Further Reading   41

3. Physiological Foundations

Muscle   46
   The Length-Tension Relation   47
   Motor Units and Recruitment   49
Proprioception   50
   Muscle Spindles   51
   Golgi Tendon Organs   53
   Joint Receptors   54
   Cutaneous Receptors   54
Spinal Cord   55
   Spinal Reflexes   55
   Servo Theory   55
   α-γ Coactivation   57
   Recurrent Inhibition   57
   Reciprocal Inhibition   58
   The Smart Spinal Cord   60
   Tuning of Spinal Reflexes   61
Cerebellum   61
   Regulation of Muscle Tone   62
   Coordination   63
   Timing   63
   Learning   65
Basal Ganglia   65
   Huntington's Disease   66
   Parkinson's Disease   66
   Theories of Basal Ganglia Function   67
Motor Cortex   69
   Force and Direction Control   71
   Whole-Body Movement   73
   Long-Loop Reflexes   74
Premotor Cortex   75
Supplementary Motor Area   76
Parietal Cortex   80
   Apraxia   81
   Cross-Modal Integration   82
Disconnections   84
Concluding Remarks   85
Summary   86
Further Reading   89

4. Psychological Foundations

Theories of Sequencing and Timing   94
   Response Chaining   94
   Element-to-Position Associations   97
   Inter-Element Inhibition   98
   Hierarchies   99

Skill Acquisition   101
   Closed-Loop Theory   101
   Generalized Programs   103
   Hierarchical Learning   106
   Mental Practice and Imagery   109
   Stage Theory   110
   Physical Changes in Skill Acquisition   112
Codes and Stores   115
   Codes   115
   Procedural and Declarative Knowledge   116
   Long-Term Memory   118
   Short-Term Memory   119
   History Effects   122
   Motor Programs   124
   The Motor Output Buffer   125
States of Mind   127
   Attention   127
   Intention   128
   Ideo-Motor Theory   129
Summary   131
Further Reading   134

II

THE ACTIVITY SYSTEMS

5. Walking

Descriptions of Walking   136
   Gait Patterns at Different Speeds   136
   Regularities in Gait Patterns   139
Neural Control of Locomotion   141
   Neural Circuits for Locomotion   143
   The Role of Sensory Feedback   146
   Descending Effects   147
   Anticipatory Postural Adjustments   150
Walking Machines   151
The Development of Walking   154
   Neonatal Reflexes   155
   Disappearance and Reappearance of Stepping   156
Models of Motor Development   158
Navigating   161
   Visual Kinesthesis   161
   Development of Visual Guidance   163
Memory   164
   Route Maps and Survey Maps   165
   Memory and Feedback   166
Summary   168
Further Reading   171

6. Looking

Blinking   174
Accommodation   177
Pupil Constriction and Dilation   177
General Features of Eye Movements   179
    Why Moveable Eyes?   179
    Physical Dynamics   180
    Activation of the Extra-Ocular Muscles   182
    Conjugate and Disjunctive Eye Movements   184
    Miniature Eye Movements   184
Saccades   187
    Saccadic Suppression   191
    Saccades and Attention   192
Smooth Pursuit Movements   194
    Optokinetic Nystagmus   195
    Vestibular-Oculo-Motor Reflex   197
Vergence Movements   200
Eye Movements and Space Constancy   201
Development and Plasticity of Oculo-Motor Control   205
Summary   206
Further Reading   209

7. Reaching and Grasping

The Development of Reaching and Grasping   214
    Direction   215
    Distance   215
    Orientation   215
    Size   216
    Functional Tuning of Grasps in Infancy   216
Visual Guidance   217
    Vision and Touch   219
    Vision for Action   221
    Eye-Hand Coordination   222
Aiming   225
    Woodworth's Pioneering Study   227
    Fitts' Law   229
    Iterative Corrections Model   230
    Impulse Variability Model   231
    Optimized Initial Impulse Model   232
Equilibrium Point Hypothesis   233
Discrete Versus Continuous Movements   237
Intersegmental Coordination   238
    Transport and Grasp Phases   240
    Hand-Space versus Joint-Space Planning   241
    Moving Two Hands at Once   244
Summary   248
Further Reading   249

8. Drawing and Writing

Drawing   254
  Planning of Strokes   254
  The Isogony Principle   257
  Two-Third Power Law   258
  Drawing Smoothly   262
Control of Writing   263
  Error Analyses   263
  Dysgraphia   263
  Reaction Time Evidence for Grapheme Selection   265
  Reaction Time Evidence for Allograph Selection   265
  Writing Size, Relative Timing, and Absolute Timing   266
  Context Effects   268
  Writing and Handedness   270
The Dynamic Dominance Hypothesis   272
Summary   273
Further Reading   275

9. Keyboarding

Reaction Time   279
  Simple Reaction Time   279
  Choice Reaction Time   280
  Stimulus-Response Compatibility   282
  Ideo-Motor Accounts of Stimulus-Response Compatibility   284
  The SNARC Effect   285
  The Simon Effect   286
  The Stroop Effect   286
  Response-Response Compatibility   287
Simultaneous and Sequential Finger Presses   288
  Simultaneous Keystrokes   288
  Sequences of Keypresses   289
  Learning Keyboard Sequences   293
  Control of Rhythm and Timing   294
  Hierarchical Time Keepers   296
  Event Timing   297
  Amodality of Timing   299
  Integration of Serial Order and Timing   300
  Adjusting the Rate of Production for Entire Sequences   301
Typing   303
  Historical Issues   304
  Units of Typing Control   306
  Typing Errors   307
  Timing of Keystrokes in Typewriting   307
  Rumelhart and Norman's Model of Typewriting   312
Piano Playing   314
Summary   317
Further Reading   321

10. Speaking and Singing

The Issues   324
Overview of the Chapter   326
The Vocal Tract and Articulatory Dynamics   328
   The Respiratory System   328
   Laryngeal Mechanisms   329
   Articulatory Mechanisms   331
   The Pharynx   332
   Vowels   332
   Consonants   333
Variability   335
   The Motor Theory of Speech Perception   336
   The Target Hypothesis   337
   Relative Positions and Acoustic Targets   339
   A Mechanism for Relative Positioning   341
   A Parallel Distributed Processing System for Coarticulation   343
High-Level Control of Speech   346
   Word Games   346
   Laboratory Studies of Speaking Speed   347
   Speech Errors   349
Brain Mechanisms Underlying Speech   353
Bird Song   354
Motor Resonance   357
Summary   359
Further Reading   362

11. Smiling

Physical Control of the Face   364
Neural Control of the Face   366
   Control of the Upper and Lower Face   366
   Volitional and Emotional Control   366
   Left-Right Differences   368
Origins of Emotional Expression   369
   Innateness and Universality   369
   Causal Connections Between Expressions and Emotions   370
   Associations Between Expressions and Emotions   371
Social Interaction   374
   Imitation in Newborns   375
   Imitation in Married Couples   375
Summary   377
Further Reading   378

III

PRINCIPLES AND PROSPECTS

12. Moving On

Integration   379
  Hitting Oncoming Balls   380
  Golf Putting   383
  Walking and Reaching   385
  Enactive Cognition   386
  More Subtle Manifestations of Cognition in Action   388
  Moving with Others   391
  Motion and Emotion   392
Individual Differences   395
Theories of Human Motor Control   397
  Dynamical Systems Theory   400
  Optimization   405
Innovations   412
  Genetics   412
  Technology   415
Concluding Remarks   418
Summary   421
Further Reading   423

References   425
Author Index   467
Subject Index   485

Acknowledgments

One reason this book exists is that a number of colleagues and students urged me to write it. I thank them for their encouragement but refrain from naming all of them here because, honestly, I don't know who all of them are. Often at conferences, young investigators who had read the first edition of *Human Motor Control* asked me when I would be coming out with a second edition. I confessed that I didn't know *if* I would be preparing a second edition, let alone *when* I would do so, but I appreciated their inquiries and felt encouraged by them.

Bruce Roberts, then at Elsevier, the parent company of Academic Press, contacted me in August 2006 and invited me to consider a second edition of *Human Motor Control*. I'm not sure what triggered Bruce's invitation 15 years after the first edition's release, but his email was welcome and reassuring. I hadn't embarked on a second edition because I was so busy with my lab research, with my responsibilities as Editor of *Journal of Experimental Psychology: Human Perception and Performance* for the 2000–2005 volumes, and with the other textbook I wrote in the interim, *MATLAB for Behavioral Scientists* (Rosenbaum, 2007). With the editing and other textbook out of the way, I felt more open to embarking on a second edition of this book. Nikki Levy helped seal the deal with Elsevier. I appreciate her patient counsel as I struggled with the decision about whether to undertake a major project like this. I also thank the people associated with Elsevier who helped with aspects of the book's production: Joanna Dinsmore, Jerome Devaraj Gnanasekar, Paul Gottehrer, and Barbara Makinster.

In the years intervening between the first and second editions of this book, I was fortunate to receive support for my research from a number of sources. I appreciate the grants I received from the National Science Foundation, the National Institutes of Health, Moss Rehabilitation Research Institute, the Research and Graduate Studies Office of Penn State's College of Liberal Arts, Penn State's Children, Youth, and Families Consortium Center, and Penn State's Science Research Institute.

I owe a great debt of gratitude to my students and colleagues who helped me continue to learn about human motor control. My graduate students at the University of Massachusetts and then at Penn State University (where I moved in 1994) were extraordinarily helpful in helping me see the many areas in which I needed to learn more about motor control. The graduate students with whom I have had the privilege of working at these two institutions were Jason Augustyn, Janey Barnes, Liana Brown, Chase Coelho, Rajal Cohen, Amanda Dawson, Jeff Eder, Cathy Elsinger, Sascha Engelbrecht, Martin Fischer, Bob Gregory, Marc Grosjean, Carrie Harp, Steve Jax, Loukia Loukopoulos, Myro Joy Lee, Esa Rantanen, Joe Santamaria, Jackie Shin, Jim Slotta, Robrecht van der Wel, and Wei Zhang.

Faculty colleagues at the two institutions likewise helped me learn about human motor control. In this regard, I am indebted to Neil Berthier, Frederick Brown, Graham Caldwell, Rich Carlson, Scott Chaiken, John Challis, Chuck Clifton, Rick Gilmore, Joe Hamil, Rachel Keen, Judy Kroll, Mark Latash, Cathleen Moore, Toby Mordkoff, Jerry Myers, Steve Piazza,

Sandy Pollatsek, Bill Ray, Keith Rayner, Bob Sainberg, Neil Sharkey, Sam Slobounov, Dagmar Sternad, Dan Weiss, Arnie Well, Michael Wenger, and Vladimir Zatsiorsky.

Individuals with whom I have collaborated on research are included in the foregoing lists but some were not. I would be remiss in not mentioning them here: Gisa Aschersleben, Adam Boltz, Peter Dixon, Robin Fleckenstein, Matt Gaydos, Scott Glover, Erin Halloran, Frouke Hermens, Chris Jansen, Peter Keller, Iring Koch, Ruud Meulenbroek, Wolfgang Prinz, Brian Rogosky, Andrei Semenov, Bert Steenbergen, Arnold Thomassen, Caroline van Heugten, Jonathan Vaughan, Matt Walsh, Jason Wark, Edmond Wascher, Florian Waszak, and Marty Weigelt. It has been wonderful to work and publish with these individuals. Much of what I have learned about human motor control is directly due to their influence.

Several colleagues helped with aspects of preparation of this second edition. Many of them were kind enough to reply to my emails in which I requested a bit more information about the whereabouts of various references and the like. For their assistance, I thank Karen Adolph, Chris Bertram, Bruce Bridgeman, Jason Friedman, Robert Full, Dexter Gormley, Ron Marteniuk, Dennis Proffitt, and Tim Welsh. I also thank Elina Mainela-Arnold for telling me about the unique gait of Icelandic horses (see Chapter 11).

The first edition of *Human Motor Control* was dedicated to my wife, Judith F. Kroll. My dedication to Judy has only deepened over the years, so I re-dedicate this second edition to her. Around the time of this writing, Judy and I celebrated our 33rd wedding anniversary, a marriage made all the more blessed by our wonderful daughters, Nora and Sarah Kroll-Rosenbaum, both of whom are successful not only in their careers (music and law, respectively), but also, and more importantly, in the way they treat others, being generous, loving people. I dedicate this book to all three of these special women in my life.

Preface

Think of all the things you did to look at this page. If you are in a bookshop, you had to enter the shop, walk down the aisles, locate the section of the bookstore that had this volume, find this book on the shelf, reach for it without yanking off other volumes, open the book, use your fingers to get to this page, and use your eyes to get to this point. For all these activities to occur, you had to draw on your knowledge of the world to make decisions about what to do, and you had to use your brain, muscles, and limbs to carry out the movements needed to bring you to your present position. How all these events came together is the subject of this book. So too are the things that make it possible to do other everyday tasks such as opening soda cans, writing notes, and singing love songs.

Motor control underlies all the activities we engage in: breathing, remaining upright if we wish, walking, reaching for objects, talking, and text messaging, to name a few. We have a vested interest in understanding how we control the motion and stability of our bodies. Many of the technologies we use and the skills we develop are embodied in the capacity to move or hold still. If we can understand how human motor control works, we can design safer workplaces, better tools, smarter robots, and more effective methods for teaching skills to others. Also, we can rehabilitate, cure, or possibly even prevent motorically expressed medical disorders.

The fact that this is the second edition of *Human Motor Control* means that the first edition was successful enough to warrant a second airing but not complete enough to stand on its own forever. The first edition was indeed successful, or at least as successful as a book on this topic can be. One reason for its success was that it conveyed the fun, excitement, and challenges of the many approaches that contribute to the field of human motor control. The second edition is meant to do the same. The many advances in the field call for an update.

As was true of the first edition of *Human Motor Control*, the second edition focuses on four core problems that lie at the heart of the field:

1. How are movements selected to achieve particular tasks when, as is almost always the case, infinitely many movements will achieve them (the *degrees of freedom* problem)?
2. How are behaviors sequenced in time (the *sequencing and timing* problem)?
3. How are perception and motor control combined (the *perceptual-motor integration* problem)?
4. How are perceptual-motor skills acquired (the *learning* problem)?

Throughout this book, these four problems will be at the heart of all that is discussed.

The organization of the second edition is similar to the organization of the book in its first incarnation. Part I, *Preliminaries*, sets the stage for the problems and approaches to be followed. Part II, *The Activity Systems*, focuses on the major functional systems that we depend on: Walking, Speaking, Smiling, and so on. The last part of the book, Part III, *Future Directions*, looks to new, exciting avenues of study, including new forms of therapy, the creation of closer ties between motor control and psychiatry, advances in genetics, new theoretical advances, and new methods for this area of study.

A great many advances have been made since the first edition appeared. Some of them are worth signaling in advance:

1. Schizophrenia and other psychiatric problems may be rooted in malfunctions of basic perceptual-motor circuits.
2. When physical actions are prepared, there is priming for the perceptual consequences that follow. This explains why, among other things, we can't tickle ourselves.
3. Our ability to understand what others say or do relies on internal modeling of the others' intentional state.
4. Robots can perform much more adroitly and with much less energy consumption than was true in the 1980's and early 1990's.
5. Advances in computational models of motor control have enabled simulated actors—sometimes called *avatars* or *simulacra*—to perform in ways that are much more like human performance than was possible before.
6. Neuroscientists have opened the "black box" of the brain, and have shed new light on neural circuits underlying action, attention, perception, and learning. Such advances have been made possible through a variety of methods that were only beginning to be developed in the early 1990's, most notably, functional magnetic resonance imaging (fMRI) and transmagnetic stimulation (TMS).
7. Major advances have been made in genetics, and these have provided new insights into the genetic bases of many motorically expressed abilities and disabilities.

Along with these developments have been others, too numerous to mention in this Preface. Suffice it to say, they will be presented in the text.

A minor change in the format of the second edition is to consolidate all the reference lists in one grand end-of-book References section. This avoids redundancy and highlights the fact that though the various topics in this book can be considered separately, all of them, ultimately, belong together.

Writing a second edition of a book affords an author the chance to atone for sins of commission and omission. The first edition had errors of both kinds. All the errors of which the author is aware have been rectified and new errors are, hopefully, few in number.

Besides these major additions, new material has been added throughout this volume and some old material that seems less critical has been removed. Of necessity, a book like this must be selective in what it includes. A number of new findings are not presented here just because of the way the story unfolded.

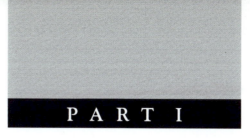

PART I

PRELIMINARIES

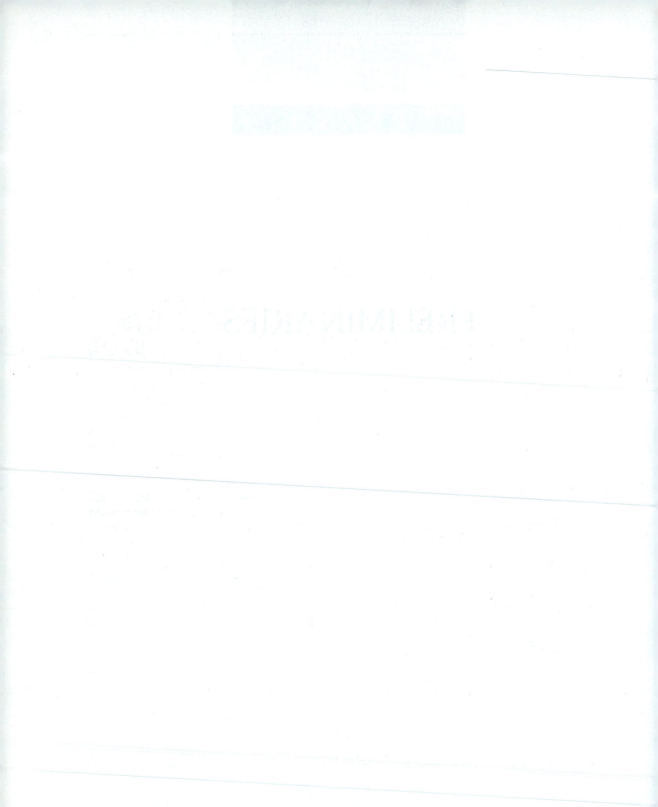

Introduction

O U T L I N E

Understanding Human Motor Control	2	Behavioral Science, Cognitive Science, and Human Factors	7
Levels of Analysis	4	Physiology, Neuroscience, Medicine, and Allied Fields	7
Fields Contributing to Research on Human Motor Control	6	Organization of the Book	7
Physics	6		
Engineering	6	Summary	9
Statistics	7		

How do we control the movements of our bodies? How do we walk, talk, sing, and smile? How do we manage to perform on the athletic field, play musical instruments, craft tools, and produce works of art? How do we learn to carry out these activities, and why are some of us better at them than others? What goes wrong when, through accident or disease, our ability to move is impaired? How can movement disabilities be restored or, better yet, prevented? And how can machines be made to carry out tasks that most people and animals perform effortlessly?

As this list of questions suggests, understanding the control of body movements can have significant effects in a wide range of endeavors. This is hardly surprising given that movements occur in all walks of life. In sports, where moving skillfully is the very essence of the activity, an understanding of motor control can permit heightened levels of competition. In the fine arts, where performance on stage or in the studio permit self-expression, understanding how movements are controlled can enhance the quality of that expression and can improve the training that leads to it. In medicine, where paralysis or lack of coordination can sabotage the quality of life, rehabilitation can be refined through deeper appreciation of the means by which the motor system functions. Finally, at home and in the workplace, where machines and other appliances are used, such devices can be made safer and more efficient through the application of principles gained through research on human motor control.

The question of how movements are controlled is just one of the questions in this field. The other major one is how we maintain stability. Holding an object steady in the face of changing wind conditions or while standing in a moving train are tasks that demand stabilization. Without muscular control, such tasks would be impossible. Because stabilization as well as movement are the jobs of the system covered here, we refer to that system as the *motor* system, not just the *movement* system or the *stabilization* system.

The word "motor" has a connotation that is worth dismissing immediately. That connotation is machinelike rigidity. Conventional motors churn away monotonously, performing the same motions over and over again. By contrast, behavior is endlessly novel, reflecting millions of years of evolution in which effective strategies developed for adaptation to ever-changing conditions.

If you doubt the sophistication of the motor system, consider the state of robots today. These devices embody much of what we know about motor control, but two-legged robots can barely walk across uneven surfaces without toppling over. Getting a robot to make a bed or fold laundry is out of the question.

The inability of robots to plan and control physical actions as flexibly as people and animals do means that people rather than robots are often called upon to perform in dangerous situations. Astronauts rather than robots typically carry out repairs in outer space. Beneath the earth, miners place themselves at risk as they pick away at unwieldy surfaces to extract coal or other minerals. On earth's surface, people defuse mines and sift through rubble after earthquakes, floods, or bomb blasts. If we knew how people control their bodies, we could endow robots with programs that enable the robots to move as people do and carry out dangerous and boring tasks that people currently do.

UNDERSTANDING HUMAN MOTOR CONTROL

What does it mean to understand human motor control? What is to be understood and what form should the understanding take? The answers to these questions are not as obvious as they might seem, for under normal circumstances, movement and stability just seem to happen. When things work well, it is easy to take them for granted. Indeed, a hallmark of skilled performance is that it occurs without the need for attention. When one thinks about performance, one's performance often suffers (Wulf, 2007).

By contrast, in abnormal circumstances, skills may be disrupted. Due to an accident or disease, the ability to move or stabilize the body may be impaired. A wide range of movement disorders afflict people, many of which will be discussed in this book. Considering these disorders and the factors that cause them can illuminate the factors that allow for normal performance. That knowledge can in turn contribute to our understanding of motor control in general.

What does it mean to understand motor control? One understands a system if one can predict and control it. We do not fully understand the weather, for example, because we cannot predict it, except at a gross level, and we cannot control the weather in any practical sense. On the other hand, we understand aeronautics well enough that we entrust our lives to airplanes traveling at breakneck speeds and at dizzying heights.

Virtually all neurologically normal individuals can control their movements reasonably well, but none of these individuals can say in detail how they achieve that control. Most adults can ride a bicycle, for example, but none can say how they do so. Even Albert Einstein would have had to think for a while before saying how he managed to cycle.

The fact that the principles of motor control cannot be easily articulated does not mean they can never be verbally expressed. The method for riding a bicycle has been written down:

> The rule observed by the cyclist is this. When he starts falling to the right he turns the handlebars to the right so that the course of the bicycle is deflected along a curve toward the right. This results in a centrifugal force pushing the cyclist to the left and offsets the gravitational force dragging him down to the right. This maneuver presently throws the cyclist out of balance to the left, which he counteracts by turning the handlebars to the left; and so he continues to keep himself in balance by winding along a series of appropriate curvatures. A simple analysis shows that for a given angle of unbalance the curvature of each winding is inversely proportional to the square of the speed at which the cyclist is proceeding [Polanyi, 1964, 49–50].

It is unlikely that Einstein drew on a verbal proposition like this one. The form of knowledge he probably relied on, and the form of knowledge that the rest of us use, is *tacit* or *implicit* knowledge (Polanyi, 1964).

By seeing that the knowledge underlying bike riding and other motor activities can be verbalized, we see that understanding motor control involves being able to state the principles of motor control. Ultimately, a theory of motor control will have to be expressed in a form that lets the theory be communicated in books such as this one and in scientific articles. In other words, it will have to verbalized. What form should that verbalized theory take?

It is possible to demonstrate one's understanding of a system by simulating it. In the case of motor control, such a demonstration can take the form of a robot that moves in a way that is indistinguishable from the way neurologically normal people do. Such a robot would pass the *Turing test* of motor intelligence. The term Turing test refers to a method of judging intelligence. The test was developed by Alan Turing, a mathematician and philosopher who helped crack the secret code used by the Nazis in World War II. Turing proposed a test for understanding verbally expressed intelligence. In the test, a human participant—call her Elana—interacts with a computer or with another person via a keyboard and display. The critical feature of the setup is that Elana does not know with whom she is dealing, a person or a computer. Based on the interactions, she tries to determine whether the individual is a computer or a person. If Elana cannot tell that she is interacting with a computer though her correspondent is in fact a machine, one can say that the designer of the computer succeeded in designing a machine that is as intelligent as a person. A Turing test of *motor* intelligence would work in similar ways. If Elana watched a robot dancing and thought it was a human being, she could say the designer of the dancing robot had captured, and truly *understood*, the control of dance.

Are we near such a demonstration? Humanoid robots developed by Mitsuo Kawato and his colleagues at the ATR Laboratories in Japan come close to passing the Turing test. One of those robots is shown in Figure 1.1. The robot shown in this figure can play air hockey as well as most people can. Even more interestingly, it does so in a way that is amazingly lifelike. If you find and watch a video of this robot on the world-wide web, be mindful that the person playing against the robot can do something the robot can't. The person can walk away, stroll down the hall, and, if he hears a child crying out for help in a room he passes, he

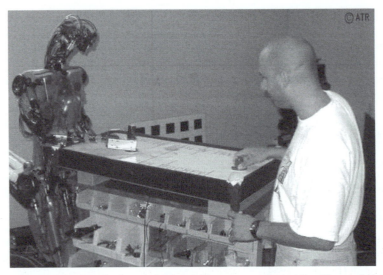

FIGURE 1.1   A humanoid robot playing air hockey with a person. From http://lasa.epfl.ch/events/events/iros03workshop/AirHockey.jpg.

can enter the room and pull the child out from the shelf and pile of books that have landed on him when he decided to climb up on his mother's bookcase. The robot, by contrast, can do just what it was programmed to do and no more.

LEVELS OF ANALYSIS

Reflecting on the air-hockey-playing robot, you might say that the lifelike performance of this robot is of only moderate interest, for human beings are made of flesh and blood, whereas robots, or at least robots like the air-hockey-playing robot shown in Figure 1.1, are made of synthetic materials. Doesn't that difference make the comparison between people and robots irrelevant to the understanding of *human* motor control?

The fact that one actor is real and the other is not does not mean that similarities between them are irrelevant. Apart from the fact that it is fun to watch a machine behave as people do, the deeper reason why robots and people are worth comparing is that different levels of analysis characterize the study of human motor control. Understanding these levels of analysis helps us appreciate why it useful to compare robots to people and animals.

David Marr (1982) proposed three levels of understanding for the study of such systems. One level of analysis that Marr identified was the *computational* level. This level, according to Marr, consists of a description, often expressed mathematically, of one or more functions that a system is supposed to achieve. The cartoon in Figure 1.2 illustrates the computational level. Here a cat prepares to jump onto a table. At some level, the cat's planning can be represented in equations and diagrams of the sorts that physicists write, although of course the cat does not explicitly use such equations anymore than people do, or, presumably, any

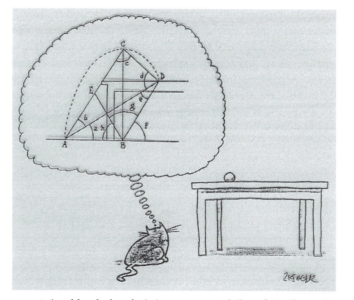

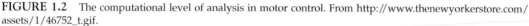

FIGURE 1.2 The computational level of analysis in motor control. From http://www.thenewyorkerstore.com/assets/1/46752_t.gif.

more than Einstein did when he rode his bicycle or carried out other physical activities. Even if equations are not used *explicitly*, they are used *implicitly* in performance. The computational level of analysis is concerned with those implicit equations.

How the cat actually jumps onto the table is left out of the computational description. The cat might crouch, leap up, prepare to land, and then use its sense of touch to check that it has landed. These behavioral and cognitive states constitute the second of Marr's levels, what can be called the *procedural* level. This term is used because it concerns events that occur in real time. (Marr actually used the term *algorithmic* level, but algorithms are *guaranteed* to work. Not all procedures do; getting a basketball to go through a net is not a sure thing, though it relies on a procedure.)

The third of Marr's levels is the *implementation* level. Here what counts is the physical stuff that permits procedures to be physically achieved. In the case of the jumping cat, the questions relevant to the implementation level are how muscles contract and relax, which brain regions become active or inactive, and so on. If the cat were robotic rather than mammalian, the relevant issues would be how the hydraulics of the actuators should be used, how the robot's battery power should be drawn on, and so on.

Having identified the three levels in Marr's triptych—the computational level, the procedural level, and the implementation level—we can now ask which of those three levels is most important in the study of human motor control. One way to address this question is to ask what would happen if any of the levels were excluded.

If the implementation level were excluded, most medical conditions involving motor control would be forgotten. No one would want that to happen, of course. We want advances in motor control to help people overcome motor-control difficulties.

If the algorithmic level were excluded, most studies of effective training procedures would be left by the wayside, as would research in the field of human factors—designing safer roads, smarter computer interfaces, and so on. Again, this is not what one would want.

Finally, if the computational level were excluded, most efforts to advance robotics would be abandoned. This, too, would be undesirable, for even if you have qualms about robots— perhaps you feel they will take over the jobs of too many people—computational work is of great importance. Thus, the understanding of human motor control requires work at all three levels. No level is more important than any other. All of the levels should be pursued and respected.

FIELDS CONTRIBUTING TO RESEARCH ON HUMAN MOTOR CONTROL

If all three levels of analysis contribute to the understanding of human motor control, one would expect fields that pursue any of the levels to contribute to this field of study. This is indeed the case, making human motor control a truly interdisciplinary area.

Physics

As mentioned earlier, physics plays a key role in the study of human motor control. This makes sense, considering that there are physical constraints on what we can do. We can only jump so high, run so fast, push so hard, and so on. Physics helps determine the factors that limit performance.

Physics can also indicate the factors that *enable* performance. A skillful baseball batter can learn how to use the momentum of her bat to maximize the force she exerts on the oncoming ball, and she can learn to hit the ball on the bat's "sweet spot," where bounce-back is maximized. Similarly, a cat preparing to jump onto a table can learn how to drop on its haunches before leaping up, exploiting elastic energy (Alexander, 1992).

Engineering

The computational style of analysis used by physicists in their theoretical work has also been used by engineers in their applied work. Men and women in engineering use physical principles to solve practical problems such as designing bridges that don't fall or designing computers that don't forget. Engineers also work on issues related to motor control such as robotics and prostheses (artificial appendages used by amputees).

One issue that engineers have worked on a great deal is how to use feedback effectively. Feedback is crucial for effective motor control, whether the performance entails standing on a moving train, chasing a fly ball, or driving an automobile. The approach to the analysis of feedback that engineers have developed is called *control theory*.

Statistics

If you take a pencil and move the tip back and forth as quickly as possible between two target points, always lifting the pencil between the hits, you will end up with a cloud of points near each target. These clouds show that, despite your best intentions, your performance is not perfect. No one's is. Everyone's performance is variable to some degree.

The study of variability as well as other features of data is the focus of statistics. Some important recent advances in the understanding of human motor control have been made possible through the application of statistics to motor control research.

Behavioral Science, Cognitive Science, and Human Factors

Researchers who study the procedural level of human motor control work in the fields of behavioral science, cognitive science, and human factors. Behavioral scientists study overt physical activity to predict and, on occasion, control behavior. Cognitive scientists are also interested in the procedural level, but are especially interested in the internal processes that allow behavior to unfold. Cognitive scientists often say they are interested in the *software* that makes behavior possible. Human factors specialists are interested in the applications of behavioral and cognitive science to practical problems such as designing easy-to-understand road signs, easy-to-use computer interfaces, and easy-to-manipulate hand tools. Scientists in these fields work in academic departments, such as departments of psychology, industrial engineering, physical education, or kinesiology, or in companies or governmental agencies. Chapter 4 provides an overview of behavioral science, cognitive science, and human factors approaches to human motor control.

Physiology, Neuroscience, Medicine, and Allied Fields

People who study the implementation level of motor control in biological systems are most often associated with physiology. Physiologists interested in motor control focus on muscle, bones, and joints, as well as the main regulator of muscle activity, the nervous system, which is the province of neuroscience. The practitioners who apply this information in the clinic are neurologists (who diagnose and treat ailments of the nervous system), orthopedists (who diagnose and treat disorders of bones and joints), physical therapists (who help restore motion and stability through behavioral rehabilitation), and prostheticians (who craft and fit artificial limbs for people with amputations). Rudiments of physiology, neuroscience, medicine, and allied fields that pertain to human motor control will be presented in Chapter 3.

ORGANIZATION OF THE BOOK

This book has three main parts. The first is introductory. It contains, besides this chapter, Chapter 2 (Core Problems), Chapter 3 (Physiological Foundations), and Chapter 4 (Psychological Foundations).

The second part is organized by activity. Within it, Chapter 5 is concerned with walking and related forms of locomotion. Chapter 6 is concerned with looking, or more specifically, the control of eye and head movements. Chapter 7 focuses on reaching and grasping. Chapter 8 treats the control of drawing and writing. Chapter 9 covers keyboarding (i.e., the control of typewriting, text-messaging, piano playing, and other finger-movement tasks). Chapter 10 covers the control of speaking and singing. Chapter 11, the last chapter in Part II, is concerned with smiling and other forms of facial expression.

The third part of the book has a single chapter, Moving On. This chapter presents new advances and new challenges that newcomers to the field may wish to take up.

You should know why the book is organized as it is and why the book has the title it has. Regarding organization, and in particular the devotion of much of the book to distinct activities (Chapters 5–11), this approach has several advantages. One is that research in motor control, like research in most fields today, has become specialized. It is not really a caricature of the field to say that there are people who work entirely on eye movements, others who work entirely on reaching and grasping, others who work entirely on speech, and so forth. The proliferation of subspecialties within motor-control research derives partly from the practical and theoretical interests of workers in the field. Practical concerns with particular tasks sometimes compel investigators to pursue particular task domains at the expense of others. A researcher working for a computer company, for example, is likely to be more interested in keyboarding than in singing. Theoretical interests also place some investigators on circumscribed research paths. Students of vision, for example, are naturally more interested in oculomotor (eye movement) control than in speech.

The second reason for devoting separate chapters to separate activities is that many of the specialty areas have developed their own problems and methodologies. The twists and turns in one area do not always map easily onto the lines of study in another area, so rather than risk losing the richness of particular areas of study, each area is paid its due by being considered on its own.

In treating the subsystems separately, it is critical that the treatment not become too parochial. Areas of common concern need to be highlighted, as does work on the coordination of different motor tasks. Being on the lookout for similarities between the motor subsystems puts one in an advantageous position for detecting differences between them. That there might be differences is a real and intriguing possibility, given that some processes may be controlled by independent modules with their own rules of operation (Fodor, 1983). If modularity applies to the motor system, different motor activities might be controlled in wholly different ways. Treating the motor activities separately makes it possible to identify those differences if they exist or note their absence if they might otherwise be expected.

Regarding the title of the book, *Human Motor Control*, many but not all of the activities that are discussed here can be carried out only by people, but many of the activities can also be carried out by non-human animals. The word "human" is included in the title even though animal research is discussed throughout the volume. Animal work is important to the understanding of human motor control (and vice versa).

The use of the term "motor control" also requires justification, for one might wonder whether there really is a system responsible for motor activity, separate from other systems responsible for perception or cognition. There is no such separate system, and no claim is made here that there is. Demarcating systems need not imply that the systems are isolated. It is helpful, if only for educational purposes, to treat motor control as a topic in its own right, just as it is helpful to analyze perceptual functions such as vision or audition on their own. Ultimately, all the seemingly separate systems work together. The extent to which they do provides clues about the integration of function that is critical for adaptive performance in everyday life.

SUMMARY

1. The study of human motor control can have practical benefits in sports, in medicine, in the home, and in the workplace.
2. Research on human motor control focuses on the control of movement as well as the control of stability.
3. Robots reflect our understanding of human motor control. Robots are still relatively primitive. They cannot exhibit the endless novelty of motor behaviors that people can exhibit.
4. The goal of studying human motor control is to understand it. A measure of understanding of human motor control is the ability to verbalize the principles of such control and the ability to simulate such control in robots. If robots act in ways that are indistinguishable from the way people act, one can say that developers of robots truly understand human motor control, at least with respect to the acts being performed by the machines they develop.
5. Different levels of analysis are pursued in the study of human motor control. These are the computational level, the procedural level, and the implementation level. The computational level pertains to abstract, typically mathematical, levels of description. The procedural level pertains to behavioral and cognitive methods used in performance. The implementation level pertains to the material substrates—the neurons, muscles, or, in the case of robots, motors, wires, and so on. All three levels are necessary for analysis.
6. Many fields contribute to the study of human control: physics, statistics, engineering, behavioral science, cognitive science, human factors, physiology, neuroscience, medicine, and allied fields.
7. This book has three sections. The first is introductory, with chapters on core problems, physiological foundations, and psychological foundations. The second section is concerned with different motor activities, with chapters on walking, looking, reaching, drawing and writing, keyboarding, speaking and singing, and smiling. The third section is concerned with recent advances and future challenges.
8. This book is called *Human Motor Control* even though research with animals is discussed and even though the system responsible for motor control is not separate from the system responsible for perception or the system responsible for learning. Distinctions between these systems are drawn for educational purposes only.

OUTLINE

The Degrees of Freedom Problem	12	*Movement Enhances Perception*	28
Whose Problem Is the Degrees		*Movement Informs Perception*	29
of Freedom Problem?	13	*Mirror Neurons*	31
Why the Term "Degrees of Freedom"?	14	**The Learning Problem**	32
Synergies	14	*Learning by Doing*	33
Relying on Mechanics	18	*Learning by Practicing Deliberately*	34
Efficiency	18	*Learning Through Specificity*	
		of Practice	35
The Sequencing and Timing Problem	20	*Learning Through Neural*	
Speech Errors	20	*Plasticity*	37
Coarticulation	22		
Timing	23	**Summary**	39
The Perceptual-Motor Integration		**Further Reading**	41
Problem	25		
Feedback	25		
Feedforward	26		

There are many ways to organize the body of knowledge comprising the field of human motor control. One is by *discipline*, taking what has been learned in the various approaches to the field, such as physics, engineering, and statistics. Another is by *method*, considering the techniques used to analyze the human motor control system, such as mathematical modeling, observation of behavior, and recording of physiological signals. Yet another approach is by *activity*, focusing on things people do, such as walking, looking, reaching, and speaking. The latter approach is taken in Part II of this book.

The present chapter follows a different way of organizing the material. It focuses on the core *problems* of motor-control research. There are four such problems, each with its own associated name.

1. The *degrees of freedom problem*: How are movements selected to achieve particular tasks when, as is almost always the case, infinitely many movements can achieve those tasks?
2. The *sequencing and timing problem*: How are behaviors ordered in time?
3. The *perceptual-motor integration problem*: How are perception and motor control combined?
4. The *learning problem*: How are perceptual-motor skills acquired?

We will consider each of these questions in turn in the remainder of this chapter. In so doing, we will sample the rich kinds of evidence in this field of inquiry.

THE DEGREES OF FREEDOM PROBLEM

Most physical tasks can be performed in an infinite number of ways. As a simple example, touch the tip of your nose. Do so now before reading further.

How did you perform this elementary task? If you are right-handed, as about 90% of people are (Hardyck & Petrinovich, 1977), you probably used your right hand. No matter which hand you used, however, you probably didn't touch some other part of your face before getting your finger to your nose. You probably also made a direct reach to your nose. You most likely did not snake your hand around the back of your head or swing your hand back and forth in a wide arc before bringing your hand nose-ward. You probably also moved at a speed that felt comfortable, neither moving your hand as quickly as possible nor at a snail's pace. You probably moved your hand such that it sped up gradually and then slowed down gradually. The peak speed of your hand was one that was neither "too fast" nor "too slow" but instead, as in the story of Goldilocks, who sought porridge that was neither too hot nor too cold and a bed that was neither too hard nor too soft, was "just right."

There are still more ways you could have performed the elementary task of touching your nose, though those methods are so farfetched it is hard even to think of them. You could have brought your arm to some unwieldy posture at the time your finger touched your nose (Figure 2.1). For that matter, you could have brought your *little* finger to your nose, or you could have brought your *forearm* to your nose, or you could have even brought your nose down to your forearm. Even more bizarrely, you could have touched your nose with your foot. The instruction with which this section began—"touch the tip of your nose"—did not prevent you from doing any of these things, but you almost certainly did none of them, nor even consider any of them before doing what you actually did.

The fact that there are many possible ways to perform a simple task like touching your nose illustrates the *degrees of freedom* problem. The term relates to the fact that there are an infinite number of ways of getting things done. When a physical task is identified, either via an overt instruction ("Touch your nose") or via a decision you make on your own ("My nose itches, so I think I'll scratch it"), the instruction does not spell out how the task should be done, but by the time you have done the task, you have, in effect, provided all the needed instructions. You have solved the degrees of freedom problem, albeit implicitly (without

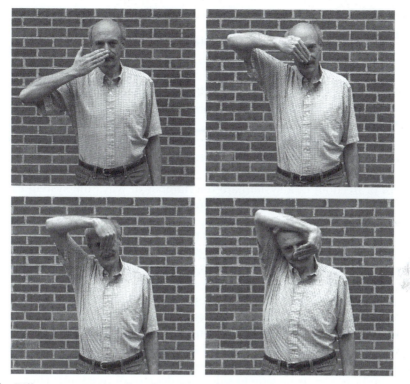

FIGURE 2.1   Different postures that allow the author to touch his nose.

conscious planning). You determined which of the infinite number of ways of possibly performing the task was the one you would perform.

Whose Problem Is the Degrees of Freedom Problem?

Is the degrees of freedom problem really a problem for us in our everyday life? To address this question, suppose your nose really itches and you have been tied up by a kidnapper. Your feet are bound together and your hands are tied behind your back. Escaping from bondage is your top priority, but if the itch really irritates you, you might do something that wasn't even mentioned before. You might hop over to the wall and rub your nose against it. Such behavior would be crazy if you could use your hands in the usual way, but if you were bound up, hopping and scratching would make perfectly good sense.

This example shows that having many behavioral options is not a curse but a blessing. If you come home with your arms filled with groceries and need to turn the light on in your apartment, you may do so with a nudge of your shoulder. You wouldn't flip the switch with your shoulder if your hands were free, however. Having many possible ways of performing a task gives you the option of performing the task in a way that makes sense at the moment. From this perspective, the degrees of freedom problem is not really a problem in the sense that it is something you need to worry about. Rather, it is an opportunity for you to adapt to changing environmental conditions. The degrees of freedom problem is only a problem for scientists interested in motor control. The problem is to understand how particular actions are chosen when many are possible.

Why the Term "Degrees of Freedom"?

Why do motor control researchers use the phrase "degrees of freedom"? Why don't they use a phrase like the "too-many-options" problem? The difficulty with the latter phrase is that there aren't really too many options. Too many in what sense? It's a good thing that tied-up hostages have the option of hopping to the wall to scratch their itchy noses that way. The fact that this option exists means it is not entirely superfluous. By extension, neither are all the other options that might be needed.

The degrees of freedom in a system are the number of ways the system can independently vary. The phrase "degrees of freedom problem" is used by motor-control researchers because generating a physical action generally involves going from many possible degrees of freedom to just the few that characterize the task that is selected. For example, the instruction "Scratch your nose" is open-ended. Few degrees of freedom are nailed down to begin with, but by the time your nose has been scratched, all the degrees of freedom have been specified.

What are some examples of actual degrees of freedom? Consider again the nose-touching example. The tip of your nose has three degrees of freedom: its x, y, and z position in space. However, the joints of your arm (excluding your hand) have seven degrees of freedom. Your shoulder can move up and down, move from side to side, and twist (three degrees of freedom); your elbow can bend and twist (two degrees of freedom); and your wrist can move up and down and can turn from side to side (two degrees of freedom). Thus, without even considering the finger, which adds still more degrees of freedom, a problem arises in determining how to bring the tip of your finger to the tip of your nose. There are more degrees of freedom in your arm than in the location to which the tip of your index finger must be brought. Consequently, there are many ways of positioning your fingertip when your finger is in contact with the tip of your nose, as shown in Figure 2.1. Similarly, there are many ways of positioning your fingertip at each spatial location on its way to your nose. Thus, the degrees of freedom problem applies to every one of those spatial locations, and it applies as well to the *timing* of the movement because the same series of locations can be occupied at different times (Figure 2.2).

These considerations indicate that the degrees of freedom problem is multifaceted. It applies to *kinematics* (positions in time) and *kinetics* (forces in time). At deeper levels, it applies to the mapping of neural activity to muscle activity. Any given series of muscle contractions and relaxations can be achieved with many different patterns of neural firing. Mathematically, the degrees of freedom problem exists whenever there is a many-to-one mapping.

Synergies

How do movement scientists address the degrees of freedom problem? One solution they have proposed is embodied in the concept of *synergies*. Synergies are interactions. An example is sexual reproduction. Neither a man nor a woman can produce a child on his or her own. Their offspring is the synergistic product of their union.

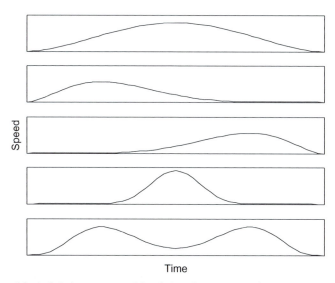

FIGURE 2.2   A few of the infinitely many possible relations between speed and time.

It has been suggested that "less sexy" interactions can play a useful role in addressing the degrees of freedom for motor control (Bernstein, 1967). The reasoning is that, in principle, synergies can reduce the number of degrees of freedom that must be independently controlled.

To understand this idea, consider the left panel of Figure 2.3. The two points in this panel have a total of four degrees of freedom. Each of the two points has two degrees of freedom; the bottom left point has an x value and a y value, and so does the top right point. By contrast, the system of two points in the *right* panel of Figure 2.3 has only *three* degrees of freedom. This is because there is a link of fixed length between the points, so if the x and y values of one of the points are known, only one other value is needed to determine the position of the other point—the angle of the link relative to the known point. This simple example (Saltzman, 1979) shows that a synergy, represented as a link between two points, can reduce the number of degrees of freedom to be managed.

What kinds of synergies exist in the motor system? Consider a commonplace, if homely, phenomenon. If you are like most people, no matter how hard you try, you probably cannot keep your eyes open when you sneeze. The interaction seems "hard-wired" in the sense that there is nothing you can do about it. This example illustrates how one kind of motor activity can automatically dictate what other activities may occur.

A more interesting phenomenon concerns wrist and elbow rotations. Try the two exercises shown in Figure 2.4. First, do the exercise shown in the top panel: Flex your elbow while flexing your wrist and then extend your elbow while extending your wrist. Repeat these two motions, going back and forth. If you are like participants in previous studies (Kots & Syrovegnin, 1966), you will find this task very easy.

Now do the exercise shown in the *bottom* panel of Figure 2.4. Flex your elbow while extending your wrist and then extend your elbow while flexing your wrist. If you repeat these two motions over and over, you will probably find this task much more difficult, again as found in previous research (Kots & Syrovegnin, 1966).

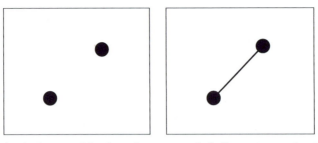

FIGURE 2.3   Reduction in degrees of freedom via a synergy. Left: Two points, each with two degrees of freedom, for a total of four degrees of freedom. Right: Two points, each with two degrees of freedom but with a rigid line between them, for a total of three degrees of freedom.

Why was the second task harder than the first? For present purposes the exact reason is less important than the fact that if there were no dependencies between the joints, one would expect the coordination of the joints to be indifferent to the phasing of their rotations. Such dependencies are dramatic, however, indicating that the behavior of one joint

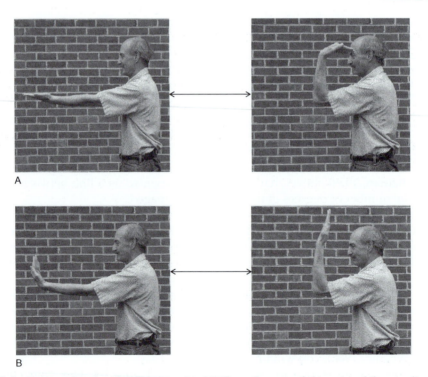

FIGURE 2.4   Two exercises that illustrate synergies. (A) The author extends his wrist while extending his elbow (left), and then flexes his wrist while flexing his elbow (right). (B) The author flexes his wrist while extending his elbow (left), and then extends his wrist while flexing his elbow (right). For most people, coordination is easier for the exercise shown in (A) than for the exercise shown in (B).

influences another's. This example shows that there are functional linkages between different parts of the body. These linkages have an effect on what movements can and cannot be done at the same time.

The foregoing example concerned coordination *within* a limb. Now consider coordination *between* limbs. As everyone knows from childhood party games, it is hard to rub your stomach while patting your head. Making circular stomach rubs corrupts your attempts at patting your head with straight up and down hand motions. Laboratory experiments have shown that such interactions are not just the stuff of children's games. In laboratory studies, it has been found that when people make rhythmic movements with their two hands, the frequency of one hand's movement affects the frequency of the other hand's movement (e.g., Franz, Zelaznik, Swinnen, & Walter, 2001).

Such interactions have ancient evolutionary origins. The fins of a fish, like the arms of a person, are coupled. Figure 2.5 shows such fishy interactions as well as a human analog (von Holst, 1939). For the human as well as the fish, the activity of one extremity affects the activity of the other extremity. The analysis of such interactions has played a major role in the study of human motor control (Amazeen, Amazeen, & Turvey, 1998; Swinnen, Heuer, & Casaer, 1994).

Do synergies actually eliminate degrees of freedom to be controlled? Typically, they do not, though they can bias the neuro-motor system to perform in certain ways rather than

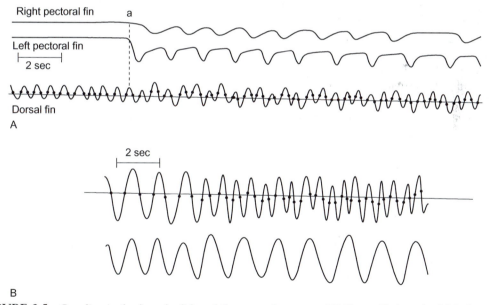

FIGURE 2.5   Coupling in the fins of a fish and the arms of a person. (A) The oscillation of a fish's dorsal fin changes when the right and left pectoral fins begin to oscillate. (B) In a person, when the right arm (upper curve) is supposed to oscillate at increasing frequencies, the left arm is affected. In both panels, the dots superimposed on the curves occupy equal time intervals. Thus variations in the dot positions along the vertical dimension indicate that the limb does not occupy the same position at the same time in the cycle. From Holst, E. von. (1973). The behavioural physiology of animal and man: The collected papers of Erich von Holst (Vol. 1). London: Methuen Ltd. With permission.

others. For example, the two exercises in Figure 2.4 show that it is more natural to flex and extend the wrist and elbow at the same time than to flex the wrist while extending the elbow, or vice versa. Nonetheless, it is still possible to flex the wrist while extending the elbow or to do the opposite, albeit with great difficulty. If synergies *prevented* the latter motions, you would unable to do them at all. For this reason, synergies can be viewed as fallback ways of performing. When these default methods are appropriate, they may be carried out because they are preferred. However, when alternate ways of performing are called for, they usually can be carried out, though not so easily or well. This is why blinking while sneezing is not a synergy. When you sneeze, you *must* blink. Blinking while sneezing is not a default option that can be overcome at will. It is a so-called hard constraint rather than a synergy. A synergy is a so-called soft constraint. It can help reduce the degrees of freedom to be independently managed but is not absolutely mandatory.

Relying on Mechanics

Other factors besides synergies are helpful in addressing the degrees of freedom problem. Another is physical mechanics. Physical properties of the body can eliminate the need to control each feature of neuro-motor control (Bernstein, 1967; Bizzi and Mussa-Ivaldi, 1989). An example comes from walking. When we walk, each of our legs goes through two main phases. One is the stance phase, when the foot is on the ground. The other is the swing phase, when the leg swings forward. Analysis of the behavior of the leg during the swing phase has shown that the forward swing can be achieved without concurrent muscle activation (McMahon, 1984). The leg's forward swing need not be planned or controlled in detail. Instead, it can be produced simply by taking advantage of the physical properties of the leg within the gravitational field. Relying on physical mechanics in this way eliminates the need to generate just the right commands at just the right time.

Another example of exploitation of mechanics also comes from walking. One of the most exciting advances in robotics has been recent the development of "passive dynamic walkers" (Collins, Ruina, Tedrake, & Wisse, 2005). These simple devices need hardly any control to achieve basic walking, at least when they walk down slopes. See http://www-personal .umich.edu/~shc/robots.html for more information.

Figure 2.6 shows some examples. Each of these simple robots consists of little more than legs and a connector between the legs. When placed on slopes and oriented in the right way, these devices walk down the slopes with gaits resembling people's. That such walking can occur as a result of mechanics suggests that human and animal walking may likewise take advantage of body mechanics. The details of every step need not be controlled; instead, walking, or at least walking in its essential form, can come "for free."

Efficiency

The third and final approach to the degrees of freedom problem relies on efficiency. The idea here is that the movements we make are usually more efficient than the movements we don't make. For example, the reason you don't snake your arm around your head to touch your nose is that the snaking movement is less efficient than the more direct movement. Apart from the fact that the snaking movement takes longer than the

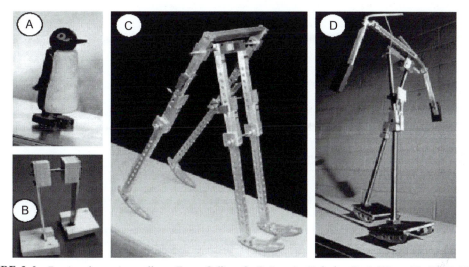

FIGURE 2.6 Passive dynamics walkers. From Collins, S., Ruina, A., Tedrake, R., & Wisse, M. (2005). Efficient bipedal robots based on passive-dynamic walkers. Science, 307, 1082–1085. With permission.

more direct path, the serpentine path gets your arm into an awkward final position. Your wrist and shoulder joints are in extreme angles at the end of the movement. Consequently, your ability to make a second response to some potential, unexpected stimulus is impaired.

In general, it is a bad idea to end a movement with the limb adopting extreme joint angles, just as it is generally a bad idea to remain near the edge of a tennis court after returning a shot to your opponent. Returning to midcourt lets you be in the best place to return the next shot. Similarly, by having your arm in the middle of its range of motion at the end of a movement, your subsequent possible movements can be maximally diverse.

People are sensitive to this fact. They deliberately adopt awkward initial postures when taking hold of objects if those initially awkward postures let them end the maneuvers in comfortable or easy-to-control final postures. For example, if you pick up an inverted glass (open end down) to pour water into it, you will probably take hold of the glass with your thumb pointing down rather than with your thumb pointing up, although the thumb-up grasp is more comfortable. Taking hold of the inverted glass with a thumb-up posture gets you into trouble if you try to pour water into the glass, for you will be in an awkward posture and it will be difficult for you to steady the glass. In the laboratory, people exhibit similar tendencies, as shown in Figure 2.7 (Rosenbaum, Vaughan, Barnes, Slotta, & Jorgensen, 1990).

Ending in a comfortable posture is one efficiency constraint. Others have been found as well. One that has received a great deal of attention is the tendency to move smoothly when going from one position to another. This tendency appears to reflect an efficiency constraint related to the avoidance of jerky movements. In more technical language, movements may reflect a constraint to minimize the mean squared rate of change of acceleration over movement time (Hogan, 1984; Hogan & Flash, 1987).

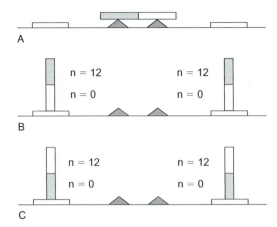

FIGURE 2.7 Experimental setup and results demonstrating the end-state comfort effect. (A) A wooden dowel with a black end and white end resting on a cradle with target disks to the left and right. (B) When the white (right) end of the dowel had to be brought down onto a target disk, 12 out of 12 participants grasped the horizontal dowel with the right thumb toward the *black* end. (C) When the black (left) end of the dowel had to be brought down onto a target disk, 12 out of 12 participants grasped the horizontal dowel with the right thumb toward the *white* end. From Rosenbaum, D. A., Marchak, F., Barnes, H. J., Vaughan, J., Slotta, J., & Jorgensen, M. (1990). Constraints for action selection: Overhand versus underhand grips. In M. Jeannerod (Ed.), Attention and Performance XIII: Motor representation and control (pp. 321–342). Hillsdale, NJ: Lawrence Erlbaum Associates. With permission.

THE SEQUENCING AND TIMING PROBLEM

A second major issue in the study of human motor control is how we control the sequencing and timing of our behaviors. When we engage in behaviors that have distinct elements, such as speaking, typing, or walking, the elements of the behaviors must be ordered correctly in time. How is such ordering achieved?

Speech Errors

Professor William Archibald Spooner, who taught at Oxford University in the late nineteenth and early twentieth century (see Figure 2.8), is alleged to have made distinctive speech errors. For example, he is reported to have said "The queer old dean" instead of "The dear old queen," and "You hissed all my mystery lectures" instead of "You missed all my history lectures." Although the authenticity of these reports has been questioned (Potter, 1980), there is no doubt that all of us make such errors from time to time. Speech errors involving the exchange of two speech sounds in analogous word positions are examples of *spoonerisms*, named after the hapless Oxford professor. The commonness of spoonerisms is reflected not just in the fact that all of us make such errors from time to time; it is also reflected in the fact (a fun fact reported here for your interest) that the word "butterfly" is actually a spoonerism. Butterflies were first called "flutter-by's," but once the "fl" and the "b" exchanged, the new name stuck.

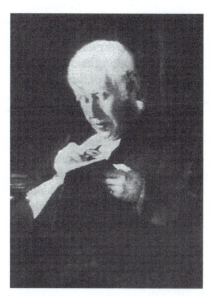

FIGURE 2.8 Professor William Archibald Spooner, after whom spoonerisms were named. From Potter, J. M. (1980). What was the matter with Dr. Spooner? In V. A. Fromkin (Ed.), Errors in linguistic performance (pp. 13–34). New York: Academic Press. With permission.

What do speech errors tell us about the control of sequencing? Suppose you said "We're going to the bootfall game," instead of the (intended) "We're going to the football game." Speech errors like this have been recorded both in spontaneous conversation (Garrett, 1982) and in the laboratory (Motley, 1980). The bootfall/football error suggests that before you said the "f" that normally goes with "football," the "b" sound was available. Furthermore, since the "b" sound exchanged with the "f" rather than, say, with the long "e" in "We're," the switch occurred in a way that was systematic. Generally, consonants only exchange with other consonants, and vowels only exchange with other vowels. Similarly, nouns tend only to exchange with other nouns, and verbs tend only to exchange with other verbs.

This birds-of-a-feather-stick-together principle suggest that there are distinct levels of representation in the planning and production of speech (Fromkin, 1980). For example, there is a level involving whole words, which respects the words' syntactic status (nouns versus verbs). There is also a level involving individual phonemes (see Chapter 10), which respects the distinction between consonants and vowels. Understanding how these levels of representation are used in speech production has been a topic of considerable interest among psycholinguists (Dell, 1986). More will be said about the modeling of speech errors in Chapter 10. For now, the important point is that the kinds of speech errors that people make indicate that speech is not simply produced by planning and then executing one utterance at a time. Rather, a plan is set up for an extended sequence of forthcoming utterances (Lashley, 1951).

Errors like those in speech also occur in other domains of performance. Perhaps you have made the mistake of throwing dirty socks into a trash can rather than into a nearby clothes hamper where you intended to throw them. Or perhaps you accidentally poured catsup into your coffee rather than on the hamburger you wanted to flavor. Errors like these tend to occur when we are distracted, but they indicate that our bodily actions, like our speech, are based on plans with distinct functional levels. Pouring the catsup into the coffee indicates that the plan for catsup pouring includes the goal of emptying the contents into a suitable receptacle. The catsup-pouring error is not based on an inability to visually distinguish coffee cups from burgers. Rather, the problem arises because an abstract description of the task to be achieved exists in the mind of the actor. In addition, the specifics of the task situation are momentarily misidentified, leading to the kinds of mistakes discussed here—so-called *action slips* (Norman, 1981).

Coarticulation

Inferences about serial order are not only based on mistakes; they are also based on accurate performance. As a case in point, look into a mirror and say, rather deliberately, the word "tulip." If you look closely, you will see that your lips round before you say "t." Speech scientists call this phenomenon anticipatory lip rounding. Like the speech errors described above, anticipatory lip rounding suggests that a plan exists for an entire word before the word is produced. If "tulip" were produced in a piecemeal fashion, with each sound planned only after the preceding sound was produced, the rounding of the lips for "u" would only occur after "t" was uttered.

Anticipatory lip rounding illustrates a general tendency that any theory of sequencing must account for—the tendency of effectors to *coarticulate*. This term, or its related noun, *coarticulation*, refers to simultaneous motions that occur in sequential tasks. In speech production, coarticulation occurs in anticipatory lip rounding, as just discussed, but it also occurs in other aspects of speech. For example, it occurs as well in nasalization. Nasalizing a speech sound occurs when the speaker allows air to pass from the lungs through the nasal cavity by lowering the velum, a fold separating the oral and nasal cavities. Nasalization often occurs before some consonants are produced. For example, in saying "Freon," nasalization occurs during the first vowel, even though nasalization is only strictly required for the /n/.

Is coarticulation just a mechanical artifact? It is not, as shown by the fact that coarticulation is language-dependent. In French, where some words can be distinguished on the basis of whether vowels are nasalized, nasalization occurs before/n/ but never so early that vowel identities, and thus *word* identities, are affected. By contrast, in English, where vowels typically are *not* distinguished by nasalization, lowering the velum often occurs in vowels, such as those in "Freon," where such lowering would not occur in French (Jordan, 1986b). Results like these indicate that a theory of coarticulation, and so a theory of sequencing in general, must account for *psychological* as well as *physiological* constraints.

Two final observations are worth making about coarticulation. One is that coarticulation is not restricted to speech. Films of typists' hands reveal that both hands move continually during typewriting (see Figure 2.9). The fingers of each hand move toward their respective keyboard targets, even when other keys are being struck (Rumelhart and Norman, 1982). More will be said about this in Chapter 9.

Similarly, in reaching for objects, it turns out that the same object is grasped differently depending on where the object will be placed. Figure 2.10 shows an experiment where this phenomenon was demonstrated (Cohen & Rosenbaum, 2004). University students were asked to grasp a standing toilet plunger and move it to a platform whose height was varied.

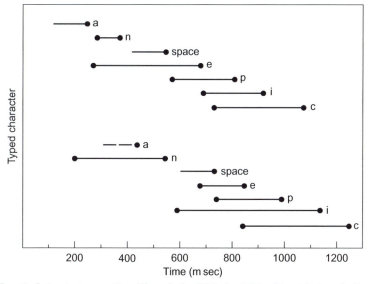

FIGURE 2.9   Coarticulation in typewriting. Though the "i" in "epic" is ultimately typed after the "e" and "p," it is initiated before either letter. Similarly, the first time "epic" is typed, the "e" is initiated before the "n" in the preceding word ("an"). The data were obtained from film records. From Gentner, D. R., Grudin, J., & Conway, E. (1980). Finger movements in transcription typing. La Jolla, CA: University of California, San Diego, Center for Human Information Processing (Technical Report 8001). With permission.

Although the starting position of the plunger was the same in all conditions, the participants took hold of the plunger low when they were going to move the plunger high and they took hold of the plunger high when they were going to move the plunger low. This behavior makes sense from the point of view of permitting comfortable or easy-to-control final postures when the plunger was brought to the target platform. This behavior shows that coarticulation applies to reaching as well as typing and talking.

Coarticulation is a blessing. Think about a typist who could move only one finger at a time. Lacking the capacity for coarticulation, the typist's typing speed would drop precipitously. Simultaneous movements of the fingers allow for rapid typing, just as concurrent movements of the tongue, lips, and velum allow for rapid speaking. Coarticulation is an effective means for increasing response speed. Similarly, being able to adjust where one takes hold of an object depending on where the object will be placed lets one complete object transports comfortably with body positions that are easy to control.

Timing

Generating movements in the right order is important, but generating movements with the right timing can be even more so. People are generally quite good at timing their movements. They can bat oncoming baseballs, coordinate dance steps with their partners, and, when playing musical instruments, start to play when the conductor gives a downbeat.

Even when there is no *a priori* reason why movements should be synchronized with perceptual events, they often are. For example, when people tap a finger in time with a metronome,

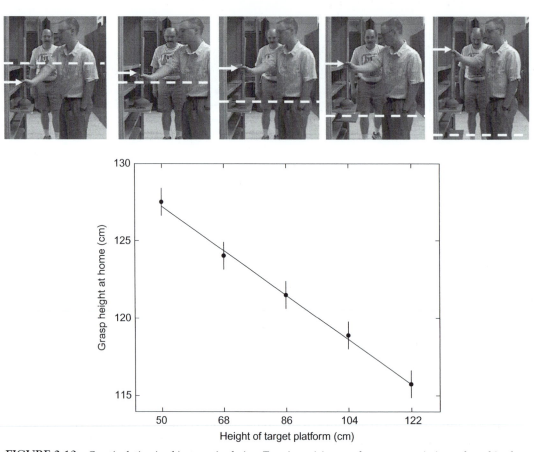

FIGURE 2.10 Coarticulation in object manipulation. Top: A participant, who gave permission to have his photo shown here, grasps a plunger on a home platform with different grasp heights (white arrows) before moving the plunger to target platforms at different heights (white dashed lines). The author, also shown here, was responsible for setting up the target platforms. Bottom: Mean grasp heights (± 1 SE) for home-to-target grasps. From Cohen, R. G. & Rosenbaum, D. A. (2004). Where objects are grasped reveals how grasps are planned: Generation and recall of motor plans. Experimental Brain Research, 157, 486–495. With permission.

their finger taps slightly lead the metronome clicks (Aschersleben & Prinz, 1995). The delays between the taps and the clicks suggest that participants try to make the feedback from their taps coincide with the sounds of the clicks. Such performance makes sense from the point of view of getting a clear error signal about timing. If the sound of the tap and the sound of the click do not coincide, the performer gets information indicating s/he has failed to synchronize perfectly. In addition, if the sound of the tap and the sound of the click are different, the participant can tell whether the tap came too early or too late.

Sometimes, feedback-based synchronization takes especially interesting, unexpected forms. In a precursor to the experiment just described, people were asked to tap the hand and foot simultaneously (Paillard, 1949). Surprisingly, the foot taps came before the hand taps by a few milliseconds. The length by which the foot led the hand was what one would expect if participants performed so as to have feedback from the toe reach the brain at the same time as feedback from the hand. It is possible to compute this expected lead time given the known speed of nerve conduction and given the known distances between the foot, hand, and brain. People tap with the foot before tapping with the hand by just the length of time that permits simultaneity of perceptual input from the two effectors. This outcome suggests that we do not strive for simultaneity of motor output, consistent with the view, advanced in the late 1800s (James, 1890), that we do not sense motor commands.

THE PERCEPTUAL-MOTOR INTEGRATION PROBLEM

Having just considered feedback-based timing, we turn to the third major problem in the study of human motor control, the perceptual-motor integration problem. The problem is how perception and motor control are combined. How does perception affect movement, and how does movement affect perception? Because we just considered this problem in connection with the use of feedback in timing, we can continue by focusing on feedback itself.

Feedback

Consider once again the task of bringing the tip of your index finger to the tip of your nose. You may have noticed that when you performed this task, your hand moved rapidly at first and then slowed down. Virtually all aiming movements proceed in this two-stage fashion. Initially, there is a rapid *ballistic* phase, and then there is a slower *corrective* phase (Elliott, Helsen, & Chua, 2001; Woodworth, 1899). Ballistic movements cannot be altered once they have been initiated. (Ballistic missiles, for example, cannot be steered once they are launched.) Ballistic movements are typically fast and cover most of the distance to the target. If the target is not reached, feedback is used to correct the error.

Correcting errors based on feedback is possible with a *negative feedback loop*, or what is also known as a *servomechanism* (see Figure 2.11). Servomechanisms have several components. One is a *reference signal*, which provides input to the loop about the target or goal state. In the case of bringing the hand to a target, the reference signal is a representation of the hand at the target—for example, a representation of the expected feeling of the fingertip on the tip of the nose. Another component is the *plant*, which is responsible for converting control signals into output (for example, moving the hand). A third component is the *comparator*, which measures the discrepancy between the sensed position of the effector and the

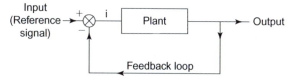

FIGURE 2.11   A negative feedback loop. From Legge, D. & Barber, P. J. (1976). Information and skill. London: Methuen. With permission.

reference signal. The comparator is used to negate error. This is why we use the term *nega-tive* feedback loop. Errors are negated in such loops.

Is there such a thing as a *positive* feedback loop? Positively! A positive feedback loop is a feedback loop in which feedback leads to larger errors, not smaller ones. You can experience a positive feedback loop if you try to cut your own hair while looking in a mirror. Things get difficult if you do this. Working in this miniature hall of reflectors, you have the disquieting experience that whenever you try to bring the scissors closer to where you want them, they only move farther away.

Why is it so difficult to control one's movements when observing them through a double mirror? The answer is that the normal mappings between movements and their visual con-sequences are reversed. Even so, it is possible to learn to adjust to this reversal in a short time (see Chapter 7). One of the most interesting problems in motor-control research is how such learning is achieved.

Some additional terms are useful in connection with feedback processing. These are *closed-loop control*, *open-loop control*, and *feedforward*. Closed-loop control occurs when feed-back returns to the comparator. Watching your hand as it approaches a visible target directly in front of you gives you the opportunity to reduce the distance between your hand and the target. If the closed feedback loop is negative, the feedback lets you reduce the distance between your hand and the target. If the closed feedback loop is positive, the feedback makes it harder for you to reduce the distance between your hand and the target.

Open-loop control occurs when feedback is unavailable. In open-loop situations, the feed-back loop is opened up and no information can get through about the success or failure of performance. An example of an open-loop task is shooting at a moving target that you can neither see, hear, nor feel. The only way you can hit the target is through dumb luck or pre-diction. If the target moves in a way you anticipate—for example, you predict it will move back and forth with some fixed frequency and amplitude in a known range of locations— you may be able to hit the target even though you are operating in an open-loop manner. If you hit the target based on prediction, you used *feedforward* control.

Feedforward

As just indicated, whenever performance is consistently accurate though feedback is removed the performer must have relied on feedforward control. The accuracy of perform-ance provides an indication of the accuracy of the performer's feedforward control.

Under open-loop conditions, a number of movement sequences can be performed sur-prisingly well. For example, monkeys deprived of sensory feedback from their limbs can walk and climb, though they do so less gracefully than monkeys with sensory feedback (Taub & Berman, 1968). Sensory feedback is eliminated in these animals by cutting the nerve fibers that transmit sensory signals from the limbs into the spinal cord. When these same nerve fibers are damaged in humans as a result of accident or disease, some movement con-trol may still be possible (Lashley, 1917). For example, a man who could not feel his body because of a disease affecting his sensory nerves could draw complex figures on command, could sequentially touch his thumb with each finger of the same hand, and could touch his nose. He could do all these things without the aid of visual, auditory, or other forms of feed-back (Marsden, Rothwell, & Dell, 1984).

Abilities such as these indicate that the gross features of some movements can be performed under feedforward control. When these same movements are performed *with* feedback, however, they are usually performed more precisely and gracefully. This outcome suggests that everyday movements reflect the combined use of feedforward *and* feedback.

Can feedforward be inferred only by removing feedback? The answer is no, as can be demonstrated through the simple act of looking into a mirror and trying to watch your eyes move. You cannot see your own eyes move, as was noted over a century ago (Dodge, 1900). If you have a friend look at your eyes while you move your eyes, he or she will have no trouble seeing your eyes dart about. This shows that eye movements are not simply too quick to be seen.

Why can't you see your own eyes move? An intriguing hypothesis (Volkmann, Schick, & Riggs, 1969; see Chapter 6) is that your brain suppresses visual inputs arising from your eye movements when your eyes jump from place to place or, said another way, when your eyes make *saccades* (the French word for jumps). There could be a distinct functional advantage of such *saccadic suppression*. Since the retinal image is smeared during saccades, the smear might serve no useful purpose for perception. Saccadic suppression could help reduce the damage to visual perception caused by such retinal smearing. Chapter 6 provides a more extensive discussion and critical evaluation of this hypothesis.

Suppression effects are not limited to eye movements. Chewing sounds are loud, yet we barely hear them. The reason is that during chewing, there is internal suppression of auditory feedback (Rosenzweig & Lehman, 1982). Similarly, during active hand movements, sensitivity to tactile stimuli is reduced (Demaire, Honoré, & Coquery, 1984). Such reduced sensitivity to self-produced actions may explain why we can't tickle ourselves (Blakemore, Wolpert, & Frith, 1998).

Feedforward helps distinguish perceptual changes due to motion arising in the external environment from perceptual changes arising from one's own motion. The disambiguation occurs by subtracting perceptual changes caused by motor commands (or internal perceptual representations leading to motor commands) from perceptual changes caused by changes in the external environment.

Support for this hypothesis came from a remarkable experiment with flies (von Holst & Mittelstaedt, 1950). The experiment was prompted by the observation that when a fly stands still and a drum with vertical stripes turns around it, the fly turns with the drum, presumably to keep itself stationary with respect to the external world. This behavior is known as the *optomotor* reflex. When the stripes are stationary, the same fly moves freely in front of them. The visual stimulus is approximately the same when the fly moves and the stripes are stationary or when the fly is stationary and the stripes move. Why does the fly turn with the stripes when the stripes turn, but seems to disregard the stripes when they are stationary?

To answer this question, von Holst and Mittelstaedt twisted the fly's head 180 degrees and glued the head in this new position (see Figure 2.12). Under this condition, the fly's behavior was, to say the least, strange. When the fly stood still and the vertical stripes were turned to the right, the fly turned to the left, and when the fly stood still and the vertical stripes turned to the left, the fly turned to the right. However, when the fly attempted to move on its own, it took a step one way or the other and kept doing this indefinitely.

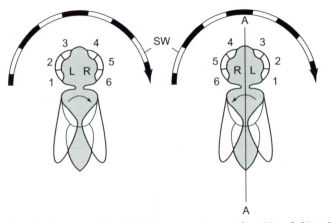

FIGURE 2.12 Behavior of a fly whose left and right eyes are in normal position (left) and whose left and right eyes have been interchanged by twisting its head 180 degrees about the longitudinal axis, A, of the body (right). Numbers designate eye segments. The arrow on the fly indicates the direction in which the fly is most likely to rotate given that the vertical stripes in front of it rotate to the right. From Gallistel, C. R. (1980). The organization of action. Hillsdale, NJ: Erlbaum. With permission.

How did von Holst and Mittelstaedt (1950) explain these results? According to the authors, the fly "expects a quite specific retinal image displacement, which is neutralized when it occurs" (p. 179). In other words, when the fly turns to the right, it has a reference signal for a retinal displacement to the left. Similarly, when the fly turns to the left, it has a reference signal for a retinal displacement to the right. Obtaining the expected retinal displacement indicates to the moving fly that the world has remained stationary. By contrast, if the fly is stationary and the retinal image moves, the shift of the retinal image indicates to the fly that it has lost its bearings with respect to the external world. Consequently, the fly turns to realign itself with its surroundings. If the eyes are spatially interchanged, as in the experiment of von Holst and Mittelstaedt, the expected and obtained retinal image displacements are reversed. The result, as von Holst and Mittelstaedt (1950, p. 179) put it colorfully, is a "central catastrophe."

Considering the behavior of the flipped-head fly shows how sophisticated the perceptual-motor system can be, and at how early a stage of evolution this sophistication took hold. Not surprisingly, internal subtraction processes of the kind proposed for the fly have also been attributed to higher animals, including people (von Holst & Mittelstaedt, 1950; Sperry, 1950; Wolpert & Flanagan, 2001). For human and nonhuman animals, the perceptual consequence of one's own actions is sometimes called *reafference*. The first person to recognize the importance of reafference and the role of feedforward in distinguishing reafference from *exafference* (perceptual input arising from outside influences) was the great German physiologist Hermann Helmholtz (1866/1962).

Movement Enhances Perception

Movement never occurs in a behavioral vacuum. We move to be able to perceive, just as we perceive to be able to move. Arguing which is more important is a red herring.

One reason why movement benefits perception is that movement allows for the transport of sensory receptors. We turn our eyes and heads so we can take in visual information from a range of locations, we walk to new locations so we can see and hear what is going on there, we use our hands so we can feel things and bring them to locations where we can look at them, smell them, taste them, and so on.

There is also a more dramatic way in which movement enhances perception. In some cases, movement actually makes it possible to see at all. The most famous case in which this principle was demonstrated involved a young woman, known in the scientific literature by her initials, D.F. (Milner & Goodale, 1995). Soon after moving into an apartment with her new husband, D.F. took a shower while her husband went out to shop for groceries. The shower's water heater malfunctioned and released carbon monoxide into the shower. D.F. fell unconscious from the fumes. Her husband returned just in time to save her.

During the recovery period, D.F. appeared, for all intents and purposes, to be blind. When she was shown familiar objects and was asked to name them, she was unable to do so, though she was able to understand and produce language, and she could name the same objects when she felt them.

The great surprise came when D.F. reached for objects (Figure 2.13). When she did so, she shaped her hand appropriately, provided her eyes were open and the room was lit. This was true even if the objects were presented at different positions in successive trials. Subsequent tests confirmed that D.F. could make appropriate use of visual information about the locations, sizes, shapes, and orientations of objects when she reached for them, even though she was unable to recognize the objects when she had to signal her recognition of them through verbal means, such as saying what the objects were. Thus, when D.F. was asked to place a card through a slot whose orientation was unpredictable, she turned the card in the appropriate manner as she brought the card toward the slot. By contrast, when she had to indicate through other means how the slot was oriented—for example, by assigning a numerical angle value to the orientation, or by turning a dial to match the orientation of the slot—she performed at chance. Her behavior contrasted markedly with the performance of normal-sighted control subjects who showed essentially perfect performance in both contexts—both when reaching for the objects and when making judgments about them.

D.F.'s performance suggests that the human brain has two systems for seeing. One is for identifying objects. The other is for interacting with objects in a physically appropriate manner. Milner and Goodale (1995) referred to these systems as the "what" and "how" systems, respectively. Other scientists had previously referred to these two systems as the "what" and "where" systems (Ungerleider & Mishkin, 1982). Regardless of the exact terms used, a deeper message from this work is that perception and motor control go hand in hand and, if you will, see eye to eye. Another lesson is that a great deal can be learned by studying patients.

Movement Informs Perception

Movement does not just make perception possible. It also influences what we perceive, often in surprising ways. Work by Dennis Proffitt and his colleagues at the University of Virginia bear this out; see Proffitt (2006) for review. In one experiment, Proffitt, Bhalla, Gossweiler, and Midgett (1995) asked university students to judge the steepness of a hill when the students stood at the base of the hill (Figure 2.14). In one condition, the students

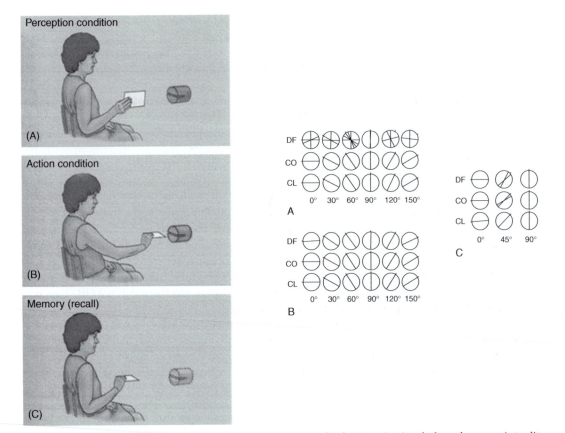

FIGURE 2.13   Left: Match card orientation to seen slit. Right: Card orientation just before placement into slit. Data from patient D.F. and two control participants, C.O. and C.L. Left panels from Gazzaniga, M. S., Ivry, R. B., & Mangun, G. R. (1998). Cognitive neuroscience: The biology of the mind. New York: W. W. Norton. Right panel from Goodale, M. A., & Milner, A. D. (1992). Separate visual pathways for perception and action. Trends in Neuroscience, 15, 20–25. M.A. Goodale & A.D. Milner In: D.J. Ingle, M.A. Goodale & R.J.W. Mansfield, Editors, Analysis of Visual Behavior, MIT Press (1982), pp. 263–299. With permission.

made the judgments while wearing a heavy backpack. In another condition, the students made the judgments without wearing a heavy weight. The hill looked steeper for the encumbered group, as indicated by the degree to which they tilted a level with their hands. However, when the same two groups gave *verbal* estimates of hill steepness (numbers rather than hand levels), the difference between them disappeared.

The latter result argues against the hypothesis that participants were responding to demand characteristics (feeling pressured by the experimenter), for it is hard to see how demand characteristics could have selectively favored greater estimates of steepness in one group than another and for one type of response than another. The positive conclusion from this work is that the steepness of the hill was apparently perceived in terms of how much effort would be needed to scale it. The hill's apparent steepness reflected its perceived *affordance* for climbing (Gibson, 1979). Perception, or at least visual perception of slant, is

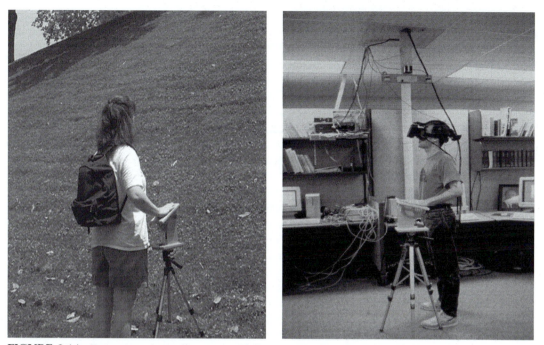

FIGURE 2.14   Estimation of visually perceived hill steepness with a hand level. Left: A participant wearing a heavy backpack. Right: A participant viewing a hill in a virtual-reality environment. Pictures kindly provided by Professor Dennis Proffitt (received April 25, 2008). With permission.

therefore *embodied*. That is, the way the environment is perceived is mediated by what we see we can do in the environment.

Two other features of the work of Dennis Proffitt and his colleagues merit attention. One is that similar effects were obtained for other perceptual features besides hill steepness. For example, Witt, Proffitt, and Epstein (2005) found that target locations that could be touched with a handheld stick were perceived as nearer when the stick could be used to touch the target compared to when the stick could not be used. Witt, Linkenauger, Bakdash, and Proffitt (2008) found that golf holes were reported to appear larger on days when golfers performed well than on days when they performed less well. Such findings extend the generality of the claim about embodied perception.

Second, virtual-reality (VR) technology was used in some of the studies. In VR, the participant is visually immersed in the environment s/he is viewing, typically through a sophisticated interface of computer technology and special head-mounted gear, such as that shown in the right panel of Figure 2.14. VR technology has proven to be a useful new tool in the study of human motor control, including studies of new ways to rehabilitate people with motor impairments.

Mirror Neurons

The final example of the tight coupling between motor control and perception comes from a chance discovery made in a neurophysiology lab in the early 1990's. Researchers at the University of Parma in Italy were recording from neurons in the brain of a macaque monkey. Between "official" recording sessions, a researcher in the lab happened to pick up a piece of food and eat it. Surprisingly, the neurons from which recordings were being taken fired vigorously upon sight of this event. Further investigation showed that the neurons fired intensely either when the monkey saw someone pick up an object and ingest it or when the monkey picked up an object and ate it itself. More generally, the neurons fired vigorously whether the same action was performed by the monkey or witnessed by the monkey. The researchers who stumbled upon this finding referred to these cells as *mirror* neurons. They used this term to refer to the fact that the neurons fired when actions animals could perform were mirrored in actions witnessed in others (for a review, see Rizzolatti & Craighero, 2004).

Do mirror neurons exist in the human brain? For ethical reasons, it is impossible to implant electrodes in the human brain to answer this question. However, there are other less invasive ways to address the question. Functional magnetic resonance imagery (fMRI) makes it possible to determine which parts of the brain become active when different tasks are performed. In fMRI studies, participants (human or animal) occupy a machine that painlessly scans the brain. fMRI scans reflect brain activity or, more specifically, blood flow to different brain areas. The more active a brain area is, the more it draws oxygenated blood to satisfy its metabolic needs. fMRI experiments have been done to test for mirror neurons, including mirror neurons in the human brain. These experiments have yielded results consistent with the hypothesis that the human brain has mirror neurons (for a review, see Rizzolatti & Craighero, 2004). Thus, people, like macaque monkeys, appear to have neurons that fire both when people perform actions and when they see others perform those same actions.

An illustrative study of human mirror neurons involved dancers watching other dancers (Figure 2.15). The dancers being watched danced either classical ballet or capoeira, a dance from Brazil (Calvo-Merino, Glaser, Grezes, Passingham, & Haggard, 2005). The dancers doing the observing were either classical ballerinas or capoeira dancers. The brain activity of the ballerinas was greater when they watched ballet movements than when they watched capoeira movements, whereas the brain activity of the capoeira dancers was greater when they watched capoeira movements than when they watched ballet movements. These differences were observed in the brain regions where mirror neurons have been found in monkeys, so the data accord with the hypothesis that mirror neurons exist in the human brain. A further suggestion of the ballet/capoeira results is that mirror neurons reflect learning.

THE LEARNING PROBLEM

We have now considered three of the four problems at the heart of motor-control research: the degrees of freedom problem, the sequencing and timing problem, and the perceptual-motor integration problem. One other problem remains to be summarized here: the skill acquisition problem. How are motor skills acquired?

In this chapter we will focus on just a handful of the most surprising and influential findings that have emerged in this area of study. This overview will give you a sense of the issues and methods that attend this domain of motor-control research. The findings to be

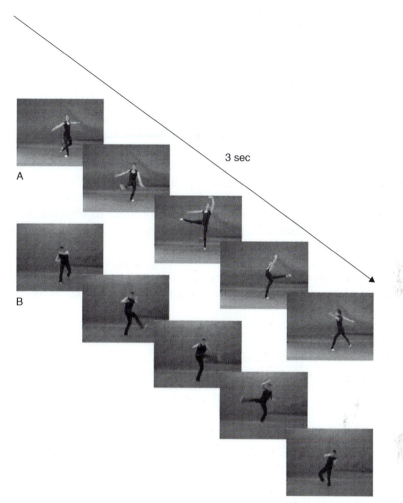

FIGURE 2.15   Moves performed in the style of ballet (A) or capoeira (B). From Calvo-Merino, B., Glaser, D.E., Grezes, J., Passingham, R.E., & Haggard, P. (2005). Action observation and acquired motor skills: An fMRI study with expert dancers. Cerebral Cortex, 15, 1243–1249. With permission.

summarized pertain to learning by doing, learning by practicing deliberately, learning through specificity of practice, and learning through plasticity.

Learning by Doing

Everyone has heard the expression "learn by doing." The phrase has a nice ring to it. You can't really learn to ride a bike by reading about it. You have to get on and try it yourself. However, there is a less trivial sense in which we learn by doing, at least when it comes to learning what perceptual changes accompany the movements we make. The only way to learn what those changes are, short of being innately equipped with knowledge of them, is to explore them via active exploration.

Held illustrated a classic experiment that made this point (Held, 1965). Two kittens were reared in darkness except when they got to spend a few minutes each day in a special environment where one kitten could walk freely and the other kitten got to ride a small gondola yoked to the kitten that was free to roam. Both kittens received essentially the same visual input, but only the kitten that could walk could actively control the visual input being received. The question was whether the kittens would exhibit the same level of visuo-motor coordination when they were later tested outside the experimental chamber.

When the kittens were later tested, only the kitten that could move freely behaved normally. The other kitten proved to be functionally blind. This was shown by holding each kitten in the air and slowly lowering each one, face down, toward a horizontal surface. Only the freely moving kitten exhibited the normal visual "placing" reaction that kittens and cats show when they are lowered to flat surfaces. The implication is that the development of normal visuo-motor coordination depended on the opportunity to correlate visual input with actively generated motor commands. When the passive cat moved its legs in the gondola, no consistent changes in visual input followed; its movements and visual perceptions were uncorrelated. By contrast, when the active cat moved its legs, the visual changes it received were directly linked to its movements, so its movements and visual perceptions could be correlated. (The two kittens were able to move equally well when they were allowed to roam freely in a dark environment.)

The gondola study shows that growing kittens, and perhaps growing children, need more than movement alone or perception alone to develop normal visuo-motor coordination. They need to be able to actively control these two kinds of experience to learn what their correlation is. Learning by doing amounts, in this view, to forming correlations between movements and perceptions.

Learning by Practicing Deliberately

In addition to learning by doing, learning is aided by practicing deliberately. Said another way, skill development is aided by practicing often and with concentration on those aspects of performance that need improvement.

This conclusion comes from a study by Ericsson, Krampe, and Tesch-Romer (1993). These authors asked whether innate talent accounts for skilled performance, as claimed by Sir Francis Galton in the late nineteenth and early twentieth century (Galton, 1979) and as still widely accepted by many athletic coaches and music teachers today. The alternative that Ericsson, Krampe, and Tesch-Romer considered was that in addition to, or instead of, sheer talent, the amount of deliberate practice one devotes to a skill accounts, to a large extent, for how well the skill develops. The results of Ericsson, Krampe, and Tesch-Romer and results of others confirmed the deliberate-practice hypothesis.

Figure 2.16 shows some results of the study by Ericsson, Krampe, and Tesch-Romer (1993). As seen here, the number of hours per week that violinists spent practicing predicted the judged quality of their performance. Having been called "talented" did not predict how well the students played as compared to the sheer amount of time they practiced. In addition, it was not just the number of hours per week the violinists spent practicing that predicted their judged quality of performance; rather, it was how they spent those practice hours. Violinists who went on to perform masterfully spent much of their time focusing on

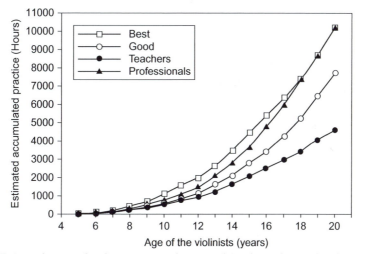

FIGURE 2.16   Estimated accumulated practice as a function of age for violinists classified as best performers, good performers, teachers, and professionals. From Ericsson, K. A., Krampe, R. T., & Tesch-Romer, C. (1993). The role of deliberate practice in the acquisition of expert performance. Psychological Review, 100, 363–406. With permission.

passages they had trouble with. Violinists who never went on to perform masterfully spent much of their time playing what they already played reasonably well.

A similar outcome applies to figure skaters. Deakin and Cobley (2003) asked figure skaters to complete diaries about their skating practice habits. The diaries revealed that elite skaters spent 68% of their practice sessions rehearsing risky moves. Lower-ranked skaters spent only 48% of their time rehearsing risky moves.

Results like these have important implications for the education of skills and for the understanding of what contributes to skill learning. In terms of the education of skills, coaches should encourage students to practice in a concerted way. The coaches should have their students focus on what needs to be improved, and the coaches should encourage their pupils to put in the time to achieve those improvements. That said, practicing with dogged determination for hours on end without a break will probably not pay off. The reason is that massed practice (i.e., practice without breaks) is generally worse than spaced practice (i.e., practice with breaks), as will be discussed in Chapter 5.

In terms of understanding the factors that contribute to skill learning, the findings of Ericsson, Krampe, and Tesch-Romer (1993) also indicate that there is a clear intellectual component to skill acquisition. Rote practice does little good as contrasted with focused exploration of alternative ways of performing.

Learning Through Specificity of Practice

Another insight that has been gained through recent research on skill acquisition is that what is learned in skill learning is often surprisingly specific. Illustrative data appear in Figure 2.17. Here basketball players made foul shots from different distances in front of a

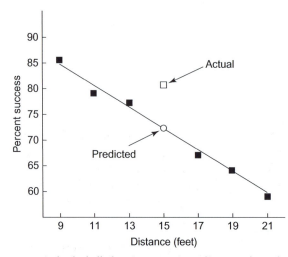

FIGURE 2.17 Percent success in basketball shooting at various distances from the basket, including the foul shot line, where the actual level of success exceeds what is predicted from a simple linear function relating success to distance. From Keetch, K. M., Schmidt, R. A., Lee, T. D., & Young, D. E. (2005). Especial skills: Their emergence with massive amounts of practice. Journal of Experimental Psychology: Human Perception and Performance, 31, 970–978. With permission.

basketball net (Keetch, Schmidt, Lee, & Young, 2005). One of the distances was the one corresponding to the normal foul shot line, where the players had made many foul shots before.

One might expect the likelihood of making a basket to decrease the farther from the basket the shooter stood. If that were the case, the likelihood of making shots from the foul line would depend only on how far the foul line happened to be from the basket. A graph showing the likelihood of making a basket as a function of shooting distance would have all the points lie on one line, including the point corresponding to the foul-line shooting distance.

The actual data were different. As shown in Figure 2.17, the likelihood of making baskets from the distance corresponding to the foul line was higher than would be expected from the best-fitting line relating hits (making baskets) to shooting distance. From this outcome, one can infer that the players learned something special about shooting from this distance. Rather than learning something general about basketball shooting that extended in a graded, uniform fashion over distances from the basket, they learned something quite specific. This phenomenon is known as *specificity of practice*.

Specificity of practice turns out to be a common phenomenon in perceptual-motor skill acquisition. A phenomenon that vividly demonstrates the phenomenon, or the belief in it, was the habit of the great concert pianist Vladimir Horowitz always to perform on his own piano. Horowitz believed in his "home piano" advantage. So too does the pop singer Tori Amos who also brings her own piano with her when she performs. Sports teams, too, benefit from playing at home. Regardless of whether the advantage accrues from friendly cheers from the fans or from familiarity with cues of the local environment, the home field advantage is a statistically reliable phenomenon (http://www.twominutewarning.com/hfa.htm).

More will be said about specificity of practice in Chapter 6. There we will consider in more detail the costs and benefits of being especially adept at performing when the conditions of performance match or do not match conditions of practice.

Learning Through Neural Plasticity

It is nice to do well when performance conditions are the same as the ones in which one has practiced, but if we could not perform what we learned in *new* environments, practice would do us little general good. A challenge in addressing the skill acquisition problem, then, is to understand the tradeoff between the capacity for generalization on the one hand and the benefit of specific training on the other. Considering this challenge leads to the fundamental question of how skills are learned at all. Here we consider the neural changes that allow for learning. Understanding those changes is one of the core problems in neuroscience as well as in motor control and related fields.

A major advance in the study of the neural basis of learning was the discovery in the 1980's of neural *plasticity*; for reviews see Buonomano and Merzenich (1998) and Kaas (1991). The discovery began with studies by Michael Merzenich and his colleagues after they found large differences in the amount of neural tissue devoted to specific functions within the brains of different animals. Classical neuroanatomy and neurophysiology would not have suggested such large differences. According to the classical view, the amount of neural tissue devoted to a given function such as touch is more or less the same in every member of a species. Merzenich and colleagues wondered why they were finding large individual differences in the amount of neural real estate devoted to various functions. These scientists hypothesized that the brain might be *plastic* or changeable. According to this view, more neural tissue comes to be devoted to often-experienced functions than to less-experienced functions.

To test this idea, Merzenich carried out a number of experiments, one of which was a bit ghoulish, though it provided unequivocal (and quite memorable) support for the plasticity hypothesis. In the first part of the experiment (not the ghoulish part), Merzenich et al. (1984) recorded from neurons in the somatosensory cortex of the owl monkey brain (see Figure 2.18). This part of the brain is responsive to touch. Within this brain region, neighboring neurons respond most vigorously to gentle touches on neighboring parts of the body. Thus, when one records from some part of the somatosensory cortex, the neurons from which one is recording fire vigorously to touch on the index finger, say. Moving the recording electrode to a neighboring site brings one to neurons that fire vigorously to touch on the *middle* finger. Moving the recording electrode a little further to a new neighboring site brings one to neurons that fire vigorously to touch on the *ring* finger.

After discovering which neurons fired in response to touch on which parts of the body, Merzenich and colleagues carried out the more ghoulish part of the experiment. They amputated the monkey's middle finger and asked what would happen to the part of the somatosensory cortex that previously responded to touch on that digit. The result was that those neurons gradually responded to touch on the adjacent fingers—the index finger and ring finger. This result provided evidence for neural plasticity. The data indicated that the neurons in the somatosensory cortex did not respond in a fixed fashion but instead responded in a way that changed with experience.

Experiment 2

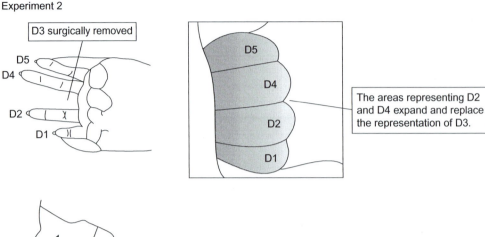

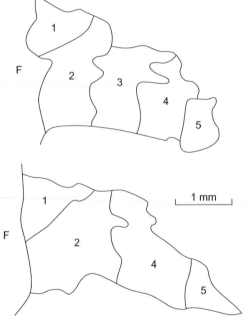

FIGURE 2.18 Neural plasticity demonstrated through amputation of a monkey's finger (digit 3). Left: Monkey's paw with third digit removed. Right: Change in responsiveness of somatosensory cortex to the five digits of the monkey when all the finger are present (top panel) and several months after the third digit was removed (bottom panel). Left panel from Kandel and Schwartz. Right panel from Mather, G. (2006). Foundations of perception. Sussex: Psychology Press.

What mechanism allowed for this change of responsiveness? One can imagine that inputs from the index finger and ring finger had always "wanted" to make contact with the middle-finger region of the somatosensory cortex. However, inputs from the middle finger had always kept those connections out. With the middle-finger input removed, that input could not prevent the index-finger and ring-finger inputs to wend their way into the middle-finger region, commandeering that region for their own purposes.

Neural plasticity has since been demonstrated with other experimental preparations. For example, another study showed that the index finger region of the somatosensory cortex is functionally enlarged when owl monkeys spent a considerable amount of time gently touching a rotating wheel to obtain a reward. Focusing on the finger led to enlargement of the brain region responsible for registering touch on that finger (Jenkins, Merzenich, Ochs, Allard, & Guic-Robles, 1990).

A similar result was obtained in humans. The amount of somatosensory cortex devoted to touch received from the tips of the left hand is enlarged in violinists compared to non-violinists, and this difference grows with practice on the instrument (Elbert, Pantev, Weinbruch, Rockstroh, & Taub, 1995). The latter result indicates that neural plasticity occurs in humans as well as monkeys. It also shows, as does the touch-training study of Jenkins et al. (1990), that neural plasticity can come about through positive means (learning), not just negative means (amputation).

In general, neural plasticity ensures economical use of the brain. No part of the brain stands idle if it can potentially serve some purpose. Contrary to the oft-quoted claim that we use only 10% of our brains—a statement that is meant to rouse us to learn—all of our brains are continually in use, with each part finding a purpose for which it is optimally suited given the nature of personal experience.

SUMMARY

1. One of the core problems in human motor control is the degrees of freedom problem. The term refers to the fact that there are generally many possible ways to complete a task, only one of which can be performed at any given time.
2. The degrees of freedom problem is a problem for researchers, not for people or animals engaged in everyday activities.
3. The degrees of freedom in a system are the ways the system can independently vary.
4. One way to reduce the degrees of freedom to be managed is to rely on synergies. Synergies are linkages between or among movement elements. An example is the difficulty encountered while trying to rub your stomach while patting your head. Synergies are soft (optional) constraints rather than hard (necessary) constraints.
5. Physics, or more specifically physical mechanics, provides another way of reducing the degrees of freedom to be independently managed. Robotic devices that walk like people do by virtue of their physical design (passive dynamic walkers) illustrate reliance on physical mechanics. This approach simplifies the motor-control problem associated with having many degrees of freedom that, in principle, need to be controlled independently.
6. Reliance on efficiency principles is a third way to reduce degrees of freedom. Two efficiency principles are, first, ending movements in comfortable postures and, second, accelerating and decelerating smoothly.
7. A second major issue in the study of human motor control is the sequencing and timing problem. The question is how elements of behavior are ordered in time.
8. One source of information about sequencing and timing comes from the analysis of speech errors. Such analyses suggest that a plan is set up in advance for an extended sequence of forthcoming utterances. Action slips (e.g., pouring catsup into one's coffee

    rather than onto one's hamburger) also provide evidence for action plans. Action slips, like speech errors, show systematic trends.

9. Another source of information about the sequencing and timing of behavior comes from analyses of coarticulation, as in rounding the lips in advance of the strict need to do so during speech. Coarticulation is also seen in typing and in reaching for and grasping objects. In typing, each finger moves toward its key target as soon as it can. In reaching and grasping, objects are taken hold of in ways that anticipate their future use.

10. Timing of behavior reflects considerable sophistication on the part of the motor-control system. Synchronization studies suggest that we care more about the synchronization of the perceptual consequences of our actions than we do about the synchronization of our efferent commands (signals to muscles).

11. The third major problem in the study of human motor control is the perceptual-motor integration problem.

12. Responding to feedback is a prime example of using perception to aid movement, and vice versa. In a *negative* feedback loop, discrepancies between desired and obtained results tend to promote error *reduction*. In a *positive* feedback loop, discrepancies between desired and obtained results tend to promote error *enhancement*.

13. Open-loop control occurs when feedback is unavailable. Closed-loop control occurs when feedback is available.

14. Feedforward control is control based on prediction. Everyday movements tend to reflect the combined use of feedforward *and* feedback.

15. Reliance on feedforward is suggested by features of performance when feedback is removed and from data indicating that perception is strongly modulated by ongoing motor activity. Perceptual inputs are interpreted differently depending on how one is moving at the time.

16. Movement enhances perception. This was shown most dramatically in the case of a woman who was unable to identify seen objects though she could reach for the objects well using her eyesight.

17. Movement informs perception. For example, the apparent steepness of a hill can change as a function of the heaviness of the backpack one is wearing when one thinks one will have to scale the hill. Such a result suggests that perception of the external environment is *embodied*, taking into account one's sense of what the environment affords for bodily action.

18. Mirror neurons are cells that fire when animals see others performing actions they can perform themselves. People also appear to have mirror neurons.

19. The fourth major problem in human motor control is understanding how motor skills are acquired.

20. One way motor skills are acquired is through learning by doing, that is, by actively exploring the effects of one's movements on the perceptual consequences those movements have.

21. Learning by practicing deliberately is another important skill-acquisition principle. Practicing long and in a focused manner is more predictive of the skill level one can attain than is "raw talent."

22. Sometimes benefits of practice are most especially clear when the conditions of performance exactly match the conditions of learning. This outcome is called *specificity*

of practice. An example is the especially high probability of basketball players making baskets when shooting from the foul line.

23. Learning is achieved through neural plasticity. Here specialized functions of brain regions change in ways that reflect personal experience. For example, a region of the brain that is initially specialized for touch of a finger will grow larger if that finger is used repeatedly in a tactile detection task. Violinists develop larger "finger areas" than non-violinists on the side of the brain encoding finger presses.

Further Reading

For a review of early work on anticipatory timing, see Schmidt (1968).

For more information about changes in motor cortex in violin players, see Munte, Altenbuller, and Janke (2002).

For an early statement about feedback control in behavior, see Miller, Galanter, and Pribram (1960). Stark (1968) offered a compendium of bioengineering studies done in the tradition of control theory. For more recent information about the use of feedback and feedforward in human perceptual-motor control, see Jagacinski and Flach (2003).

A book that made the case, early on, for viewing action as a means of governing perception was written by Powers (1973).

Latash (2008b) provided a book-long treatment of synergies.

Daniel Wolpert and his colleagues (http://www.wolpertlab.com/) have championed the role of feedforward control (e.g., Wolpert & Flanagan, 2001).

For a popularized treatment of feedforward control mechanisms in relation to itch, see Gawande (2008). The patient described in this article had an itch on her head that was so intense she literally scratched through her skull.

If you are curious to see how findings from perceptual-motor control studies can be extended to solve the world's political problems, see Gilbert (2006).

A book that reproduced classic articles on the core problems of action was compiled by Gallistel (1980).

Neural plasticity has received press in connection with phantom limbs. Here, patients who have lost a limb through amputation still feel the limb. Oddly, the patients may feel that the absent limb is being touched when another part of the body is being palpated. Ramachandran and Blakeslee (1998) wrote a book about this phenomenon and its roots in neural plasticity. One of the patients they described felt his absent arm being touched when pressure was gently applied to his face. Where the arm was felt to be touched depended on where on the face the gentle pressure was applied. Ramachandran and Blakeslee (1998) explained this phenomenon by noting that incoming sensory signals from the arms and face go to closely neighboring regions of the brain (within the somatosensory cortex). After loss of the arm, inputs from the face encroach onto the region that normally receives inputs from the arm. When the arm area is activated, higher centers interpret the activation as coming from the arm itself.

Another book about neural plasticity, written for a general audience and with an emphasis on the uplifting possibilities of this newfound brain malleability, is Doidge (2007).

Physiological Foundations

OUTLINE

Muscle	46	**Basal Ganglia**	65
The Length-Tension Relation	47	*Huntington's Disease*	66
Motor Units and Recruitment	49	*Parkinson's Disease*	66
		Theories of Basal Ganglia Function	67
Proprioception	50	**Motor Cortex**	69
Muscle Spindles	51	*Force and Direction Control*	71
Golgi Tendon Organs	53	*Whole-Body Movement*	73
Joint Receptors	54	*Long-Loop Reflexes*	74
Cutaneous Receptors	54	**Premotor Cortex**	75
Spinal Cord	55	**Supplementary Motor Area**	76
Spinal Reflexes	55		
Servo Theory	55	**Parietal Cortex**	80
α-γ Coactivation	57	*Apraxia*	81
Recurrent Inhibition	57	*Cross-Modal Integration*	82
Reciprocal Inhibition	58		
The Smart Spinal Cord	60	**Disconnections**	84
Tuning of Spinal Reflexes	61	**Concluding Remarks**	85
Cerebellum	61		
Regulation of Muscle Tone	62	**Summary**	86
Coordination	63	**Further Reading**	89
Timing	63		
Learning	65		

Movements are made in response to a variety of signals. Some come from the external environment—a traffic light changing from red to green, the sound of a car horn, a thumbtack stepped on accidentally. Others come from the internal environment—a suddenly remembered appointment, an impulsive thought, a deep sentiment. Meanwhile, some movements are automatic while others are deliberate. Withdrawing one's hand from an unexpectedly hot stove is automatic. Giving a downbeat to a symphony orchestra is usually more deliberate.

No matter what the signal or context for movement, virtually all movements involve a large number of muscles (see Figure 3.1). These muscles act on our behalf but not with our deliberation. If we had to think about what our muscles do, we would be unable to move skillfully. Given that we move as skillfully as we do, the main challenge in the study of motor physiology is to understand how, from a physical standpoint, we can move and maintain positions as adaptively and effortlessly as we do.

The nervous system allows for skilled motor performance by relying on a set of linked special-purpose mechanisms. At the lowest levels are sensory receptors and muscle fibers. These structures are connected through a variable number of synapses, or gaps, between neurons. Some of the connections involve only a single synapse (monosynaptic connections). Other connections involve many synapses (polysynaptic connections). Because only a few synapses are required for some sensori-motor loops, some motor responses to sensory inputs are extremely rapid and automatic. The patellar tendon tap, the procedure in which the tendon below your knee is tapped by a physician, is a familiar example.

Pathways running through the spinal cord allow for communication between the peripheral and central nervous systems. Ascending spinal pathways allow afferent (incoming sensory) signals from the periphery to reach the brain. Descending spinal pathways from the brain allow efferent (outgoing motor) signals from higher centers to reach the periphery, where they excite or inhibit motor neurons and excite or inhibit interneurons (neurons that synapse onto other neurons).

The brain contains a neural network consisting of 10^{12} to 10^{14} neurons, each of which may have 10^4 or more synaptic connections. The brain is not anatomically homogeneous. Even to the naked eye, distinct brain regions can be discerned (see Figure 3.2). Through dissection and other neuroanatomical techniques, one can see a number of cell types and patterns of connectivity in the brain.

By recording the activity of neurons in different brain regions and by studying the effects of lesions in various brain sites, it has been found that there are important functional distinctions among brain centers. Some of these centers are primarily devoted to hearing, others are mainly dedicated to vision, others are mainly devoted to smell, and so forth. In the domain of motor control, some centers are involved in relatively low-level aspects of the control of movement and posture, such as the direction and force of single limb movements. Other centers are involved in higher-level aspects, such as the planning of extended sequences of movements. The notion that different parts of the nervous system provide different levels of control provides a helpful didactic principle for reviewing motor neuroscience. To a large extent, it is the principle around which this chapter is organized.

Some disclaimers should be offered for the review to follow. The review is not meant to be an exhaustive treatment of motor physiology or neuroanatomy. Knowing about these topics is important for a complete understanding of motor neuroscience, but this book is mainly about the psychology of human motor control. Therefore, the more modest aim of this chapter, vis-à-vis neuroscience, is to convey a sense of the major principles of this approach. The Further Reading section at the end of the chapter provides pointers to more information.

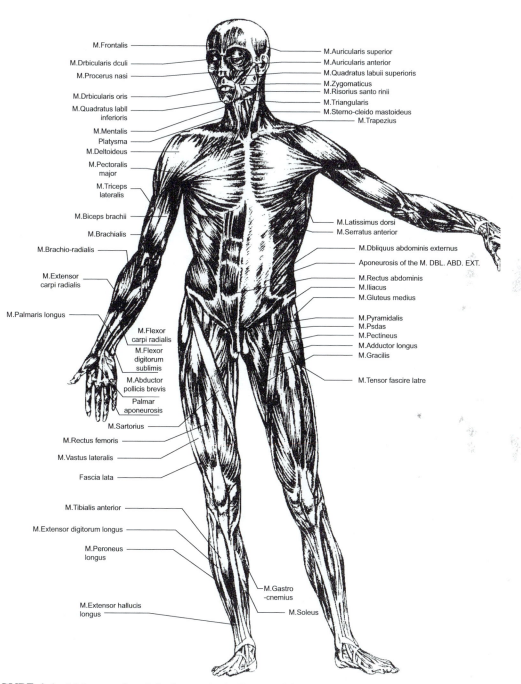

FIGURE 3.1 Major muscles of the human body. Reprinted from Anatomy for artists. Milan: Vilencia. With permission.

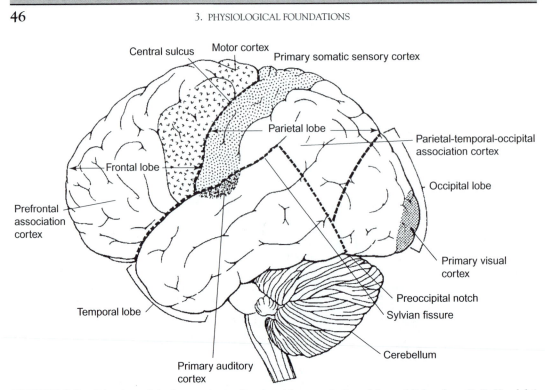

FIGURE 3.2   Side view of the human brain. Reprinted by permission of the publisher from E. R. Kandel & J. H. Schwartz (eds.), Principles of neural science (2nd ed.), p. 214. Copyright © 1985 by Elsevier Science Publishing Co., Inc.

MUSCLE

Muscles produce force by contracting. They contract in response to a neurotransmitter, acetylcholine, released by motor nerves at the neuromuscular junction. When a muscle's receptors for acetylcholine are damaged, as in the disease *myesthenia gravis*, muscle contraction is impaired and weakness can result (Drachman, 1983).

Whereas muscles *contract* in response to nerve impulses, they *stretch* or *lengthen* only mechanically, through the action of opposing muscles or external loads. This is a very important principle, which was not always appreciated, as seen below.

In the third century B.C.E., the Greek thinker Erasistratus proposed that muscles fill with spirits sent through the nerves (McMahon, 1984). According to Erasistratus, when muscles fill, their girth expands but their length decreases, much as a balloon changes shape when it fills with air. Not until 1663 was it understood that muscles simply shorten. In the decisive experiment, a frog's muscle was placed in an air-filled tube and the nerve running to the muscle was pinched. The muscle contracted in response to the nerve stimulation, but the volume of air in the tube remained constant (Needham, 1971). Had the muscle expanded, the volume of air in the tube would have shrunk. The fact that it did not poked a hole in the "balloon theory" of muscle contraction.

It took nearly 300 years to appreciate how muscle contraction works. With the development of the electron microscope and the polarizing light microscope, it became possible to see that when muscles shorten, two types of protein filaments, actin and myosin, slide past each other, forming tiny interlocking cross-bridges. The cross-bridges allow for the buildup of muscle force (Pollack, 1983).

The Length-Tension Relation

The formation of cross-bridges between actin and myosin affects macroscopic as well as microscopic features of muscle performance. If a single muscle, excised from an animal, is stretched to different lengths, it resists the stretch with more tension as the muscle is stretched more and more; see Figure 3.3(A). This is a result of the mechanical properties of the muscle as shown by the fact that the muscle responds this way even when it receives no nerve stimulation. A mechanical spring behaves in the same way. In an ideal spring, the relation between tension and stretch from the spring's resting length is linear; this relation is known as Hooke's law. As a practical matter, the relation between spring tension and spring stretch is nonlinear, and the same is true of muscle.

As shown in Figure 3.3A, if the experiment with the stretched muscle is repeated and the nerve to the muscle is stimulated, the total tension the muscle produces is greater than the tension produced when the muscle is stretched without added stimulation (the "passive" condition). The total tension curve ("active + passive") has a somewhat different shape from the "passive tension" curve. The passive tension curve rises monotonically, but the total tension curve has a dip. The difference between the two curves is due to actively developed tension in the muscle—the amount of tension resulting from neurally driven contraction. As seen in Figure 3.3A, the active-tension curve is an inverted-U-shaped function of length.

What accounts for the inverted-U shape of the active tension curve? The shape reflects the strength of actin-myosin cross-bridges formed at different muscle lengths (Figure 3.3B). When muscle is very short, there is too much overlap among the filaments to allow much tension to build. When muscle is very long, there is too little overlap for appreciable tension to develop. At intermediate muscle lengths, however, many cross-bridges can be formed and tension can be maximized (Huxley, 1974; McMahon, 1984).

Length-tension relations have effects on everyday activities. At extreme joint angles, when muscles tend to be maximally stretched or maximally contracted, the forces that can be produced are smaller than when muscles are neither maximally stretched nor contracted, as typically occurs at intermediate joint angles. This is why greater force can be generated when the joint is in the middle of its range of motion than at either end of its range of motion. A practical consequence of this principle was described colorfully by Rothwell (1987):

> As every hero in a gangster movie knows, the way to make the villain release his grip on the gun is to flex the wrist forcibly to reduce the power of the finger flexors. The gun will thereupon fall dramatically to the floor, to be kicked neatly away by the hero's foot. The importance of this example is that the nervous system must somehow take into account the length-tension relationship of muscle during normal movement, in this instance by extending the wrist when a maximal flexor force is required [Rothwell (1987, p. 24)].

Keeping the joints near the middle of their ranges of motion not only allows for greatest power in isometric force production. It also allows for maximal rates of oscillation (Rosenbaum, van Heugten, & Caldwell, 1996).

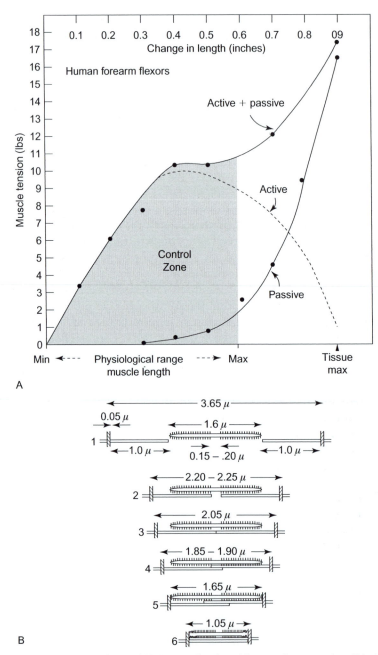

FIGURE 3.3   The length-tension relation. (A) Tension developed by muscle contraction ("Active") estimated by subtracting tension in passively stretched muscle ("Passive") from tension in driven muscle ("Active + passive"). From Brooks, V. B. (Ed.) (1981). Handbook of physiology, Section 1, Vol. II, Part 1. Baltimore: Williams & Wilkins. With permission. (B) Presumed basis for the relation: Active tension is greatest when there is maximum overlap between filaments (2 and 3), and it decreases if the overlap is less (worst case in 1) or if the filaments collide (worst case in 6). 1 corresponds to the right-hand side of the graph in A; 6 corresponds to the left-hand side. From Rothwell, J. C. (1987). Control of human voluntary movement. London: Croom-Helm. With permission.

Motor Units and Recruitment

The muscles fibers within a muscle group are innervated by motor neurons. Any given muscle fiber is innervated by just one motor neuron. A motor neuron and the muscle fibers it innervates are called a *motor unit*.

The muscle fibers within a motor unit usually have similar mechanical properties. Such mechanical homogeneity may simplify the recruitment of motor units. For a given task, the motor units to be recruited can be the ones that are mechanically best suited to the task. Similarly, tasks with different mechanical demands may call for the recruitment of different motor units. Swinging the leg or maintaining stance, for example, are carried out with different motor units (Loeb, 1985).

The number of muscle fibers in a motor unit varies from effector to effector. In the hand and eye, fewer than 100 muscle fibers occupy a motor unit; in the lower leg, a single motor unit may contain as many as 1,000 muscle fibers (Buchthal & Schmalbruch, 1980). Generally, the larger the number of muscle fibers in a motor unit, the less precise the associated movements.

Activation of a motor unit is all or none. It is impossible to voluntarily activate some but not all of the muscle fibers within a motor unit. In this sense, the motor unit is the most basic unit of motor control. On the other hand, it is possible to voluntarily recruit some motor units but not others. With feedback, such as visual or auditory signals concerning the activity of single motor units, people can learn to activate just one motor unit at a time (Figure 3.4).

When movements are produced without overt feedback about the activity of single motor units, motor units tend to be recruited in an orderly fashion (see Figure 3.5). The

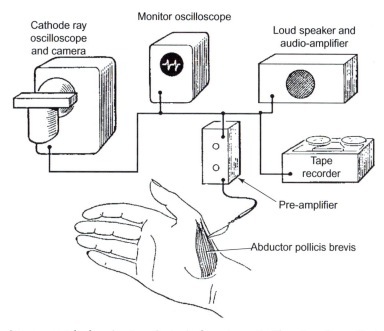

FIGURE 3.4 Arrangement for learning to activate single motor units. The setup shown illustrates the original technology used. From Basmajian, J. V. (1974). Muscles alive: Their functions revealed by electromyography (Third Edition). Baltimore: Williams & Wilkins. With permission.

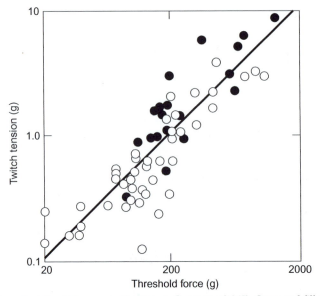

FIGURE 3.5   The size principle of Henneman, Somjen, & Carpenter (1965). Open and filled circles correspond to data obtained from the same subject at different times. From Brooks, V. B. (1986). The neural basis of motor control. New York: Oxford University Press. With permission.

first activated motor units are usually the ones whose muscle fibers are smallest and least forceful. As recruitment continues, the motor units that turn on have larger and more forceful muscle fibers. This orderly relation is called the *size principle* (Henneman, Somjen, & Carpenter, 1965).

What is the physiological basis of the size principle? Small motor neurons have low thresholds for generating action potentials (neural firings), whereas large motor neurons have high thresholds for generating action potentials. Thus weak inputs to the motor neuron pool can produce action potentials in small motor neurons. As the strength of input grows, larger motor neurons begin to fire owing to their increasing thresholds for activation.

The size principle has several functional advantages for motor control. One is that large forces are not produced when they are unnecessary; recruitment can stop when the appropriate forces have been generated. The size principle also has a computational benefit. Because hundreds or even thousands of motor units may be involved in the activation of a muscle group, the number of possible recruitment orders can be very large—larger in fact than the number of neurons in the brain (Enocka & Stuart, 1984). Thus a regular recruitment order based on size helps reduce the degrees of freedom problem at this low level of control.

PROPRIOCEPTION

Information about the position and motion of the limbs is provided both by the overt consequences of our actions, perceived primarily through the eyes and ears, and also from sensory receptors within the muscles, tendons, joints, and skin. Information provided by the latter receptors is called *proprioception*. Proprioceptive information specifically related to movement is called *kinesthesis*. In this section, we will rely on the term proprioception as an umbrella term for all internal sensing of position, whether position stays constant or changes over time.

Muscle Spindles

Only some of the muscle fibers within a muscle group are powerful enough to move or stabilize a limb. These large-diameter muscle fibers are called *extrafusal fibers* (or extrafusals). In parallel with the extrafusal fibers, and attached to them, are *muscle spindles*. Muscle spindles contain small muscle fibers called *intrafusal fibers* (or intrafusals). The intrafusals that make up a muscle spindle are connected to a single extrafusal, as shown in Figure 3.6. The midsection of the muscle spindle contains the spindle's cell nuclei, which are housed in either a nuclear bag fiber or a nuclear chain fiber.

A sensory nerve fiber—the Ia afferent—is wrapped around the central region of the nuclear bag fiber as well as the central region of the nuclear chain fiber; the part of the Ia afferent surrounding the spindle is called the primary ending. The Ia afferent responds primarily to differences between the length of the extrafusal and the intrafusal, as well as changes in this length difference over time (Matthews, 1972). When an extrafusal fiber contracts relative to an intrafusal fiber, Ia activity diminishes, but when an extrafusal fiber stretches relative to an intrafusal, Ia activity increases. The increase in Ia activity results in signals being sent to the spinal cord, where they can trigger reflex responses.

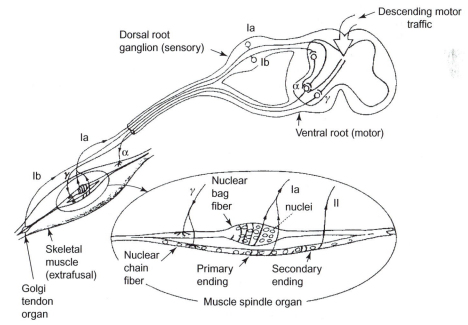

FIGURE 3.6 Muscle proprioceptors and their basic circuitry. From McMahon, T. A. (1984). Muscles, reflexes, and locomotion. Princeton, NJ: Princeton University Press. With permission.

Another sensory fiber—the group II afferent—is wrapped around the peripheral region of the nuclear chain fiber, in what is called the secondary ending. Like the Ia, the activity of the group II afferent diminishes when the extrafusal contracts relative to the intrafusal. Conversely, the activity of the group II afferent increases when the extrafusal stretches relative to the intrafusal. In general, the group II afferent is less sensitive than the Ia (Matthews, 1972; Rothwell, 1987).

For some time, it was thought that muscle spindle discharge does not contribute to the conscious perception of muscle stretch. This belief was prompted by the claim that awake patients undergoing routine operations on the ankle literally could not tell when someone was pulling their leg (Gelfan & Carter, 1967). In this study, the investigators pulled on the long tendon of the toe muscles to determine whether patients could tell that their tendons were being pulled. They could not. The same result was obtained for the wrist. The long tendons of the finger muscles were tugged and again patients seemed unaware that this manipulation was being carried out. These findings appeared to rule out a contribution of muscle spindle activity to the conscious perception of muscle stretch.

Matthews and Simmonds (1974) later repeated this procedure and found that patients could in fact detect muscle and tendon stretch quite well. In another study not involving surgery Goodwin, McCloskey, and Matthews (1972) applied vibration to the biceps muscle. Vibration applied to muscle stimulates muscle spindles. Goodwin, McCloskey, and Matthews reasoned that the vibration would activate muscle stretch receptors, so if subjects sensed muscle stretch, they would be able to perceive the limb as being more outstretched than it really was. This is just what happened. As shown in Figure 3.7, when subjects positioned the non-vibrated arm so it matched the perceived position of the vibrated arm they overestimated the angle of the elbow joint; the subjects' eyes were closed in this procedure. In a control condition, when subjects were asked simply to match the position of the non-vibrated arm with the other arm, they could do so nearly perfectly. Thus, subjects could accurately match the positions of the two arms. The systematic errors observed in the vibration condition suggested that muscle stretch can in fact be perceived.

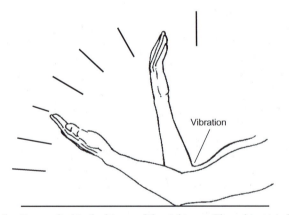

FIGURE 3.7   Effect of vibration applied to the biceps of the right arm. The subject tried to match the felt position of the right arm with the position of the left arm. The scale marks 10 degree divisions. From Rothwell, J. C. (1987). Control of human voluntary movement. London: Croom-Helm. With permission.

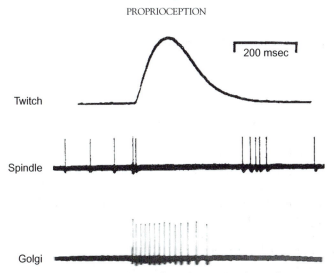

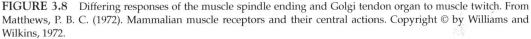

FIGURE 3.8 Differing responses of the muscle spindle ending and Golgi tendon organ to muscle twitch. From Matthews, P. B. C. (1972). Mammalian muscle receptors and their central actions. Copyright © by Williams and Wilkins, 1972.

Golgi Tendon Organs

Muscles attach to other anatomical structures—bone or skin—through tendons. Attachments of muscle to skin permit, among other things, changes in facial expression. Dimples, it turns out, are a cute by-product of tendon-to-skin attachments.

Within tendons are sensory receptors called Golgi tendon organs. These receptors have distinct afferent fibers (Ib fibers) whose response characteristics are, to a first approximation, the opposite of muscle spindles' (see Figure 3.8). When a muscle twitches—that is, when it undergoes a rapid, single contraction—its muscle stretch receptors usually fire less than before the twitch. By contrast, Golgi tendon organs fire *more* when the twitch begins and usually stop firing when the twitch is over (Matthews, 1972).

For some time, it was believed that the exclusive role of Golgi tendon organs is to signal dangerously high muscle tensions. This belief was fostered by the impression that Golgi tendon organs have high thresholds for firing, supposedly because it took a great deal of muscle tension to activate Ib afferents (Rothwell, 1987). More detailed study revealed, however, that tendon organs are in fact quite sensitive to muscle tension. For example, Ib afferents actually respond to induced muscle tensions of a tenth of a gram or less (Binder, Kroin, & Moore, 1977; Houk & Henneman, 1967).

The threshold for responding to Golgi tendon organ input is modulated by the brain. Patients with reduced communication between the spinal cord and brain due to brain damage may show a symptom that is specifically related to the processing of Golgi tendon organ inputs. In such patients, or at least those with lesions of upper motor neurons, tugging on the arm shows it to be rigid; the muscle has very high tonus. However, if the tugging force is increased, the arm suddenly lets go. This sudden release following earlier sustained resistance to stretch is called the *clasp knife* response, by analogy to the tendency of a jackknife to resist opening during gradually increasing force, but then to release. The clasp knife response is due to the Golgi tendon organ's exceeding an unusually high threshold in the patients who exhibit this anomoly. The absence of the clasp knife response in neurologically normal individuals is likely due to low thresholds for muscle contraction in response to stretch of the Golgi tendon organs.

Joint Receptors

Sensory endings in the joint provide another source of proprioceptive information. Skoglund (1956) reported that individual joint receptors respond preferentially to different joint angles (see Figure 3.9). Because it also appeared in this study that joint receptors adapt very slowly, continuing to fire for a long time after a joint angle is assumed, Skoglund proposed that joint receptors supply information about static limb position only. Later work called this view into question. Clark and Burgess (1975) and Grigg (1976) found that joint receptors actually adapt quickly, though these receptors mainly fire at extreme joint angles, as if signaling that the body is approaching a not-very-useful position (Rothwell, 1987).

Cutaneous Receptors

When movements are made, the skin surface deforms. Standing creates pressure sensations in the soles of the feet, and rubbing one's hand on a table produces sensations of displacement over the skin surface. The sensory receptors that respond to mechanical

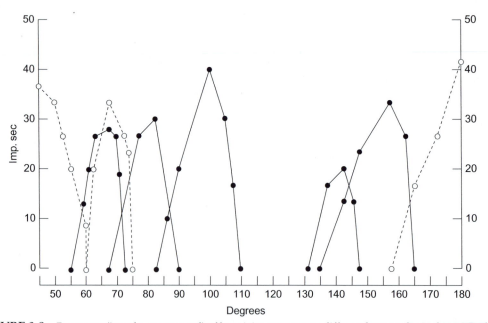

FIGURE 3.9 Responses (impulses per second) of knee joint receptors to different knee angles in the cat. Each set of connected points corresponds to a single receptor. Filled points and solid lines are from one cat. Unfilled points and dashed lines are from another cat. From Skoglund, S. (1956). Anatomical and physiological studies of knee joint innervation in the cat. Acta Physiologica Scandinavica, 36, (Supplement 124), 1–101. With permission.

deformation of the skin are called *mechanoreceptors*. Other skin receptors transmit signals that are coded as temperature-related or painful.

Damage to cutaneous mechanoreceptors can have disruptive effects on performance. Patients with damage to the pressure sensors in the soles of the feet have difficulty maintaining balance if their eyes are closed (Romberg's sign). Similarly, fine manipulations with the hands and fingers, performed without visual feedback, become difficult if mechanoreceptors in the skin of the hand or fingers are damaged (Rothwell, 1987).

An indication of the tightness of the coupling between mechanoreceptor activity and motor control is the rapidity with which people can respond to tactile stimuli. In lifting a small object with the fingers, the grip may tighten 80 ms after the object has slipped very slightly (Johansson & Westling, 1988).

There has been relatively little research on the role of cutaneous receptors in motor control. In the area of robotics, however, increasing attention has been paid to touch because of the need for precise sensing of mechanical disturbances in machine assembly and related tasks. Robots that place nuts on screws perform better if equipped with sensitive touch sensors than if they are not so equipped (Brady et al., 1986). The Steinway piano company has found that equipping robot piano polishers with tactile sensors enhances the robots' polishing performance (Amato, 1989).

SPINAL CORD

Spinal Reflexes

As was seen in Figure 3.4, Ia and Ib afferents project to the spinal cord. The Ib afferent, from the Golgi tendon organ, synapses onto an interneuron, which synapses onto a motor neuron, which in turn stimulates the extrafusal muscle to which the tendon is attached. Thus, the Ib afferent from the Golgi tendon organ ultimately has an inhibitory effect on the extrafusal muscle to which the tendon is attached. The inhibitory effect reduces the muscle tension sensed by the tendon organ.

In contrast to the Ib afferent from the tendon organ, the Ia afferent from the muscle spindle synapses directly onto the motor neuron for the spindle's extrafusal fiber. This monosynaptic connection allows for the most famous of all reflexes—the simple *reflex arc*. When impulses arrive from the Ia, the motor neuron for the extrafusal is excited. This causes the extrafusal to contract, which in turn relieves the stretch on the spindle. When the stretch is relieved, the Ia quiets down and the reflex contraction subsides.

Servo Theory

Recall that the muscle spindle contains a muscle fiber—the intrafusal. The intrafusal has a dedicated motor neuron, the so-called γ (gamma) motor neuron. The extrafusal also has a dedicated motor neuron, the α (alpha) motor neuron. Why does the muscle spindle contain a contractile fiber with its own motor neuron, the γ?

A provocative answer was suggested by Merton (1972), who hypothesized that the spindle-extrafusal system works like a servo device (see Chapter 2). Suppose an intrafusal fiber is made to contract through the effect of a γ motor neuron, but the adjacent extrafusal fiber does not contract because its α motor neuron has not been activated. The intrafusal will shorten, but because the intrafusal is very small, its contraction will be too weak to move the limb. On the other hand, because the intrafusal shortens while the extrafusal does not, the central, noncontractile portion of the muscle spindle will stretch, causing the Ia to fire. The firing of the Ia will cause the α motor neuron to fire, and the α motor neuron will then cause the extrafusal fiber to contract. In essence, then, the signal from the γ motor neuron to the intrafusal fiber becomes amplified. The entire system acts as a servo, much like the system that enables a driver of a 2-ton automobile to turn the car by rotating the steering wheel with one finger.

What might be the advantage of this method of control? Amplifying the effect of the intrafusal does not reduce effort, for the same degree of effort must ultimately be expended regardless of whether the extrafusal is turned on directly, via immediate stimulation of the α motor neurons, or indirectly, via the γ loop. The main advantage of the γ loop is that it could promote efficient load compensation. If the extrafusal were stretched during a contraction caused by the imposition of an unexpected load (for example, if the arm bumped against an object), there would be a discrepancy between the length of the intrafusal and the length of the extrafusal. If such a discrepancy arose, the stretch receptor would fire, causing the extrafusal immediately to contract to counteract the stretch. Having the γ loop provides an effective means of rapidly compensating for load disturbances.

Despite the attractiveness of the servo hypothesis, it ran into an obstacle. The damage came from a study in which fine electrodes were used to record the activity of muscle spindle afferents as well as extrafusals during isometric flexion of the index finger (Vallbo, 1970). As seen in Figure 3.10, action potentials from the spindle afferents occurred *after* the onset of electromyographic (EMG) activity in the extrafusal muscle, not before. This result directly

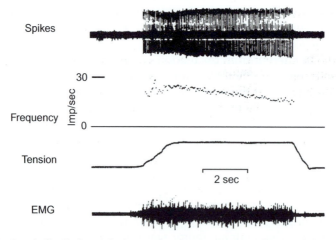

FIGURE 3.10   Muscle spindle discharge during weak voluntary isometric flexion of the index finger. Top trace: Directly recorded spindle afferent activity. Second trace: Instantaneous frequency of spindle afferent action potentials (in impulses per second). Third trace: Muscle tension. Fourth trace: Muscle EMG. From Vallbo (1970). With permission.

contradicts the servo model's prediction that spindles would become active *before* extrafusals, not after.

In hindsight, there may be a good reason why the servo model was disproved. If motor neurons could only be activated after γ motor neurons turned on, delays would always occur before extrafusal contraction began (Vallbo, 1970). Such delays might be maladaptive when rapid responses are required.

α-γ Coactivation

Why did spindle afferents fire at all in Vallbo's (1970) experiment? Contraction of the extrafusal should have relieved stretch on the muscle spindle, so spindle afferents should have stopped firing, not started firing, when the extrafusal contracted. The firing of the spindle afferents implies that the length of the muscle spindle relative to the extrafusal decreased. This means that the spindle contracted. Spindle contraction is caused by γ motor neuron activity, whereas extrafusal contraction is caused by α motor neuron activity. The simultaneous activation of the spindle afferent and extrafusal must have come about, therefore, because the α and γ motor neurons came on at about the same time. This simultaneity of activation of α and γ motor neurons is called α-γ coactivation.

Why does the nervous system rely on α-γ coactivation? The simplest reason may be that turning on these motor neurons at different times would require a mechanism to select and control the delays. The cost of such a mechanism, in terms of number of neurons or neural connections, might be prohibitive. This fact, coupled with the fact that α-γ coactivation allows for rapid compensation for imposed loads, has led to general acceptance of the coactivation model.

Recurrent Inhibition

As was seen in Figure 3.6 the spinal cord is the site of communication between Ia afferents and α motor neurons as well as between Ib afferents and α motor neurons. A number of other spinal circuits allow for communication among neural elements involved in muscle activation and proprioception. One such circuit allows motor neurons to inhibit themselves—a phenomenon called *recurrent inhibition*. Recurrent inhibition is achieved with a neuron, the *Renshaw* cell, that inhibits the motor neuron that excites it (see Figure 3.11). The inhibitory effect of the Renshaw also extends to nearby motor neurons (Baldissera, Hultborn, & Illert, 1981).

A likely reason for recurrent inhibition is that modulating the activity of Renshaw cells can affect the sensitivity of motor neurons. If Renshaw cells are activated by supraspinal (brain) centers, the Renshaw cells will exert a greater inhibitory effect on motor neurons. Consequently, more activation must be supplied to the motor neurons to get them to produce a desired level of activity. On the other hand, if Renshaw cells receive little or no activation from supraspinal centers, or if they are actively inhibited by supraspinal centers, relatively little excitation is needed to drive the motor neurons. Modulating the level of Renshaw cells can therefore influence the level of excitation needed to drive motor neurons. This can be a useful tool for moving at the slightest provocation or for refraining from moving unless it is essential.

Descending influences

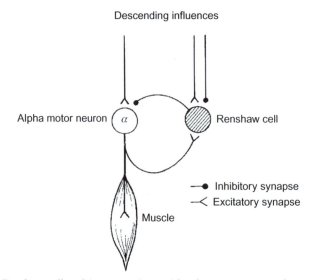

Alpha motor neuron α Renshaw cell

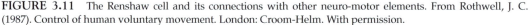

—● Inhibitory synapse
—< Excitatory synapse

Muscle

FIGURE 3.11   The Renshaw cell and its connections with other neuro-motor elements. From Rothwell, J. C. (1987). Control of human voluntary movement. London: Croom-Helm. With permission.

Inhibiting Renshaw cells may also allow coarsely graded descending signals to have more finely graded motor effects than would be the case otherwise (Baldissera et al, 1981). Suppose descending signals can only take on values of 10, 30, 50, 70, and 90 (arbitrary units). If Renshaw cells reduce these signals by a factor of 2, the possible signal strengths are 5, 15, 25, 35, and 45. If the Renshaw cell reduces the signals by a factor of 10 rather than 2, the possible signal strengths are 1, 3, 5, 7, and 9. Greater resolution of signal strengths is possible when the Renshaw cell reduces signals by a factor of 10 rather than 2 because when the Renshaw cell reduces signals by a factor of 10, differences of 2 can be discriminated, whereas when the Renshaw cell reduces signals by a factor of 2, the smallest differences that can be discriminated are of size 5.

Reciprocal Inhibition

Another form of interaction within the spinal cord is *reciprocal inhibition*. Reciprocal inhibition can be demonstrated as follows (McMahon, 1984). Flex your elbow and stiffen it, as in Figure 3.12A. Place your other hand around your upper arm. You should be able to feel the biceps and triceps muscles harden, reflecting their contracted state. Now ask a friend to push upward against your hand (Figure 3.12B). You should feel your biceps briefly "soften" as the upward force is applied. When this occurs, the biceps has become momentarily inactive.

The spinal circuit underlying this effect is shown in Figure 3.12C. When the upward force is applied to the hand, the triceps stretches and stretch receptors within the triceps are activated. Afferent fibers from the stretch receptors in the triceps project to interneurons in the spinal cord, which inhibit motor neurons of the opposing muscle (the biceps).

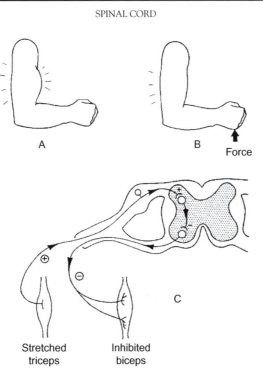

FIGURE 3.12 Reciprocal inhibition. (A) Co-contraction of the biceps and triceps while holding the elbow at 90 degrees. (B) The biceps is deactivated when an upward force is applied to the forearm. (C) The underlying mechanism. Plus sign denotes an excitatory effect. Minus sign denotes an inhibitory effect. From McMahon, T. A. (1984). Muscles, reflexes, and locomotion. Princeton, NJ: Princeton University Press. With permission.

Reciprocal inhibition is not restricted to the biceps and triceps of the human arm. It is a general phenomenon in which the stretch of one muscle inhibits the activity of the opposing muscle. Reciprocal inhibition prevents muscles from working against each other when external loads are encountered. The physiological properties of reciprocal inhibition have been studied in detail (Jankowska & Lindstrom, 1971).

It is worth emphasizing that reciprocal inhibition does not occur between motor neurons directly. Biceps motor neurons do not inhibit triceps motor neurons, for example. If inhibition existed between motor neurons of opposing muscle groups, it would be difficult or even impossible to activate the biceps and triceps simultaneously, as in the first part of the exercise you just performed. Co-contraction of opposing muscles is widespread (Marsden, Obeso, & Rothwell, 1983). It allows joints to stiffen, which is an efficient means of resisting perturbations—for example, when one prepares to catch a heavy object dropped from overhead (Lacquaniti & Maioli, 1989).

Stiffening a joint by contracting the muscles around it can be a more efficient means of resisting load perturbations than activating only a single muscle and relying on stretch reflexes to counteract loads that may be encountered (Hasan, 1986). Keeping a medium level of stiffness may be an optimal means of moving a limb through an entire trajectory. Small changes in the relative stiffness of the muscles can create a series of equilibrium positions to which the limb is driven over time (Hasan, 1986). More will be said about relative stiffness and equilibrium positions in Chapter 9.

The Smart Spinal Cord

All of the facts discussed so far in this section on the spinal cord pertain to reflexes and their top-down control. The circuits that have been discussed are relatively simple, possibly leaving one to think that the spinal cord is not very smart. One might imagine that the spinal cord may only manage single muscles but not achieve useful coordination of muscle groups. This view would be uncalled for, however, because it turns out that the spinal cord is much smarter than one might expect, notwithstanding its relatively low position within the central nervous system.

Studies of spinal frogs show this intelligence vividly, as demonstrated in research with spinal frogs (i.e., frogs whose spinal cords have been surgically disconnected from the frogs' brains). Neurally driven activity in muscles below the spinal cut must be attributed to the spinal cord alone.

Fucson, Berkenblit, and Feldman (1980) studied the behavior of spinal frogs (Figure 3.13). These experimenters applied a bit of irritating chemical to the skin of these frogs and filmed the reactions that followed. Fucson, Berkenblit, and Feldman found that their spinal frogs displayed the same behavior as physiologically normal frogs. As in normal frogs, the spinal frogs' hindlimbs moved to approach the irritation site. The wiping motions were remarkably accurate. Especially interesting was the fact that even when the initial positions of the frog's hindlimb varied and the location of the touch was unpredictable, the wiping reflex still worked well. From this outcome, one can conclude that the frog's spinal cord is very smart indeed.

The coordination required for the frog's wiping reflex is similar to the coordination required for bringing the tip of one's finger to the tip of one's nose, the simple activity that occupied our attention in Chapter 2. The frog's ability to bring its toe directly to an irritated patch of skin implies that within the frog's spinal cord are mechanisms capable of relating body positions to one another within a single spatial map. Attributing this capability to the

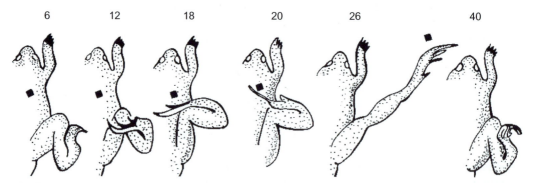

FIGURE 3.13 Wiping reflexes in the spinal frog evoked by chemical stimulation (black square). The numbers at the top are film frame numbers. The movement was filmed at 48 frames per second. From Berkenblit, M. B., Feldman, A. G., & Fucson, O. I. (1986). Adaptability of innate motor patterns and motor control. Behavioral and Brain Sciences, 9, 585–638. With permission.

frog's spinal cord is not to trivialize the computations. The fact that spinal frogs can perform the wiping reflex implies that the transformations of sensory signals from the skin and limb into a spatial map and the subsequent translation of these spatial coordinates into motor commands are phylogenetically ancient achievements.

Tuning of Spinal Reflexes

The spinal cord normally works *with* the brain, not independently of it. As noted by James (1890) and Sherrington (1906), spinal cord activity is regulated by the brain so that, among other things, muscle tone can be increased in preparation for movement. The increase in muscle tone is caused by lowering of reflex thresholds and is especially high when individuals are highly aroused, for example, after drinking large quantities of coffee or while being in a fearful state. Muscle tone can also be elevated by relatively unemotional anticipation of coming movement demands. Enabling such anticipation, tendon and muscle stretch reflexes are augmented following a warning signal for an impending movement-demanding stimulus; the augmentation can last for several seconds (Brunia, 1999).

Reflex tuning can be fairly specific, as shown with the Hoffman reflex, or H-reflex. Here, researchers electrically stimulate the sensory nerve coming from a muscle or tendon and measure the ensuing muscle activity. In one H-reflex experiment, participants were presented with a warning tone followed by a signal to move (Prochazka, 1989). If the H-reflex was triggered during the interval between the warning signal and the subsequent "go" signal, the reflex was stronger than usual. The increase was greatest in the muscles that were primarily responsible for the upcoming movement. A similar effect can be obtained by asking participants merely to *imagine* moving one leg or the other. The H-reflex is amplified in the leg that is imaginally prepared for action (Bonnet, Decety, Jeannerod, & Requin, 1997).

The preceding examples all refer to the tuning of short-latency reflexes. There is also evidence for tuning of long-latency reflexes (i.e., reflexes mediated by the brain as well as the spinal cord). For example, Koshland and Hasan (2000) found that when participants' limbs were perturbed prior to execution of planned movements, long-loop reflexes both hastened and strengthened movement in the intended direction; this was true regardless of the direction of the applied perturbation. That this effect was based on tuning of long-loop reflexes rather than short-loop (spinal-only) reflexes was evident from the latencies of the responses; the responses came too late to be plausibly ascribed to short-loop reflexes.

CEREBELLUM

In the preceding sections, we focused on spinal mechanisms. Now we look up, so to speak, to the brain. The brain's principal roles in motor control are, in the short run, to govern motor output based on perceptual information and intentional states. In the long run, the brain's principal role in motor control is to acquire perceptual-motor skills.

In the sections that follow, we will concentrate on the ways these short- and long-run roles are achieved by six brain centers that play a role in human motor control: the cerebellum, the basal ganglia, the motor cortex, the premotor cortex, the supplementary motor cortex, and the parietal cortex (see Figure 3.2). Other areas of the brain also contribute to the control of movement and stability, albeit more indirectly. Focusing on the six areas that are discussed here is not meant to imply that only these areas are important for human motor control. With 7/8 of the brain devoted to motor control, according to Sir John Eccles, winner of the Nobel Prize for Physiology or Medicine in 1963, we would be remiss in relegating any part of the brain to outcast status when it comes to motor control or, for that matter, any function.

More than half the neurons in the human brain reside in the cerebellum (Ito, 1984). The anatomy of the cerebellum has been studied in great detail, but a review of that anatomy is unimportant for present purposes (but see Ito, 1984; Llinas, 1981; or Schmahmann, 2000). Instead, we will consider the main motor-control functions served by the cerebellum, those being the regulation of muscle tone, coordination, timing, and learning.

Regulation of Muscle Tone

The cerebellum receives input from muscle spindles and Golgi tendon organs as well as centers for vision, hearing, touch, and balance. When the cerebellum is damaged, muscle tone (the slight tension continually present in the muscles) is impaired.

In cats, disconnecting the cerebellum from the spinal cord results in *decerebrate rigidity*, a syndrome in which the limbs become extremely rigid (see Figure 3.14). The source of decerebrate rigidity in cats is elevated sensitivity of the muscle spindle system. The stretch receptors become acutely sensitive to extrafusal stretch, causing extrafusals to contract more than usual (Matthews & Rushworth, 1958).

In human and non-human primates, damage to the cerebellum results in abnormally low muscle tone or *hypotonia*. Anatomical differences between the feline and primate nervous system account for the fact that cerebellar damage leads to rigidity in cats and flaccidity in primates (Gilman, Bloedel, & Lechtenberg, 1981).

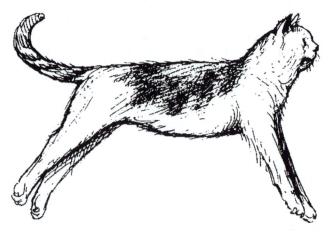

FIGURE 3.14 Decerebrate rigidity in the cat. From Oxford University Press, Brain, Symposium on the Cerebellum: (3) The Influence of the Cerebellum upon the Reflex Activities of the Decerebrate Animal; Lewis J. Pollock, et al.; October 1927. With permission.

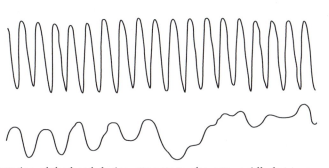

FIGURE 3.15 Orientation of the hand during attempts to alternate rapidly between a palm-up and a palm-down position in a patient with unilateral cerebellar damage. Top trace: Performance by the unaffected hand. Bottom trace: Performance by the affected hand. From Holmes, G. (1939). The cerebellum of man. Brain, 62, 1–30. With permission.

Coordination

Cerebellar damage often takes the form of coordination difficulties—a syndrome known as *ataxia*. The incoordination can take several forms. Maintaining steady balance while standing can be compromised (Nashner, 1976; see also Chapter 5). Walking heel to toe may become all but impossible. Speech may become slurred (*dysarthria*), and nystagmus eye movements (see Chapter 6) may be damaged. Visually guided hand movements may also deteriorate. In attempting to point to a target, cerebellar patients may significantly overshoot the target (*hypermetria*), although the overshoots are usually followed in such patients by a series of homing-in movements. Once the arm comes to rest, the arm may oscillate noticeably. Because this oscillation usually occurs just before or after purposeful movements, it is sometimes called *intention tremor*.

Cerebellar insult can also mar the production of sequences of movements. Alternating between palm-up and palm-down hand gestures, for example, may break down (see Figure 3.15). The mental effort required for such tasks may also increase. Normally, a task like turning the hand back and forth between a palm-up and palm-down posture (supinating and pronating the hand, respectively) can occur automatically. This same task takes much more concentration in cerebellar patients, one of whom reported, "I have to think out each movement . . . I come to a dead stop in turning and have to think before I start again" (Holmes, 1939).

Timing

Closely related to difficulties of movement sequencing are difficulties in movement timing. Overshooting targets during aiming movements (*hypermetria*) can be viewed as a timing problem (Eccles, 1977). The timing of muscle contractions is also impaired after cerebellar damage. A task in which such impairment has been observed is step-input tracking. Here, a target jumps from one position to another, typically on a computer screen, and the subject is supposed to keep the computer's cursor aligned with the target. Hallet, Shahani, and Young (1975a, b) set up a step-input tracking task in which subjects made flexion movements about the elbow to keep a cursor aligned with the target. Elbow angle was recorded electronically

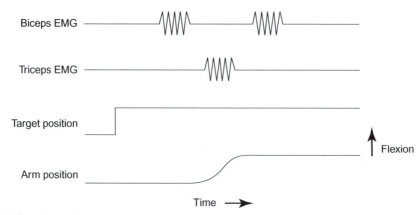

FIGURE 3.16 Idealized EMG activity in the biceps and triceps during rapid flexion of the elbow in a step-tracking task. From Hallett, M., Shahani, B. T. & Young, R. R. (1975a). EMG analysis of stereotyped voluntary movements in man. Journal of Neurology, Neurosurgery, and Psychiatry, 38, 1154–1162. With permission.

and was then represented by the cursor's position on the screen. The subject's task was to keep the cursor aligned with the target by flexing and extending the elbow. In normal individuals (Hallet, Shahani, & Young, 1975a), a characteristic triphasic pattern of EMG activity was recorded from the biceps and triceps (see Figure 3.16). First the agonist became active, then the antagonist became active, and then the agonist became active again. (An agonist is a muscle that promotes a movement, whereas an antagonist is a muscle that opposes a movement.) This pattern of EMG activity was not present in cerebellar patients (Hallet, Shahani, & Young, 1975b). For them, the first agonist burst was significantly prolonged, or both the first agonist burst and the antagonist burst were significantly prolonged.

Alcohol has similar effects in neurologically normal individuals. Like patients with cerebellar damage, normal individuals who have ingested large amounts of alcohol show elevated reaction times, behaviors reminiscent of hypermetria, and intention tremor, as well as abnormally timed EMG patterns in step-input tracking tasks (Marsden, Merton, & Morton, 1977). It is no wonder, then, that cerebellar patients appear, to the untrained eye, to be intoxicated. The similarities between the effects of alcohol and the effects of cerebellar damage suggest that the cerebellum may be a brain center that is especially strongly affected by alcohol or a site where the effects of alcohol are especially apparent.

Different parts of the cerebellum may affect different stages in the production of timed responses. This statement follows research by Ivry, Keele, and Diener (1988) that focused on rhythmic finger-tapping in patients with presumed lesions in the lateral or intermediate regions of the cerebellum. The patients were asked to tap at a rate of about 2 cycles per second. By recording the timing of patients' finger taps, Ivry, Keele, and Diener used statistical properties of the inter-tap times to estimate the temporal variability associated with two basic processes underlying tapping performance: (1) waiting to initiate each response and (2) executing each response when the waiting period was over. Ivry, Keele, and Diener found that patients with damage to the lateral region of the cerebellum exhibited higher than normal variability in the timing process but essentially normal variability in the execution process. By contrast, patients with primary damage to the intermediate region exhibited higher than normal variability in the execution process but essentially normal variability in the timing process. More will be said about this in Chapter 8.

Other studies corroborate the view that the lateral and intermediate regions of the cerebellum may be associated with different aspects of motor control. Neurons in the lateral cerebellum become active well in advance of EMG activity, whereas neurons in the more medial zones of the cerebellum become active only during movements or shortly after movements have been performed (Schwartz, Ebner, & Bloedel, 1987). This finding fits with the hypothesis that the lateral cerebellum is primarily involved in aspects of motor control that pertain to the planning or programming of movement, whereas the intermediate or medial regions are primarily involved in movement execution.

Learning

The cerebellum is not only important for performing behaviors; it is also important for learning them. Damage to the cerebellum interferes with motor learning. For example, cerebellar damage interferes with adaptation of the vestibular ocular reflex (VOR), the mechanism that allows for the automatic compensatory eye movements that keep the eyes on a stationary visual target when the head turns. Adaptation of the VOR has been studied by fitting volunteer subjects with prisms that reverse the right and left visual fields. Over time, the direction of eye rotation relative to head rotation reverses. In animals with lesions of the cerebellum this reversal never happens (Robinson, 1976).

The cerebellum also appears to be involved in learning skillful limb movements. Gilbert and Thach (1977) recorded from climbing fibers within the cerebellums of monkeys who were trained to resist loads applied to the wrist. As the resistive movements became more coordinated, there was an accompanying change in the firing patterns of the cerebellar fibers.

Learning to anticipate visual stimuli in reaction time tasks also appears to be based on cerebellar changes (Sasaki, Gemba, & Mizuno, 1982). Cerebellar neurons fire before movements are made in response to anticipated visual signals, and lesions of the cerebellum reduce the capacity for visuo-motor anticipation. Cerebellar activity also turns out to be proportional to the degree of error made while learning to use a computer mouse with a novel rotational transformation (Imamizu et al., 2000).

Results like these have encouraged the development of detailed computational models of cerebellar learning (Albus, 1981; Ito, 1984; Llinas, 1981; Marr, 1969). Analysis of the cerebellum as a perceptual-motor learning device has long been an active research area in neural and cognitive science (Churchland, 1986; Imamizu et al., 2000; McCormick & Thompson, 1984).

BASAL GANGLIA

The basal ganglia are a set of interconnected structures in the forebrain. The roles played by the basal ganglia in motor control are suggested by the behavioral disruptions that follow damage to these structures and by changes in their levels of activity when different tasks are performed.

Huntington's Disease

A dramatic behavioral syndrome attributable to basal ganglia degeneration is Huntington's disease. This malady manifests initially as occasional clumsiness and forgetfulness. Gradually, Huntington's patients fall prey to uncontrollable ballistic movements (*chorea*), an inability to reason (*dementia*), and finally death. The choreiform movements of Huntington's disease can be grotesque. The patient's arms and legs may flail wildly. The patient's face can become a mask of contorted expressions. In the late stages of the disease, the patient must be tied down.

The physiological change that occurs in Huntington's disease is damage to the dendrites within the basal ganglia that are responsible for the production and uptake of a neurotransmitter, gamma-amino-butyric acid (GABA). The cause of this physiological change is genetic, as established through a study of the family histories of Huntington's patients on the East Coast of the United States. Almost all the patients descended from a single family that migrated to Salem, Massachusetts from England in 1630 (Côté & Crutcher, 1985). Seventeenth century Salem was known for its "witches"—individuals whose bizarre behavior led to their being accused of possession by the devil. These people were probably victims of Huntington's disease.

The growth of expertise in genetics in the twentieth and twenty-first centuries has made it possible to determine the specific chromosomal defect that causes Huntington's disease. It has become possible to identify the defect in still-healthy individuals. For individuals in families with a history of the disease, determining whether or when to be tested for the chromosomal abnormality can be an agonizing personal decision (Brody, 1988).

Parkinson's Disease

Another motor disorder associated with damage to the basal ganglia is Parkinson's disease. Named after James Parkinson, a London physician who described the syndrome in 1817, Parkinson's disease has several signs. One is a shuffling gait. Another is shaking motion at rest (*resting tremor*). Another is slowness in the initiation of movements on command (*akinesia*). Yet another is slowness in the completion of ongoing movements (*bradykinesia*). In clinical examination, Parkinson's patients often display high resistance to tugging on the limb (*rigidity*). Normal individuals, by contrast, typically display only moderate resistance to passive manipulation (a sign of normal muscle tone).

The cause of Parkinson's disease is a deficit of a neurotransmitter, *dopamine*. Lower than normal amounts of dopamine have been found in autopsy studies of the brains of Parkinson's patients. A drug, L-DOPA, that elevates brain dopamine levels can help Parkinson's patients, but it may do so only temporarily and with unpleasant side effects. Another drug, deprenyl, appears to be more effective. Rather than boosting dopamine levels directly, it retards the action of enzymes that break down dopamine too rapidly. Administration of deprenyl can delay the onset of Parkinson's disease by several months (Fackelmann, 1989). Another treatment for Parkinson's disease is transplantation of dopamine-producing tissues (for example, from the adrenal gland) into the basal ganglia. The effectiveness of this procedure remains controversial.

Two additional methods that have been pursued to treat Parkinson's disease are deep brain stimulation (DBS) and genetic therapy. In DBS, electrodes are implanted in the brain,

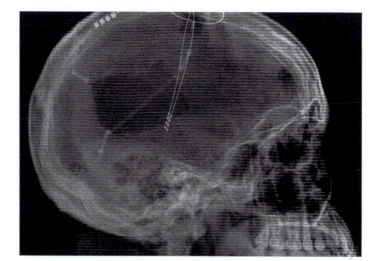

FIGURE 3.17   Deep brain stimulation (DBS) of the thalamus used for treatment of Parkinson's disease. From Kluger, J. (September 10, 2007). Rewiring the brain. Time, Volume 170, Number 11, 46–47. With permission.

and sites that would normally receive neurotransmitter stimulation receive electrical stimulation instead. This method has shown promise, as demonstrated by its presentation in popular outlets like *Time* magazine (see Figure 3.17).

The other new method that has been pursued for treatment of Parkinson's disease is genetic therapy (Kaiser, 2007). The idea here is to introduce genes that tend to stimulate neurons that can calm neural activity antithetical to the production of dopamine. This approach likewise shows promise as treatment regiment for Parkinson's disease, a malady which afflicts about 1.5 million Americans (Kaiser, 2007). Gene therapy is likely to become a more-and-more widely used treatment method in medicine.

Theories of Basal Ganglia Function

In view of the unfortunate consequences of basal ganglia disease, what can we say are the functions served by this set of neural structures? From the outset, it is important to observe that while the basal ganglia are involved in motor control, they may serve non-motor functions as well. Patients with basal ganglia disease don't just have difficulty performing movement sequences; they also have difficulty recalling sequences of symbols (Côté & Crutcher, 1985; Gunilla, Oberg, & Divac, 1981). Also, as mentioned earlier, dementia is one of the symptoms of Huntington's disease. That this is true should not be surprising in view of the fact that the basal ganglia appear to be important in learning and maintaining skills, as shown in neuroimaging of the two main structures of the basal ganglia, the caudate and putamen (Grafton, Hazeltine & Ivry, 1995; Poldrak, Prabakharan, Seger, & Gabrieli, 1999).

One hypothesis about the role of the basal ganglia in motor control is that the structures in this neural constellation contribute to the activation or retrieval of movement plans (Marsden, 1982). Consistent with this hypothesis, neurons in some basal ganglia structures (the globus pallidus and the zona reticulata of the substantia nigra) have been found, in monkeys, to discharge before voluntary movements of the arm or leg and before chewing or licking movements (Iansek & Porter, 1980). Similarly, Parkinson's patients have difficulty beginning voluntary movements. For example, they may have difficulty starting to walk when asked to do so, although, paradoxically, they may start walking with no difficulty in a different intentional context—when asked simply to leave the room. Visual stimuli can also be effective in helping Parkinson patients start to walk. Figure 3.18 shows that the placement of markers on the floor at regularly spaced intervals can help Parkinson's patients locomote in a nearly normal fashion. Providing the markers can be nearly as effective as L-DOPA medication (Forssberg, Johnels, & Steg, 1984).

Besides serving to retrieve or initiate movement plans, the basal ganglia may serve to scale the amplitudes of movements. Basal ganglia disease may disrupt the overall size and timing of movements in such tasks as handwriting, reaching, grasping, and manual positioning (Brooks, 1986). The pallidum appears to be the structure within the basal ganglia that is mainly responsible for this scaling function.

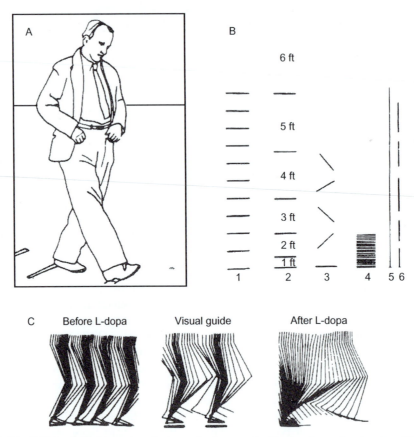

FIGURE 3.18   Walking in Parkinson's patients can be improved with visual cues for stepping. (A) Parkinson's patient walking on a floor with stripes. (B) Positions of stripes that are most helpful (1), somewhat helpful (2), and unhelpful (3–6). Time-lapse diagrams of shuffling gait before medication, after medication, and with visual guidance but no medication. From Brooks, V. B. (1986). The neural basis of motor control. New York: Oxford University Press. With permission.

A final function served by the basal ganglia pertains to perceptual-motor integration. Cells in the caudate nucleus of the basal ganglia have been found, in sedentary cats, to respond to light brushing of the face, but to respond at different levels if the same stimulus is applied during mouth or head movements (Manetto & Lidsky, 1989). Manetto and Lidsky (1989) suggested that the basal ganglia may be a site where perceptual inputs are gated by motor activity.

MOTOR CORTEX

So far in this chapter, we have moved up from the lowest, or most primitive, levels of the motor system to the higher, more phylogenetically advanced levels. Now we turn to the phylogenetically highest levels—those occupying the cerebral cortex. First, we will consider the motor cortex, then we will consider the premotor cortex; next we will turn to the supplementary motor area, and finally we will look at the parietal association area.

The motor cortex was the first brain area in which evidence was obtained for localization of function. In 1870 two German physiologists, Fritsch and Hitzig, applied voltage to the part of the brain that is now known as the motor cortex, thanks to their pioneering work. In the dogs in which they applied the stimulation, Fritsch and Hitzig observed muscle twitches immediately after the electrical stimuli were applied. Which muscles twitched depended on where the stimulating electrodes were placed. When an electrode was turned on in one spot, muscle activity occurred in one part of the dog's leg; when an electrode was turned on in a nearby site, muscle activity occurred in a nearby part of the same leg, and so on. Based on these observations, Fritsch and Hitzig suggested that muscles are represented discretely and topographically in the brain. Topographic representations preserve the spatial organization of objects being represented even if the relative sizes of the objects are not preserved.

It happens that Fritsch and Hitzig's hypothesis about topographic representation of the body in the brain was anticipated in the mid-nineteenth century by Hughlings Jackson, a British neurologist. Jackson arrived at this conclusion by watching the gradual spread of focal epileptic seizure activity from one body part to the other in people experiencing epileptic seizures. Jackson hypothesized that during an epileptic attack, one brain site after the other falls prey to the electrical "storm" comprising a seizure. Seeing this orderly spread of epileptic activity, Jackson reasoned that distinct areas of the brain control the musculature of distinct body parts and that adjacent brain sites control adjacent body parts.

Fritsch and Hitzig's conclusion, based on experimental stimulation of the brain, confirmed Jackson's conjecture, based on clinical assessment. A valuable lesson from this series of events is that careful observation of behavior can lead to important insights about the brain.

Showing that electrical stimulation of the dog's brain agreed with Jackson's hypothesis about the human brain did not seal the deal on human brain function. It remained to be shown that electrical stimulation of the human brain would yield results analogous to those obtained in dogs, whereupon Jackson's hypothesis would be confirmed. The critical test was provided by two Canadian neurosurgeons, Penfield and Rasmussen (1950), who treated severe epilepsy in the principal way available at their time, by cutting nerve tracts within the brain to reduce the spread of seizure activity. Before lesioning any brain site, Penfield and Rasmussen determined whether the site was vital for cognitive or behavioral functions.

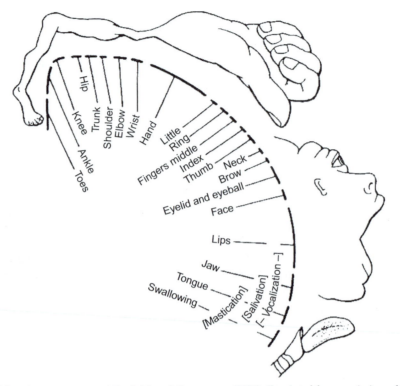

FIGURE 3.19   The motor map of Penfield and Rasmussen (1950). Reprinted by permission of the publisher from Voluntary movement, by C. Ghez, in Principles of neural science (2nd ed.), pp. 487–501. Copyright © 1985 by Elsevier Science Publishing Co., Inc.

To test each area, Penfield and Rasmussen placed stimulating electrodes in that area and observed what happened when the electrode was turned on. Like Fritsch and Hitzig, they stimulated one area, observed any muscle response that followed, then stimulated a neighboring area, observed the resulting muscle activity, and so on. By repeating this procedure, these neurosurgeons developed a "motor map" of the body (see Figure 3.19). The map revealed that neighboring parts of the musculature are controlled by neighboring sites in the motor cortex. The map showed that some body regions are more amply represented than others. The fingers and lips take up a larger portion of motor cortex than do the thighs or torso. Presumably, the great precision with which the mouth and hands can move is attributable to the larger amount of motor cortex dedicated to the oral and manual regions as compared to the thigh and torso regions.

Penfield and Rasmussen, like Fritsch and Hitzig, found that stimulation of the motor cortex triggered muscle twitches. Elicitation of twitches by stimulation of the motor cortex is what one might expect from a center that activates muscles but is not involved in organizing complex programs for extended movement sequences. A way to test this hypothesis further is to determine when the motor cortex becomes active relative to the onset of movement. If the motor cortex becomes active immediately before movement, but other areas become active significantly earlier, this outcome would be compatible with the hypothesis that the motor cortex is a trigger center rather than a planning center for movement.

Recordings of the electrical activity of the brain from the scalp bear out the trigger interpretation. Deecke, Scheid, and Kornhuber (1969) recorded brain potentials from people asked to move the right index finger at will. By recording when various brain areas became active before the movement, Deecke et al. found that there was a reliable increase of electrical activity in the motor cortex about 50ms before the first sign of electrical activity in the finger muscles. Earlier activity was recorded in other brain sites. Deecke et al. called the burst of electrical activity in the motor cortex the *motor potential*. Because 50ms is a very short delay prior to EMG activity, the shortness of the delay supports the hypothesis that the motor cortex is one of the last sites in the brain to be activated before movements begin, a kind of "launch pad" for the issuance of motor commands.

Why, from a neuroanatomical perspective, are such short delays observed between motor cortex activity and EMG activity? In primates, many neurons of the motor cortex make monosynaptic connections with spinal motor neurons, especially motor neurons of the finger muscles (Phillips & Porter, 1977). Such connections presumably allow for the precision of hand and finger movements. In agreement with this view, some motor cortex neurons actually synapse onto just one motor unit (Asanuma, 1981). This and related results have been taken to suggest that at least some motor cortex neurons control individual muscles rather than entire movements (Evarts, 1967; Kakei, Hoffman, & Strick, 1999).

Force and Direction Control

Although the motor cortex is primarily related to muscle activity rather than more global aspects of movement, it has been possible to relate motor cortex activity to two features of movement, force and direction. In a classic series of studies on force and direction control, Evarts and colleagues (see Evarts, 1981) showed that neurons of the motor cortex discharge selectively depending on the direction and force of movements that monkeys are about to perform. In one experiment, monkeys turned a handle back and forth. A weight attached to the handle assisted or resisted one of the directions of movement. Recordings of individual neurons in the motor cortex showed that the cells' discharge frequency increased with the force required to turn the handle. If flexion was assisted by the weight, so that low force was required, the discharge frequency was low, but if flexion was resisted by the weight, so that high force was required, the discharge frequency was high. The cells began to discharge before movement-related EMGs were observed, indicating that the cells were involved in some aspect of the preparation or triggering of movement. The cells were also active or silent depending on whether the forthcoming movement required flexion or extension, suggesting that the cells were directionally tuned.

Later experiments shed more light on the role of the motor cortex in the control of direction and other aspects of movement. In experiments by Georgopoulos and colleagues (Georgopoulos, Schwartz, & Kettner, 1986; Georgopoulos, Lurito, Petrides, Schwartz, & Massey, 1989), monkeys made hand movements toward each of a number of targets spaced around a starting point (see Figure 3.20). Discharge rates of individual neurons were found to depend on the direction of movement, but none of the neurons fired uniquely to a particular direction. Thus, one motor cortex neuron fired the most when the monkey's paw moved

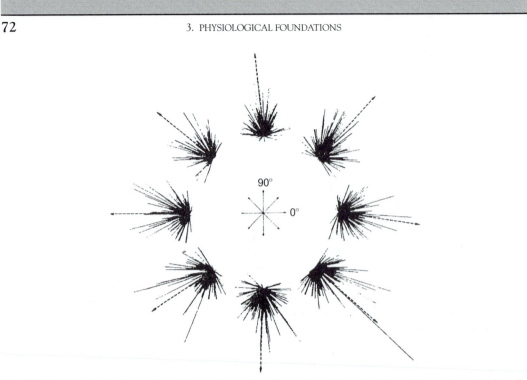

FIGURE 3.20   Population coding in the motor cortex. The sunburst at each of the eight positions displays the amount of activity of over 200 neurons when a monkey made a movement toward a target at a radial position corresponding to the radial position of the sunburst (for example, toward 4 o'clock in the case of the sunburst at the 4 o'clock position). The length of each sunburst corresponds to the amount of activity from one neuron. The arrow extending from each sunburst indicates the population vector of the entire ensemble. From Georgopoulos, A. P., Kalaska, J. F., & Massey, J. T. (1981). Spatial trajectories and reaction times of aimed movements: Effects of practice, uncertainty, and change in target location. Journal of Neurophysiology, 46, 725–743. With permission.

in the 45 degree direction, fired less when the monkey's paw moved in the 35 degrees or 55 degree direction, and fired still less when the monkey's paw moved in the 25 degree or 65 degree direction. Another motor cortex fired most when the monkey's paw moved in the 55 degree direction, less in the 45 degree or 65 degree direction, still less in the in the 35 degree or 75 degree direction, and so on. Every direction studied was found to have a cell that fired most vigorously to it, but no cell fired uniquely to a single direction. In addition, none of the cells responded differently depending on the *amplitude* of movement, an outcome that fits with the view that direction and amplitude are separable components of motor control (Gordon & Ghez, 1994; Rosenbaum, 1980).

Given that none of the cells studied by Georgopoulos et al. (1986) uniquely coded a particular direction, how could movements be made in specific directions? The answer, according to Georgopoulos et al. (1986), was embodied in one of the most influential concepts in neuroscience, the *population coding* hypothesis. According to the population coding hypothesis, at least as applied to the control of movement direction, the direction in which a limb is commanded to move represents a weighted sum of the directions signaled by the population of cells in the motor cortex. This computational scheme is surprisingly powerful and may be used in other brain systems as well—for example, in systems underlying visual perception (Erickson, 1984).

How does population coding work? Suppose a cell in the motor cortex responds with strength 100 (arbitrary units) when receiving a signal from perceptual or volitional centers calling for a movement in that cell's preferred direction. However, that same cell responds with one less unit of strength for each degree of angular departure from that preferred direction. Thus, the cell might respond with strength 100 for a 90 degree movement, 99 for a 91 degree or 89 degree movement, 98 for a 92 degree or 88 degree movement, and so on. Another cell specialized for an 80 degree movement might respond with strength 100 to a signal calling for an 80 degree movement, 99 to a signal calling for a 79 degree or 81 degree movement, 98 to a signal calling for a 78 degree or 82 degree movement, and so on. Suppose a signal to the motor cortex calls for a movement of 85 degrees. Each of the cells described above responds with strength 95, yielding a net output of 95 + 95 = 190. If another direction were called for, say 90 degrees, the cell specialized for 90 degrees would respond with strength 100 and the cell specialized for 80 degrees would respond with strength 90, so the net output would again be 190. Thus, the same strength of output would be possible for the 85 degree movement and the 90 degree movement, even though the 85 degree direction had no specialized cell. The system as a whole would be robust if a given cell, or if a few cells, died. All that would happen if some cells succumbed is that directional accuracy would be compromised in proportion to the number of absent cells (Sahrmann & Norton, 1977).

One of the most exciting features of the population coding hypothesis is that it does not require an overseer who makes an executive decision about how the animal should move. Instead, the movement that is carried out is just the weighted sum of the "votes" cast by the relevant neurons. It is heartening to see that such a method works as well as it does because, apart from the fact that it satisfies one's affinity for democracy, it is preferable theoretically to have a system in which no intelligent executive is required than to have a system in which the services of an intelligent executive are enlisted. As soon as a decider is postulated, one runs into the infinite regress problem of determining how that decider knows what to do (the "homunculus" problem of psychology).

Whole-Body Movement

The task studied in most of the experiments by Georgopoulos and his colleagues was directing one hand to a seen target. Being able to move the hand to a seen target is an important achievement, but that achievement pales in comparison to generating a whole-body movement. Data obtained by Graziano, Taylor, and Moore (2002) indicate that the motor cortex includes cells that code adoption of entire body positions.

Graziano, Taylor, and Moore (2002) applied electrical stimulation to sites in the motor cortex, as other researchers had done before, but in contrast to previous researchers, Graziano and colleagues let their electrical stimulation last a relatively long time—500 ms rather than 50 ms, as used in the classic studies of Penfield and Rasmussen (1950). The rationale given by Graziano, Taylor, and Moore for their use of long-duration stimuli was to provide stimuli whose durations would be more physiologically realistic than the very brief bursts used before.

Stimulating the motor cortex for these relatively long durations led to an intriguing result. As shown in Figure 3.21, monkeys in which the stimulation was applied moved to characteristic

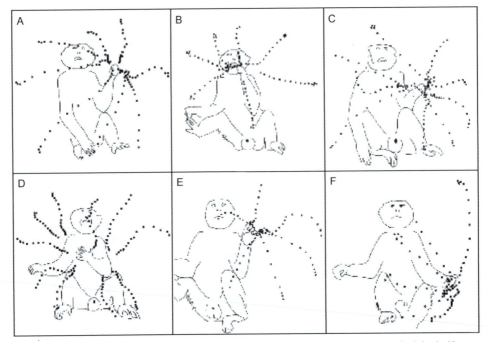

FIGURE 3.21 Adoption of characteristic postures when electrical stimulation was applied for half a second to the motor cortex of a monkey subject. Panels A–F correspond to conditions in which stimulation was applied to different brain sites. Dotted paths show motions to the same characteristic postures from the postures the monkey happened to be in when the stimulation was applied. From Graziano, M. S., Taylor, C. S. R., and Moore, T. (2002). Complex movements evoked by microstimulation of precentral cortex. Neuron, 34, 841–851. With permission.

postures no matter what postures they were in to begin with. For example, if stimulation was applied to a given site of the motor cortex, the monkey adopted an "apple-eating" posture no matter where its arms were at the moment the stimulation was given. If the stimulation was applied to another site of the motor cortex, the monkey adopted a "hitch-hiking" posture no matter where its arms were at the time of stimulation, and so on for other postures. Careful analyses of the functional properties of the motor cortex neurons that were stimulated for these long periods indicated that some but not all of neurons could be described as "posture neurons" (i.e., neurons that seemed to control adoption of characteristic body positions). Other neurons coded movement amplitudes, movement directions, and/or movement speeds (Aflalo & Graziano, 2007). Aflalo and Graziano (2007) found, however, that of these factors, the one that was coded predominantly by the neurons was final postures. This finding has important implications for a theory of motor control described in the last chapter of this book.

Long-Loop Reflexes

Besides triggering movements, the motor cortex also receives feedback from the movements it triggers. Neurons of the motor cortex receive sensory feedback from the muscle fibers they innervate (Asanuma, 1981), allowing for tight coupling between efferent and afferent functions.

Some of the earliest evidence for such a feedback loop came from an experiment in which people were asked either to resist or not resist a tug on the wrist (Hammond, 1956). Depending on the instruction, the EMG response was either large or small. However, the instructionally influenced component of the EMG came after another EMG response, which was essentially unaffected by instruction and had a very short latency after the tug. This first response was automatic and was probably based entirely on spinal circuits. By contrast, the delayed response was likely to have been mediated by pathways between the spinal cord and motor cortex. A finding that buttresses this hypothesis is that the delayed response was seldom seen in patients with lesions in the spinal path that relays sensory signals to the cerebral cortex (Marsden, Merton, & Morton, 1973). In addition, neuronal firing rates were found to increase in the motor cortex immediately after external loads were imposed on cortically driven muscles, as tested in a similar experimental setup (Cheney & Fetz, 1984).

A feedback loop involving the motor cortex has clear utility. Such a loop can alter thresholds for movement in response to different inputs and thereby permit adaptive responding. A number of studies have supported the hypothesis that neuro-motor responsiveness within the motor cortex can be significantly affected by expectancy or "set" (Bonnet & Requin, 1982; Evarts & Tanji, 1976).

In the experiment of Evarts and Tanji (1976), monkeys were trained either to resist or assist an externally imposed muscle stretch. If the movement was primarily achieved with the triceps, then when the triceps was stretched by the external load, there was an immediate increase in the firing rate of triceps-related motor cortex neurons. The magnitude and latency of this initial response was approximately the same regardless of the instructed response stretch. However, about 40 ms later, the same neurons discharged differently depending on the instructional context. Either the rate increased when the stretch was to be assisted (with increased triceps activity) or it decreased when the stretch was to be resisted (with increased biceps activity). Surveying the two main results of this experiment, we can conclude that the first response was automatic, being triggered by pathways running directly from the muscle spindles to the motor cortex, whereas the second response was not automatic, being affected instead by the animal's volitional state.

PREMOTOR CORTEX

The motor cortex mainly projects to the distal musculature (especially the fingers). By contrast, the area just anterior to the motor cortex, the premotor cortex, mainly projects to the proximal musculature. Efferent fibers from the premotor cortex primarily serve to innervate motor neurons of the trunk and shoulders (Wiesendanger, 1981). The premotor cortex also receives inputs from the posterior parietal cortex, an area important for spatial orientation. These anatomical features, taken together, suggest that the premotor cortex plays a role in orienting the body and readying the postural muscles for forthcoming movements.

Recordings from neurons in the premotor cortex corroborate this hypothesis. Weinrich and Wise (1982) recorded from premotor cortex cells in monkeys who performed a task in which a warning light indicated the likely direction of a forthcoming movement. During the interval between the warning signal and the go signal, a number of cells in the premotor cortex fired vigorously and then stopped firing after the go signal appeared. The cells may have therefore helped establish the postural set for the forthcoming task, providing input to the postural muscles to allow those muscles to remain poised for the required movement.

Besides helping to establish postural sets for forthcoming movements, the premotor cortex also helps select movement trajectories. In monkeys, lesions of premotor cortex often result in an inability to redirect the paw around the back of a transparent object to reach a food reward. Even with visual feedback indicating that the object is in the way, monkeys with premotor cortex lesions seem unable to recognize the possibility of guiding the paw through an alternate, indirect route (Wiesendanger, 1981).

The premotor cortex is also involved in cross-modal sensory integration, as shown by Graziano and colleagues (Graziano & Gross, 1994; Graziano & Cooke, 2006), who found cells in the premotor cortex tuned to positions of visual stimuli relative to parts of the body. Such cells fired most vigorously when objects were presented at particular distances and directions relative to the hand. Other premotor cortex cells studied by Graziano et al. fired most vigorously when objects were presented at particular distances and directions relative to the face.

Having such cells confers a clear adaptive benefit. If a pebble is flying through the air and is rapidly approaching one's hand or face, it helps to have neurons that directly signal where that missile is in relation to the body. When those neurons fire, one is alerted to take the necessary defensive strategy: withdraw the hand if the hand is about to be struck or withdraw the face (or head) if the face is in the line of fire.

The foregoing results show that the premotor cortex plays a role in integrating visual and tactile input. Another series of studies reveals another kind of interplay between these two senses that may likewise be mediated by the premotor cortex. This series of studies concerned the *rubber hand illusion.*

If you are a participant in an experiment on the rubber hand illusion, you lay your hand on a table and then look down at it. Unbeknownst to you, however, the hand you are seeing is not your own. Rather, it is a rubber hand, of the Halloween-store variety, presented to you via mirrors. The rubber hand and your hand cannot occupy the same place, of course, which is used to advantage by the experimenter interested in examining what happens if you *feel* your own hand being tapped while *seeing* the rubber hand being tapped at the same time. If, hypothetically, the touch signals and the sight signals merge into one integrated experience, then a strange thing should happen: You should begin to feel your hand where the rubber hand is. Just such an illusion has been reported (Botvinick & Cohen, 1998). Subsequent studies have shown that it is possible to elicit the rubber hand illusion with touch alone.

SUPPLEMENTARY MOTOR AREA

Located dorsal to the premotor cortex (closer to the scalp than the premotor cortex) and anterior to the motor cortex (closer to the forehead than the motor cortex) is the supplementary motor area (SMA). This structure is involved in the high-level planning and production of complex movement sequences (Wiesendanger, 1987). Several findings support this conclusion.

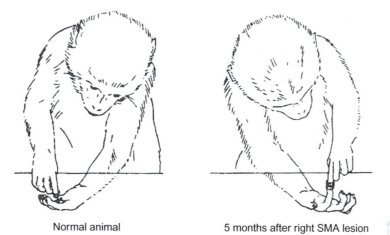

Normal animal   5 months after right SMA lesion

FIGURE 3.22 Unilateral lesion of the supplementary motor area disrupts cooperative behavior of the two hands, even if the monkey receives visual feedback. Normally, the monkey can push a morsel of food out of the hole and catch it with the other hand, but not after the lesion. From Brinkman, C. (1981). Lesions in supplementary motor area interfere with a monkey's performance of a bimanual co-ordination task. Neuroscience Letters, 27, 267–270. Copyright © by Williams and Wilkins, 1981. With permission.

First, monkeys with damage to the SMA have difficulty carrying out complex finger sequences as well as tasks requiring bimanual coordination, such as pushing a morsel of food from a hole and catching it with the other hand (Brinkman, 1984; see Figure 3.22).

Second, people with damage to the SMA have difficulty with the high-level control of movement. Such individuals may develop the weird phenomenon of the *anarchic hand*. Here, environmental stimuli trigger movements that may be at odds with, or completely unrelated to, the person's intentions. The sight of a doorknob, for example, may trigger a reach-and-grasp movement (Frith, Blakemore, & Wolpert, 2000). Dr. Strangelove, the fictional military general whose insanity led him to foment nuclear attacks, displayed the anarchic hand, as the actor Peter Sellers memorably demonstrated in the 1964 anti-war movie bearing that general's name.

A third source of evidence for the high-level control of movement by the SMA comes from studies in which electrical activity of the SMA was monitored during periods preceding spontaneously generated movement. Significant levels of activity could be detected over the SMA as long as 1 s before movement began (Deecke et al., 1969). Centers responsible for high levels of control are likely to become activated long before the inception of movement, so this outcome accords with the hypothesis that SMA plays a role in planning rather than simply triggering movements. Recall that the motor cortex, by contrast, becomes active only 50 ms or so before muscles are activated.

A fourth source of evidence for the planning role of the supplementary motor cortex comes from brain imaging studies. In an early investigation of this kind, volunteers were injected with radioactive xenon (dissolved in a saline solution) that was then carried through the bloodstream to the brain for purposes of positron emission tomography (PET). The procedure was carried out for diagnostic purposes—for example, to determine the location of a suspected brain tumor. Because areas of the brain that are metabolically active tend to draw more blood than areas that are less metabolically active, the amount of blood flow in a given area, as indexed by the amount of radioactive xenon carried to it, reveals how active that brain region is. PET scans showed that the SMA is active when people imagine carrying out sequences of finger movements and when the same people actually perform the same sequences (see Figure 3.23). By contrast, the motor cortex only "lights up" in PET scans when those same finger sequences are actually performed (Roland, Larsen, Lassen, & Skinhoj, 1980). This pattern of results lends further support to the view that the SMA is involved in high-level movement planning or representation (Wiesendanger, 1987).

Finger movement sequence (performance)

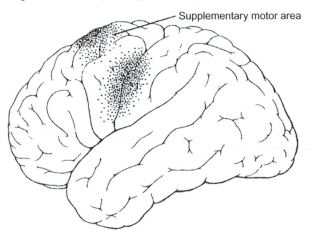

Supplementary motor area

Finger movement sequence (mental rehearsal)

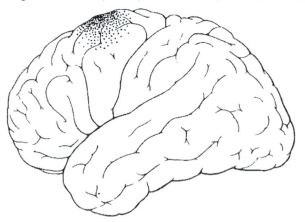

FIGURE 3.23 Cerebral blood flow during physical performance of a finger sequence (top panel) and during mental rehearsal of the same finger sequence (bottom panel). Reprinted by permission of the publisher from Voluntary movement, by C. Ghez, in Principles of neural science (2nd ed.), pp. 487–501. Copyright © 1985 by Elsevier Science Publishing Co., Inc.

The latter line of work was extended in a study that received worldwide attention (Owen et al., 2006). The discovery concerned a young woman who had been in a car accident. She sustained severe traumatic brain injury and afterwards was completely immobile. Her brain waves and other physiologic signs indicated that she had entered a coma after the accident. Later, however, she awoke, albeit without opening her eyes or giving any other indication that she knew where she was, could hear others, and so on. The hint that she was actually awake came from recordings of her brain activity. These showed that her brain went through normal sleep-wake cycles. Because she alternated between sleep and waking but was otherwise paralyzed, she was said to be in a vegetative state.

Another way of describing this woman's condition is Kafkaesque. Here, reference is made to the great fiction author, Franz Kafka, who wrote about people trapped in terrible situations, such as a salesman who woke only to discover that he had been transformed into an insect. The Kafkaesque description of this young woman is that she was "locked in." According to this way of describing her condition, she was fully aware of what was being said around her, was completely conscious, and fully desirous of expressing herself. Meanwhile, however, she was imprisoned in her own body.

Contemplating this state of existence is troubling, to say the very least. It raises a significant scientific question: Can one actually have thoughts when one is totally paralyzed? A radical behaviorist would say no: Thought is nothing but movement. A cognitivist, on the other hand, would say yes: Thoughts exist autonomously and are expressed through movement.

These two possible answers to the scientific question feed back to a troubling ethical question: Should someone in a vegetative state be "let go"? It would be hard to say yes to this question if the cognitive view were correct.

Using functional magnetic resonance imagery (fMRI) rather than PET, Owen et al. (2006) peered into the brain of this young woman and reached a startling, if not chilling, conclusion. As shown in Figure 3.24, they found that when the young woman was asked to imagine playing tennis, her SMA lit up in just the same way as occurred in neurologically normal control subjects. Similarly, when the young woman was asked to imagine walking through her home, other brain areas lit up that were the same as the areas that lit up in neurologically normal controls given the same house-touring instructions. Owen et al. (2006, p. 1402) summarized their results as follows:

> These results confirm that, despite fulfilling the clinical criteria for a diagnosis of vegetative state, this patient retained the ability to understand spoken commands and to respond to them through her brain activity, rather than through speech or movement. Moreover, her decision to cooperate with the authors by imagining particular tasks when asked to do so represents a clear act of intention, which confirmed beyond any doubt that she was consciously aware of herself and her surroundings. Of course, negative findings in such patients cannot be used as evidence for lack of awareness, because false negative findings in functional neuroimaging studies are common, even in healthy volunteers. However, in the case described here, the presence of reproducible and robust task-dependent responses to command without the need for any practice or training suggests a method by which some noncommunicative patients, including those diagnosed as vegetative, minimally conscious, or locked in, may be able to use their residual cognitive capabilities to communicate their thoughts to those around them by modulating their own neural activity.

From the perspective of determining what the SMA does, the results obtained by Owen et al. (2006) confirm that the SMA plays a role in representing extended sequences of actions. Beyond this, the data show that mental activity can indeed occur without external movement, consistent with the cognitive but not the behaviorist view. Clinically, the data of Owen et al.

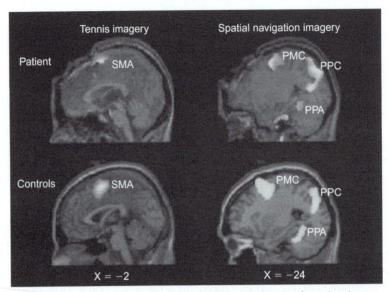

FIGURE 3.24   Functional magnetic resonance imagery (fMRI) of the brains of a patient in a vegetative state (top row) and of neurologically normal controls (bottom row) while imaging themselves playing tennis (left column) or walking through their homes (right column). The lit up areas are the supplementary motor area (SMA), lateral premotor cortex (PMC), posterior parietal cortex (PPC), and parahippocampal gyrus (PPA). From Owen, A. M., Coleman, M. R., Boly, M., Davis, M. H., Laureys, S., & Pickard, J. D. (2006). Detecting awareness in the vegetative state. Science, 313, 1402. With permission.

encourage the belief that it will be possible someday to help people leading lives befitting a Kafka novel escape their nightmare existences, if indeed their existences have this nightmarish quality.

PARIETAL CORTEX

The three parts of the cerebral cortex that we have considered so far—the motor cortex, the premotor cortex, and the supplementary motor cortex—occupy the frontal lobes, cerebral structures that lie anterior to the Sylvian fissure. The parietal cortex lies posterior to the Sylvian fissure and anterior to the parietal-occipital sulcus (see Figure 3.2). Damage to the parietal cortex often results in deficits of spatial attention and an inability to perform activities requiring spatial facility, such as drawing diagrams or building three-dimensional block structures (Luria, 1973). Cells in this region respond selectively to signals presented at locations to which movements will be made. The same cells may be quiet when stimuli are presented at the same locations and when no movements are made to them or when the same movements are made in a seemingly purposeless way (Mountcastle, Lynch, Georgopoulos, Sakata, & Acuna, 1975). This set of results suggests that cells in the parietal cortex code spatially relevant behavioral intentions.

Apraxia

Damage to the parietal cortex also results in *apraxia*. First identified in the early twentieth century by the neurologist Hugo Liepmann, apraxia is a "disturbance of motor behavior that cannot be attributed to muscular weakness, incoordination, or sensory loss, or to lack of attention or the incomprehensibility of directions to act" (Freeman, 1987, p. 30). Apraxic patients have difficulty carrying out tasks such as lighting a cigar, putting on a hat, or opening a lock with a key. Because they can carry out the individual components of these acts and can understand verbal instructions, as demonstrated through independent tests, the difficulties these patients experience stem from a breakdown in the retrieval of movement plans or the enactment of those plans once they are retrieved.

Liepmann identified two kinds of apraxia. One is *ideational apraxia*—a breakdown in the ability to access the "ideas" or "memory representations" for motor acts. A patient with ideational apraxia cannot pantomime the use of an object when asked to do so but can manipulate the object successfully when it is physically present (Heilman, 1973). Such a patient cannot swing an imaginary hammer when asked to demonstrate hammering, but when given a hammer can use it properly. Another sign of ideational apraxia is an inability to sequence complex chains of acts. Preparing a cup of coffee or opening a can and emptying its contents may be impossible. The inability to sequence tasks correctly can have dire consequences. One ideational apraxic almost lost her life when she misordered the tasks of turning on a gas stove, lighting a match, and blowing out the match (Miller, 1986).

Difficulties like these result from an inability to access concepts for sequencing, not just an inability to perform the sequences. That the difficulty is conceptual was demonstrated in a study in which ideational apraxics were asked to arrange photographs of related tasks in the correct order—for example, pictures of someone looking up a telephone number, picking up the receiver, and dialing the number. The patients could not perform this task correctly (Lehmkuhl & Poeck, 1981).

Another kind of apraxia identified by Liepmann is *ideomotor apraxia*. This form of apraxia represents a breakdown in the translation of memory representations into motor commands. The problem is not that the memories cannot be accessed; rather, the problem is that once the memories have been accessed they cannot be realized. A symptom of ideomotor apraxia is the inability to imitate what someone else is doing, though the patient can say or otherwise indicate what action he or she is supposed to perform (DeRenzi, Motti, & Nichelli, 1980).

Liepmann ventured a hypothesis about the neurological disconnections that underlie apraxia. In arriving at the hypothesis, he was struck by the fact that apraxia was far more common in people with right-side hemiplegia (paralysis of the right side of the body) than in people with left-side hemiplegia (paralysis of the left side of the body). Because each side of the body is primarily controlled by the contralateral (opposite) hemisphere, Liepmann inferred that the left hemisphere houses the plans that cannot be accessed or realized.

Liepmann had another insight as well. He saw that if plans for movement are in the left hemisphere and the left hand is mainly controlled by the right hemisphere, then when the left hand is used to carry out motoric plans, those plans must somehow be passed from the left hemisphere to the right. Liepmann proposed that the *corpus callosum*, the main pathway linking the left and right hemispheres, might be the conduit for this information. According

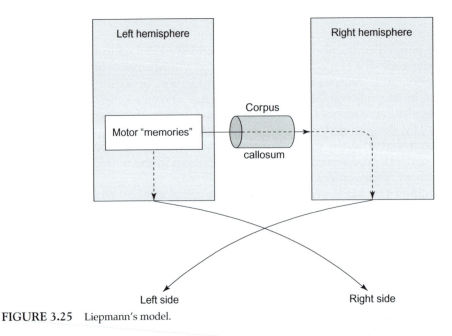

FIGURE 3.25   Liepmann's model.

to this model, signals from the left hemisphere pass through the corpus callosum to the right hemisphere and from there to the left side of the body (Figure 3.25). Postmortem examinations of apraxic patients have largely confirmed this hypothesis (Freeman, 1984; Heilman & Roth, 1985; Miller, 1986).

Cross-Modal Integration

The parietal cortex is sometimes called the association area of the brain. This term refers to the fact that associations appear to be made in this region of the brain, often between disparate sources of information such as sights and sounds, sights and touches, or movements and their sensory consequences. Because these various sources of information are of different kinds or "modes," the parietal cortex is said to participate in *cross-modal integration*. (We saw earlier that the premotor cortex also participates in this kind of integration.)

To see how this plays out in specific studies, consider what happens when you make a saccadic eye movement from one position to another. If your eyes are open and the saccade is made in illumination, the image of the external environment shifts. Somehow, however, you appreciate that the shift of the image of the external environment on your retina was due to your eye movement and not to external motion. Thus, if you were visiting the mountains and an image of a mountain jumped across your retina, you would appreciate that it is more likely that your eye jumped than that the mountain did. It turns out that neurons in the parietal cortex are involved in solving this problem.

Figure 3.26 shows the setup for the relevant experiment (Duhamel, Colby, & Goldberg, 1992). Here, recordings were made from neurons in the parietal cortex. Before the saccades were made by the monkeys in this experiment, the monkeys' parietal neurons responded to

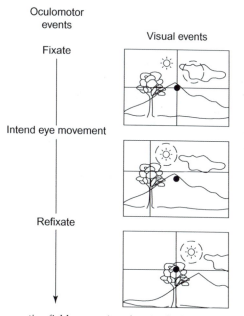

FIGURE 3.26   Change in the receptive field properties of parietal cortex neurons in a monkey as it looks at one location (top panel), prepares to direct its gaze to another location (middle panel), and then brings its gaze to that new location (bottom panel). The dot shows the current gaze location, the dashed circle shows the receptive field of the neural pool whose activity is recorded along with the monkey's eye position, and the crosshairs are centered on the presumed frame of reference of the cortical representation. From Duhamel, J-R, Colby, C. L., & Goldberg, M. E. (1992). The updating of the representation of visual space in parietal cortex by intended eye movements. Science, 255, 90–92. With permission.

stimulation of one part of the visual scene. However, as the time of the saccade approached, the neurons' receptive fields shifted to the part of the visual scene that would have the same position relative to the line of gaze *after* the forthcoming saccade as the original receptive field had relative to the line of gaze *before* the saccade. Thus, if the neurons' receptive field first included the image of the *cloud* in Figure 3.26, the same neurons' receptive field changed to include the image of the *sun* once the next saccade was prepared. The reason the sun was picked up was that it happened to occupy the same position relative to the forthcoming gaze as the cloud did during the initial gaze. Duhamel, Colby, and Goldberg showed that the neurons' visual receptive fields shifted in a manner consistent with the cartoon in Figure 3.26. These neurons participated in a circuit whose frame of reference for coding visual input shifted to accommodate forthcoming eye positions.

Because the parietal cortex engages in cross-modal integration and spatial attention, damage to the parietal cortex may result in deficits in these functions, but either function may be recruited to aid the other. Individuals with damage to the parietal cortex sometimes show spatial neglect, ignoring the side of space contralateral to the damaged parietal cortex. However, this spatial hemi-neglect can be ameliorated by capitalizing on the parietal lobe's penchant for cross-modal integration.

Brown, Kroliczak, Demonet, and Goodale (2008) made good on this possibility by showing that patients who ignored the side of visual space feeding their damaged parietal cortices were more likely to see an object in the neglected field if their hands were near the visual stimulation sites than if their hands were far from the visual stimulation sites. The benefit of hand proximity was not due to seeing the hand, for the hand could not be seen. In this instance, then, out of sight did not mean out of mind. Having the one hand near the visual stimuli gave the hemi-neglect patients a better feel for what visual stimuli were out there.

A similar, intriguing discovery was made by Taylor-Clarke, Kennett, and Haggard (2002). This team of investigators showed that people's ability to discriminate between two versus one touched location on the skin was enhanced by seeing the arm where the touch was applied. This surprising benefit was obtained even though the stimulation sites were not visible themselves. A control condition showed that the improvement in tactile discrimination was not due to spatial orienting (looking in the direction of the touches).

DISCONNECTIONS

The review has focused so far on the roles played by different parts of the brain in human motor control and related functions. Mindful of the functions served by different brain regions, we must not forget that the different parts of the brain must work together to enable functionally adaptive, goal-directed actions. Linkages between brain areas have to work properly to ensure that the various players in the neural orchestra play a symphony.

We have already encountered one example of a problem associated with a damaged connection between brain areas. As mentioned in the last section, apraxia can be brought on by a malfunctioning corpus callosum, a neural structure whose raison d'etre appears to be connecting different brain regions.

Another disconnection syndrome is associated with a neural bridge between two areas that have long been known to play important roles in language. One of those areas, *Wernicke's area*, plays an important role in language *comprehension*. The other, *Broca's area*, plays an important role in language *production*. The *arcuate fasciculus* bridges these two sites.

As might be expected from the descriptions of Wernicke's and Broca's areas, damage to the bridge between them leads to problems with the transition from understanding language to generating language. A task as mundane as repeating word for word what one is hearing becomes severely compromised in people with damage to the arcuate fasciculus (Geschwin, 1965).

Disconnections between other areas have been noted as well, and the effects of those disconnections have been linked to other sorts of problems. A particularly intriguing hypothesis concerns the problems that arise from disconnections between the frontal region of the brain and the parietal region. According to Frith, Blakemore, and Wolpert (2000), schizophrenics may have damage to these connections and that damage compromises the schizophrenics' appreciation of the sources of action-related perceptual inputs. As is well known, schizophrenics may hear voices that others do not hear. It may be that the voices they hear are their own, generated subvocally but without appropriate monitoring of the voices' source. By this line of argument, schizophrenics may lack a normal sense of agency for the actions they perform. Without a memory trace of having just willed an action, perceptual signals generated by the schizophrenics' own actions may come to be ascribed to the external environment.

Delusions may arise from a breakdown in the processing of feedforward signals. Consistent with this hypothesis, schizophrenics are less likely than normal controls to be aware of the fact that a moving hand they are watching on a video monitor is not in fact their own (Daprati et al., 1997).

CONCLUDING REMARKS

Motor neuroscience is a dynamic field in which breakthroughs have been made and will, in all likelihood, continue to be made. We have merely skimmed the surface of this exciting area of study.

Before ending the chapter, it is worthwhile to consider some ideas that were not broached earlier and also to emphasize some ideas that bear further stress. First, it is important to realize that any given motor act is made possible by the collective effects of many brain centers, acting simultaneously and sequentially. As indicated in the foregoing review, at different times relative to the production of a single motor act, different brain areas become active (Deecke et al., 1969). Thus, a motor act is the product of the orchestrated activity of many brain centers. If those centers are not properly connected, problems can arise.

Second, there is redundancy in the roles served by different brain areas. Sometimes an area that reliably becomes active when a particular act is performed is not active when that act is performed in other contexts. For example, though the motor cortex projects to the arms, the arms can sometimes move when the motor cortex is silent. This point became apparent in a laboratory where a monkey was trained to make a controlled lever movement (Fetz, cited in Ghez, 1985). One day the monkey became agitated and banged the lever back and forth. In this emotional state, the monkey's motor cortex became less active than normal. This surprising result implies that the monkey's arm could be driven by structures other than the motor cortex. Thus, there are multiple routes to the production of arm and other movements. The notion that there are multiple paths for the production of single motor acts was recognized as long ago as 1906, when Sherrington, one of the first physiologists to study reflexes (and for which he received the Nobel Prize), referred to the motor unit as the final common pathway (Sherrington, 1906).

A third general point about motor neuroscience is that the centers we have considered are not the only ones involved in motor control. The centers we have concentrated on are usually regarded as major motor centers, but other centers also come to play a role. Indeed, all areas of the brain are involved either directly or indirectly in the generation of behavior. This means that a complete theory of motor neuroscience will probably amount to a complete theory of the brain. By the same token, studying the neural basis of motor control is likely to shed light on brain organization at large.

The final point to be discussed in this chapter concerns the source of intentions. Movements are made in response to perceptual input and intentional states. But where do intentional states come from? This question is profound, and if any area of study can answer it, the investigation of the neural substrates of voluntary movement and stability may be it.

Two studies already conducted in this context provide an indication of the kind of answer that may emerge. One was the investigation, already cited, of the electrical activity of the human brain prior to voluntary movement (Deecke et al., 1969). Recall that motor potentials recorded in the motor cortex occurred 50 ms prior to the first sign of finger EMGs (Deecke et al, 1969). This same study revealed that as long as 1.5 s before the same EMGs, there was diffuse activity over virtually the entire cerebral cortex. As the time of finger movement approached, the recorded brain activity became more and more focused, concentrating ultimately on the motor cortex. The timing of this early brain activity (the pre-movement potential) gave a hint of when intentions arise—at least 1.5 s before simple movements. As for *where* intentions arise, the topography of the pre-movement potential suggested that intentions originate in the collective activity of neurons dispersed widely throughout the brain.

Another study that yielded a similar result had people provide an estimate of when they first decided to produce a simple voluntary movement (Libet, Gleason, Wright, & Pearl, 1983). The time estimates were consistently late. Participants estimated the initial decision as occurring a half second after pre-movement potentials were recorded from their own brains. A possible interpretation of this result is that people are poor at estimating when things happen inside their heads, but there is a problem with this account. In a control condition, Libet et al. found that the same subjects accurately, or more accurately, estimated when a sensory stimulus was presented. Apparently, then, people only become aware of their own intentions some time after a significant amount of neurological activity allows the intentions to coalesce. Some have said this outcome indicates that intentions are illusory (Wegner, 2002). Another possibility is that intentions are not illusory, but the formation of intentions, which are coherent psychological states, arise through a coalescing of diffuse neural activity. Many small events must often come together for some large event to occur. Tornados exist, for example, through the many small climatic events that lead to their formation. Saying that tornados are illusory could lead to a whirlwind of unfortunate consequences.

SUMMARY

1. The central aim of motor neuroscience is to understand how the physical makeup of the nervous system and musculo-skeletal system allows for the adaptive control of posture and movement. Specialized mechanisms allow motor control to be carried out in such a way that attention to the detailed properties of muscle activity is generally unnecessary.
2. Muscles contract when they are stimulated at the neuromuscular junction. Muscles stretch when they are subjected to mechanical loads.
3. The tension developed by muscle during active contraction is an inverted-U-shaped function of muscle length. The shape of the function is due to the strength of actin-myosin bridges at different muscle lengths.
4. A motor neuron and the muscle fibers it innervates comprise a motor unit, the most basic element of motor control. It is impossible to voluntarily contract some but not all of the muscle fibers within a motor unit. With feedback, however, it is possible to activate a single motor unit. Motor units tend to be recruited in an orderly size-dependent fashion. Units containing small muscle fibers are generally activated before units containing large muscle fibers.

5. Muscle spindles are attached to the large muscle fibers (extrafusals) that produce adequate force to move a limb. Muscle spindles contain small fibers (intrafusals) that also contract. The sensory nerve fibers attached to muscle spindles respond to differences in the length of the muscle spindle relative to the extrafusal. These sensory fibers serve as muscle stretch receptors. The signals they produce can be consciously perceived.

6. Sensory receptors in muscle tendons (Golgi tendon organs) tend to fire when muscle tension increases. The response properties of Golgi tendon organs are roughly opposite the response properties of muscle spindles. Golgi organs fire when muscles contract, whereas stretch receptors fire when muscles lengthen.

7. Sensory receptors in the joints fire primarily at extreme joint angles. They may provide a warning signal about awkward or dangerous postures.

8. Sensory receptors in the skin (cutaneous receptors) are vital for precise manipulation, particularly when other forms of feedback, such as vision, are absent. They may also be important for balance.

9. Spinal circuits provide the neurological basis for perceptual-motor communication in the peripheral motor system. The simplest spinal circuit is the reflex arc. Here, muscle contracts immediately in response to stretch.

10. According to the servo theory of muscle activation, extrafusals contract via a stretch reflex triggered by the earlier activation of intrafusals. The timing of muscle spindle discharge and extrafusal activity suggested, however, that intrafusals and extrafusals are generally activated simultaneously. Such coactivation permits rapid correction for unexpected loads.

11. Motor neurons not only activate muscles; they also excite Renshaw cells, which inhibit the motor neurons themselves. This seemingly paradoxical effect has functional advantages. It provides a way of modulating and finely grading the amount of input that suffices to activate motor neurons.

12. Reciprocal inhibition exists between stretch receptors from one muscle and the motor neurons responsible for activating opposing muscles. Reciprocal inhibition prevents muscles from working against each other during responses to muscle stretch.

13. The cerebellum regulates muscle tone, coordination, timing, and learning. If the cerebellum is disconnected from the spinal cord, muscle tone is adversely affected. Coordination deficits following cerebellar damage take the form of poor balance (*ataxia*), slurred speech (*dysarthria*), reaching too far (*hypermetria*), and oscillation in conjunction with purposeful movements (*intention tremor*). The sequencing of repetitive movements also becomes difficult and requires more attention than usual. Timing difficulties associated with cerebellar damage take the form of abnormal durations and phase relations of EMG patterns, as well as abnormal variability of otherwise rhythmic behavior. The cerebellum's role in learning is suggested by the inability of animals with cerebellar damage to adapt eye-head coordination after wearing reversing prisms, by changes in cerebellar activity related to the development of limb coordination, and by the need for the cerebellum in tasks requiring adaptation to visuo-motor rotations.

14. The roles of the basal ganglia in motor control are suggested by behavioral consequences of basal ganglia disease. In Huntington's chorea, patients make wild,

uncontrollable movements. In Parkinson's disease, patients exhibit shuffling gait, shaking motion at rest (*resting tremor*), slow movement initiation (*akinesia*), slow movement execution (*bradykinesia*), and muscle rigidity. The basal ganglia appear to play a role in initiating movements, modulating the global scaling of movement amplitudes, regulating perceptual-motor interactions, and learning.

15. Brief, localized electrical stimulation of the motor cortex triggers muscle twitches. Which muscles twitch depends on where the stimulation is applied. Varying the stimulation site allowed investigators to develop "motor maps." These maps are organized topographically, with neighboring regions representing neighboring musculature. Regions of the maps devoted to the face and hands are typically larger than those devoted to other parts of the body.

16. Neurons of the motor cortex generally fire just before movements are made. The discharge of motor cortex cells is related to the force and direction of movement. Different cells are tuned to different directions of movement, but individual cells respond to a whole range of directions and to a degree that declines as the called-for direction departs from the cell's preferred direction. The output of the entire population of motor cortex neurons is a weighted sum of the individual neuron's activity levels (population coding).

17. Motor cortex neurons receive sensory feedback from the muscles they drive, allowing for cortically mediated responses to muscle stretch. Because these responses have relatively long latencies, they are called *long-loop reflexes*. The immediate responses of motor cortex neurons to muscle stretch are independent of volitional state. The more delayed responses depend on expectancies or set.

18. Electrical stimulation of motor cortex neurons lasting longer (500 ms) than the stimulation used in traditional studies (50 ms) can yield body positions that depend on where the stimulation is applied.

19. The premotor cortex plays a role in orienting the body and readying the postural muscles for forthcoming movements. It also plays a role in selecting movement trajectories and in relating positions of visual stimuli to parts of the body. The latter result illustrates cross-modal integration, which is also illustrated by phenomena such as the rubber hand illusion, where people can be led to feel their hand at a different place from where it actually is.

20. The supplementary motor area (SMA) is involved in the planning of extended sequences of movements. Regardless of whether a person performs a finger sequence or imagines it, the supplementary motor area "lights up" when viewed with positron emission tomography (PET) or functional magnetic resonance imagery (fMRI). fMRI studies have revealed that a so-called vegetative state may actually mask the ability to comprehend instructions and imagine performing instructed tasks. Damage to the SMA can result in the *anarchic hand*, a syndrome in which the hand acts without the person being able to control it.

21. The parietal cortex contains cells whose discharge properties are related to the behavioral relevance of spatial locations. In general, this brain region is crucial for spatially directed behavior.

22. Damage to the parietal cortex can result in apraxia, an inability to perform purposeful motor acts when the perceptual, cognitive, and motoric components of the acts are

otherwise intact. The incidence of apraxic symptoms in the left and right hand suggests that the memory representations for learned movement sequences are generally stored in the left hemisphere. The right hand receives motor commands directly from the left hemisphere, and the left hand receives motor commands from the right hemisphere after that hemisphere has received signals from the left hemisphere via the corpus callosum.

23. The parietal cortex plays a role in integration of sensory inputs from different modalities, as can be crucial for interpreting sensory inputs correctly when they accompany different motor acts. Thus, the visual receptive fields of neurons in the parietal cortex may change in tandem with saccadic eye movements.

24. Surprising illusions can also rise from cross-modal sensory integration. For example, holding the unseen hand near a visual stimulus in a region of space that is generally ignored can help draw attention to that visual stimulus. This fact might prove useful in the treatment of spatial hemi-neglect, a syndrome in which people with damage to the parietal cortex ignore the contralateral side of space.

25. Connections between brain areas are just as important as individual brain areas themselves. When those connections are impaired, performance can suffer. For example, damage to the arcuate fasciculus, a bundles of nerve fibers joining Wernicke's area, which plays a role in language comprehension, and Broca's area, which plays a role in language production, can lead to breakdowns in the capacity to repeat what is said.

26. Delusions of control in schizophrenia may stem from disconnections between the frontal region of the brain and the parietal region. These disconnections may be associated with schizophrenics' failing to appreciate that they themselves generate actions that produce perceptual effects. As a result, the schizophrenics may "hear voices" because they may not appreciate that they have generated the subvocal speech themselves.

27. Every motor act is the product of the collective activity of many brain centers. The formation of intentions is a prime example.

Further Reading

Journals presenting research on or related to motor neuroscience include *Brain, Cortex, Experimental Brain Research, Journal of Neurophysiology, Journal of Neuroscience, Nature, Nature Neuroscience, Nature Reviews Neuroscience, Neuroimage, Neuron, Neuropsychologia, Science,* and *Spinal Cord.*

A number of books provide in-depth reviews of motor neuroscience. Useful texts include Brooks (1981, 1986), Jeannerod (1988), Gazzaniga (2004), Kandel, Schwartz, and Jessell (2000), Latash (2008a), and Rothwell (1987).

Motor neurons can die off. The famous baseball player Lou Gehrig developed a disease in which his motor neurons died, causing him to become paralyzed and, finally, to die. This disease came to be called Lou Gehrig's disease. It is also known as amyotrophic lateral sclerosis (ALS) or motor neuron disease. For an overview of the history of ALS, including cutting-edge approaches to its treatment, see Aebischer and Kato (2007).

For discussion of exceptions to the size principle of motor neuron recruitment, see Desmedt (1981).

This chapter discussed the role of the frog spinal cord in motor control (Fucson, Berkenblit, & Feldman (1980). Additional work on the computational prowess of the frog's spinal cord is described by Bizzi, Mussa-Ivaldi, and Giszter (1991). These investigators showed that electrical stimulation of the frog's spinal cord causes force fields to develop in the frog's hindlimb. Which forces developed depended on where the stimulation was applied and which combination of sites was stimulated.

Brief mention was made here of muscle-stiffness control. Additional studies indicate that the motor system can selectively stiffen muscles to prevent movements in particular directions either while attempting to maintain steady postures or while making movements (Burdet, Osu, Franklin, Milner, & Kawato, 2001; Darainy, Towhidkhah, & Ostry, 2007; Franklin, Liaw, Milner, Osu, Burdet, & Kawato, 2007; Popescu, Hidler, & Rymer, 2003). Regulating stiffness or impedance (Palazzolo et al., 2007) is an active area of research in human motor control.

The cerebellum has come to be recognized as a seat of emotion as well as motor control. See Schmahmann, Anderson, Newton, and Ellis (2001) and Schutter and van Honk (2005).

The homunculus of Penfield makes for a catchy cartoon (Figure 3.19), but the detailed organization of the motor cortex is not quite as tidy as the cartoon would suggest. A given area of the motor cortex is likely to represent a blend of neighboring body regions, not just a single area (Schieber, 2001). Whether this integration reflects inputs to muscle synergies for controlling a given target effector remains to be seen.

Schieber and his colleagues have done other important research on the functional properties of the motor cortex. Davidson, Chan, O'Dell, and Schieber (2007) demonstrated plasticity for connections between motor cortex and α motor neurons depending on task experience. This is an example of neural plasticity of the kind discussed in Chapter 2.

The population coding hypothesis has been used to account for drawing behavior in monkeys (Schwartz, 1994) and has been used to account for data from a task in which monkeys were invited, via a clever experimental procedure, to "change their minds." This experiment was based on the possibility of recording from many neurons of the motor cortex simultaneously and determining where, at any moment, the population vector as a whole was "pointing." The direction implied by the summed activity of motor cortex neurons was estimated at successive times to find out how the implied direction changed in a task where a monkey learned that if a light appeared at a point along the perimeter of a circle, the movement that would have to be performed (to obtain a sip of fruit juice) would have to be directed to a point 90 degrees counterclockwise from the original stimulus (Georgopoulos et al., 1989). The direction of the neuronal population vector shifted steadily from the original stimulus location to the final target location, as if the monkey performed a mental rotation similar to that studied in research on human visual imagery (Shepard & Cooper, 1982).

The population coding account of motor cortical activation of movement has been challenged with respect to its mathematical claims (Mussa-Ivaldi, 1988) and with respect to the interpretation of what movements factors are actually represented (Scott, Gribble, Graham, & Cabel, 2001).

Transmagnetic stimulation (TMS) has been used to study the role of the motor cortex and other brain structures (Figure 3.27). In TMS, a brief magnetic pulse is applied to the participant's scalp with his or her permission

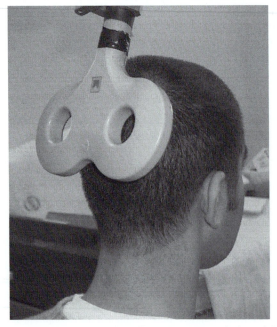

FIGURE 3.27   Transmagnetic stimulation. From http://www.princeton.edu/~napl/images/r_TMS.jpg.

and after all appropriate safeguards are taken to minimize risk. Underlying brain regions are activated or de-activated, often resulting in observable muscle activity or other behavioral or other cognitive or emotional changes. Studying the effects of the magnetic pulses can provide a window into the state of the nervous system when the pulses are applied. For reviews, see Rossini et al. (1994) and Walsh and Cowey (2000).

Prefrontal cortex, a region of the brain anterior to the premotor cortex, plays a role in demarcating boundaries between action sequences (Fujii & Graybiel, 2003) and the formation of plans for behavior (Zillner, 2008).

Damage to the basal ganglia can result in Parkinson's disease, the most common of all neurological disorders. A primary symptom of Parkinson's disease is resting tremor. But resting tremor is just one of a spectrum of tremor types that characterize human motor control. Another type is intention tremor, which was mentioned here in connection with cerebellar damage. Tremor does not only arise in disordered states, however. Even at rest, tremor is manifested in neurologically normal individuals, as you can see for yourself by holding a sheet of paper on your upturned palm with your arm outstretched. The paper will jitter no matter how relaxed or healthy you may be. Reviews of research on tremor can be found in Cohen (2008) and Elble and Koller (1990).

Apraxia was discussed briefly in this chapter, principally in connection with classical work on it. For more recent work, see papers by Buxbaum and her co-workers (e.g., Buxbaum, 2001; Buxbaum, Sirigu, Schwartz, & Klatzky, 2003; Pavese & Buxbaum, 2002).

This chapter discussed brain imaging of a young woman in a vegetative state (Figure 3.24). For more information about efforts to communicate with individuals who are "locked in," see Kubler, Kotchoubey, Kaiser, Wolpaw, and Bierbaumer (2001).

For more information about movement-related shifts in frames of reference, similar to the material discussed in connection with Figure 3.26, see Salinas and Their (2000).

To learn more about phenomena related to the rubber hand illusion, see Botvinik (2004), Ehrsson, Geyer, and Naito (2003), Ehrsson, Spence, and Passingham (2004), and Ehrsson, Holmes, and Passingham (2005).

The research by Libet, Gleason, Wright, and Pearl (1983) on the estimation of intention-formation times in the brain has been followed up by a number of investigators, among them Brass and Haggard (2007), Waszak et al. (2005), and Keller et al. (2006).

4

Psychological Foundations

O U T L I N E			
Theories of Sequencing and Timing	94	*Long-Term Memory*	118
Response Chaining	94	*Short-Term Memory*	119
Element-to-Position Associations	97	*History Effects*	122
Inter-Element Inhibition	98	*Motor Programs*	124
Hierarchies	99	*The Motor Output Buffer*	125
Skill Acquisition	101	**States of Mind**	127
Closed Loop Theory	101	*Attention*	127
Generalized Programs	103	*Intention*	128
Hierarchical Learning	106	*Ideo-Motor Theory*	129
Mental Practice and Imagery	109	**Summary**	131
Stage Theory	110		
Physical Changes in Skill Acquisition	112	**Further Reading**	134
Codes and Stores	115		
Codes	115		
Procedural and Declarative Knowledge	116		

This chapter, in contrast to the last, presents a level of description a bit removed from the physical basis of movement. The level of description is psychological, meaning that the structures and processes of interest are considered without explicit reference to their physical realization. Instead, they are considered with respect to their functional properties. This does not mean that the psychological approach disregards physical bases for motor control or other functions. Psychologists appreciate that physical factors underpin the functions they wish to analyze, but they feel that those functions can be studied on their own terms.

The chapter has four parts. The first is concerned with theories of sequencing and timing. Historically, the sequencing and timing problem has been a focus not just of "motor psychologists" but also of psychologists working outside the field of motor control, not to mention non-psychologists. This merging of approaches makes the sequencing and timing problem an ideal starting point given what was discussed in the last chapter. The present chapter will mainly look at sequencing rather than the control of timing per se. Timing will be taken up in more detail in Chapter 9, Keyboarding.

The second part of the chapter will be concerned with theories of skill learning. This topic has also been pursued by investigators both inside and outside the field of motor control. Diverse approaches have been taken to the skill-learning problem, and important advances have been made in this area in recent years. Some of those advances were introduced in Chapter 2. They will be elaborated upon in this chapter, and other important topics will be covered as well.

The third part of the chapter will be concerned with the memory systems and forms of mental representations that are used in human motor control. Motor control, both in humans and in animals, relies on procedural rather than declarative knowledge. This distinction is one of the most important in psychology. A variety of memory systems also play a role in human motor control. These memory systems differ in their durability and in the roles they play. An overarching question about the memory systems underlying motor control is whether they are similar to the memory systems underlying perception. For example, are there buffers for the maintenance of about-to-be-issued motor commands, just as there are buffers for the maintenance of sensory information?

The fourth part of the chapter will be concerned with states of mind. Here we will focus on attention, intention, and the so-called ideo-motor theory of action.

THEORIES OF SEQUENCING AND TIMING

Much of the work in psychology that bears on motor control has been concerned with the sequencing and timing problem. Recall from Chapter 2 that the nub of this problem is to discover how the elements of a movement sequence are ordered in a series. Hence, this issue has also been called the *serial order* problem (Lashley, 1951). When one says "happy birthday," for example, what is the nature of the memory representation that allows the sounds of this phrase to be arranged as they are? In this section, we will consider four historically important answers to this question: response chaining, element-to-position associations, inter-element inhibition, and hierarchies.

Response Chaining

The oldest proposed solution to the sequencing and timing problem is that the stimulus produced by a movement triggers the next movement in the sequence (Figure 4.1). This hypothesis was popularized by William James (1890), who suggested that as connections between stimuli and responses become stronger with practice, movement sequences are produced more rapidly and smoothly as a result.

It is difficult to introduce this *response chaining* theory without treating it as a straw man. So many arguments have been leveled against it that the amount of space devoted to its destruction usually exceeds the amount of space devoted to its introduction. Nevertheless,

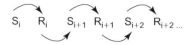

FIGURE 4.1   Response chaining theory. Stimulus i triggers response i, which triggers stimulus i + 1, which triggers response i + 1, and so on.

it is worth discussing the arguments against the theory because a considerable amount of work has been incited by it. In addition, a critical review of the arguments provides a potentially enlightening way of gaining familiarity with psychological argumentation.

One problem with response chaining concerns timing. Suppose it takes 100 ms to initiate a movement in response to feedback from the immediately preceding movement. If movements can be produced more quickly than once every 100 ms, response chaining theory can be rejected. This argument was presented in a famous article by the American physiologist Karl Lashley (1951). The article is worth reading today because of its historical importance as a manifesto for cognitive psychology (Rosenbaum, Cohen, Jax, van der Wel, & Weiss, 2007). Lashley argued that the very high speeds at which movement sequences can be performed rule out response chaining. For example, pianists produce arpeggios so quickly that one cannot take seriously the proposition that each keystroke is produced in response to feedback from the keystroke just before it.

There is a difficulty with this argument, however. It is hard to know how long it takes to respond to feedback. Suppose it takes 80 ms rather than 100 ms. Then if responses can be produced at a rate of once every 80 ms, response chaining theory need not be rejected. No matter how quickly responses can be produced, a proponent of chaining theory might argue that feedback works more quickly than was previously supposed (Adams, 1976).

Another difficulty with Lashley's (1951) timing argument is that one can imagine that a movement may not be produced in response to feedback from the immediately preceding movement but rather in response to feedback from an earlier movement. Even if the delay between movement $n - 1$ and movement n is too short for feedback from movement $n - 1$ to trigger movement n, movement n might be triggered by feedback from movement $n - 2$ or $n - 3$, and so on (Figure 4.2).

Another challenge to response chaining theory pertains to a logical problem. Suppose that instead of saying "happy birthday," one says, "happy birthright." According to response chaining theory, when one says "birth," the next syllable should be uniquely triggered. However, the same utterance can be followed by different outputs, as this example shows. Having multiple outputs after a given output is problematic for the theory.

A counterargument that can be proposed is that there may be subtle differences in the first syllable of "birthday" and "birthright" which trigger "day" or "right." If one's measure were sensitive enough, one might be able to identify those differences, or so the argument goes. This is a tricky argument to make, however, because it can never be falsified. The

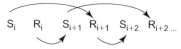

FIGURE 4.2   Response chaining theory with delays. Stimulus i triggers response i + 1, which triggers stimulus i + 1, which triggers response i + 2, and so on.

argument is metaphysical—beyond the reach of actual observation—rather than scientific—within the reach of actual observation, and so does not belong in scientific discourse.

Another argument that can be raised against response chaining theory concerns the effects of interrupting feedback. If feedback is eliminated, then according to response chaining theory, it should be impossible to carry out well-ordered sequences of movements. A number of studies have shown, however, that movement sequences *can* be performed reasonably well even if sensory feedback is interrupted. For example, Lashley (1917) found that a patient with damage to the sensory nerves leading from the patient's legs could still make voluntary leg movements. Other examples will be presented later in this book.

Are these results devastating to response chaining theory? The problem with the feedback-interruption studies is that they rule out a particular version of response chaining theory, a version that assumes sensory feedback provides the necessary trigger for forthcoming movements. If one does not interpret the theory this way, the ability to move despite the elimination of feedback limits the scope of the theory but not its basic assumptions (Adams, 1984).

Response chaining theory can be viewed more abstractly as simply implying a series of "forward associations": Response n triggers response $n + 1$, which triggers response $n + 2$, and so on. Each trigger is made possible by an associative link, though the physical nature of the link need not be specified. (Remember that a psychological theory need not make commitments about physical implementation.) If the theory is viewed in these abstract terms, the fact that movements can be carried out without sensory feedback need not be viewed as devastating to the theory. Similarly, if the theory is viewed as saying that forward associations exist entirely within the central nervous system rather than requiring external sensory feedback, then again it is not damaging to the response chaining claim that movements can continue even if sensory feedback is stopped.

An abstract theory of this sort was once proposed for the sequencing of speech (Wickelgren, 1969). The theory held that a word like "pin" is represented by elements with information about each linguistically distinct sound element or phoneme in the word (see Chapter 10). According to the theory, "pin" is represented as $\{_{\#}p_i, {}_{p}i_n, {}_{i}n_{\#}\}$, where the subscripts denote preceding and following elements, and # denotes a word boundary. Once $_{\#}p_i$ has been activated, the next element to be called for is $_{p}i_n$, because its core element, i, is designated by the right-hand subscript of $_{\#}p_i$. Furthermore, the left-hand subscript of $_{p}i_n$ indicates that p is the preceding phoneme.

One problem with this theory, aside from determining who writes and reads the subscripts, is the logical one raised earlier. Why wouldn't pin be replaced willy-nilly by pit, for example? The string for pit, $\{_{\#}p_i, {}_{p}i_t, {}_{i}t_{\#}\}$, has the same initial element as the string for pin. Activating $_{\#}p_i$, therefore, does not uniquely specify the following element.

A second problem is that there are rules for pronunciation that generalize beyond familiar utterances. When children are presented with a picture of a novel creature with an unfamiliar name (for example, a "wug") and are asked to say what they see when shown two wugs, they pronounce the final s as a z rather than as a hard s, in accord with English phonology (Berko, 1958). How can children produce phonologically lawful utterances for words they never heard? According to chaining theory, or the version of it proposed by Wickelgren (1969), a distinct string for "wugs" would be needed, but where that string comes from is unclear. More worrisome, distinct strings would be needed for every possible utterance, which would surely tax the storage capacity of human memory (MacNeilage, 1970).

Rule-governed behavior is not limited to language production. It is also displayed by people in nonlinguistic contexts and by animals. In one demonstration of rule-governed behavior in animals (Hulse, 1978), rats were trained on a maze-running task where, in successive experimental trials, they received more and more reinforcement or less and less reinforcement no matter how well or how poorly they did. In blocks of trials where more reinforcement was given, running speed increased, but in blocks of trials where less reinforcement was given, running speed decreased. When the rats were transferred to a new maze, similar either to the one in which reinforcement grew more generous or similar to the one in which reinforcement grew less generous, running times were faster or slower, respectively. Thus, the rats seemed to induce a rule.

Similar results have been obtained with other species and with rats in other experimental contexts, supporting the conclusion that animals pick up lawful relations among events, even if the relations are not realized physically in the environment (Hulse, Fowler, & Honig, 1978). This capacity for apprehending rules and for behaving according to them is difficult to accommodate with chaining theory—so hard, in fact, that no one has been able to resurrect chaining theory in the face of rule-governed behavior. For this reason, even the most ardent defenders of response chaining theory have admitted that "response chaining . . . is dead" [Adams, 1984, p. 20].

Element-to-Position Associations

Other theories of serial order have done only marginally better, but it is worth mentioning these other theories to provide a sense of the range of theories that have been proposed.

One of those theories holds that sequencing is represented by associations between response elements and serial positions (Figure 4.3). "Happy birthday," for example, might be represented by a link between /ha/ and 1, a link between /pi/ and 2, and so forth. This system can account for the fact that when people try to recall previously learned word lists, they accidentally substitute words from similar list positions. For example, when trying to recall the second word from one list, they may substitute the second word from another list (Fuchs & Melton, 1974). This phenomenon is easy to account for with element-to-position associations: The correct position-association is activated, but the correct element is not.

An appealing feature of element-to-position theory is that it can be generalized to provide an account of timing. Suppose one wants to play three notes on the piano, but with different rhythms. The timing as well as the serial ordering of the notes can be defined by associating the notes with tags for different times (Rosenbaum, 1985). An F# played as a half note followed by a G played as a quarter can be represented by associating F# with Time 1 and G with Time 3 (arbitrary time units), but if F# is to be played as a quarter note followed

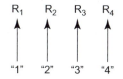

FIGURE 4.3 Element-to-position associations. Response R1 is the first response because it is associated with "1," response R2 is the second response because it is associated with "2," etc.

by G played as a quarter, then F# can be associated with Time 1 and G can be associated with Time 2. There is a problem with this theory, however. Like chaining theory, it fails to account for rule-governed behavior. In addition, the theory begs the question of how times or serial positions should be marked. What is Time 1, for example? When one is born? And how does one account for the fact that it is possible to speed up or slow down overall rates of performance?

Inter-Element Inhibition

Whereas element-to-position theory assumes that there are abstract elements (sequence position tags) to which response elements are associated, the next theory to be discussed says that sequencing is represented solely in terms of connections among the elements of the sequence itself (Estes, 1972). In this respect, the theory is like response chaining, but in contrast to response chaining, it assumes that there are inhibitory as well as excitatory links between elements.

The main ideas in inter-element inhibition theory are shown in Figure 4.4. Here, Element 4 is defined as the fourth element because it receives inhibitory connections from three other elements, Element 3 is defined as the third element because it receives inhibitory connections from two other elements, and so on. All the elements are activated simultaneously by a high-order element. The element that is output first is the one with the least inhibition (Element 1). Once Element 1 has been executed, it no longer inhibits the other elements, leaving Element 2 as the element with the least inhibition, so it is produced next. Once Element 2 is produced, it stops inhibiting the remaining elements, allowing Element 3 to be produced next. Finally, Element 4 remains and is executed last.

This theory has much to recommend it. By relying on inhibitory connections among elements, it does not beg the question of how serial position is represented (unlike the element-to-position model). Moreover, inhibitory connections are physiologically realistic. The utility of the theory has been demonstrated in a successful model of typewriting control (Rumelhart & Norman, 1982), discussed in some detail in Chapter 9.

On the other hand, concerns can be expressed about the inter-element theory (Rosenbaum, 1985). One is that it is unclear how a sequence can be initiated. When the elements of a sequence receive excitatory input, why don't all the elements fire at once? Inhibition must build up among the elements to ensure that they are produced in the order implied by their inhibitory connections. This means that some additional mechanism must delay simultaneous

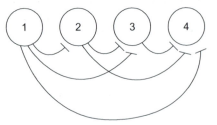

FIGURE 4.4   The interelement inhibition model of Estes (1972). From Estes, W. K. (1972). An associative basis for coding and organization in memory. In A. W. Melton & E. Martin (Eds.), Coding processes in human memory (pp. 161–190). Washington, D. C.: V. H. Winston. With permission.

production of the elements until enough inhibition has built up. From this it does not follow that the theory is fatally flawed, only that the theory needs elaboration.

A second concern is that the same elements are sometimes produced in different orders. It is possible to say "villain" and "anvil," for example, or "bad" and "dab." In the theory, to allow for such reversals, one would have to invert inhibitory connections between sequence elements. Thus, inhibition from d to b in "dab" would be replaced with inhibition from b to d in "bad." Some other mechanism would then be needed to determine how the inhibitory connections should be set up. One would be left with the underlying question of how that determination was made and what mechanism achieved the reordering.

A way around this problem is to allow for multiple representations of sequences containing the same elements. There could be a "dab" sequence apart from a "bad" sequence, for example. Since "dab" and "bad" mean different things, this might be tolerable. However, one would ultimately need as many representations of a phoneme as there are words containing it. Every word with a b, for instance, would need its own inhibitory pattern. Thus, the b representation would be replicated thousands or even millions of times. This seems uneconomical, though that sense does not prove that multiple representations do not exist.

The final problem with inter-element theory is the same problem that bedevils all the other theories discussed so far: It cannot easily account for rule-based behavior.

Hierarchies

The final theory of serial order to be reviewed here is the one that has fared the best. It assumes that elements of response sequences are organized hierarchically. The distinguishing feature of hierarchical organization is that it has distinct levels of control.

The concept of hierarchy is familiar to anyone who has looked at a company's organizational chart. The company is hierarchical if there is a president at the highest level, vice-presidents at a lower level, department heads at a still lower level, and so forth. When the president issues a command, it is interpreted by the vice-presidents, who delegate authority to department heads, and so on. In some hierarchies, the president issues commands directly to department heads or workers at lower levels. Likewise, feedback to someone at a given level may come from individuals at the next level down or from individuals more than one level down. In all such cases, the system can be considered hierarchical because it has distinct tiers of control.

A considerable amount of evidence suggests that hierarchical models provide a useful explanatory framework for understanding motor control. In the context of the sequencing and timing problem, a hierarchical model does much better than any other model discussed so far.

Consider the finding that has been most troublesome for the other models—the importance of rules. In hierarchical models, a rule can be viewed as a function applying to any of a large number of possible instances. The function can be assumed to occupy a high level in the hierarchy, and the sequences to which the rule applies can be assumed to occupy, or be represented at, lower levels.

To make this more concrete, consider the task of learning a sequence of numbers, such as 3, 2, 4, 3, 5, 4, 6, 5, and so on. This sequence is easy to learn, particularly if it is presented in chunks: [3, 2], [4, 3], [5, 4], [6, 5]. A simple set of rules describes this sequence: Start with an

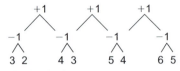

FIGURE 4.5   Tree diagram for an easily chunked sequence.

input number, $n = 3$, subtract 1 to get an output number, then repeat this procedure again, incrementing the input number by 1 each time the procedure is repeated.

Note that the foregoing description refers to a repeated procedure. In models of sequence learning, such procedures have been represented hierarchically, for example, with tree diagrams (Figure 4.5). An indication that such sequences are used is that when sequences are hard to describe hierarchically they are hard to learn, but when they are easy to describe hierarchically they are easier to learn (Jones, 1981; Restle, 1970; Simon, 1972).

A corollary of this finding is that when people are asked to recall previously learned material, their recall indicates that they have formed hierarchical codes. Consider the following list of letters: FB, ICI, AKG, BTW, A. This list is hard to learn. But if the boundaries between the letters are shifted, the list becomes much easier: FBI, CIA, KGB, TWA (Bower, Clark, Lesgold, & Winzenz, 1969). In the second segmentation, the sequences are familiar, or were at the time the study was done: TWA stood for Trans-World Airways, the KGB was the security arm of the Soviet Union, and the FBI and CIA were, as they are today in the United States, the Federal Bureau of Investigation and the Central Intelligence Agency. In terms of a hierarchical model, each sequence makes contact with an already-learned high-level unit (a familiar three-letter sequence). The availability of these already-learned units facilitates learning.

A study of chess players supports the idea that learning is facilitated by the availability of pre-existing, high-level units (deGroot, 1965). Expert and novice chess players were shown displays of chess pieces. Later they were asked to recall the positions. When the pieces were organized sensibly, as in a game, the experts recalled the positions better than the novices did, but when the pieces were organized randomly, there was no difference between the recall levels of the experts and the recall levels of the novices (deGroot, 1965). Apparently, then, the experts benefited from exposure to the previously learned configurations. The experts had in memory hierarchically structured representations of chess piece configurations.

In further support of this interpretation, when experts recreated chess configurations and their placements of pieces on the board were timed, it was found that pieces belonging to a meaningful group were usually set down on the board in rapid succession. Once a meaningful configuration was completed, there was often a longer delay until the next configuration began (Chase & Simon, 1972). These results are consistent with a hierarchical model. They suggest that information is being accessed or "unpacked" in groups or "chunks" (Miller, 1956). Similar timing effects have been observed in studies of rapid keyboarding (see Chapter 9), which suggests that access to hierarchically organized information applies to memories subserving motor control as well as memories subserving more symbolic activities like chess playing.

SKILL ACQUISITION

In the preceding section, we considered the memory representations underlying the sequencing of behavior. In this section, we consider how movement sequences are learned. The treatment will be brief, owing to this book's focus on motor control rather than motor learning. Learning cannot be ignored in the study of motor control, of course, because what is learned must be suited to the kinds of movements that can be made. Furthermore, the movements that can be made are determined to a large extent by what can be learned. However, attempting a comprehensive treatment of all of motor learning would result in a section as long as the volumes already devoted to this topic (e.g., Holding, 1989; Magill, 1989; Schmidt & Lee, 2005).

Closed-Loop Theory

Adams (1971) proposed that motor learning proceeds through the refinement of perceptual-motor feedback loops. Consider the task of reaching for a glass. According to Adams, when one has little experience with this task, a crude first movement is made toward the glass, perceptual feedback indicates that the movement was not effective, then subsequent movements are performed to reduce the error between the perceived position of the hand and the perceived position of the glass. As practice continues, the perceptually defined reference condition for each hand position along the trajectory toward the glass becomes better suited to completion of glass grabbing. Adams called this perceptually defined reference condition the *perceptual trace*. He argued that learning reflects the development of more adaptive perceptual traces as well as more adaptive capacities for generating movements that reduce errors between perceptual traces and actual outcomes. Adams called this view *closed-loop* theory. Recall from Chapter 1 that closed-loop control relies on feedback-based correction.

According to closed-loop theory, feedback should help people perform tasks more effectively. Feedback does, in general, aid skill acquisition. People learning new tasks who are explicitly told about their performance usually do better than people who are not told how well they have done. Such explicit, verbal feedback is called *knowledge of results* (KR).

In one of the earliest demonstrations of KR, Thorndike (1927) showed that blindfolded subjects could learn to draw a line of fixed length if they were told "right" or "wrong" after each trial but not if they were told nothing (the no-KR condition). Closed-loop theory accounts for this result by saying that subjects developed an increasingly well-formed perceptual trace in the KR condition but not in the no-KR condition.

Although closed-loop theory seems to provide a reasonable account of skill acquisition, it runs into problems. That it does so is not to undermine the importance of Adams' (1971) contribution, for had he not proposed closed-loop theory, many important findings in the field, sought at first to test his theory, might not have been obtained.

One problem with closed-loop theory is that it ultimately reduces to a response chaining theory. Each movement, or component of a movement, is assumed to be triggered by a perceived error. Yet many movement sequences can be performed effectively when feedback is removed. As will be seen in Chapter 5 (Walking) and Chapter 7 (Reaching and Grasping), complex movements can often be performed effectively without proprioceptive, visual, or other forms of feedback.

A second difficulty with closed-loop theory is that it applies in a much more straight-forward way to simple, one-dimensional movements than to more complex movements. In bringing one's hand toward a glass, for example, it is plausible that the distance between the hand and the glass is reduced over time through an error-correction strategy. But if the task is to say "happy birthday," it is hard to see how each utterance is initiated for the sake of correcting an error. Thus, the scope of the theory is limited (Schmidt, 1988).

A third difficulty with closed-loop theory is that it predicts incorrectly that the more KR a learner receives, the more effectively he or she will perform. In fact, this is not always the case. Consider the data in Figure 4.6, which come from an experiment in which people were trained to reproduce target movements with the arm (Winstein & Schmidt, 1989). For some subjects, KR was given on 100% of the trials, but for other subjects KR was given on every other trial (the 50% group). During training, the performance levels of the two groups did not differ, and in an immediate retention test in which KR was withheld, there was hardly any difference between the groups. However, in a delayed retention test, given a day later, the 50% group did *better* than the 100% group. This surprising result constitutes disap-pointing KR for Adams (1971). More disappointing is the fact that similar results have been obtained by other investigators (Ho & Shea, 1978; Johnson, Wicks, & Ben-Sira, 1981, cited in Winstein & Schmidt, 1989).

These things having been said, it is important not to dismiss the theory entirely. There is, in fact, a reason to be more receptive to the tenets of closed-loop theory than might be imag-ined given the results just reviewed. This is the finding concerning specificity of practice, broached in Chapter 2 (see Figure 2.17). Recall from Chapter 2 that in a study of basketball shooting, Keetch, Schmidt, Lee, and Young (2005) found that people who spent many hours

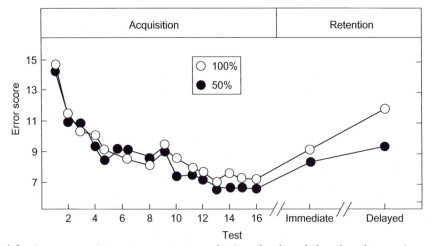

FIGURE 4.6   Average error in target movement reproduction when knowledge of results was given on 100% or on 50% of the trials. Each data point corresponds to a 12-trial block. From Winstein, C. J. & Schmidt, R. A. (1989). Sensorimotor feedback. In D. H. Holding (Ed.), Human skills (Second Edition) (pp. 17–47). Chichester: John Wiley & Sons. Copyright © 1989. Reprinted by permission of John Wiley & Sons, Ltd.

practicing shooting foul shots from the foul line were more successful at landing baskets from the foul line than would be expected by generalizing their success rates at neighboring distances. Keetch et al. referred to shooting from the foul line as an "especial" skill. According to these authors, shooting from the foul line benefited from specificity of practice. This interpretation is consistent with Adams' closed-loop theory. In fact, Adams' theory provides a clue as to what may have made specificity of practice at the foul line so "especial." For Adams, shooting baskets from a particular spot on the court helps learners develop a strong perceptual trace as well as effective methods for reducing errors in performance relative to that strong perceptual trace. Therefore, his theory predicts especial skills.

Evidence from another experiment provides further support for this view. Proteau, Marteniuk, and Lévesque (1992) studied performance in a repetitive aiming task. Participants brought a hand-held stylus to a target as quickly as possible over and over again. As expected, participants got better as they practiced more. Their movement times decreased and they still managed to reach the target. The result of the experiment that fit with Adams' closed loop theory was that the more participants practiced the task, the more their performance suffered from removal of visual feedback. This is a surprising outcome from a perspective different from Adams'. If one thought, contra Adams, that participants became *less* dependent on visual feedback as they practiced the aiming task, then one would expect that the more participants practiced the task, the *less* their performance would suffer from the removal of visual feedback. The fact that removal of visual feedback (turning off the lights after the hand left the start block) led to *more* disruption of performance suggests that participants in this study became more dependent on visual feedback with practice, not less so. They performed as if they were attempting to acquire specific perceptual inputs, as Adams' closed-loop theory predicted. When those perceptual inputs were disrupted, performance suffered.

Generalized Programs

Whereas one may say that Adams' closed-loop theory does a good job of explaining specificity of practice, one also needs a way of explaining skill generalization. Someone who is good at shooting baskets from the foul line will still be able to shoot baskets from other places on the court. It is not the case that a fictional basketball player who has spent his or her entire life shooting from the foul line will, when escorted to some other place on the court, have absolutely no idea what to do there.

A theory that does a better job than closed-loop theory in accounting for generalization says that learners form *schemas* or *generalized programs*. A schema is a knowledge structure that can be instantiated in different ways depending on the values of its underlying variables or parameters. A generalized program is a schema for a procedure. It has parameters that affect the forms that actions take.

An advantage of the schema or generalized-program view is that it provides a way of accounting for the endless variability and novelty of performance (Bartlett, 1932). It also provides a way of accounting for consistency in the movement patterns that are produced—for example, the consistency of a writer's script (Glencross, 1980). Consistency, according to the theory, derives from the use of the same generalized program in different circumstances. Variability, by contrast, derives from the modifiability of parameters within the same generalized program.

The capacity for setting parameters in a generalized program reduces the number of distinct programs that must be held in memory (Schmidt, 1975, 1976). Instead of having to store a memory for every possible sequence, only a core set of programs needs to be maintained. Setting the parameters of the program allows the program to be tailored according to immediate task demands.

An experiment on choosing between movement sequences indicates how parameter setting might work (Rosenbaum, Inhoff, & Gordon, 1984). College students were asked to perform a finger-tapping sequence with the left hand or right hand. The hand to be used was indicated by a visual signal (an X or O) that appeared on a computer screen (see Table 4.1). In one condition, the left-hand sequence and the right-hand sequence were mirror images of one another. For example, the subject was asked to tap the index finger, then the middle finger, and then the middle finger again, performing each sequence either with the left hand or right. In another condition, the two sequences were *not* mirror images of one another. The second tap was performed with the middle finger of one hand or with the index finger of the other hand. As shown in Table 4.1, the time to perform the first response in the required sequence (always an index finger tap) was shorter when the sequences were mirror images than when they were not.

This result can be explained with a parameter-setting model. Suppose the choice between mirror image sequences is achieved with a generalized program consisting of an ordered set of finger tap instructions as well as a parameter corresponding to the left or right hand. A verbal statement of such a program might be the following:

1. Sequence = Hand(Index, Middle, Middle)
2. If the signal is X, then Hand = Left; if the signal is O, then Hand = Right.
3. Perform the Sequence.

Statement 2 denotes the decision to be made to choose the right- or left-hand sequence. The decision cannot be made until the choice signal is identified.

If the choice to be made is between two sequences that are not mirror images, an additional decision is required:

1. Sequence = Hand(Index, Finger, Middle)
2. If the signal is X, then Hand = Left and Finger = Middle; if the signal is O, then Hand = Right and Finger = Ring.
3. Perform the Sequence.

TABLE 4.1 Mean Choice Reaction Times to Select Each of Two Types of Finger Sequence When the Other Possible Finger Sequence Was a Mirror Image or Nonmirror Image of the Sequence to Be Performed[*]

	Finger Sequence	
Relation	Index-Index-Middle	Index-Middle-Middle
Mirror	434 + 15	441 + 15
Nonmirror	492 + 10	491 + 7

[*]Times are in milliseconds, as are estimates of + 1 standard error of estimate of the mean. Adapted from Rosenbaum, D. A., Inhoff, A. W., & Gordon, A. M. (1984). Choosing between movement sequences: A hierarchical editor model. Journal of Experimental Psychology: General, 113, 372–393. With permission.

Note that in this second case, the value of a finger parameter as well as the value of a hand parameter must be specified. If specifying the extra parameter takes extra time, one has a way of explaining the shorter choice time for the mirror image sequences.

Other experiments support the conclusion that choices between movement sequences are sped up when the sequences can be distinguished by a small number of parameters. Heuer (1982) showed that choosing between left- and right-hand movements takes less time if the movements have the same spatio-temporal form than if they have different spatio-temporal forms. These results, and others like them, are easily explained in terms of parameter setting within generalized programs (Rosenbaum, 1987a, b, 1990).

Besides making predictions about choice reaction times, generalized program theory also makes a surprising prediction about skill learning. It predicts that variable practice should lead to better transfer than consistent practice (Schmidt, 1975). Consistent practice is practice on just one task. Variable practice is practice on a range of related tasks.

Suppose one practiced equally on tasks 1, 2, 4, and 5, where the tasks varied along some continuum, such as the required duration of a lever movement. If later on, task 3 were tested for the first time, then according to generalized-program theory, the task would be performed well because it was the average of the other practiced tasks. Suppose, on the other hand, that one had only practiced task 2. Performance on task 3 would then be worse according to the theory because the task average was centered on 2 rather than 3. This prediction is surprising because more practice occurred close to 3 when only 2 was practiced than when the whole range of tasks was practiced. All practice was just one step away from 3 in the consistent-practice condition (2 only), but only two out of the four practice experiences were one step away from 3 in the variable-practice condition.

The data on the effects of consistent versus variable practice have generally upheld the prediction that variable practice should lead to better performance than consistent practice. For reviews, see Johnson (1984), Newell (1985), and Schmidt and Lee (2005). In one successful study (Carson & Wiegand, 1979), children either practiced throwing a beanbag of a single weight to a target or practiced throwing beanbags of different weights to the same target. Later, when the children threw a beanbag with a weight that had not been previously experienced, the group exposed to several beanbags did better than the group exposed to only one.

In another study, subjects were trained on a task in which a tennis ball was grabbed, then several barriers were knocked down with the hand, and then the ball was placed in a final location (Shea & Morgan, 1979). The goal was to minimize the time for the entire series of actions. One group of subjects (the blocked group) practiced the task with the barriers occupying a fixed set of locations within a block of trials. Another group of subjects (the random group) practiced the task with the barriers occupying a number of different locations within a block. As seen in Figure 4.7, during acquisition, the blocked group outperformed the random group, but in a later transfer test the random group outperformed the blocked group. This result is similar to the "beanbag" results described above. Both studies suggest that exposure to a range of tasks leads to better long-term retention than does exposure to a single version of a task.

What causes the benefit of variable practice? One possibility is that subjects form an "average" representation of the experiences they have and the average is generally more stable when the instances are randomly presented than when they were not. Suppose that

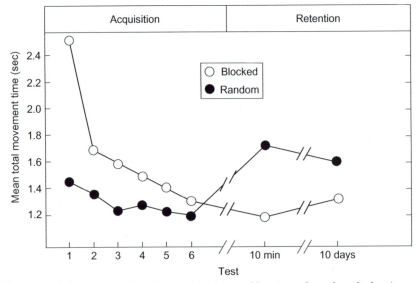

FIGURE 4.7 Mean total movement time for a series of manual barrier strikes when the barriers were either in a single set of locations in each block of acquisition trials (Blocked) or in varied locations (Random). From Shea, J. B. & Morgan, R. L. (1979). Contextual interference effects on acquisition, retention, and transfer of a motor skill. Journal of Experimental Psychology: Human Learning and Memory, 5, 179–187. Copyright © 1979 by the American Psychological Association. Adapted with permission.

one must learn the average of a series of numbers from 1 to 8, and the numbers are presented in a random order (without replacement) such that the first eight numbers are 7, 2, 4, 6, 3, 8, 1, 5. The running average for this series (i.e., the average of the numbers up to each point in the series) is 7, 4.5, 4.3, 4.75, 4.4, 5.0, 4.43, 4.5. By contrast, suppose the numbers are presented in blocked fashion, and only 1 and 8 are presented in the first eight positions: 1, 1, 1, 1, 8, 8, 8, 8. The running average for this series is 1, 1, 1, 1, 2.4, 3.33, 4.0, 4.5. In this second series, the running average is less stable than in the first, blocked, series, though the running average ends up the same (4.5) in the two cases. The greater stability of the running average in the unblocked case could lead to its being learned better.

Hierarchical Learning

Schemas and generalized programs are intuitively attractive concepts, but they are hard to identify and their internal structure is difficult to probe. Hierarchical structures, on the other hand, are structured in a clearly defined way, with levels containing fewer and fewer elements per level the higher one goes. In addition, it is easy to imagine how a hierarchy might emerge in the course of skill acquisition. Low-level units could promote the formation of higher-level units, which in turn could promote the formation of still higher-level units.

Hierarchical learning was first proposed in the late nineteenth century (Bryan & Harter, 1897). Curious about the training of telegraph operators, Bryan and Harter suggested that students of Morse code first hear dots and dashes automatically, then hear words (sequences of dots of dashes) automatically, and then hear sentences (sequences of words) automatically.

A similar course of development presumably also applies to *sending* Morse code (Leonard & Newman, 1964).

It is possible to formalize Bryan and Harter's description to make it a bit more precise. Suppose one must be exposed to a sequence of events some number of times to have it form a memory unit. Because there are 26 letters in the alphabet but more than 26 words, any given letter is likely to be experienced more often than any given word. It should therefore take longer to form word units than letter units. Furthermore, if the formation of memory units speeds up the processing of the elements of those units, then as units are formed at higher levels, the time to process their elements should decrease, but each such decrease should be observed less and less often over the course of practice.

This line of reasoning can be used to account for the change in performance speed that typically occurs with continued practice on a task. A representative curve is shown in Figure 4.8A. The curve shows how the rate of rolling cigars in a factory changed over the course of years at the job. The time needed to roll cigars decreased and then appeared to level off (Crossman, 1959). The data points could be fit with a curve described by the equation

$$T = a/P^b, \tag{4.1}$$

where T denotes the time to complete the task, P denotes the number of practice trials, and a and b are nonnegative empirical constants (numbers, typically fitted from obtained data, greater than or equal to 0). This equation is sometimes called the power law of learning (Newell & Rosenbloom, 1981). It has that name because P is raised to a power, namely, b, because the equation has been found to hold over such a wide range of observations that it can be considered a law, and because its domain of application is learning Equation 4.1 can be converted to the equation for a straight line by taking the logarithm of each side of the equation:

$$\log T = \log(a/P^b) = \log(aP^{-b}) = \log a - b(\log P). \tag{4.2}$$

Recall that the logarithm of a number is the exponent to which some base value is raised to yield that number. Because log a and b are constants, Equation 4.2 describes a straight line, as seen in Figure 4.8B. The straight line in Figure 4.8A and the curved line in Figure 4.8B are mathematically equivalent, but the straight-line representation helps one see that improvement never stops, provided P continues to grow. The implication is that an old dog can learn new tricks, or at least get faster on tricks it has practiced, if it continues to practice. For a discussion of this implication and the possibility that an alternative mathematical expression might provide a better fit to the data, see Heathcote, Brown, and Mewhort (2000).

As mentioned above, the relation described in Equations 4.1 and 4.2 is called a law because it has been found to hold in a wide range of circumstances. It applies not only to cigar-rolling times, but also to reading times for inverted and reversed text (Kolers, 1976), to times taken to justify mathematical proofs (Neves & Anderson, 1981), and even to the time for a very prolific writer, Isaac Asimov, to write books (Ohlsson, 1992). The fact that the power law applies to perceptual-motor activities and intellectual activities suggests that

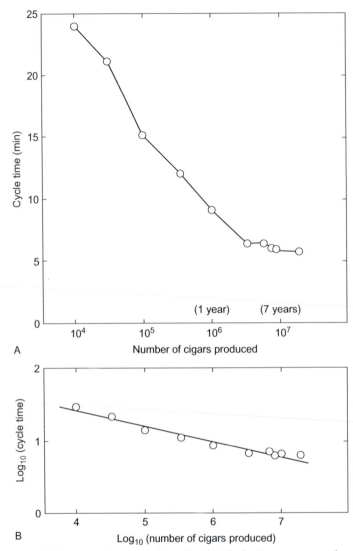

FIGURE 4.8   Time to roll cigars as a function of practice. (A) Cycle time versus number of cigars produced. (B) Same data plotted on log-log coordinates. From Posner, M. I. (1967). Characteristics of visual and kinesthetic memory codes. Journal of Experimental Psychology, 75, 103–107. With permission.

skill learning is, at some level, the same for activities that vary in "how perceptual-motor" or "how intellectual" they are (Rosenbaum, Carlson, & Gilmore, 2001; Schmidt & Bjork, 1992).

Consistent with the view that the power law of learning reflects hierarchical skill learning, it has been shown that people benefit from accessing high-level memory units during the course of practice (MacKay, 1982, 1987). An experiment by MacKay and Bowman (1969) illustrates this approach. Participants who were fluent both in English and in German recited a sentence in one language, attempting to say it more and more quickly with practice. With

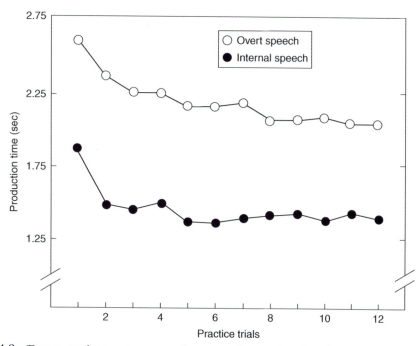

FIGURE 4.9 Time to produce sentences overtly or covertly as a function of practice. From MacKay, D. G. (1982). The problem of flexibility, fluency, and speed-accuracy trade-off in skilled behavior. Psychological Review, 89, 483–506. Copyright © 1982 by the American Psychological Association. Adapted with permission.

practice, their speaking rate increased, as shown in Figure 4.9. The participants then switched to a sentence in the other language. Recitation speed continued to improve, but only if the new sentence had the same meaning as the sentence recited before. If the new sentence had a different meaning, improvement was less rapid, regardless of whether the new sentence was in the same language as the first sentence.

MacKay and Bowman (1969) explained this result by saying that learning proceeds much as Bryan and Harter (1897) assumed, through the formation of higher-level units. The highest-level unit for a sentence is its meaning. Thus, if subjects practice saying a sentence over and over again, a unit corresponding to the meaning of the sentence may be formed. Later, when the subject switches to another sentence, if the same meaning can be activated, the new sentence can be learned quickly because its meaning has been acquired.

Mental Practice and Imagery

If learning is hierarchical, it should be possible to improve on a task by practicing it mentally. The reason is that mental practice should help form or refresh high-level units that are activated when the task is later carried out. Partly to test this prediction, and partly because it may be a useful practical tool for improving skill, mental practice has become a popular research topic. In general, mental practice has been found to be more effective than no practice at all but less effective than "the real thing" (Feltz & Landers, 1983; Richardson, 1967a, b).

A judicious mixture of mental and physical practice can significantly reduce the amount of physical practice needed to achieve a given level of performance (McBride & Rothstein, 1979).

MacKay (1981) tested the value of mental practice in the speeded recitation task described above (see Figure 4.9). Besides asking participants to recite sentences overtly, he also asked them to do so covertly. While beginning each covert recitation, the participants pressed a button, recited the sentence silently, and then pressed the button again when the sentence was over. When the times between button presses were later compared with the times to say the same sentences aloud, the times in the two conditions declined with practice in almost the same way, as would be expected if practice strengthened high-level units as well as low-level units. Had there been no high-level units or if only low-level units could be strengthened by practice, practice on the covert task would not have led to the improvements that were observed.

Can MacKay's results be explained without appealing to mental practice? Suppose MacKay's subjects made small, inaudible movements with their mouths. The improvements they showed could then be attributed to low-level effects rather than learning at high levels of a skill hierarchy. It has been found, in fact, that when people are asked to imagine making movements, significant EMG activity occurs in the associated musculature (Hale, 1982; Jacobson, 1931).

MacKay (1981) did not measure articulatory EMGs, but it is doubtful that subvocal speech could have accounted for his results. As mentioned earlier, MacKay found that subjects exhibited perfect transfer from one language to another only if the meaning of the sentence was preserved, making this a high-level effect *par excellence*. Second, other studies of mental practice have yielded results that do not support the view that muscle activity is essential for learning. Minas (1978) examined the effects of mental practice in a task where balls of different weight were thrown into a sequence of bins. Mental practice facilitated sequencing (getting the balls into the right bins at the right times) but mental practice did not facilitate force modulation (propelling balls of different weight into the correct bins). If subjects had made subtle arm movements during the rehearsal period, they would have been able to control the forces and sequencing of their throws. The fact that only sequencing benefited from mental practice suggests that mental practice was truly mental and not just an artifact of muscular change. Recall as well from Chapter 3 that during mental rehearsal of motor tasks, the supplementary motor cortex but not the motor cortex is active, but during overt performance, the supplementary motor cortex and motor cortex are both active (Roland, Larsen, Lassen, & Skinhoj, 1980). Thus, the brain respects the difference between mental practice and physical practice advocated here.

Stage Theory

When one learns a new skill, one has the sense of progressing through distinct stages. Paul Fitts (1964), a pioneer in the field of skilled performance, suggested that there are three principal stages of skill acquisition. During the initial *cognitive* phase, one learns the basic procedures to be followed, often using verbal cues. Talking to oneself is common at this early stage, and a considerable amount of attention is also usually required in this early stage.

The second stage represents a transition from reliance on verbal, conscious control to more automatic control. Fitts (1964) called this the *associative* phase. He chose this term because he believed that during this stage the learner tries out various task components and associates them with the success or failure that follows. Through this associative process, task components that contribute to success are preserved, whereas task components that contribute to failure are eliminated. Feedback about performance is especially important during this phase (Johnson, 1984).

In the third stage, the *autonomous* or *automatic* stage, behavior is performed quickly and consistently with little conscious involvement. Performance at this stage is possible even when one engages in other tasks. Professional pianists playing at cocktail parties, for example, can engage in conversations while going on with their renditions of well-learned tunes. Skilled typists can repeat what is said to them while they type (Shaffer, 1975), and with enough training, adults who have had extensive practice reading and writing can read intelligently while simultaneously writing down and even categorizing words presented to them at the same time (Spelke, Hirst, & Neisser, 1976).

As a historical note, the first research that documented such abilities was conducted by Gertrude Stein for her doctoral dissertation at Harvard University in the late 1800's. This was one of the first theses in experimental psychology and certainly one of the few by a woman in the early days of this field. Gertrude Stein's dissertation was done under the supervision of William James, whose contributions were mentioned earlier (see Chapter 2). Of special note, Gertrude Stein became one of the most famous intellectuals in the first half of the twentieth century. She was well known for her writings, including her oft-quoted phrase, "A rose is a rose is a rose." Her Paris salon was frequented by major luminaries, including the painter Pablo Picasso, who painted a portrait of her.

Returning to automization, another important feature of this late stage of skill acquisition is that performers shift from continual to intermittent reliance on feedback. This shift was demonstrated in a study (Pew, 1966) in which participants tried to keep a dot in the middle of a screen as the dot moved unpredictably to the left or to the right (see Figure 4.10).

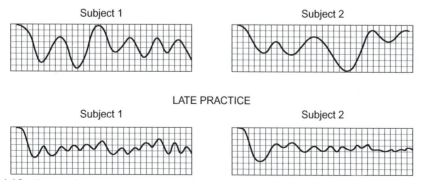

FIGURE 4.10 Error in keeping a cursor centered on a screen (vertical axis) versus time (horizontal axis) for two subjects, early and late in practice. From Pew, R. W. (1966). Acquisition of hierarchical control over the temporal organization of a skill. Journal of Experimental Psychology, 71, 764–771. Copyright © 1966 by the American Psychological Association. Reprinted with permission.

Participants learned that pressing a left button caused the dot to move to the left and pressing a right button caused the dot to move to the right. At first, the participants made one button press and waited to observe its effect, then they made another button press and waited to observe its effect, and so on. Later, they produced rapid sequences of responses, with such short delays between the presses that, in all likelihood, they did not generate corrective responses to individual button presses but instead anticipated the effects of their responses and chunked their series of button presses together, timing the presses to ensure that the dot stayed closer to the center of the screen for longer periods than was the case when practice began.

Physical Changes in Skill Acquisition

So far in this discussion of skill learning, we have focused on theories of skill acquisition that emphasized changes in memory representations and changes in cognitive strategies for perceptual-motor coordination. Conveniently, given these concerns, the measures we have considered have been ones that are the bread and butter of human experimental psychology, namely, response speed and accuracy. Yet performance also becomes more graceful and more physically efficient over the course of learning. Other measures are needed to capture these physical changes.

Figure 4.11 shows a tennis champion's two arms. The arm used for hitting the ball became larger than the other arm because of the stresses placed on the muscles and bones through years of play. Presumably, this tennis player's arms were not different before he started playing. The illustration shows that adaptation to ongoing, repetitive movement demands can be physical.

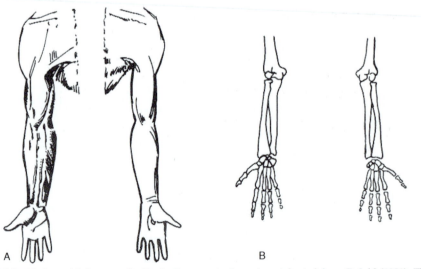

FIGURE 4.11   Right and left arms of a Davis Cup tennis champion. Adapted from E. Jokl (1981). The human hand. International Journal of Sport Psychology, 12, 140–148. With permission.

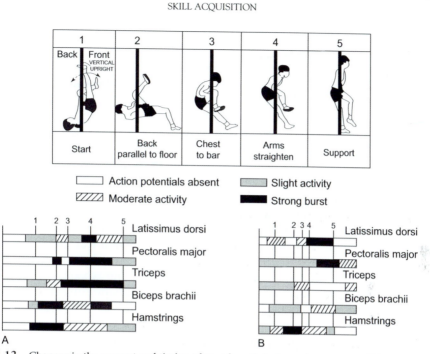

FIGURE 4.12 Changes in the amount and timing of muscle activity in novice gymnasts (A) and practiced gymnasts (B) while performing the five maneuvers shown in the top panel. Numbers in the bottom panels correspond to the five maneuvers. From Kamon, E. & Gormley, J. (1968). Muscular activity pattern for skilled performance and during learning of a horizontal bar exercise. Ergonomics, 11, 345–357. With permission.

Other skill-related changes can be attributed to improvements in timing, tuning, and coordination. Figure 4.12 summarizes the results of a study of gymnastic performance in novice and skilled gymnasts (Kamon & Gormley, 1968). With practice, the gymnasts' movements became more refined, and the efficiency of muscle activity likewise improved. Strong bursts of activity generally had shorter and shorter durations, and the number of times a given muscle reached maximum activity levels diminished. Greater skill in this case meant greater efficiency. Counterproductive or unnecessary movements fell away and, to the extent that the activity analyzed in this study was representative of others, one would expect such movements to fall away in other tasks as well.

Besides varying the timing of muscle events, skill learners also alter patterns of inter-limb coordination. Recall from Chapter 2 that one of the central problems for the motor system is the degrees of freedom problem, the problem of regulating the many degrees of freedom responsible for achieving a task. Nicolai Bernstein (1967), the Russian scientist who first formulated the degrees of freedom problem, suggested that novice performers try to reduce the complexity of the problem by locking joints, and then, with experience, letting the joints move more freely. The transition that Bernstein (1967) predicted was observed by a team of Russian investigators (Arutyunyan, Gurfinkel, & Mirskii, 1968), who analyzed the motion and stability of people learning to shoot handheld pistols. These investigators found that novice shooters first held their wrists and elbows rigid, but later they unlocked their wrists and elbows, allowing their firing accuracy to improve. Unlocking the wrist and elbow allowed the arm to compensate for motion in the hand and also allowed the hand to compensate for motion in the arm. Variability in the position of the gun barrel was therefore reduced through these newly allowed counterrotations of the hand and arm.

A similar shift from the locking to the unlocking of joints has been observed in learning to write with the nonpreferred hand (Newell & van Emerick, 1989) and also in learning to use a ski simulator (Vereijken, Whiting, & Beek, 1992); see Figure 4.13. However, other studies have not found this same progression of unlocking mechanical degrees of freedom. Why this is so has confounded researchers in the field, leading them to suggest that different motor tasks recruit biomechanical degrees of freedom in different ways (Buchanan & Kelso 1999; Buchanan, Kelso, DeGuzman, & Ding 1996; Newell 1996, Newell & Vaillancourt, 2001). One hopes that someday it will be possible to predict, with more specificity, which biomechanical degrees of freedom are linked and which are unlinked over the course of learning.

Another challenge is to develop a psychological theory of the mechanisms by which effectors come to be coupled or decoupled and the way relevant learning is internally represented. Some have expressed doubts about whether such a model can ever be developed (Fowler & Turvey, 1978). The author's view is that there is no reason why such a model cannot emerge. Indeed, one approach has appeared that holds promise in this regard. This approach is embodied in the concept of the *uncontrolled manifold* (Scholz & Schöner, 1999). The idea is that in a hypothetical control space, co-variation between or among values on certain dimensions may matter to the success of a task, whereas variation along one or more other dimensions may matter little. According to this view, motor skill learning entails, at an abstract descriptive level, exploration of the effects of occupying different positions in the control space. This geometric metaphor provides one way of visualizing the changes that occur in the internal representation of tasks to be controlled.

Another possible approach, not mutually exclusive with the uncontrolled manifold hypothesis, is to pursue a model that is more explicitly hierarchical. One could assert that effectors are first controlled independently, and then a higher-level control element is formed

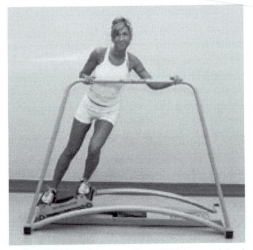

FIGURE 4.13   Ski simulator like the one used by Vereijken, Whiting, and Beek (1992). From http://www.ski-training.nl/contents/media/skiinfitnesszaal4_web.jpg.

that enables motion in one effector to be compensated for by motion in other segments. An advantage of pursuing such a model is that one might then have a model that applies to all of skilled behavior. This would help make good on the suggestion that learning of motor skills is no different, at a deep level, from learning of other kinds of skills (Rosenbaum, Carlson, & Gilmore, 2001; Schmidt & Bjork,1992). Encouraging work along these lines has been pursued by Latash, Scholz, and Schöner (2007).

CODES AND STORES

Having broached the question of how learning is achieved and internally represented, we can next ask what modes of coding and storing information are brought to bear in initiating movements. An overarching theme is that there are distinct modes of storing and coding information for motor control, just as there are distinct modes of storing and coding information for other aspects of perception and cognition.

With respect to storage, information occupies different memorial states. Information in memory may be permanent and not currently attended to (*long-term memory*), or it may be the subject of current awareness (*working memory*). Information in working memory may have been retrieved from long-term memory or may have been taken in through the senses and still be in a relatively fragile state where it is not yet consolidated in long-term memory and so occupies so-called *short-term memory*. If the information has *just* arrived through the senses, it may be in an even more fragile state, provided it is still in raw sensory form. The most fragile form of sensory memory has been called *iconic memory* for visual information (Neisser, 1967; Sperling, 1960) and *echoic memory* for auditory information (Darwin, Turvey, & Crowder, 1972). A tactile form of sensory storage has also been hypothesized (Bliss, Hewitt, Crane, Mansfield, & Townsend, 1966).

The memory states just referred to need not be equated with distinct storage compartments. Thus, it need not be the case that there is a separate "box in the head" corresponding to working memory. Rather, the contents of working memory may simply be parts of long-term memory that are most highly active. Likewise, the contents of the sensory buffer may simply be the most recently activated parts of long-term memory, activated by sensory inputs.

Research into the structure of the information-processing system has largely ignored motor function, with motor control often being added as an afterthought, if at all, in many information-processing models. Apart from the possible reasons for this neglect (Rosenbaum, 2005; Whiting, 1989), a major question for students of motor control is whether the sorts of models that have been proposed for information intake also apply to information output. This will be an important question in the discussion to follow. Along the way, we will consider another important concept from cognitive psychology, the concept of *codes*.

Codes

Information is experienced in distinct codes or representational formats. Although internally stored information is ultimately represented in the form of neural activity, codes or representational formats can be meaningfully considered not just because they characterize differences in subjective experience (phenomenology) but also because they turn out to have important functional consequences for memory and performance.

A first demonstration that there are distinct memory codes was the finding that people make different sorts of mistakes when recalling information to which they were exposed either a short time ago or a relatively long time ago. Shortly after seeing letters, people tend to substitute letters that *look* like the letters, but later they substitute letters that *sound* like the letters they saw (Conrad, 1965). This pattern of results—visual confusions early and acoustic confusions later—suggests that the information is first represented in visual form and then is represented in acoustic form, possibly because the reader sounds out the letters for him- or herself. Finding that there is a shift from visual coding to phonological coding led to the phonics method of teaching reading, which has largely supplanted the "whole-word" method, which emphasizes recognition of each word as a visual whole (Rayner, Foorman, Perfetti, & Pesetsky, 2001).

A great deal of research has been done on memory codes (Posner, 1978). Codes have been identified for most of the sensory modalities (see Posner, 1978) as well as for more abstract spatial dimensions (Baddeley & Lieberman, 1980) and for abstract meaning (Kroll & Potter, 1984). Whether there are distinct motor codes is a question that will be taken up later in this chapter.

Procedural and Declarative Knowledge

Perhaps the most fundamental distinction that has been drawn in the study of forms of memory representation is between procedural and declarative knowledge (Squire, 1987). Because motor control involves the physical enactment of procedures, it is worth considering this distinction in some detail. A way to do so is to review the case of a neurological patient known in the literature by his initials, H.M.

When H.M. was a young man he had severe epilepsy. To alleviate his seizures, he underwent a surgical procedure involving bilateral removal of the hippocampus, a structure in the forebrain. Soon after H.M.'s surgery, which involved removal of his left and right hippocampus it became apparent that as a result of the operation, he suffered a significant memory impairment. He could not learn new lists of words. When later asked to recall the lists or indicate whether he recognized them, his performance was no better than chance. H.M. was also unable to recognize people who visited him each day to test him on these word lists.

A first interpretation of H.M.'s difficulty was that he could not form new memories. According to this view, the regions of H.M.'s brain that were lesioned were the areas that allow for the transformation of information from a short-term fragile form to a long-term permanent form. This interpretation came into question, however, when it was found that H.M. could learn new perceptual-motor skills (Scoville & Milner, 1957). For example, he could learn mirror tracing, where the task is to trace a complex path while viewing the path through a mirror (Figure 4.14). The task is hard at first, but with practice gets easier. H.M. improved on mirror tracing at the same rate as normal individuals, yet each day when the task was presented to him, he denied ever having seen it before.

This striking outcome suggests that the human brain is organized in such a way that it stores different kinds of information in different ways (or perhaps in different locations). The brain respects the distinction between "knowing how" and "knowing that," or, to use

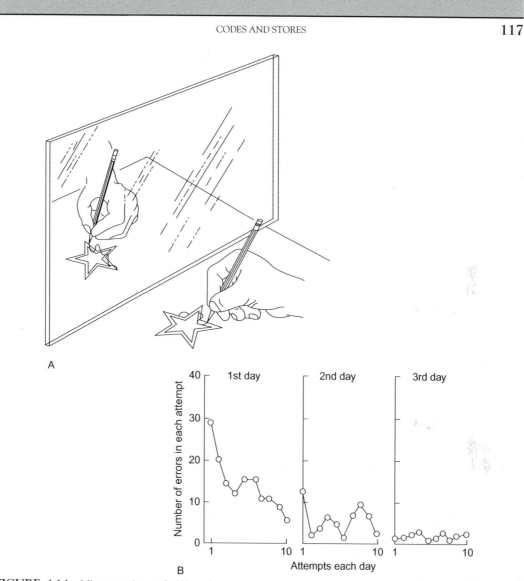

FIGURE 4.14 Mirror tracing task (A) and improvement on mirror tracing task as a function of number of attempts on the first, second, and third days of testing in patient H.M. (B). While the hand is tracing the shape (a star in this instance) it can only be seen in the mirror. Errors are made when the pencil goes outside the shape's borders. From Smith and Kosslyn (2008), p. 200. With permission.

the terms with which we began this section, procedural and declarative knowledge (Squire, 1987). Procedural knowledge consists of implicit instructions for the performance of a series of operations, for example, riding a bicycle. As often as not, it is difficult or even impossible to verbalize procedural knowledge. Declarative knowledge consists of facts that can be stated verbally, such as propositions about persons, places, things, and events—for example, "Christopher Columbus discovered America in 1492."

The fact that information is coded in procedural form does not mean it can never be articulated. Otherwise, it would be a vain hope for researchers concerned with skill to think they could ever articulate the nature of skill knowledge. Physicists know, for example, that the rule for riding a bicycle is to turn the handle bars so the curvature of the bike's trajectory is proportional to the angle of its imbalance divided by the square of its speed, as mentioned in Chapter 1 (Polanyi, 1964). Most bicyclists cannot state this proposition spontaneously when asked how they manage to ride their bikes. However, at some level, the information summarized in the proposition is embodied in the neural networks that allow cyclists to ride as they do.

Long-Term Memory

Let us consider the parallels that have been drawn between characteristics of the information-processing systems underlying motor production and characteristics of the information-processing systems underlying symbolic inputs. First consider long-term memory. Recall that long-term memory is the relatively permanent repository of previously learned material, the "place" where material can reside without being attended to. Although there is debate about how much information can be held in long-term memory and over how long a period of time it can be retained there (Loftus & Loftus, 1980; Penfield & Roberts, 1959), there is no question that the capacity of long-term memory is vast.

One form of long-term memory that is said to be especially resistant to forgetting is motor skill information. Once one learns how to ride a bicycle, for example, one never forgets how to do so—at least according to popular belief. There has been little research on the long-term retention of motor skills, though the few studies that have been done accord with the lore. In one study (Fleishman & Parker, 1962) it was reported that subjects who learned a three-dimensional tracking task retained their ability to perform the task, even over a 2-year period (Figure 4.15). Whatever decrement there was upon returning to the task after 2 years was overcome within the first two trials.

The few other studies that have been reported on long-term retention of motor skills have been concerned with shorter lags between initial learning and later testing. Little or no skill loss has been observed in tasks to which subjects return after intervals of 21 days (Ryan, 1965), 12 weeks (Meyers, 1967), or 1 year (Ryan, 1965). An anecdote from one of the foremost authorities on skill learning and retention is also worth quoting:

> My father started me skiing when I was 4 years old, and I skied every winter until I was 15, whereupon I stopped completely for 14 years. When I returned after this retention interval ... it seems safe to say that I was skiing as well as I ever did, and that by the end of the day I was skiing better [Schmidt, 1988, p. 500].

Recent work has shown that long-term memory of movement patterns affects the perception of movement patterns. An example of this effect was described in Chapter 2 in connection with mirror neurons (Figure 2.15). In that study, dancers' brain activity depended on whether they watched dance moves they had learned themselves.

The way observers mentally partition observed sequences of actions likewise reflects their long-term experience with those actions. Illustrative data appear in Figure 4.16. Here, people varying in their experience playing tennis indicated how they mentally partitioned observed phases of a tennis serves. Based on statistical inference techniques, the authors of this study

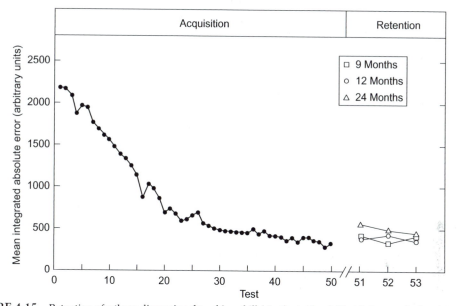

FIGURE 4.15   Retention of a three-dimensional tracking skill (similar to the skill of flying an airplane) 9 months, 12 months, or 24 months after a series of 50 6-minute practice periods. From Fleishman, E. A. & Parker, R. F., Jr. (1962). Factors in the retention and relearning of perceptual motor skill. Journal of Experimental Psychology, 64, 215–226. Copyright © 1962 by the American Psychological Association. Adapted with permission.

(Schack & Mechsner, 2006) determined that individuals with a great deal of tennis-playing experience had more structurally elaborate mental representations of the observed serves than did low-level players or non-players. The results of this study, shown in Figure 4.16, bear out the hypothesis discussed earlier in this chapter, that skill acquisition is associated with the formation of ever more elaborated hierarchical structures.

Short-Term Memory

Whereas the preceding discussion concerned long-term memory for movements, the discussion in this section concerns memory for just-experienced movements. The question is whether the retention of just-experienced movement information is similar to retention of just-experienced symbolic information. Michael Posner, a leading investigator in the fields of cognitive psychology and cognitive neuroscience, suggested that it is.

Posner (1967) investigated the codes used in short-term memory for movement. His subjects traced a straight line with one hand, moving from a home position to a final target position. The movement was performed with or without visual feedback. After the movement was completed, subjects tried to reproduce the movement either immediately or after a delay. Two delay conditions of equal duration were used. In one, subjects had no specific instruction. This was the "unfilled interval" condition. In the other, subjects classified numbers. This was the "filled interval" condition. Posner found that when visual feedback was unavailable, accuracy of reproduction was worse following the filled interval than following the unfilled interval, which in turn was worse than when reproduction was tested with no

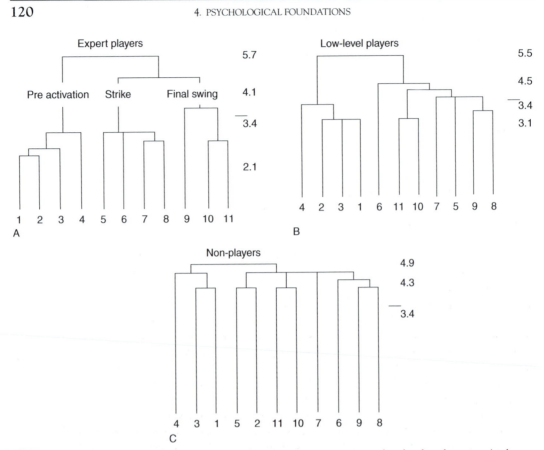

FIGURE 4.16 Inferred mental representations of tennis serves among expert, low-level, and non-tennis players. From Schack, T. & Mechsner, F. (2006). Representation of motor skills in human long-term memory. Neuroscience Letters, 391, 77–81. With permission.

delay. When visual feedback was available, accuracy of reproduction was as good following unfilled intervals as in the immediate-test condition, though it was worse when the interval was filled than unfilled. Having visual information therefore helped safeguard the information from forgetting. This outcome supports the hypothesis that there are distinct codes for stored movement information.

What aspect of movement was most important in the experiment just described? Was it the distance to be covered or the location of the final position? Efforts to answer this question have yielded dramatic results. Laabs (1973) found that location reproduction was relatively unaffected by the duration of an unfilled retention interval but distance reproduction was substantially affected by the duration of the retention interval. Laabs experimentally dissociated distance and location by independently varying the amplitude of the movement and its starting and ending locations. Other investigators replicated Laabs' findings; see Smyth (1984) for an excellent review.

What accounts for the superiority of location reproduction over distance reproduction? An intriguing possibility is that movements are produced with reference to locations rather than to distances. This would help explain the superiority of location reproduction, provided one assumes that recall improves if it recreates the means by which information is stored. Consistent with this idea, memory for positioning movements is better when subjects select the movements they will later reproduce than when their hands are passively manipulated by someone else (Kelso & Stelmach, 1976; Paillard & Brouchon, 1968).

Kelso and Holt (1980) provided evidence for the view that movements are produced through location specification. In their study, subjects were temporarily deprived of proprioceptive feedback from the fingers of one hand by wearing a blood-pressure cuff. At the start of each trial, the subject rotated the extended index finger to a position of his or her own choosing. The finger was then returned either to the original starting position or to a different starting position. The subject's task was to bring the finger back to the *location* that was reached before or to cover the same *distance* that was reached before. Subjects reproduced locations more accurately than distances.

How could subjects bring the finger to the correct final location when feedback was removed? Answering this question in detail would distract us from the questions at the focus of the present discussion, but the question will be taken up in Chapter 7, in the section on the equilibrium-point model of motor control. For now, the important point is that movements may be generated with respect to target locations rather than with respect to target distances. This may explain why location reproduction is generally better than distance reproduction. We remember better what our nervous systems care about. With respect to the theme of codes for motor memory, the results of Kelso and Holt (1980) support the view that there are distinct codes for motor memory. Location and distance, or variables associated with these variables, may be functionally distinct.

Another study of memory for movement (Smyth & Pendleton, 1989) provides additional support for the functional distinctiveness of location and distance. The question posed in Smyth and Pendleton's study was whether movement information and spatial information are represented differently. *A priori*, the answer is not obvious, for movements usually have spatial components. Furthermore, spatial tasks, such as pointing to a series of locations, have motor elements.

To test for a dissociation of spatial and motor codes, Smyth and Pendleton asked subjects to watch someone perform a sequence of hand gestures they would have to reproduce immediately afterward. In one condition, while watching the hand gestures, the subjects repeatedly squeezed a handheld tube. In another condition, while watching the hand gestures, the subjects continually tapped four plates in a clockwise order. In a control condition, the subjects watched the gestures without performing a concurrent task. Reproduction of the hand gestures was as accurate following the finger-tapping task as in the control condition, but was worse following the squeezing task.

One can interpret this result by suggesting, as Smyth and Pendleton did, that the squeezing task drew upon a motor code, whereas the spatial tapping task drew upon a spatial code. The selective interference between squeezing and learning hand gestures may have occurred, therefore, because the hand gestures were coded primarily in motoric form.

A challenge to this interpretation is that the squeezing task may have simply been more demanding than the tapping task. The difficulty of squeezing may have been sufficient to impair learning of any kind. To test this possibility, Smyth and Pendleton (1989) conducted a second experiment in which subjects watched someone tap out a spatial pattern with a finger. While watching, subjects performed the same concurrent tasks as in the first experiment—simply watching the to-be-performed movements, squeezing a tube, or tapping in a clockwise order. This time, reproduction of the observed pattern was adversely affected by the tapping task, not by the squeezing task. Thus, there was selective interference depending on the nature of the task. These results, taken as a whole, suggest that spatial codes and motor codes are distinct.

History Effects

The studies just reviewed tell us about people's abilities to reproduce movements they have just learned. Another approach to the study of short-term motor memory is to ask how people's recent performance influences their ongoing performance. History effects of this sort can suggest that performers remember what they just did and that their memories affect what they do next.

An illustration of this approach is to consider a study in which college students were asked to perform series of repetitive motor responses, where the responses to be performed in a production cycle were either identical to or different from responses in previous production cycles (Rosenbaum, Weber, Hazelett, & Hindorff, 1986. One task was repeating the first n letters of the alphabet over and over again as quickly as possible for 10 seconds. This task was performed under the requirement that speakers always alternate between stressed and unstressed utterances. As seen in Figure 4.17, the mean number of letters produced was higher when n was even than when n was odd.

The source of difficulty in the odd-n case was that a given letter was produced with varying stress levels in successive production cycles. When n equaled 3, for example, the sequence to be produced was AbCaBcAbCa . . ., where capital letters denote stressed letters and lowercase letters denote unstressed letters. Note that each letter alternates between stressed and unstressed form. By contrast, when n equaled 4, the sequence to be produced was AbCdAbCd . . . . In this case, each letter was always stressed or was always unstressed. The greater difficulty encountered in the odd-n case can be explained by saying that each time the subject got ready to produce a letter, he or she accessed a still-active memory trace from its last production. If the stress level from the last production matched the stress level of the next production, the trace could serve as a "ready-to-run" program. However, if the necessary stress of the letter did not match its previous value, the stress level had to be altered, and this extra task, by hypothesis, took extra time. According to this account, mapping a new parameter (such as a new stress level) to a letter name slows performance. As the delay between successive productions of a letter increases, the strength of the association between the stress level and the letter name diminishes. This can explain why as n increased, the difference between odd and even values of n grew smaller. The slowing of performance in this context was called the *parameter remapping* effect. The term referred to the fact that having to remap parameters, such as accents to letters, slows performance.

The parameter remapping effect is not restricted to reciting letters. It is also observed in finger tapping, violin bowing (Figure 4.18), hand-path trajectory formation for aiming (Jax & Rosenbaum, 2007; van der Wel & Rosenbaum, 2007), phasing of finger wiggling by the two hands (Kelso, 1984), and reaching for objects (Joseph, 1999; Rosenbaum & Jorgensen, 1992;

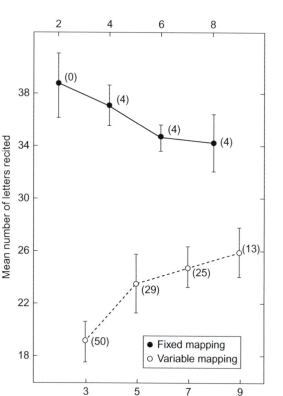

FIGURE 4.17 The parameter remapping effect, indexed by mean number of letters recited in 10 seconds as a function of list length (number of letters recited from the beginning of the alphabet). Number of errors is given in parentheses. From Rosenbaum, D. A., Weber, R. J., Hazelett, W. M., & Hindorff, V. (1986). The parameter remapping effect in human performance: Evidence from tongue twisters and finger fumblers. Journal of Memory and Language, 25, 710–725. With permission.

Smith, Thelen, Titzer, McLin, 1999; Spencer, Smith & Thelen, 2001). From the perspective of short-term or working memory, history effects like these suggest that the information guiding production of movements remains active in memory for some time after the movements have been produced. Were this not the case, it would not matter if responses were produced in the same way or in different ways in successive production cycles.

What functional advantage might arise from having a system that exhibits history effects like these? A possible answer is that preserving features of recently performed movements may facilitate preparation of forthcoming movements. Only those features that distinguish forthcoming movements from their predecessors would have to be specified. This method of preparing forthcoming movements is likely to be more efficient than a method that requires each movement to be programmed entirely "from scratch" (Rosenbaum, 1980, 1983; Rosenbaum, Cohen, Jax, van der Wel, & Weiss 2007).

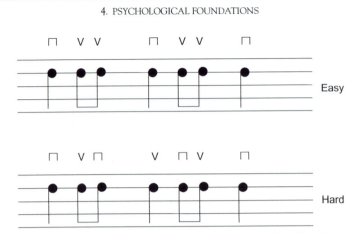

FIGURE 4.18   Parameter remapping effect demonstrated through easy and hard bowing patterns. The inverted-U shape denotes down bowing direction. The caret denotes up bowing direction.

Motor Programs

A word used in the last sentence—"programmed"—was the subject of intense debate among students of human motor control in the 1980's and 1990's. Earlier than this, in the late 1960's, the motor program was associated with the control of ballistic movements. Keele (1968) defined the motor program as "a set of muscle commands that are structured before a movement sequence begins, and that allows the sequence to be carried out uninfluenced by peripheral feedback" (p. 387). Keele wrote this definition when the major issue in the field was the extent to which skilled movement depends on sensory feedback. Keele reasoned that if a movement sequence can be performed skillfully even when sensory feedback is unavailable, one can conclude that the sequence was centrally controlled. For him, the word "program" designated the set of commands within the central nervous system that allowed for such control.

A number of complaints arose about the programming concept (Kelso, 1981 Meijer & Roth, 1988). One was that sensory feedback has an effect on movement. Much of the grace and subtlety of movement that is present when feedback is available deteriorates when feedback is withdrawn. Kelso and Meijer and Roth argued from this outcome that the motor program, as defined by Keele (1968), had limited utility.

The problem with this challenge is that a careful reading of Keele's (1968) definition shows that though a motor program may allow a movement sequence to be carried out uninfluenced by peripheral feedback, it does not require peripheral feedback to have negligible effects.

Consider a conventional computer program. Such a program is designed to carry out procedures differently depending on what input it receives. Thus, a conventional computer program is not immune to feedback; quite the opposite is true. The analogy to computer programs is a second source of dissatisfaction with the motor program concept. The nervous system is quite different from a computer, the argument goes, so the term "program" is misleading.

Clearly, there are differences between the nervous system and most modern computers. Most computer systems today rely on serial processing, whereas one of the most important features of the nervous system is that it relies on parallel processing. Moreover, the individual processing elements of a computer are very fast, whereas the individual processing elements of the nervous system—neurons—are comparatively slow. Nevertheless, computers are likely to change dramatically in the next few years. Indeed, there is a concerted effort to make them more brain-like. When this happens, the complaint that human motor programs aren't like computer programs may no longer apply. The implication to be drawn is that the word "program" may be offensive in large part because of the current state of technology.

A third complaint about motor programs is related to the use of the term "muscle commands." Use of this term led to the reproof that information guiding movement is more abstract than commands for muscle contractions (Tuller, Turvey, & Fitch, 1982). Indeed, as was seen in the last chapter, only some efferent signals directly activate motor neurons; efferent signals also influence gains in feedback loops, for example. In addition, as will be seen later in this book, there is reason to doubt that information governing movement and stability is defined with respect to the activity of particular muscles or muscle groups (Klapp, 1977b). These observations having been made, the larger point is that difficulties with a particular term ("muscle commands") used by just one author (Keele, 1968) need not rule out the underlying concept of a motor program, which can be defined here as a functional state that allows particular movements, or classes of movements, to occur. For the author of this book and other investigators who subscribe to the cognitive approach to the study of motor control (i.e., an approach that does not shun memory representations or memory codes), understanding these functional states—that is, understanding motor programs—is arguably the single most important aim in the study of motor control (human or otherwise).

The Motor Output Buffer

If there are sensory buffers for the maintenance of just-received sensory signals, are there analogous structures for the maintenance of to-be-generated motor commands? Are there, in short, motor output buffers?

Several studies bear on this question. In one of the first (Henry & Rogers, 1960), people were asked to carry out a series of manual tasks as quickly as possible after hearing an auditory signal. The independent variable was the number of tasks in the series. In one condition, subjects simply lifted the hand from a key after the signal came on. In another condition, they lifted the hand and immediately reached out and grabbed a tennis ball. In a third condition, a still more complicated series of movements was required, though the first movement was, again, lifting the hand from the start key. Subjects were aware before the auditory signal what tasks would have to be performed. Thus, in principle they could fully prepare for the tasks ahead of time.

Suppose an index of full preparation is a fixed, minimal reaction time. If subjects could fully prepare all the tasks they would have to perform, one would expect the first movement in the series always to have that fixed, minimal time. The same outcome would be expected if subjects could only prepare the first movement, no matter how many movements had to be made. Henry and Rogers (1960) found, instead, that reaction time increased with the number of movements to be performed. On the basis of this finding, they proposed that after the "go" signal was heard, commands for the forthcoming series had to be "loaded" into a buffer—or into what these authors called a "memory drum." According to the model, the more commands were needed, the longer the loading time. The memory drum model is equivalent to saying there is a motor output buffer, a limited-capacity store for low-level motor commands.

Alternative interpretations of Henry and Rogers' (1960) findings are worth considering. One is that the kinematics of the first movement changed depending on the movements to follow. If that were the case, the observed reaction-time effect would be an artifact of the kinds of first movements subjects chose to carry out in the three conditions of the experiment.

Another possibility is that the components of the forthcoming sequence inhibited each other, as in Estes' (1972) theory discussed earlier in this chapter. According to this account, reaction time increased as inhibition increased.

Still another possibility is that all the instructions were fully loaded into the motor output buffer before the go signal was presented (assuming for now that there is a motor output buffer), and the contents of the buffer had to be searched for the instruction associated with each movement. As more instructions occupied the buffer, the search time increased and reaction time grew (Sternberg, Monsell, Knoll, & Wright, 1978).

Based on Henry and Rogers' (1960) experiment, it is impossible to tell which of these explanations best accounts for the experiment's outcome. However, other studies, following Henry and Rogers', have yielded systematic effects of task complexity on reaction time with other sorts of responses (Klapp, 1977a; Rosenbaum, 1987a; Sternberg et al., 1978). These results cast doubt on the first-movement-different hypothesis and strengthen the other, more centrally based hypotheses, all of which share the assumption that there are limits on the number of movements that can be programmed in advance. Such limits would be expected if there were a limited-capacity buffer for forthcoming motor commands.

If the motor output buffer has a limited capacity—that is, if it can only store a limited number of instructions concerning forthcoming movements—one should be able to demonstrate that when one "spills the contents" of the buffer, its contents are indeed very small. A method has been developed for this purpose. It requires subjects to stop responding when a signal is presented (Ladefoged, Silverstein, & Papcun, 1973; Slater-Hammel, 1960). In one such study (Logan, 1982), typists were instructed to stop typing as soon as they heard a tone. The typists generally performed only a single keystroke after the tone sounded. If the contents of the motor output buffer had consisted of instructions for more than one keystroke—say, instead, the motor output buffer contained instructions for an entire multi-letter word—the entire word would have been typed when the stop signal came on. The fact that typists generally produced only one keystroke after the stop signal suggests that the capacity of the motor output buffer is no greater than one keystroke's worth of motor instructions. That it is so small need not be a bad thing. Sometimes it is good to be able to stop what one is doing immediately.

STATES OF MIND

The preceding major section of this chapter was called Codes and Stores because it concerned the formats (codes) used to represent information and the properties of the memory systems (stores) used to house that information. In this section, we look at states of mind for movement. We consider the role of attention and intention in motor control as well as the importance of mental representations for movement goals. Those mental representations turn out to be perceptually rich, highlighting the value of considering motor control jointly with perception. As stated in Chapter 1, it makes little sense to debate whether motor control or perception is more important. The two systems work together. The unification of perception and motor control culminates, theoretically, in the proposal that the initiation of voluntary movement relies on anticipation of desired perceptual effects. This concept, embodied in the so-called ideo-motor theory of action control, is the final topic to which we turn in this chapter. First, however, we direct our attention to attention itself.

Attention

It takes a great deal of attention to carry out unpracticed complex tasks. A familiar example is shifting gears in driving. Someone just learning to coordinate the clutch, brake, gas pedal, and stick of a standard-transmission vehicle cannot hold a conversation while shifting from one position to the next. With practice, however, the same individual can listen to and speak with others, adjust the radio, glance into the rearview mirror for a makeup check, and so on. It is inadvisable to do any of these things while gear shifting or, for that matter, while driving at all, because driving, like other complex perceptual-motor tasks, requires attention. On the other hand, the amount of attention driving takes is vastly smaller after a great deal of practice than after a paucity of practice. This fact was mentioned earlier in connection with the stage theory of Fitts (1964).

From the fact that less attention is needed to carry out a practiced task, one should not conclude that no attention is required to carry out a task once it has been practiced. The conclusion should be avoided not just to avoid illogic (it doesn't follow that no attention is required); it should also be avoided because doing so can literally save one's life. Studies of simulated driving have shown that talking on a cell phone while driving impairs driving as much as drinking several beers (Strayer & Drews, 2007).

Nowhere is the problem of distraction more at the focus of attention than in the cultivation of elite performance, whether in athletics or in the arts. A gymnast who might be able to perform the most awesome vaults and somersaults in practice might "choke" in competition. Similarly, a singer who can produce the most iridescent arias in rehearsal may clam up in the concert hall. Tendencies to fold up under pressure can be due to the allocation of too much attention to the wrong aspects of performance. Directing attention away from the task to be performed, as in thinking extraneous thoughts like "What are they thinking about me?," can divert precious cognitive resources from features of the task that are important for successful performance.

Ironically, directing too much attention to a highly practiced task may also hurt performance (Beilock, Bertenthal, McCoy, & Carr, 2004, Wulf, Hoss, & Prinz, 1999). Beilock et al. (2004) showed that directing attention to the way a task is performed can help the task if it is unpracticed, but can hurt performance if it is highly practiced. This outcome firms up the hypothesis that a great deal of attention to the way a task is performed is needed early in skill learning, making more attention helpful rather than harmful at that stage, but that little attention is needed late in skill learning. In fact, too much attention to the method of performance becomes harmful rather than helpful in the later stage.

Other studies of the role of attention in motor control have contributed to our understanding of the relation between these two functions. How people direct their attention has surprisingly subtle effects on motor performance. For example, when people perform a task that has been used widely to understand the underpinning of coordination—swinging two handheld pendulums back and forth at tempos they prefer—the timing of the swings depends on whether the participants attend to the left hand or to the right (Pellecchia, Shockley, & Turvey, 2005; Temprado, Zanone, Monno, & Laurent, 2001). Such results suggest that there is an intimate relation between attention and motor control. One influential group of investigators has even proposed that attention is nothing more than readiness to act (Rizzolatti & Craighero, 1998; Rizzolatti, Riggio, & Sheliga, 1994).

Intention

Physical actions let you express your intentions. You intend to press an elevator button and you do so, you intend to pour catsup and you do that, you intend to see a candidate get into office and you vote for him or her, and so on. To the extent that this seems like a simple cycle—intend, act, intend, act, . . .—the study of motor control can be as much about the investigation of intentions as it is about the control of the body per se. What makes the investigation of intentions, or intentional states, so interesting is that even with the objective and sensitive measures available to students of motor control, understanding the status of intentions can quickly become complicated.

Consider the game of Ouija (pronounced "wee-jee").The Ouija player rests his or her hand on an object (the Ouija) that can slide across a board with very little pressure. With targets nearby, a player can direct the object to targets corresponding to his or wishes. "Who is the boy you have a crush on?" one player asks another. After the Ouija has traveled to "B," then to "E," and then to "N," the active player's crush is revealed. The fun of Ouija is that players deny that they themselves moved the Ouija. Rather, they aver that it was moved by the unconscious mind or ethereal spirits.

Regardless of how one thinks of the unconscious or of spirits, behaviors such as playing Ouija reveal a thin veil rather than a thick wall between intentions and actions. Our thoughts are quickly and easily manifested in our behavior. Thus, it is hard to conceal what one thinks because fleeting expressions on our faces betray our feelings (Ekman & O'Sullivan, 1991). Likewise, slight twitches of the muscles in the arm and shoulder correlate with forthcoming directions of pointing movements (Cohen & Rosenbaum, 2007). Tiny occasional ocular saccades also betray where one plans to direct one's gaze (Engbert & Kliegl, 2003).

So sensitive is motor behavior to one's state of mind that deliberately attempting to suppress movements can, ironically, exaggerate the movements one is trying to suppress

(Wegner, Ansfield, & Pilloff, 1998). Trying not to think of elephants causes one, ironically, to think of little else (Lakoff, 2004).

The question of how intentions are formed is one of the most alluring but also one of the most elusive topics in psychology. One method that has been used to explore this question has been to ask people to indicate when they first become aware of intentions that they manifest behaviorally. As shown in seminal work by Libet, Gleason, Wright, and Pearl (1983), times when people first become aware of their own intentions *follow* the first clear signs that those intentions have formed in their brains. Much debate has swirled around the significance of this finding, and investigators have argued about the optimal methods to use in pursuit of this interesting empirical question, which ultimately is directed to the profoundly important question of where and how intentions arise in the first place.

Ideo-Motor Theory

In studies of the so-called *kinesthetic illusion*, which were popular in the nineteenth century, people held a weighted pendulum as still as possible, but the pendulum still moved for longer and in more varied directions than if it were simply suspended from an inert beam. Even if the arm was externally supported, the handheld pendulum continued to swing, demonstrating that the effect stemmed from muscular activity in the arm and not just from the participant's swaying to and fro in a manner unrelated to the pendular support (e.g., trying to stay steady on one's feet). The swinging of the pendulum was also strongly affected by the availability of vision (Chevreul, 1833, cited in Easton & Shor, 1976).

These phenomena suggested a direct link between mental states and muscular activity. Appreciating this connection, Carpenter (1852) coined the phrase *ideo-motor* to refer to the idea that every thought—conscious or unconscious—spawns a commensurate action.

The ideo-motor principle was popularized by James (1890), but fell out of favor during the reign of behaviorism (Thorndike, 1911). Later it was revived (Greenwald, 1970) and then received a strong boost from Wolfgang Prinz and his colleagues at the Max Planck Institute for Psychological Research in Munich and Leipzig, Germany (Hommel, Musseler, Aschersleben, & Prinz, 2001).

It is important to be clear about what is claimed in ideo-motor theory. The core claim is that every thought—conscious or unconscious—has a commensurate action. Taken literally, this claim is hard to believe, or at least hard to prove. Thinking of pressing an elevator button may easily produce a corresponding action, but what does thinking of the odor of baked cookies inspire, action-wise? Sniffing may follow and there may even be a dash to the kitchen. But these physical actions may also follow the thought of the odor of sautéed mushrooms. One can suggest that the physical actions for baked cookies and for sautéed mushrooms differ in some minute, not-so-obvious way, but the actions for going to the kitchen for sautéed mushrooms are very different if one has the thought while sitting in one's lounge chair or while standing atop a ladder. Thus, action differences are unlikely, in themselves, to resolve the problem.

The problem of associating actions with thoughts is compounded if one considers complex thoughts such as ruminating about tax reform. If every thought has a corresponding action, does it follow that every action has a corresponding thought? If you see someone's leg bouncing up and down beneath a table during a conversation, are those bounces part of what the person is thinking? Possibly, but it is unclear how a rigorously framed theory of thought can incorporate leg motions unless such motions are the subject of the thoughts themselves. The easier solution to this quandary is to allow that while some actions may have direct sources in particular thoughts, others may not. The latter actions might be called involuntary. This terminology may be helpful because it rescues us from the "tax reform" problem raised above: No matter how one feels about different tax packages, one must ultimately do something physically if one wants to affect the policy that is adopted—voting for the candidate one prefers, writing an email to the relevant economists, and so on. Each of these physical behaviors probably has a proximate cognitive source (a thought that gives rise to the necessary physical behaviors), but not all physical behaviors have discernible cognitive origins.

With these philosophical points behind us, we can consider briefly some of the evidence that has been adduced for ideo-motor theory. A great deal of research has been done on this topic in the past few years, most of it from Wolfgang Prinz's group, fine reviews of which have appeared (Hommel et al., 2001; Knoblich, Thornton, Grosjean, & Shiffrar, 2006).

The work that has been done in connection with ideo-motor theory has been pursued along several lines. One follows from the idea that if there is a mental representation of the perceptual consequences of a forthcoming behavior, the time to produce the behavior should be shorter when the signal for the behavior shares features with those anticipated perceptual consequences than when it does not.

Table 4.2 shows how this logic plays out. The table provides a conceptual overview of the kind of experiment that helped Greenwald (1970) reinvigorate ideo-motor theory. Participants either spoke or drew a letter depending on which condition they were in at the time. Meanwhile, the signal indicating which letter was supposed to be produced was either auditory or visual. Ideo-motor theory predicted that reaction times should be shorter to say a letter in response to a heard letter than in response to a seen letter. It also said that reaction times should be shorter to write a letter in response to a seen letter than in response to a heard letter. Just this sort of interaction was observed (Greenwald, 1970), and qualitatively similar results were obtained in other tasks (Hommel et al., 2001).

Another line of work on ideo-motor theory relied on imitation. The underlying idea is that watching another's actions should activate the corresponding actions in oneself. An impressive body of evidence has supported the idea that people are not only highly prone to imitate others but also that they are prone to imitate others in ways that imply sophisticated cognitive machinery when they do so.

TABLE 4.2   Conceptual Overview of Research Described by Greenwald (1970), Where Short and Long Reaction Times (RTs) Were Obtained with Different Combinations of Input and Output Modalities, in Support of Ideo-Motor Theory. From Greenwald, A. G. (1970). Sensory feedback mechanisms in performance control: With special reference to the ideo-motor mechanism. Psychological Review, 77, 73–99. With permission

Output Modality	Input Modality	
	Auditory	Visual
Vocal	Short RTs	Long RTs
Written	Long RTs	Short RTs

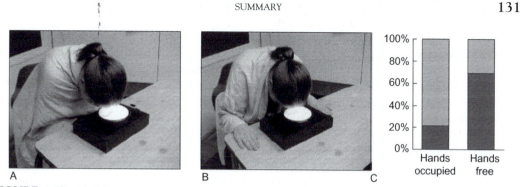

FIGURE 4.19 Model turning on a light with hands occupied (A) and with hands free (B) and the likelihood of infants later turning on the light with their foreheads after seeing the model either with hands occupied or with hands free (C). From Gergely, G., Bekkering, H., & Kiraly, I. (2002). Rational imitation in preverbal infants. *Nature*, 415, 755. With permission.

Figure 4.19 illustrates this point. Here, babies, tested one at a time, watched a model turn on a light by depressing a switch with her forehead (Gergely, Bekkering, & Kiraly, 2002). In one condition, the model's hands were free, but in another condition, the model's hands were beneath the table where the model was sitting. The question was how the baby would later turn on the light, having watched the model turn on the light with hands free or hands occupied. If the babies merely imitated the physical behavior they saw, they should have always used their foreheads, for that is how the switch was physically activated. But if the babies analyzed the *reason* for the model's physical behavior, they should have used their foreheads less when the model's hands were occupied than when the model's hands were free. As shown in the right side of Figure 4.19, babies performed in a way that indicated they analyzed the reason for the model's behavior.

This outcome tells us that babies are capable of smart imitation. They not only recognize how others behave but also, within limits, why.

SUMMARY

1. The psychological approach to human motor control focuses on the functional control of movement and stability—what might be called the software rather than the hardware of human motor control.
2. Four issues lie in the spotlight of the psychological approach to human motor control. These are (a) sequencing and timing, (b) skill learning, (c) memory systems and forms of mental representations, and (d) states of mind, including attention, intention, and the so-called ideo-motor theory of action.
3. Historically, an important theory of sequencing and timing (also known as serial ordering of behavior) is embodied in the concept of *response chaining*. The idea is that the stimulus produced by a movement triggers the next movement in the sequence. According to the theory, differences in successive stimuli give rise to differences in successive responses. One difficulty with the theory is that successive movements often occur too quickly for any one movement to be elicited by sensory feedback from the

preceding movement. A second difficulty is that the same output can be followed by different outputs on different occasions. A third difficulty is that interrupting sensory feedback does not always interrupt movement. Counterarguments can be raised to these challenges, and elaborations of the response chaining theory can be proposed to surmount the challenges. Nonetheless, the theory is damned by the fact that behavior reflects sensitivity to rules.

4. Another theory of sequencing holds that associations are formed between the elements to be produced and markers or tags for their serial positions; this is the *element-to-position* theory. If the markers are regarded as time tags, the theory potentially explains timing. The theory has problems, however, including the fact that it cannot explain sensitivity to rules.

5. A third theory of sequencing says that elements of a sequence inhibit each other; this is the *inter-element inhibition* theory. The more inhibition an element receives, the later it occurs. Despite its apparent physiological plausibility, this theory encounters problems in implementation and storage. In addition, like the two theories summarized above, it neglects the capacity for rule-governed behavior.

6. The *hierarchical* theory of serial order is more successful. It provides a framework for understanding rule-governed behavior and accurately predicts which sequences will be easy or hard to learn. The hierarchical theory also provides a basis for understanding aspects of response timing.

7. Turning to the skill learning problem, Adams (1971) proposed a *closed-loop* theory in which learning reflects the development of perceptual goals along with means of satisfying those perceptual goals. The theory has problems but may provide an account of results favoring specificity of practice. The latter results indicate that with a great deal of practice on a task, performance may become more and more reliant on specific feedback associated with the task's completion.

8. An alternative theory of skill development is that the learner forms generalized programs. These are instructions for procedures that can be instantiated in various ways depending on the values taken on by the program's internal variables or parameters. Evidence for the setting of these variables or parameters has been obtained in choice reaction time experiments. The finding that variable practice can lead to better long-term retention than consistent practice also supports a prediction of the theory.

9. Another theory of skill learning focuses on hierarchical learning. It says that low-level memory units promote the formation of higher-level memory units. Such a hierarchical theory can account for the power law of learning, which relates speed of performance to amount of practice. The theory can also account for the observation that transfer from one task to another, such as speeded recitation of a sentence in one language followed by speeded recitation of a sentence in another language, is aided by the presence of high-level memory units common to both tasks (for example, a common meaning for the two sentences).

10. Hierarchical learning theory predicts that mental practice and imagery can aid learning. The reason is that mental practice and imagery can strengthen high-level memory units. Mental practice has been shown to aid learning of motor tasks, though not as much as physical practice. It is doubtful that the benefits of mental practice derive only from subtle muscle activity.

11. A stage theory of skill learning was proposed by Fitts (1964). According to the theory, skill learning has three main stages. First, there is a cognitive stage, during which basic procedures are learned and their execution is, in general, highly attention-demanding. Then there is an associative stage, during which one tries out different task components and associates them to task success. Third, there is an automatic stage, during which the task can be performed with less deliberate attention, often with intermittent rather than continuous reliance on feedback.

12. Skill acquisition is often accompanied by physical changes. For example, besides seeing increases in speed and accuracy of movement as skill develops, one also sees increases in grace and efficiency of performance. One way such improvements occur is that degrees of freedom become freed up with practice. Learning to couple and decouple effectors may be an important part of motor learning. A challenge is to model how such learning occurs. One possibility is that the learning may be done through hierarchical learning. Another is that it may be done by discovering which factors matter a lot to task success and which do not (the uncontrolled manifold hypothesis).

13. Distinct modes of storing and coding information exist for human motor control, as is true of other aspects of human perception and cognition. Storage may last for varying amounts of time, being in long-term memory (the longest amount of time), in working or short-term memory, or in a buffer (the shortest amount of time).

14. Information may also be subjectively coded in different forms, such as visually or acoustically. For example, seen letters are initially coded visually and later are coded acoustically.

15. Procedural knowledge is different from declarative knowledge. Declarative knowledge can be expressed as propositions (verbal statements) about persons, places, and things. Procedural knowledge usually cannot be expressed propositionally. Procedural knowledge underlies sequences of operations, including those used in perceptual-motor performance. The distinction between procedural knowledge and declarative knowledge was confirmed in psychology and neuroscience by the finding that a patient who had undergone bilateral removal of the hippocampus could not learn new facts but could learn new skills.

16. Long-term memory for skills is resistant to forgetting. Well-learned skills show little decrement following retention intervals of weeks, months, or even years. Another benefit of learning skills to a high level of proficiency is that highly practiced performers of a task can form more hierarchically complex memory representations of observed performances of the task than can less practiced performers.

17. Short-term memory for movements is usually better for voluntarily selected movements than for passively induced movements. Locations to which one has moved are generally remembered better than distances that were covered, suggesting that location information and distance information may be coded differently. Movement information may itself have a different representational format from spatial information.

18. History effects exist in human motor control. One demonstration of history effects is that when a series of responses is produced over and over again as quickly as possible, the speed of responding is higher when the responses are identical over repetitions than when the responses change over repetitions. This result implies that traces of previously performed responses persist in working memory. Forthcoming responses may therefore

be prepared by altering those features or parameters of the trace that distinguish the previous version of the response from the version needed next.

19. Motor programs are functional states that dispose the organism to carry out particular movements or classes of movements.

20. Just as there may be buffers for just-received sensory information, there may be buffers for forthcoming motor commands.

21. Two lines of evidence suggest that the human memory system is severely limited in its capacity to store instructions for immediately forthcoming motor responses (an indication of a buffer). First, the time to initiate movement sequences increases with sequence complexity. Second, when people are instructed to interrupt ongoing sequences of rapid responses as quickly as possible, they can stop immediately without producing extended series of responses.

22. A great deal of attention is needed to carry out unpracticed tasks. Ironically, however, directing a great deal of attention to a highly practiced task can hurt its quality. The susceptibility of motor performance to attention is also demonstrated in the rather subtle effects that attention can have on movements.

23. Intentions underlie voluntary behavior, but sometimes, involuntary features of behavior betray intention in the making. A question that has inspired much debate is when people first become of their intentions.

24. The ideo-motor theory says that every thought—conscious or unconscious—has a commensurate action. Consistent with the view that such action-initiating thoughts have perceptual contents, it has been found that the time to produce a behavior is shorter when the signal for the behavior shares features with the behavior's anticipated perceptual consequences than when it does not. Another line of work on ideo-motor theory has relied on imitation. Watching another's actions activates the corresponding actions in oneself.

Further Reading

For an exploration of the hierarchical control of behavior, see MacKay (1987).

For more about research leading to the memory drum theory of Henry and Rogers (1960), see Fischman, Christina, and Anson (2008).Leading researchers in the field of behavioral timing are Russell Church of Brown University (e.g., Church, 2003, 2006), Richard Ivry of the University of California, Berkeley (e.g., Ivry, 1996), Warren Meck of Duke University (e.g., Meck, 2003), and Alan Wing of Birmingham University and Peter Beek of Free University, Amsterdam (Wing & Beek, 2002). A classic compendium of relatively early work on timing was edited by Gibbon and Alan (1984).

For more research on the question of when intentions are formed and when they are recognized as having been formed by the actors in whom the intentions arise, see Haggard and Libet (2001), Haggard and Cole (2007), Waszak et al. (2005), and Keller et al. (2006).

Several textbooks in cognitive psychology now include chapters on motor control (Glass, 2004; Smith and Kosslyn, 2007; Willingham, 2004).

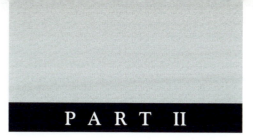

PART II

THE ACTIVITY SYSTEMS

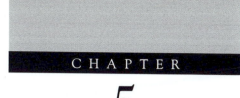

CHAPTER

5

Walking

OUTLINE

Descriptions of Walking   136
     Gait Patterns at Different Speeds   136
     Regularities in Gait Patterns   139

Neural Control of Locomotion   141
     Neural Circuits for Locomotion   143
     The Role of Sensory Feedback   146
     Descending Effects   147
     Anticipatory Postural Adjustments   150

Walking Machines   151

The Development of Walking   154
     Neonatal Reflexes   155
     Disappearance and
       Reappearance of Stepping   156

Models of Motor Development   158

Navigating   161
     Visual Kinesthesis   161
     Development of Visual Guidance   163

Memory   164
     Route Maps and Survey Maps   165
     Memory and Feedback   166

Summary   168

Further Reading   171

There are several reasons for beginning our survey of motor activities with an analysis of walking. When human newborns are supported beneath their shoulders, they exhibit a stepping pattern similar to that seen in walking adults (André-Thomas & Autgarden, 1966). The capacity for walking therefore appears to be innate (Grillner, 1981). Nevertheless, the form that walking takes at any given time depends on the terrain on which one treads and the speed with which one wishes to reach one's destination. These features illustrate ways in which ongoing feedback interacts with built-in neural capacities. We will address this issue at many points in this book.

Another striking feature of locomotion is that it takes many forms. Trotting, galloping, strutting, creeping, limping, and swimming with various strokes all belong to the same broad performance class as walking. All these behaviors are characterized by rhythmic, alternating activity of limbs on opposing sides of the body, usually carried out for purposes of propelling the body forward. Because walking is representative of all locomotory activities, this chapter is called Walking, thoughwalking will not be the only form of locomotion to be described.

Walking and related forms of locomotion are remarkably flexible. Based on incoming perceptual information, one can speed up or slow down, turn, step up, step down, and even walk backward. The ease with which one can switch from one of these behaviors to another points to a sophisticated mechanism for selecting and initiating different patterns of locomotion. Because the patterns are usually selected automatically on the basis of sensory input, it is reasonable to hypothesize that there are direct links between perception and locomotion. The research to be described here bears this out.

The flexibility of walking is not entirely dictated by the external environment, however. Through internal decisions, people can readily adopt different gaits, including stylized, theatrical patterns such as limping, marching, and dancing.The fact that different walking styles can be adopted at will implies that walking can come under voluntary control and does not have to be performed in a fixed fashion in response to immediate sensory input. Different levels of walking control exist, therefore. How these levels are coordinated is another issue we will consider.

DESCRIPTIONS OF WALKING

To understand how walking is controlled, it is important to describe walking accurately. We have already noted some features of walking that can be observed without sophisticated technology. Walking takes many forms, it is responsive to the structure of the external environment, it can be consciously controlled, and it is innately programmed. Another feature is that, as a result of trauma or disease, walking may become impaired, leading to, or stemming from, lack of coordination, weakness, or paralysis.

With these preliminaries in mind, let us begin our review of walking research with a description of how the legs move when animals or people cover distances at different speeds.

Gait Patterns at Different Speeds

In the late nineteenth century, the American photographer Eadweard Muybridge (1887/1957) set out to resolve a controversy of his day: When horses trot, do all their legs leave the ground at once? Muybridge set up the first time-lapse camera system to address this question (see Figure 5.1). His pictures revealed that all of a horses' feet do indeed leave the ground during trotting (panels 4 and 5, and 9 and 10). His pictures also showed that when a horse walks or trots, it uses different gait patterns. During walking, the horse adopts a three-legged stance (panels C and D of Figure 5.1), where during trotting, such a stance is never adopted; three legs are never on the ground at once.

Do people also change gait patterns when they change speed of locomotion? Figure 5.2 shows that they do. During walking there are periods when both feet are on the ground, but during running there are periods when only one foot is on the ground (Alexander, 1984).

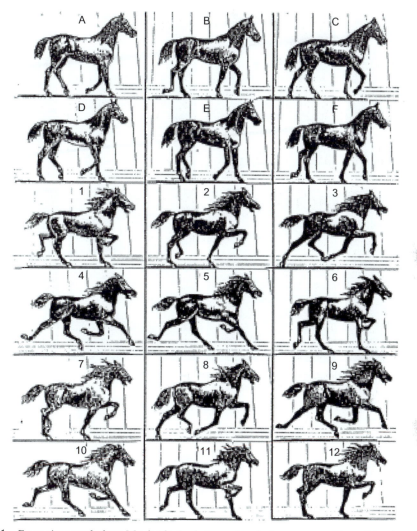

FIGURE 5.1 Engravings made from Muybridge's photographs of a horse engaged in walking (panels A–F) and trotting (panels 1–12). Reprinted from Scientific American, October 19, 1878.

Why does the pattern of gait change with speed of locomotion? Why don't we always walk over all the speeds we need or always run even when we needn't hurry?

An answer was provided by the British biomechanist R. McNeil Alexander (Alexander, 1984). Alexander introduced the simplified walker shown in Figure 5.3. This person's leg is assumed to be perfectly straight when his or her foot is on the ground, at which time the person's center of mass is also highest. When the person steps forward, his or her center of mass descends in an arc whose radius equals l, the normalized length of the person's leg. If the person moves the foot downward with velocity v, the acceleration of the center of mass is v^2/l. This quantity cannot exceed the acceleration due to gravity, g, unless the person

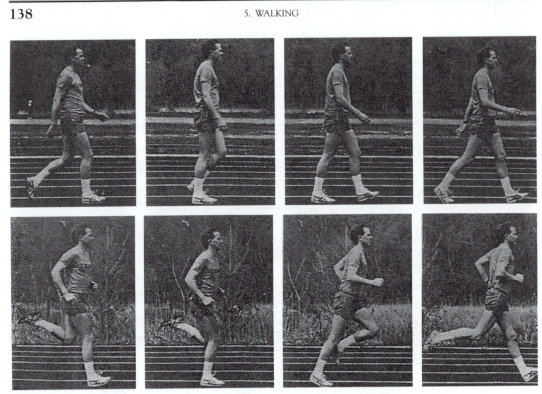

FIGURE 5.2　Stages of walking and running. Reproduced from Alexander (1984).

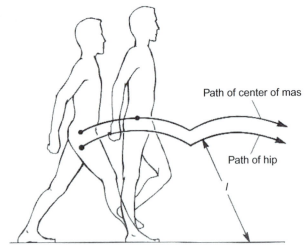

Path of center of mas

Path of hip

l

FIGURE 5.3　A simplified model of walking. From Alexander (1984).

deliberately pulls his or her foot downward at an exceptionally high rate, which would counter the goal of moving forward. Thus v^2/l must be less than or equal to g. Equivalently,

$$v \le \sqrt{gl} \tag{5.1}$$

Because g is about $10\,\text{m/s}^2$ and the length of the leg of a typical adult is about $0.9\,\text{m}$, Equation 5.1 implies that it is impossible to walk more quickly than about $2.5\,\text{m/s}$, which is the approximate transition speed from walking to running for most people (Alexander, 1984).

Why does running enable one to proceed more quickly than $2.5\,\text{m/s}$? The reason is that running is a series of controlled *leaps*, whereas walking is a series of controlled *falls*. Leaps are possible during running because the elastic recoil of the leg muscles and tendons enables the runner to "bounce" back after his or her foot strikes the ground.

If the shift from walking to running is due to physical factors, the power requirements for walking should exceed those for running at or above speeds where walking gives way to running. The actual power requirements have been estimated from measures of oxygen consumption and carbon dioxide release (Margaria, 1976). As seen in Figure 5.4, estimated power requirements do in fact become greater for walking than for running at around $2.5\,\text{m/s}$. The power requirements for bicycling are the least at this speed because during cycling the center of mass of the body remains at nearly constant height, so the mechanical energy of the body does not fluctuate between potential energy and kinetic energy in each stride, as is true in walking or running.

Regularities in Gait Patterns

There is considerable regularity in the characteristics of individuals' gaits. This has been shown through a perceptual demonstration devised by a Swedish psychologist, Gunnar

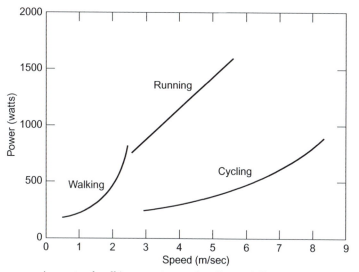

FIGURE 5.4 Power requirements of walking, running, and cycling at different speeds. From Alexander (1984).

Johannson (1973), following earlier work by Mayer (1895/1972). Johannson filmed people with a small number of luminous dots attached to their clothing. When the film was viewed later, only the lights could be seen; the actor's body and surroundings were invisible. Those viewing the moving dots had an unmistakable and immediate impression of a person in motion. Observers could see people walking, dancing, and running, and could even distinguish among their friends as well as between males and females whom they didn't know (Cutting & Proffitt, 1981). The ability to see people in motion is present at an early age. Infants between 4 and 6 months old are more likely to look at moving light patterns from someone running in place than to look at the same number of lights moving randomly (Fox & McDaniel, 1982).

For such perception to be possible, there must be regularity in the gait patterns that people and animals display (Blake & Shiffrar, 2007; Cutting, 1986). Some of those regularities are identified here.

One is that the time that a leg swings between successive footfalls (the swing phase) changes only slightly with walking speed whereas the time that the foot remains on the ground (the stance phase) increases with the time spent in each step (see Figure 5.5). This principle is remarkably widespread in the animal kingdom. It is seen in cockroaches (Pearson, 1976), lobsters (Macmillan, 1975), cats (Goslow, Reinking, & Stuart, 1973; Miller & Van der Meeche, 1975), dogs (Arshavsky, Kots, Orlovskii, Rodionov, & Shik, 1965), and humans (Herman, Wirta, Bampton, & Finley, 1976; Shapiro, Zernicke, Gregor, & Diestel, 1981). The swing phase has an approximately constant duration because the foot is flung forward in a ballistic fashion, with much of its trajectory being determined by gravity alone (McMahon, 1984).

Another kind of regularity that has been observed in analyses of gait concerns the time-varying angles of the knee and hip. During normal running, the angles of a runner's knee and thigh co-vary systematically. This relationship is shown in Figure 5.6 in a so-called angle-angle diagram (Enoka, 1988). Such diagrams are useful for therapeutic purposes. They allow clinicians to determine the nature of gait disorders and chart progress in therapy (Shumway-Cooke & Woollacott, 2006). The angle-angle diagram shown on the right panel of Figure 5.6 comes from a person with a below-knee amputation, wearing a foot prosthesis. The person's gait is still imperfect, as seen by comparing the left and right panels of Figure 5.6. Comparisons like this provide objective means of evaluating the effectiveness of different prosthetic designs.

A similar sort of analysis allows for the evaluation of gait in patients with cerebral palsy and other neurological damage. In one application (Teitelman, 1984), small lights were temporarily and painlessly attached to the lower extremities of patients with cerebral palsy. The positions of the lights were recorded as the patients walked. The time-varying angular changes of the knee, hip, or ankle were then analyzed to determine whether those changes differed from the patterns observed in normal individuals. By simultaneously recording the electromyographic activity of the leg muscles, it was possible to determine whether abnormalities in the pattern of joint angles were due to misordering of the activation of the leg muscles. Informed by such results, it was then possible to determine whether surgical rearrangement of the leg muscles was advisable. The results were often positive (Teitelman, 1984).

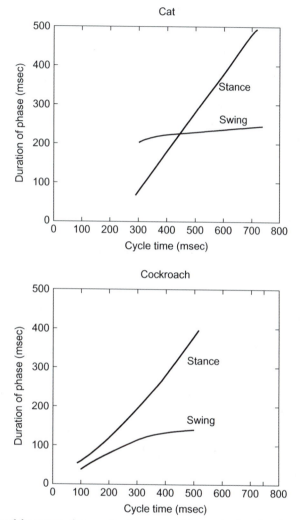

FIGURE 5.5   Duration of the stance phase and swing phase of the cat (top) and cockroach (bottom) as a function of cycle time. From The control of walking by K. R. Pearson. Copyright © (1976) by Scientific American, Inc., 235 (6), 72–86. All rights reserved.

NEURAL CONTROL OF LOCOMOTION

How does the nervous system activate and de-activate muscles in the proper temporal order to control gait? Consider the activity of the muscles in one leg of a walking cat. Figure 5.7 shows that there are orderly patterns of muscle activity within the cat's leg during a step cycle. During the swing phase the flexors are active and the extensors are inactive, but during the stance phase the flexors are inactive and the extensors are active. This

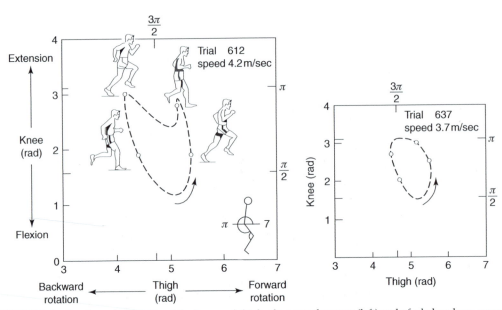

FIGURE 5.6 Angle-angle diagram of the knee and thigh of a normal runner (left) and of a below-knee amputee (right). There is less flexing of the knee joint in the amputee than in the normal individual. From Enoka, R.M., Miller, & Burgess (1982). Below-knee amputee running gait. American Journal of Physical Medicine, 61, 66–84. Copyright © by Williams & Wilkins, 1982. With permission.

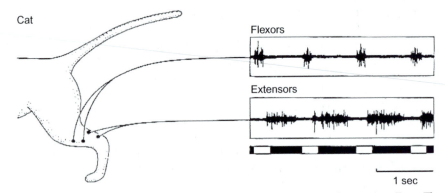

FIGURE 5.7 Extensor and flexor activity of the hind limb of the cat during locomotion. From The control of walking by K. R. Pearson. Copyright © (1976) by Scientific American, Inc., 235 (6), 72–86. All rights reserved.

sequence of electromyographic activity accounts for the distinct types of motion observed in the swing phase and the stance phase of cat locomotion. In the swing phase, when the flexors are active, the leg is retracted and pulled forward toward the next footfall. In the stance phase, when the extensors are active, the leg is pushed down so the body can advance.

Some of the earliest research on the neural regulation of leg muscle activity came from the British physiologist Charles Sherrington (1906), who was knighted and received a Nobel prize for his research on this and related topics. Sherrington severed the cat's spinal cord, separating it from the brain, and observed that rhythmic activity in the legs still occurred. From this observation he inferred that the spinal cord can produce rhythmic movement without input from the brain. Sherrington believed that the spinal cord generates rhythmic movement through a reflex arc in which sensory feedback from one burst of muscle activity serves as the stimulus for the next burst. Locomotion, according to this view, is the culmination of this reflex chain.

The reflex chain hypothesis came into question in 1911, when another British physiologist and a former student of Sherrington, Graham Brown, performed an experiment similar to Sherrington's. Graham Brown severed the spinal cord of the cat to see what locomotion abilities remained, but unlike Sherrington, Graham Brown also eliminated sensory feedback to the spinal cord by cutting the dorsal roots (see Chapter 4). When he did this, he observed that rhythmic contractions of the leg muscles continued. Because the rhythmic contractions occurred without input from the brain and without sensory input from the muscles, Graham Brown inferred that the spinal cord must have produced the series of efferent signals on its own. This outcome contradicted Sherrington's reflex chain hypothesis.

Graham Brown's discovery had enormous theoretical significance, for it implied that sensory feedback contributes less to movement than Sherrington had suggested. Given the revolutionary impact of Graham Brown's finding, it was important to be sure that the procedure for eliminating sensory feedback was effective. Cause for concern was fueled by the discovery, a number of years later, that some sensory feedback is transmitted through the ventral roots of the spinal cord as well as through the dorsal roots (see Grillner, 1981).

Later research vindicated Graham Brown (Cohen, Rossignol, & Grillner, 1988; Grillner, 1981). In one procedure, called *fictive locomotion*, the spinal cord was functionally isolated by severing its connections to the brain and brain stem. Moreover, the dorsal roots were cut below the level of the spinal transection and the muscles were completely paralyzed to ensure that no feedback from the muscles could infiltrate the spinal cord via the ventral roots. Paralyzing the muscles was achieved with curare, a neuromuscular blocking agent. The activity of the ventral roots of the isolated spinal cord was then recorded to see what signals, if any, still emerged from the isolated cord.

The result was dramatic: The spatial and temporal distribution of bursts recorded in the ventral roots was similar to that seen in behaving animals. Thus, the fictive locomotion procedure indicated that there are central pattern generators within the spinal cord. Studies by other investigators confirmed that central pattern generators are widespread (Delcomyn, 1975).

A host of questions is suggested by these findings: How are rhythm generators neurally organized? Are they situated within individual neurons (what some investigators call pacemaker cells) or are they emergent functions from interconnections among several neurons? How are they affected by sensory input? What is the brain's role in locomotion? Each of these questions is taken up in the next sections.

Neural Circuits for Locomotion

Because the mammalian spinal cord is a complex structure, neurophysiologists interested in the control of locomotion have worked with animals with simpler neural circuitry. One such animal is the cockroach, whose neural circuitry for locomotion was studied in considerable detail by Pearson (1976). Gait patterns of the cockroach are similar to those of the cat in that different sequences of footfalls occur as the cockroach modulates its speed of locomotion. In addition, the duration of the cockroach's stance phase varies with the gait being performed, although the duration of its swing phase is essentially constant. Finally, when electrodes are used to record muscular activity in the leg of the cockroach, flexor activity is observed during the swing phase and extensor activity is observed during the stance phase, as in mammals. These similarities between locomotion in the cockroach and locomotion in other species are remarkable in and of themselves. They suggest that the problem of locomotion may be solved in common ways among animal species whose evolutionary divergence points came at different times in history. The similarities also make the cockroach an appropriate model system in which to investigate the neural circuitry underlying locomotion in mammals, including human beings.

Figure 5.8 shows a neural circuit for cockroach locomotion hypothesized by Pearson (1976). The circuit is known as a flexor burst generator. The circuit is assumed to periodically excite flexor motor neurons and to periodically inhibit extensor motor neurons. The periodicity of the flexor burst generator arises from mutual inhibitory influences among interneurons excited by central command neurons that tonically (continually) activate the extensor motor neuron. When the common exit point for the flexor burst generator (interneuron 1) is turned on, it activates the flexor motor neuron as well as an interneuron that inhibits the extensor motor neuron. Thus, the flexor motor neuron is normally off but is turned on by the flexor burst generator. Similarly, the extensor motor neuron, which is normally on, is turned off (indirectly) by the flexor burst generator. Because the flexor burst generator produces bursts of approximately constant duration, the activation time of the flexor motor neuron is approximately constant, which can explain why the duration of the swing phase is approximately fixed. By contrast, the extensor motor neuron is always on, except when it is inhibited, and the length of time the extensor motor neuron has an outward effect depends

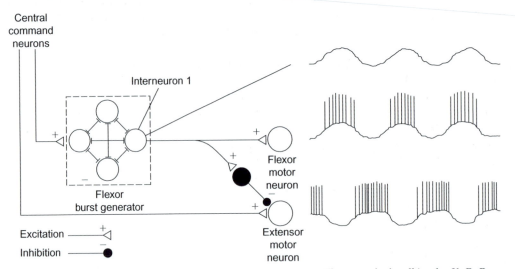

FIGURE 5.8   Hypothesized circuit for cockroach locomotion. From The control of walking by K. R. Pearson. Copyright © (1976) by Scientific American, Inc. 235 (6), 72–86. All rights reserved.

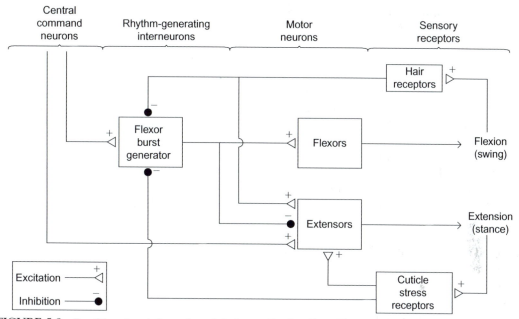

FIGURE 5.9 Possible network for cockroach limb coordination. From The control of walking by K. R. Pearson. Copyright © (1976) by Scientific American, Inc., 235 (6), 72–86. All rights reserved.

on the duration of the step cycle. This aspect of the model helps explain why the duration of the stance phase changes with the duration of the step cycle.

As satisfactory as this theoretical circuit may be for explaining the control of a single leg, it cannot account for the coordination of multiple legs. The circuit must be elaborated to account for multi-leg coordination. Figure 5.9 shows such an elaborated circuit. Two features are added to account for coordination of multiple limbs. One is inhibition between flexor burst generators for adjacent limbs, which can account for the fact that the cockroach never steps with adjacent legs simultaneously. The other is sensory inhibition, sent from a receptor on each leg to that leg's flexor burst generator. The receptor that Pearson (1976) suggested was one that responds to mechanical loading of the leg. The receptor is activated during the stance phase of the step cycle. As the cockroach pushes forward and the load on the leg is reduced, the receptor's activity diminishes and the flexor burst generator that it normally inhibits stops being inhibited so that flexor burst generator can produce the next period of flexor activity, giving rise to the next swing phase.

Although this model was proposed quite some time ago, it is still apt today. Two lessons can be learned from the model. One is that one need not posit a single pacemaker cell to understand how rhythmic activity can occur. An entire group of cells can also yield such activity, which is a good thing, because one would not want to have just one pacemaker cell for controlling the movement of a limb. Should that one cell die, one would be paralyzed.

A second lesson of Pearson's (1976) model is that the sequencing of leg movements may be modulated by sensory feedback. The control of locomotion is achieved through an interplay of central pattern generators and sensory influences. As seen below, this view has received wide support.

The Role of Sensory Feedback

With the exception of Pearson's proposal about the role of feedback in the control of cockroach locomotion, none of the results presented so far forces the conclusion that sensory feedback has an impact on walking. The reason is that the other results indicate that even when the spinal cord receives no sensory input, it still generates highly organized patterns of efferent signals. Consider the following facts, however.

Patients with *tabes dorsalis*, a disease of the dorsal roots of the spinal cord, have great difficulty walking (Kalat, 1984). Similarly, when sensory feedback is eliminated from "spinal" animals (animals whose spinal cords have been separated from the brain), overall speed of locomotion is reduced, though the basic sequencing of steps is preserved (Carew, 1985).

Second, in fictive locomotion (described above), the time intervals between neural bursts recorded at the ventral roots for the extensor and flexor muscles are significantly longer than in chronic spinal cats whose muscles still work and in whom feedback enters the spinal cord (Grillner, 1981).

These two results imply that sensory feedback does make some contribution to walking movements. How then can we account for the findings, reviewed earlier, suggesting a wholly central basis for the control of locomotion?

The contribution of sensory feedback can be appreciated by considering a study by Taub and Berman (1968). Prior to their work, it was generally accepted that monkeys with deafferented limbs cannot walk or manipulate objects, for when the limbs on one side of the body were deafferented, those limbs were not used. Taub and Berman (1968) went on to do something surprising. They severed the dorsal roots of *both* sides of the monkey's spinal cord and discovered that the monkeys would then use their limbs, though the monkeys did so more slowly and more awkwardly than when feedback was available. Taub and Berman's (1968) finding suggested that animals deprived of sensory feedback prefer not to generate movements that normally involve that feedback. However, when the animals have no choice, then, all else being equal, they can move, at least in a rudimentary fashion. This outcome indicates that sensory feedback is not absolutely necessary for locomotion (or reaching), but it is useful for the tuning of movements. The picture that emerges is that the nervous system has central programs for movement patterns, but the exact way those programs are used depends on information supplied to them from the sensory apparatus (Keele, 1968, 1981).

A related hypothesis is that if sensory feedback interacts with central pattern generators, then the way sensory information affects locomotion (or any centrally programmed motor activity) should depend on the motor system's current state. This prediction has been supported in theoretical and experimental work.

Theoretically, as seen earlier in Pearson's (1976) model of cockroach walking, feedback can affect the phase relations of the legs. If the flexor burst generator for a given leg receives inhibitory signals from that leg's load sensor, the burst generator does not fire and so does not inhibit neighboring burst generators. Consequently, the swing phase can be initiated.

Experimental work has shown that when a cat is prevented from extending its hind leg, its leg immediately flexes, but this occurs only if the hind leg is prevented from extending at a critical point in the stance phase (Grillner, 1981). A related phenomenon was reported by Forrsberg, Grillner, and Rossignol (1975). In their experiment, the top of a cat's paw was touched with a rod during the swing phase or during the stance phase of the step cycle. Though the stimulus was the same in both cases, the cat's response was different. If the stimulus was applied during the swing phase, there was an enhanced flexion response, as if the animal was raising its paw above an unexpected obstacle. By contrast, if the stimulus was delivered during the stance phase, there was an enhanced extension response, as if the animal was trying to ensure its foothold. Thus, the same stimulus had opposite effects depending on when it was applied. This outcome implies that the nervous system enables adaptive, context-dependent reactions through centrally programmed neural changes. The human nervous system does so as well, for similar observations have been made in humans while walking or standing still (Nashner, Woollacott, & Tuma, 1979).

Descending Effects

If context affects responsiveness, one might expect the brain to play an important role in walking control. What is that role? Is it just that the brain sends signals down to the spinal cord telling the spinal cord each and every step to trigger? It is conceivable that the brain plays some such role, for otherwise the effect of spinal cord injury in cases where the brain can no longer communicate with the spinal cord would be less devastating.

Figure 5.10 shows a setup that has proven useful for studying the more subtle nature of the brain's control of, or involvement with, the spinal cord (Nashner, 1976; Nashner & McCollum, 1985). Subjects were asked to stand on a platform that could undergo a variety of sudden displacements. The platform could slide back, causing the subject to tilt forward, or it could tilt up toward the subject's face, causing the subject to sway back. The important feature of this pair of platform maneuvers was that both of them stretched the gastrocnemius muscle (the large muscle group on the back of the lower leg). In general, stretching the

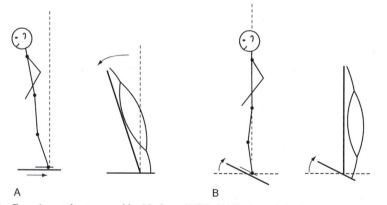

A   B

FIGURE 5.10 Experimental setup used by Nashner (1976). (A) Backward displacement of the platform induces a reflex response that *stabilizes* posture. (B) Upward displacement of the platform induces a reflex response that *destabilizes* posture. Reprinted by permission of the publisher from Posture and locomotion, by T. J. Carew, in Principles of neural science (2nd ed.), pp. 478–486. Copyright © (1985) by Elsevier Science Publishing Co, Inc. With permission.

gastrocnemius gives rise to a single reflex response—contraction of that muscle. However, the fact that gastrocnemius contraction followed both types of platform movement created an interesting problem. When the platform tilted back, the body tilted forward, so when the gastrocnemius contracted, the effect was to oppose body sway, and that helped stabilize the body. Conversely, when the platform tilted up, the body tilted back, which promoted backward tilt, and that destabilized the body. Could subjects turn off the reflex when it had untoward consequences? The answer was that the reflex continued to operate when it had a stabilizing effect, but when it had a destabilizing effect the reflex was attenuated (see Nashner & McCollum, 1985; Shumway-Cook & Woollacott, 2006).

Did the brain attenuate the destabilizing reflex? Several lines of evidence indicate that it did in this experiment and does so more generally. One line of evidence is that patients with damage to the cerebellum are less able than normal subjects to inhibit the reflex when its effect is destabilizing (Shumway-Cook & Woollacott, 2006). Likewise, patients with vestibular damage exhibit abnormal responses when subjected to platform rotations (Allum & Pfaltz, 1985). Finally, in normal individuals, detailed studies of their muscle responses following experimentally induced postural perturbation indicate that the vestibular system coordinates the distribution of restoring forces over widely distributed sites in the body (Shumway-Cook & Woollacott, 2006). An important conclusion from these studies is that whole configurations of muscles are activated in response to postural disturbances (Shumway-Cook & Woollacott, 2006). Such muscle synergies can be controlled by the brainas, shown by the fact that they can be elicited by electrical stimulation of the motor cortex (Humphrey, 1986; Massion, 1984).

The brain also affects the selection and control of gait patterns (Shik, Severin, & Orlovky, 1966). Shik et al. (1966) cut the spinal cord of the cat at different levels, and for each level determined what stepping patterns could be performed when cats were placed on a treadmill. When the spinal cord was cut below the brain stem (causing the spinal cord to be isolated from the brain stem and higher brain structures), coordinated gait could still occur. This outcome corroborates the results described by Graham Brownand Grillner (1981). When the spinal cord was left connected to the brain stem but the brain stem was disconnected from higher brain centers, distinct patterns of gait could be elicited by electrically stimulating the mesencephalic locomotor region (see Figure 5.11). As the strength of electrical stimulation increased and as the speed of the treadmill increased, the pattern of gait changed from walking to trotting to galloping. Similar effects were obtained by injecting L-DOPA (a precursor of dopamine) into the same brain stem region (Shumway-Cook & Woollacott, 2006).

Other studies have provided information about how the brain controls the speed and direction in which an animal walks or runs (Freed & Yamamoto, 1985). Animals can be made to run clockwise or counterclockwise when dopaminergic cells in the substantia nigra are electrically stimulated. Whether the animal runs clockwise or counterclockwise depends on which hemisphere receives the stimulation. Recall from Chapter 3 that the substantia nigra is an area involved in the production of dopamine. A consequence of reduced dopamine production in the substantia nigra is Parkinson's disease. Parkinson's patients also have trouble initiating gait, often shuffling their feet when trying to walk forward or when trying to turn (Kalat, 1984).

Speed and direction of locomotion also appear to be controlled, at least in part, by the nucleus accumbens (see Chapter 4). The amount of dopamine in this structure has been

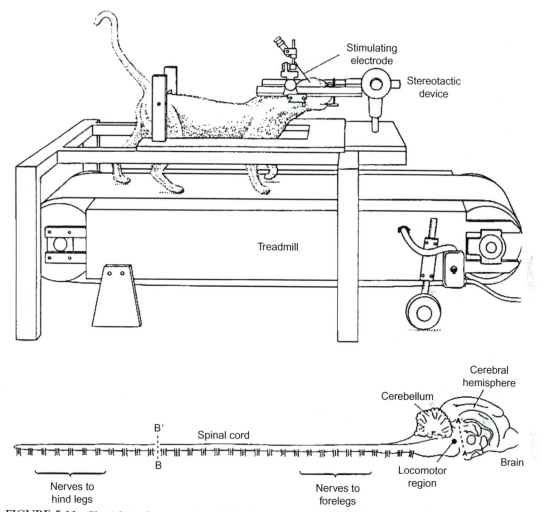

FIGURE 5.11 Physiological preparation of Shik, Severin, and Orlobsky (1966). Dashed lines between A and A′ and between B and B′ show transection locations. From Pearson (1976.) The control of walking. Scientific American, 235 (6), 72–86. With permission.

shown, in treadmill-running rats, to be related to the speed and direction of movement. The caudate nucleus, another basal ganglia structure, plays a role in the regulation of posture. Depending on the degree of lateral or vertical curvature of a treadmill in which a rat is running, the amount of dopamine in the caudate nucleus (contralateral to the lateral direction of turning) increases or decreases.

Another important role played by the brain in the control of walking is visual guidance. When cats are required to walk over a perfectly even surface, relatively little neural activity is recorded in the cortico-spinal tract (see Georgopoulos & Grillner, 1989). However, when cats are required to walk over uneven terrain, the level of activity in the cortico-spinal tract increases markedly (Georgopoulos & Grillner, 1989). Transection of the cortico-spinal tract eliminates the capacity for climbing a ladder—another task requiring visually directed limb positioning.

These observations are interesting, not just for shedding light on the control of locomotion but also for understanding the control of reaching and grasping (see Chapter 7). The cortico-spinal tract is active during manual aiming tasks. This suggests that the neural systems underlying the control of locomotion and the control of reaching and grasping (see Chapter 7) rely on overlapping neural fields (Georgopoulos & Grillner, 1989). Everyday observation suggests that they should, of course, because many locomotion tasks, particularly among animals, require grasping as well as propulsion. Squirrels and monkeys must grab hold of tree branches while clambering. Little research has been done on the coordination of reaching and walking. Some of this research is described in the last chapter of the book. Not surprisingly, people are good at coordinating their simultaneous reaching and walking behavior (Carnahan, McFadyen, Cockell, & Halverson, 1996; Marteniuk & Bertram, 2001; Rosenbaum, 2008; van der Wel & Rosenbaum, 2007).

After all this discussion, how can we summarize the brain's role in the control of locomotion? The brain can be said to play a moderating role. Without the brain's involvement, the neural activity that occurs in the spinal cord is associated with pattern generators whose activity can be modulated over short periods and with short latencies by sensory feedback. However, spinal neural activity can also be influenced by inputs from higher centers. These higher centers take longer to affect the spinal cord than do direct afferent inputs to the spinal cord, but they can affect larger decisions like which gait to use and which response to make to particular forms of stimulation.

Anticipatory Postural Adjustments

That the brain affects locomotion in the manner just described is further supported by an important line of investigation that has not been mentioned yet. This work concerns *anticipatory postural adjustments*, or APAs. APAs occur when people (and animals) prepare, usually unconsciously, to undergo postural perturbations. The postural perturbations can come from outside, when one expects to be pushed by an external source such as a dropping ball or a linebacker from an opposing football team, or from within, when one prepares to perform some physical action. Self-initiated actions, like externally derived actions, introduce forces and torques that require counteracting forces and torques to restore postural equilibrium.

A way to get a sense of these perturbing effects is to stand on a sensitive scale and watch the weight indicator change as you lift your arm or, for that matter, your little finger. Even when you try to stand perfectly still, the weight indicator changes, indicating that perfect stillness while standing is illusory.

Careful analyses of the properties of the mini-motions made on scales or on other suitable recording devices have revealed that these tiny motions are surprisingly complex (e.g., Zatsiorsky & Duarte, 2000), they are affected by ongoing visual tasks (Stoffregan, Hove, Bardy, Riley, & Bonnet, 2007), and they are affected by ongoing cognitive activities (Pellecchia, 2003); but see Stoffregan et al. (2007).

Even if postural adjustments are relatively insensitive to upcoming arithmetic differences, they reveal marked sensitivity to upcoming mechanical perturbations. The adjustments are not perfect, for if they were, one would not see the needle on one's scale change when one lifts a paper clip. Still, the adjustments are good enough to keep one balanced and, in most cases, to leave one oblivious to how much the nervous system does to maintain postural equilibrium. So fundamental to the maintenance of balance is motor activity that it is incorrect to say that the only job of the motor system is to help us move; the other is to steady us as we do so (Belen'kii, Gurfinkel, & Pal'tsev, 1967).

Much of what we have learned about preparation for postural perturbations has been acquired by recording electromyographic (EMG) signals from muscles involved in postural support. This work has shown that when one makes a fast voluntary movement, there are antecedent, compensatory changes in the background activity of the leg and trunk muscles. Such early EMG changes constitute the APAs referred to at the start of this section. APAs have been observed prior to voluntary arm, trunk, and leg movements and in situations where loads are applied to or removed from the upper extremities, usually with advance knowledge on the part of the subject. For reviews of this work, see Latash (2008a,b). Insofar as all of APAs reflect expectations about upcoming postural demands, they show that the brain tunes postural reflexes in an adaptive way, at least when everything is working properly.

WALKING MACHINES

As discussed in Chapter 1, an effective way to test one's understanding of a biological control system is to simulate it in an artificial device. In this regard, it is instructive to consider the efforts that have been made to build machines that can walk. Walking machines are valuable for scaling uneven terrain (for example, in military and exploratory missions) or in carrying passengers who cannot walk themselves.

In deciding how to build such machines, it has been useful to identify the essential conditions that any walking system must satisfy. Raibert and Sutherland (1983) listed five such conditions:

1. It must regulate its sequence of footfalls.
2. It must not tip over.
3. It must distribute the load and lateral forces acting on the legs among all the legs.
4. It must ensure that the legs do not move beyond their travel limits. For example, it is usually imperative for the legs not to bump into each other.
5. It must ensure that chosen footholds provide adequate support. Choosing footfalls is primarily a visual task since it is usually best to decide before stepping whether a surface will support the body.

Building a walking machine is a difficult engineering problem. In the nineteenth century, a patent was issued for a rudimentary walking machine, similar to modern walking toys (see Raibert & Sutherland, 1983). Not until the 1960's, however, was a machine built that was capable of walking more or less on its own. This was a four-legged, electrically driven walking device constructed in 1966 at the University of Southern California. The usefulness of this device was limited by the fact that it was too small to be ridden by a human drive. At the same time, it was too unsophisticated to be controlled without a person on board (McMahon, 1984).

A much larger four-legged walking machine was built in 1968 at General Electric (McMahon, 1984). It was the size of an elephant but was extremely hard to control. A human driver sat atop the contraption and was supposed to instruct the back legs how to move by moving his or her own legs. At the same time, the human driver was supposed to instruct the front legs how to move by moving his or her own arms. The task proved unmanageable for the driver, so this artificial walking elephant was left standing in its stall.

A more successful device, designed in the early 1980's, had six rather than four legs (Figure 5.12). Six is the smallest number of legs that provide a consistently stable base of support during locomotion, because with a six-legged walker, it is possible to alternate between one tripod (three-legged) stance and another. Three is the smallest number of legs needed for static balancing. Think of a three-legged piano stool, which can stand on an even

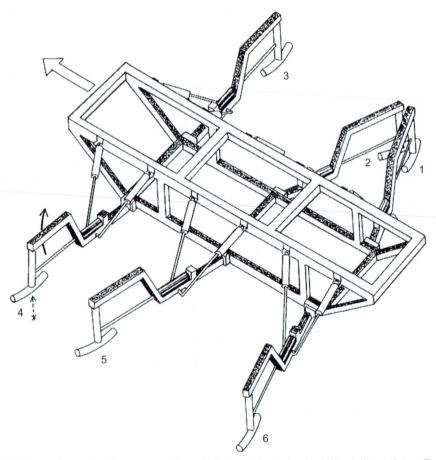

FIGURE 5.12   Six-legged walking machine. From Raibert and Sutherland (1983). Machines that walk. Scientific American, 248, No. 1, 44–53. With permission.

surface without any active control system. The balance problem is significantly easier for a six-legged walking device than for a walking device with four or fewer legs. Conceivably, this is why insects have six legs.

The six-legged device shown in Figure 5.12 was built in such a way that each of its legs was equipped with a pair of hydraulic actuators. Each actuator received input from a computer that responded to feedback from the machine's legs. The computer allowed for release of a fixed amount of oil to one or the other actuator for any given leg. Only one actuator for a leg received oil at any given time, so there was a kind of reciprocal inhibition between each leg's actuators, much as there is between the muscle antagonists of a biological limb (see Chapter 4). The decision about where the machine should tread and how quickly it should tread was left to a human operator who sat atop the machine. When the driver selected a path, the computer determined which legs were free to move and where the next step should be taken. The machine could turn, walk forward and back, and could tilt up or down or to one side or the other. An important feature of the control system was that some of the adjustments made by the machine were entirely passive. The actuators acted as passive hydraulic circuits, like the shock absorbers of a car, so compensations for elevations or depressions in the ground were achieved, within limits, without any involvement of the computer or human operator. Thus, the computational burdens of guiding the machine were reduced by exploiting the machine's physical structure.

In the years since the development of this walking machine, there has been significant progress in the design of machines capable of moving through the natural environment, and not just on smooth roads, for which legs are but a nicety, but also through brush, over rocks, and even through mud. This advance has been enabled by reliance on mechanics to help simplify the control problem, as with passive dynamic walkers like the one shown in Figure 2.6. In addition, there have been dramatic advances in the development of walking machines made possible by the incorporation of knowledge gained through the study of animal locomotion in its myriad forms (Cruse, Kindermann, Schumm, Dean, & Schmitz, 1998; Dickinson et al., 2000).

Research on animal locomotion has shown that Nature has evolved all sorts of tricks for dealing with the demands of moving through a wide range of challenging environments—on sand, on ice, on tree trunks, in choppy water, in turbulent wind, and so on. This research has revealed an amazing repertory of neural and physical solutions to the problem of propelling animal bodies forward, backward, up, and down, not to mention holding still in conditions that challenge stationarity (e.g., in severe winds or in thrashing waves). The neural solutions that have materialized take the form of reflex circuits that are astonishing for their quickness and adaptability. The physical solutions that have appeared take the form not just of *reflexes*, but also of *preflexes*. These are mechanical dispositions of animal bodies, or parts of animal bodies, to respond to perturbations adaptively based entirely on mechanical properties. Studies of insects, reptiles, birds, amphibia, and mammals have revealed a stunning spectrum of structural designs that permit immediate mechanical responses to perturbations (Dickinson et al., 2000). Because the responses are mechanical rather than neural, they permit virtually instantaneous responses without the need for neural computation. Engineers have capitalized on such information to build devices capable of locomotion with minimal supervisory control -- for example , a robot "cockroach" equipped with rotating "flapper" legs that enable the robot to tool around on its own through slush, mud, and thickets (Figure 5.13).

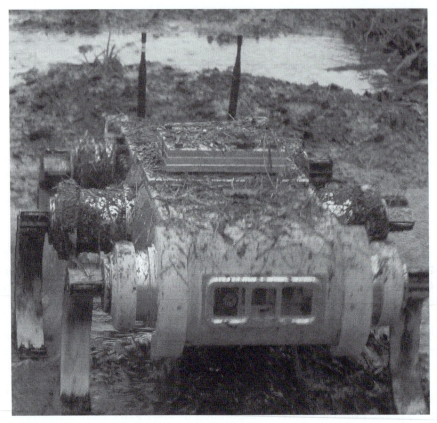

FIGURE 5.13   A cockroach-inspired robot, roughly the size of a bread box, making its way through mud on a trip that also included trudging through weeds, climbing over rocks, stepping over railroad tracks, and righting itself after nearly toppling over. Photograph kindly provided by Professor Robert Full, University of California, Berkeley, July 7, 2008.

THE DEVELOPMENT OF WALKING

Machines that walk do so through human craft. Adult humans and animals that walk do so based on growing and learning. As mentioned earlier in this chapter, walking patterns are innate. Newborn colts and calves can stand up and walk within the first minutes of life. Human infants in their first day of life exhibit stepping movements when held beneath their shoulders, provided their feet can touch the ground (Andre-Thomas & Autgarden, 1966). Some people have been so impressed by the newborn's capacity for stepping that they have encouraged newborns to swim. When held in water, healthy newborns can exhibit impressive coordinated arm and leg movements (McGraw, 1939). Moving on from there, a healthy, typically developing baby is said to go through a series of motor milestones (Shirley, 1931): The baby first lifts its head, then supports its body on its arms, next turns over, then sits up, then crawls, then walks with assistance, and finally walks alone, toddling at first and later walking in full. In the next sections, we ask what accounts for this progression.

Neonatal Reflexes

One way to develop an account of the development of walking is to note that several characteristic behaviors or, as they are classically called, "reflexes," come into play during walking. Some of these behaviors appear in infancy but not in later life (Easton, 1972). The disappearance of these behaviors signal neurological changes that allow for more mature forms of motor behavior.

Consider some of the reflexes exhibited by infants (Figure 5.14). One is the startle reflex, which is triggered by unexpected noise or changes in bodily position, particularly changes in body position that create a sensation of falling. The baby's arms and legs move symmetrically, first outward, then upward, then inward. The hands open and clench, as do the legs.

Another infantile reflex, the tonic neck reflex, is an asymmetrical pose adopted by newborns up to about 16 weeks of age. The baby's head and arm extend to one side. On the opposite side, the arm and leg flex. The functional significance of the tonic neck reflex has been widely discussed. One hypothesis is that it enables the infant to observe its own hand, thereby facilitating the development of hand-eye coordination. Although the tonic neck reflex disappears during development, it may remain available later in life (see Figure 5.15), providing a built-in pattern that can be called upon as necessary (Easton, 1972).

The righting reflex occurs when the infant is pulled up to a sitting position. When the righting reflex is exhibited, the infant attempts to keep its head erect. The head may flop forward or back due to poor coordination or weakness.

When pressure is applied to the palm of the baby's hand or foot, the fingers or toes curl up as if to grab the object. Because this grasp reflex is seen in the feet as well as the hands, it may be a throwback to a time when our pre-human ancestors dwelled in trees.

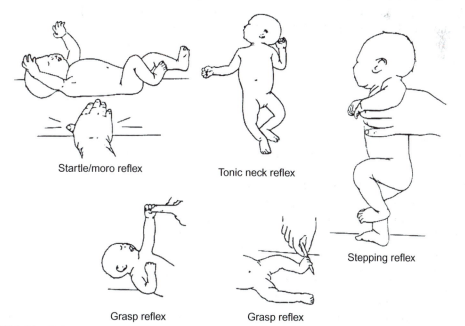

Startle/moro reflex   Tonic neck reflex   Stepping reflex

Grasp reflex   Grasp reflex

FIGURE 5.14   Reflexes seen in the human infant.

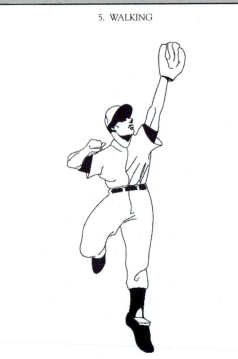

FIGURE 5.15   Catching a fly ball can result in a pose strongly resembling the tonic neck reflex of infancy.

The Babinski reflex is another involuntary response to stimulation of the bottom of the feet. Named for the neurologist who first described it, the foot pulls up, the toes fan out, and the big toe is raised. The Babinski reflex disappears during normal development. Its presence in older children or adults is generally taken as a sign of neurological damage.

The crawling reflex occurs in babies who have not yet learned to walk. As its name implies, this reflex is an alternating pattern of extensions and flexions of the arms and legs, performed with the belly on the ground.

The so-called swimming reflex is essentially the same as the crawling reflex, except that it occurs in water. An additional reflex is called upon when a baby is placed in water. If the baby's face happens to be momentarily submerged, the baby rarely chokes or aspirates water. This implies that babies can inhibit their breathing. Other, more sophisticated, means of coordinating breathing and movement have also been documented (Bramble & Carrier, 1983).

Another reflex seen in babies has already been mentioned, the stepping reflex. The stepping reflex is present in newborns but usually disappears by around 4 weeks of age, only to reappear at 8 months to 1 year. The reasons for the disappearance and reappearance of stepping in infants have been debated. The debate is informative and is reviewed below.

Disappearance and Reappearance of Stepping

Why does stepping disappear and then reappear in human infants? According to one view, the reasons are cognitive (Zelazo, 1983), but according to another view, the reasons are physical (Thelen, 1983).

The departure point for the cognitive hypothesis is that the reappearance of stepping coincides with the emergence of cognitive sequencing abilities. At around 1 year of age, babies can recognize sequences of lights, as indicated by measures of smiling, vocalization, pointing, or changes in heart rate (Kagan, 1971). Zelazo (1983) suggested that because walking requires sequential control of behavior, the control of walking only becomes possible when cognitive sequencing has been achieved.

Why, then, is stepping possible at an earlier age? According to the cognitive account, the baby's mind is taken up with other things during development, causing the primitive stepping reflex to fall away only to be relearned later. Consistent with this hypothesis, leg movements are facilitated by learning. When babies are rewarded for kicking by letting their kicks activate an attractive mobile, more kicks occur (Rovee & Fagan, 1976; Thelen & Fisher, 1983). Furthermore, when babies are encouraged to practice stepping, walking may develop somewhat earlier than when no practice is employed.

Now consider the alternative to the cognitive account. Thelen (1983) attributed the reemergence of stepping to physical changes. She was skeptical of the psychological view because walking is possible in animals that have limited cognitive abilities (such as insects), because walking develops even in people who are profoundly retarded, and because decerebrate animals (animals with the cerebral cortex disconnected from their lower nerve centers) can still walk. Thelen also noted that reclining infants can kick throughout the first year of lifeand that the kinematic patterns of their kicks are virtually indistinguishable from the kinematic patterns of normal stepping movements (Thelen, Bradshaw, & Ward, 1981). Finally, 2- to 8-month-old infants can step remarkably well when held upright in water (Thelen, 1983), as shown in Figure 5.16. These findings indicate that the *capacity* for sequential stepping does not actually disappear between 2 and 8 months of age. The baby's nervous system can generate sequences of muscle commands required for stepping behavior all through the first year of life.

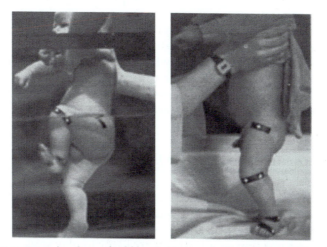

FIGURE 5.16 Leg movements in a 2-month-old boy held up on dry land (left) or held up in water (right). From Thelen, E. & Fisher, D. M. (1982). Newborn stepping: An explanation for a "disappearing" reflex. Developmental Psychology, 18, 760–775. With permission.

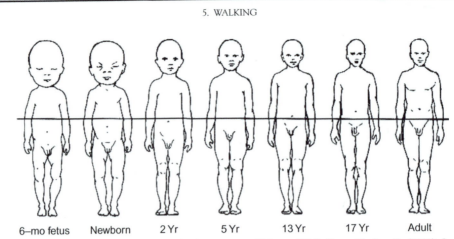

6–mo fetus   Newborn   2 Yr   5 Yr   13 Yr   17 Yr   Adult

FIGURE 5.17 Developmental changes in body structure (Palmer, 1944). From Thelen, E. (1983). Learning to walk is still an "old" problem: A reply to Zelazo. Journal of Motor Behavior, 15 (2), 139–161. With permission.

So why is stepping not generally observed in more mature babies, or more specifically, between 2 and 8 months of age? Thelen's (1983) answer is that the baby's legs are simply not strong enough to support its body. As seen in Figure 5.17, the baby's center of gravity is high above its legs, and this creates a mechanical disadvantage for the legs, a problem that is only aggravated by the fact that the legs are weak at this age. As the baby's legs get stronger and as the body's center of gravity descends, the mechanical demands of supporting the body decline and the possibility of walking returns.

From Thelen's work, we can learn a useful general lesson about the analysis of motor behavior: In attempting to explain behavioral phenomena, although it can help to look to the inner world of the mind, it is also important to look first to established laws of physics. Physical relations can often explain behavioral phenomena. Looking for physical relations does not dilute the importance of cognitive accounts. On the contrary, such accounts become more credible when possible physical accounts (i.e., accounts based on traditional mechanics and biomechanics) have been exhausted. This point was emphasized for the study of perception by James Gibson (1979), who argued that ecological optics can eliminate the need to postulate problem solving in perception (Purves & Lotto, 2003; Rock, 1983). In the author's view, a balanced approach that embraces both perspectives is more appropriate than an approach that allows only one approach.

MODELS OF MOTOR DEVELOPMENT

How can we explain the changes that occur in motor development, especially in the domain of balance and locomotion? Three principles related to neural development have been proposed, and a fourth principle has been proposed about behavioral exploration. All these principles deserve mention, as all of them are likely to play some role.

One principle related to neural development is that nerve fibers in the central nervous system undergo myelination, the process by which axons come to be coated with the fatty substance that allows for speeded neural transmission (see Chapter 3). Once this coating has formed, finer coordination becomes possible (Yakolev & Lecours, 1967).

A second principle related to neural development is that cortical centers take over or inhibit functions that were performed by subcortical centers (McGraw, 1943). This assumption explains why reflexes seen in young infants, such as the tonic neck reflex and the grasp reflex, are supplanted by other, more flexible behaviors. It also explains why primitive reflexes such as the Babinski reflex are seen in patients with cortical damage. Similarly, tonic flexion of the extremities, seen in some patients with cerebral palsy, may result from abnormal cortical inhibition of lower motor centers. Finally, postures adopted during sleep in normal adults are similar to those exhibited by babies, as if during sleep, inhibitory influences of the higher brain centers are turned off.

The third principle related to neural development is that neural maturation proceeds in a cephalo-caudal (head-to-tail) and proximal-distal (medial-to-peripheral) direction (e.g., Woollacott, Debu, & Mowatt, 1987). This principle accounts for the fact that refined movements occur early in the proximal musculature (such as the mouth) and only later occur in the distal extremities (such as the feet and fingers). Thus, while stepping may wax and wane developmentally, rooting (the tendency of the head to turn toward a stimulus that affords sucking) and sucking are highly developed from birth and remain strong from that point onward. Functionally, the advantages of cephalo-caudal and proximal-distal maturation are readily apparent: It is more important for survival to be able to eat or drink than to play the piano or kick a soccer ball.

The fourth principle relates to behavioral exploration. The idea is that while neural maturational changes may play a role in motor development, behavior itself contributes to the behaviors that unfold. The idea here is that babies, and for that matter children and adults, are capable of exploring the environment in physically creative ways. The discovery of affordances in the environment (i.e., finding things the environment lets one do) promotes the discovery of ever-richer behavioral opportunities.

Among the first scientists to appreciate the latter point were Goldfield, Kay, and Warren (1993), who studied babies in "jolly jumpers" (Figure 5.18). When a baby is placed in a jolly jumper, the baby occupies a secure seat hanging from a beam via two elastic bands. Crucially for the jolliness of the jumping experience, the seat is at a height that lets the baby plant his or feet on the ground. Once the baby gets the hang of it, she can do more than drag her feet on the floor. She can firmly plant her feet on the ground and, at just the right moment, provide an emphatic "umph" to lift herself upward for the next cycle of happy bouncing.

Babies get good at this. As shown in Figure 5.18, jolly-jumping infants learn to increase the amplitudes of their jumps, achieving bigger jumps without increasing the jump periods but instead decreasing the variability of the bounce periods. Thus, babies learn to get more "bang for the buck" as they hang in these fun contraptions. They do so through behavioral exploration, relying on trial and error to find out what movements are most helpful and when those movements should be made. Neural maturation in any of the senses outlined above is not what accounts for the greater efficiency of performance that is manifested over the course of practice with the jolly jumper. Instead, learning about the jolly jumper itself, or more aptly about the baby-plus-jolly-jumper as a unified mechanical system, is what allows babies to exploit the system more and more efficiently.

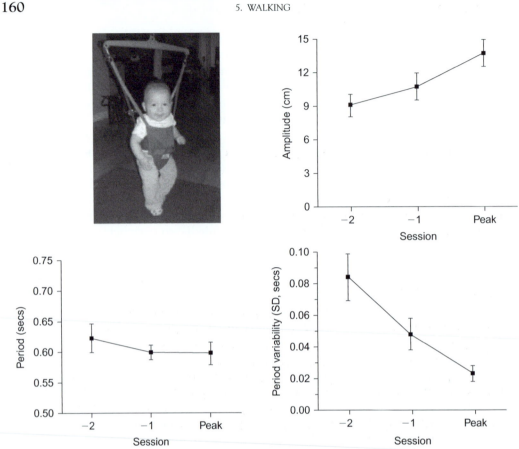

FIGURE 5.18   Jolly jumping. Top left: A baby in a jolly jumper. Top right: Jump amplitude as a function of session. Bottom left: Jump period as a function of session. Bottom right: Period variability as a function of session. Sessions defined relative to session of peak performance. Photo from http://www.decio.com/blog/uploaded_images/ruby-jumper-750342.jpg. Graphs from Goldfield, E. C., Kay, B. A., & Warren, W. H. (1993). Infant bouncing: The assembly and tuning of action systems. Child Development, 64, 1128–1142. With permission.

This way of looking at motor development has been emphasized in work by Karen Adolph (2008) and her colleagues at New York University. Focusing on the period of development when babies learn to crawl and toddle, Adolph showed, as Thelen (1995) had proposed earlier, that babies are not governed by rigidly unfolding maturational schemes. Rather, babies exhibit impressive problem-solving abilities as their bodies change, enabling them to tune their motor behavior to the affordances of the environments in which they find themselves.

Figure 5.19 illustrates this point. When confronted with a slope, babies do not invariably perform some maturationally dictated behavior. Rather, they do different things, any one of which has a reasonably good chance of getting them safely to the bottom of the slope. They may scoot down on their behinds, slide on their bellies feet first, or slide on their bellies hands first. What they do is what seems best at the time. Being able to recognize what seems best and engaging in that behavior is nontrivial. Harking back to a theme of Chapter 1,

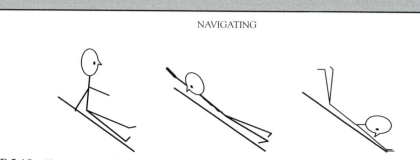

FIGURE 5.19 Three means of descending a slope. From Adolph, K. (2008). Learning to move. Current Directions in Psychological Science, 17, 213–218. With permission.

where we discussed the current state of robotics, robots cannot do anything remotely similar to babies when it comes to electing different slope-descending maneuvers. We are years away from having robots that can exhibit the same behavioral creativity that babies do.

NAVIGATING

The final topic to be covered in this chapter is navigation. Navigation can be defined as the adaptive control of whole-body motion in the external environment. Navigation depends on perception and memory as well as motor control. Perception is needed to determine the physical properties of the environment through which one moves; see, for example, Fajen and Warren (2003). Memory is needed to recall where sites are located and what kinds of actions are afforded by the objects and terrain being encountered. Motor control is needed to carry out the physical actions that are ultimately selected. In this section, we will consider the role of perception in locomotion, focusing primarily on vision. After that, we will turn to the role of memory.

Visual Kinesthesis

As you move through the environment, the pattern of light impinging on your retina (the light-sensitive portion of the back of your eye) varies. The variation varies with the layout of the visual world, with the conditions of illumination, and with the manner in which you travel. Assuming that you can normally respond to visual input remarkably well, it has been suggested, as implied earlier in this chapter, that the visual system evolved so as to respond instantly to the geometric properties of optical input (Gibson, 1950, 1966, 1979). The central idea is that the physical layout of the external environment is directly specified by the optical array emanating from it. Said another way, the light rays bouncing off objects in the external world and coming to the eye directly specify the physical properties of those objects. The visual system, in this theory, need not decipher the structure of the external world by piecing together bits of visual evidence, as some have argued. Rather, according to this theory of *ecological perception*, the optic array contains adequate information to make the structure of the external environment immediately and unambiguously apparent.

To appreciate the promise of this theoretical position, it is useful to consider David Lee's "swinging room" (Lee & Aronson, 1974; Lee & Lishman, 1975). This is not a discotheque; instead, it is a large inverted moveable box made up of four walls and a ceiling (see Figure 5.20).

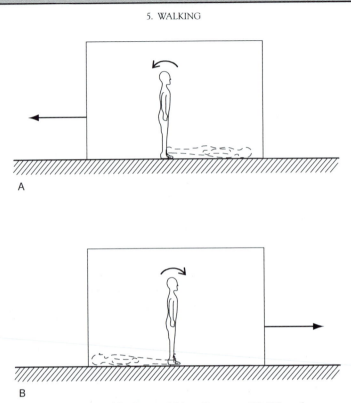

A

B

FIGURE 5.20　The swinging room used by Lee and his colleagues. (A) When the room approaches, the subject sways back to avoid falling forward. (B) When the room recedes, the subject sways forward to avoid falling
backward. From Lee, D. N. & Thomson, J. A. (1982). Vision in action: The control of locomotion. In D. J. Ingle,
M. A. Goodale, & R. J. W. Mansfield (Eds.), Analysis of visual behavior (pp. 411–433). Cambridge, MA: MIT. With
permission.

When one stands inside this contraption, the question is how the person will respond. Will s/he
stand perfectly still or will s/he sway in relation to the motion of the surroundings?

The answer is that s/he sways. Moreover, the sway correlates with the sway of the room.
When the wall approaches the subject, the subject sways backward. When the wall recedes
from the subject, the subject sways forward.

The reason subjects sway as they do can be found by considering the optical flow associated with various postural states. When the wall of the swinging room approaches, the image
of the wall on the subject's retina grows. Such an increase in retinal image size also occurs
when one falls forward. Thus, subjects sway backward when the wall approaches because
the visual input received from an approaching wall specifies forward falling, and backward
swaying counteracts this illusory fall. Similarly, when the wall of the swinging room recedes,
the image of the wall on the subject's retina shrinks, as occurs when one falls backward.
Thus, subjects sway forward when the wall recedes because the visual input received from a
receding wall specifies backward falling, and forward swaying counteracts this illusory fall.

As logical as this explanation is, it may not fully convey the immediacy and cogency
of one's perceptual experience in the swinging room. To appreciate what that perceptual

experience is like, recall your feelings when you watched a movie filmed from a descending roller coaster or from an automobile speeding around a hairpin curve. If you ever saw such a movie and can recall how you felt while watching it, you know how compelling the experience of visually induced motion can be.

Lee and his colleagues argued that the swinging room creates just this sort of perceptual experience. Going further, they argued that the body sway elicited in the swinging room illustrates several more subtle points. One is that kinesthesis (the perception of body movement) is not governed entirely within the body but can also be governed from outside through vision. To capture this idea, Lee and his colleagues, like Gibson before, used the term *visual kinesthesis*.

A second conclusion that can be drawn from the swinging room studies is that the effect of visual kinesthesis is so powerful it gives rise to overt physical responses. In the movie theater, you may feel like you are being swung around in your seat while watching a chase scene. By recording body sway, Lee and his colleagues showed that such movements actually occur.

The third point to be drawn from the swinging room research is that there is a regular relation between external input and the kinesthesis that accompanies it. One reliably sways backward or forward when the front of the room approaches or recedes, respectively, because optical flow directly provides information about the actor's interaction with the external world (Cutting, 1986; Gibson, 1950, 1966, 1978; Lee & Thomson, 1982). Thus, optic flow provides direct information about one's bearings in the environment.

It is possible to characterize in precise mathematical terms the relations between optical flow and the actor's place in the external world. According to Lee (1976), the inverse of the rate of expansion of the retinal image of an object equals the time remaining until contact is made with the object. Said more simply, if an object is approaching, its image on the retina expands, and the closer the object is to the eye, the higher the rate at which its retinal image expands (assuming constant velocity of object approach). At higher retinal image expansion rates, the less time remains until impact. The beauty of this formula is that optical information alone specifies time-to-contact. Behavioral evidence from birds (Lee & Reddish, 1981) and people (Lee, Young, Reddish, Lough, & Clayton, 1983) suggests that the visuo-motor system may in fact rely on this formula, or some analogue thereof, to regulate behaviors when time-to-contact matters.

Development of Visual Guidance

How does navigation develop? If visual input can directly specify how one is moving through the environment, one might expect very young children to rely on visual guidance during locomotion. Lee and his colleagues (Lee & Aronson, 1974; Lee & Lishman, 1975) tested this hypothesis by studying toddlers' responses to the swinging room. The result was dramatic. Unlike adults, whose body sway was somewhat amplified by the to and fro motion of the walls around them, toddlers sometimes were literally knocked off their feet when they tried to stand in the swinging room.

An implication of this result is that toddlers are sensitive to the same visual cues as adults. In fact, they may be even more sensitive, for they have less experience relying on their own proprioceptive input to control their standing behavior. Toddlers have a much harder time standing with their eyes closed than adults do. When adults try to stand on one foot or stand in an awkward posture, they sway more strongly in the swinging room than when both of their feet are planted firmly on the ground (Lee & Thomson, 1982).

Even if vision helps specify the nature of one's position in the environment, the question remains of how the ability to coordinate visual and motor information changes developmentally. Some of the most influential research on this topic has been done with animals, in part because it is possible to influence animals' experience in ways that cannot be done ethically with children.

As discussed in Chapter 2, pairs of kittens were linked to one another such that one kitten could walk freely while the other rode a small gondola that was transported through the same restricted visual environment by its partner (Held, 1965). The important feature of the experimental environment was that both kittens received essentially the same visual input, but later only the freely moving kitten displayed normal visuo-motor coordination. As discussed in Chapter 2, this result suggested that only the active kitten learned to correlate its movements ensuing visual changes. This study suggests, then, that kittens—and perhaps children—need more than movement alone or perception alone to develop normal visuo-motor coordination. They need to be able to actively correlate the two kinds of experience.

To evaluate this claim further, it is worth considering an alternative interpretation of the gondola study results. Perhaps the active kittens were simply more interested in their surroundings than the passive kittens were. Thus, the passive kittens paid less attention to their perceptual experience than the active kittens did. Several experiments discredited this hypothesis (Hein, 1974). In one, kittens were allowed to see with one eye while moving freely and to see with the other eye while being transported in the gondola. Only the eye that could see during active movement could later aid locomotion; the other eye was effectively blind. Apparently, then, each eye, or its corresponding brain region, learned on its own. If the kittens simply were more motivated when they could move freely, the sheer opportunity for free movement would have allowed both eyes to develop properly.

In another experiment, kittens wore a collar that prevented them from seeing their feet or torso. These kittens could later avoid obstacles but could not reach for objects as well as normally raised kittens. A similar result was obtained with monkeys and, in a study of pointing, with people. The results as a whole suggest that the mere opportunity to move in a lighted environment does not ensure normal visuo-motor coordination. What matters instead is the opportunity to correlate actions with accompanying perceptual changes.

MEMORY

Walking is rarely aimless. One usually walks to a goal, which is often a remembered site. Clearly, a complete understanding of walking requires a theory of spatial memory.

The history of research on spatial memory parallels the history of research on the neural control of walking. Early on, when walking was thought to be controlled by reflex chains, a number of investigators also thought there might be no spatial memory per se, only familiar sequences of ambulatory responses. The idea was that when one walked to work, for example, the first step somehow triggered the second, the second step somehow triggered the third, and so on.

Such a theory is not very satisfying. One can take a step from one's house and go to work or to any of a number of other places. Thus, a given a footstep cannot uniquely specify what other steps will follow (Lashley, 1951). If one supposes that the first step that leads to work is slightly different from the first step that leads, say, to the beach, this merely begs the question of how those minute differences arose.

Another problem with the reflex chaining account stems from the fact that it predicts that an animal's ability to get to a location will be impaired if the animal's normal actions for getting there cannot be employed. Thus, if a rat has learned to run a maze and the maze is flooded, reflex chaining predicts that the rat should be unable to swim to the spot where it previously found food. Similarly, if a rat has learned to run a maze from a fixed starting point, reflex chaining predicts that the rat should have great difficulty getting through the maze when placed in a different starting position.

Experiments on maze-running rats have disconfirmed these predictions (Tolman, 1948). Rats placed in a familiar maze but in an unfamiliar start location found their way to the usual reward location more quickly than rats placed in an unfamiliar maze. The rats also proceeded effectively to the usual goal sites of familiar mazes if the mazes were suddenly flooded, showing that they could switch to swimming to the reward site. These results argue against reflex chain theory. They also argue against any theory that suggests animals learn paths to particular locations solely in terms of the movements made to those locations. More abstract representations are needed.

Route Maps and Survey Maps

Tolman (1948) suggested that such abstract representations do in fact exist, and he was careful to distinguish between two possibilities regarding their nature. One possibility was that the representations were route maps. Such maps embody the series of locations through which one must pass to get from point A to point B. A typical route map might be described by instructions such as, "Drive down to the firehouse and make a right, then make a left at Smith's Drug Store, and then make a left at the schoolhouse."

Route maps can be contrasted with survey maps, which, like conventional cartographic representations, specify spatial relations among points of interest but not necessarily with information about the means of traveling between those points. Survey maps usually afford greater flexibility than route maps because they allow one to reach desired locations independently of the position from which one starts and independently of the means by which one travels.

That route maps are actually used was shown in some striking demonstrations of maze-running behavior in rats (Olton, 1979). After several thousand occasions in which rats ran from one point to another to get food in a maze, they passed right over the food if it was suddenly placed along the way to the familiar feeding site. Even more dramatically, if the maze had elevated arms rather than arms enclosed within walls, the rats actually ran over the ends of the arms if the normal arm extensions were suddenly removed.

People are also prone to make these sorts of errors. When one alters a habitual travel regimen (for example, driving home from work) to make an unusual detour (say, to pick up

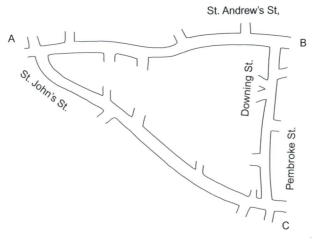

FIGURE 5.21   Map of the intersections whose angles were estimated from memory by the subjects in Moar and Bower's (1983) study. From Moar, I., & Bower, G. H. (1983). Inconsistencies in spatial knowledge. Memory & Cognition, 11, 107–113. Reprinted by permission of the Psychonomic Society, Inc.

some groceries), the detour may not always materialize (Norman, 1981). These examples show that travel from one point to another can become so automatized that a route map rather than a survey map may be used. Thus, a route map may be used not only when one is first learning the layout of an area but also when one is traversing a very familiar path.

Perhaps because survey maps are abstract, they are subject to distortion. Moar and Bower (1983) asked people in Cambridge, England to estimate, from memory, angles of three street intersections (see Figure 5.21). Although each intersection had an angle of less than 90 degrees, when the Cambridgians estimated each angle individually, they exhibited a strong bias towards 90 degrees. This outcome suggests that all three intersections could not have been represented in a single survey map, for if they had been, they would have formed an impossible triangle. Moar and Bower hypothesized that subjects maintained separate representations of the intersections in their memories. The maps were connected through some overarching scheme that did not explicitly or accurately represent their spatial relations.

Memory and Feedback

The subjects in Moar and Bower's (1983) study may have misrepresented street intersections in memory, but they clearly did not fall off the sidewalk when actually turning street corners. The perceptual input one receives while moving through the environment helps one adjust the detailed characteristics of one's movements and probably also helps one update one's spatial memory. There has been relatively little research on this important topic, although some of the studies that have been done provide some useful information about it.

Lee, Lishman, and Thomson (1982) filmed long jumpers as the jumpers ran toward the spot from which the jump was executed (the jump board). The variability of step

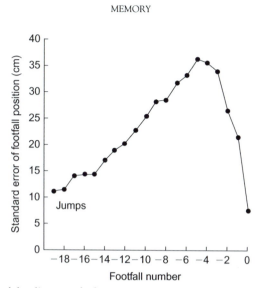

FIGURE 5.22 Variability of the distance of a long jumper's footfalls as a function of number of footfalls from the jump board (footfall number 0). From Lee, D.N., Lishman, J.R. & Thomson, J. (1982). Regulation of gait in long jumping. *Journal of Experimental Psychology*, 8, 448–459. Copyright © 1982 by the American Psychological Association. Reprinted by permission.

positions was small in the early part of the run, increased dramatically, and then returned to a small value around the launch point (see Figure 5.22). A plausible interpretation of this result is that the jumpers first ran in a routine fashion, effectively being impervious to the detailed characteristics of the visual feedback they received. Then they relied on visual feedback to adjust the positions of their feet. This adjustment phase allowed them finally to get their feet into the stereotyped positions needed for effective jumps. By this account, the jumpers did not rely exclusively on memory or on visual feedback, but instead, as they ran down the runway, they shifted from one mode of control (memory) to another (visual feedback). This example illustrates how locomotion, though it is fundamental to motor activity, depends on a complex interplay of memory, perception, and motor commands.

Further support for this conclusion comes from research on a less specialized form of locomotion, the simple act of walking itself. One would expect walking to be slower in cluttered environments than in uncluttered environments. With rocks or rubble in the road, one must mind one's step. But if one's walking is slower on a cluttered path than on an uncluttered path, this could be due to perception, cognition (decision making), or changes in walking itself.

To the best of the author's knowledge, no systematic research has been done to systematically assess the relative contribution of these three variables. One reason may be that relatively few investigators with a cognitive bent have studied the control of locomotion. For many such researchers, the study of locomotion, and indeed, the study of human motor control, may seem beneath them, perhaps because they see their research as being about intellectual activities rather than the activities of blue-collar workers, or perhaps because, like philosophers of mind over the centuries, they see their task as one that involves understanding how we come to know the world, in which case *perception* seems to be the thing to study, not physical action, though physical action reveals what we know just as assuredly as perception does (Rosenbaum, 2005).

Some research, however, has demonstrated that there is a clear cognitive contribution to the control of walking. Several studies have shown that walking is slowed or made more variable by simultaneously carrying out mental arithmetic tasks (Hausdorff, Balash, & Giladi, 2003; Mulder, Berndt, Pauwels, & Nienhuis, 1993) or word generation tasks (Haggard, Cockburn, Cock, Fordham, & Wade, 2000). These studies have all used visually guided walking through the environment, so the combined effects of dealing with the terrain, dealing with one's movements, and dealing with heightened cognitive challenges were not teased apart.

An obvious way to evaluate the interactions of cognition and walking control per se is to perform the simple experiment of asking how mental arithmetic performance (e.g., subtracting by 7's) or word generation is affected by walking on a treadmill or riding a stationary bike. Such a study would help determine whether the slowing of walking that accompanies mental arithmetic is due to difficulties with visuo-spatial processing or difficulties with movement control. If the difficulties are due to visuo-spatial processing, mental arithmetic or word generation should be no slower or more variable if they are done while sitting still or while using a treadmill or stationary bike. Likewise, using a treadmill or stationary bike should be no slower or more variable if they are carried out with extra cognitive tasks added to them. On the other hand, if the locus of the interference is in movement control per se, using a treadmill or stationary bike should be adversely affected by the addition of cognitive challenges. It would be surprising if mental arithmetic or word generation interferes with merely moving one's legs, just as it would be surprising if merely moving one's legs interfered with mental arithmetic or word generation. Future experiments can reveal whether the actual outcome will be surprising or not.

SUMMARY

1. Walking and other forms of locomotion are innate, yet different gaits can be adopted in response to sensory input and internal decisions. These observations invite three questions: What neural mechanisms underlie basic ambulatory patterns? How is locomotion influenced by sensory feedback? What is the role of high-level (brain) control?
2. Distinct gait patterns characterize different locomotion speeds. The reason for the switch from walking to running as one speeds up can be traced to the fact that walking is a series of controlled *falls* whereas running is a series of controlled *leaps*. Walking faster than about 2.5 m/s would require one to fall more quickly than gravity allows.
3. Gait patterns are so regular that it is possible to visually recognize walking patterns when only a few lights, affixed to walkers' joints, are visible. One regularity of gait is that the step cycle of each leg is made up of a stance phase, whose duration varies with gait, and a swing phase, whose duration is roughly constant. There are also typical time-varying changes in the angles of the knee and hip that are easily seen in angle-angle diagrams and that can be used for diagnosing gait disorders and their treatment.

4. Rhythmic activity of the leg muscles can occur in cats whose spinal cords are disconnected from the brain, implying that the brain is unnecessary for the generation of basic walking patterns. When sensory feedback to the spinal cord is also eliminated and the leg muscles are prevented from moving, the spinal cord still displays rhythmic activity of the sort underlying locomotion, suggesting that the spinal cord has central pattern generators. This suggestion has been confirmed with fictive locomotion, where the spinal cord is isolated and its endogenous neural activity is recorded from the ventral roots.

5. Although locomotion relies on central pattern generators, it is also affected by sensory feedback. The timing of walking movements differs when sensory feedback is present or absent. In addition, the same sensory input has different effects on behavior depending on when it occurs in the step cycle. These effects have been explored both in behavioral experiments and in theoretical neural network modeling work.

6. Further evidence that sensory feedback modulates central pattern generators comes from disruptions in walking when sensory feedback is disrupted, as in tabes dorsalis (a disease of the dorsal roots of the spinal cord), in "spinal" animals (animals whose spinal cords have been separated from the brain), and in fictive locomotion (where the spinal cord is surgically isolated and internal neural activity is recorded). Additionally, bilateral removal of sensory afferents relevant to locomotion does not disrupt the main features of locomotion, though the grace of locomotion is impaired.

7. Not only does sensory feedback affect the expression of central pattern generators;, but ccentral pattern generators also affect how sensory feedback is responded to. Different responses are made to the same feedback depending on the phase of locomotion when the feedback is delivered.

8. The brain modulates reflex responses to postural disturbances. This has been shown by studying responses to shifts of a platform on which people stand. The stretch reflex of the gastrocnemius muscle can be attenuated when this reflex destabilizes the body in this experimental context. The ability to attenuate the reflex is impaired in patients with vestibular damage.

9. Structures in the brain also help govern transitions from one gait pattern to another. Varying the intensity of stimulation in the brain stem helps produce different gait patterns. The cortico-spinal tract is also active during stepping movements requiring precise visuo-motor coordination. Because many of the same brain sites are also active during visually guided manual reaching, it appears that locomotion and reaching share common control mechanisms. In general, the brain modulates spinal cord activity.

10. The role of the brain in tuning spinal cord activity is further demonstrated through anticipatory postural adjustments, or APAs. These arise when one expects a perturbing force or torque. APAs are typically manifested as increases in the activity of leg and trunk muscles that stabilize the body.

11. By drawing on information about the kinematics and physiology of biological locomotion, scientists have developed machines that can walk. In devising such devices, scientists have found it useful to articulate the conditions that all walking system must satisfy. Among these are the need to maintain stability and the need to prevent collisions among the legs. An insight that has emerged from the design of artificial walking systems is that the complexity of locomotion control can be reduced

by exploiting the physical properties of the walking system. Recent advances in robotics have been made possible by designing robots that rely on *preflexes* (mechanically given responses to perturbations) as well as reflexes.

12. Babies exhibit a number of triggered behaviors or "reflexes." These include the startle reflex, the tonic neck reflex, the righting reflex, the grasp reflex, the Babinski reflex, the crawling reflex, the swimming reflex, and the stepping reflex.

13. The stepping reflex is present in newborns but usually disappears by around 4 weeks of age, only to reappear at 8 months to 1 year. The reasons for the disappearance and reappearance of stepping in infants have been debated. One explanation is that the reappearance of stepping coincides with, and is dependent on, the emergence of cognitive sequencing skills. Another explanation is that stepping is temporarily absent for physical reasons only, having to do with the size of the body and the relative weakness of the legs. The physical explanation appears to be correct. A lesson learned from this outcome is that it is useful to attend to physical causes of behavior as well as, and generally before, attending to psychological causes.

14. Four principles provide a useful way of conceptualizing motor development. One is that nerve fibers become myelinated. The second is that cortical centers inhibit subcortical centers. The third is that development proceeds in a cephalo-caudal (head-tail) and proximal-distal (medial-peripheral) direction. The fourth is that active exploration exposes babies to ever-richer behavioral possibilities.

15. Babies in jolly jumpers learn to exploit the mechanics of the jolly jumper system, thereby engaging in active exploration. The same can be said of babies who use a variety of behavioral strategies for descending slopes. These abilities reveal physical problem-solving skills that modern robots cannot yet emulate.

16. One of the main challenges in locomotion is to respond adaptively to visual information about the surroundings. Responses to visual information may be based on properties of the optical flow to which one is exposed. A dramatic demonstration favoring this hypothesis is that body sway can be induced by having a subject stand in a room with a stable floor and moving walls. The observed body sway is closely related to the sway of the room, giving rise to the proposition that vision and kinesthesis are so closely interwoven that one can speak meaningfully of *visual kinesthesis*. An example of the potential informativeness of visual kinesthesis is the relation between the rate of expansion of the retinal image of an object and the time to contact the object.

17. During development, the ability to respond adaptively to visual input depends on the opportunity to actively correlate perceptions with actions.

18. In addition to perception, memory for the environment is also important for control of navigation. It is unlikely that internal maps of the surroundings reduce to memorized sequences of muscle movements, for it is possible to get to a target location in a familiar area from a variety of starting positions and through unfamiliar means (for example, swimming in a suddenly flooded maze).

19. When possible, people develop abstract spatial maps (survey maps) of their surroundings. In learning about a new place, however, or in covering the same path many times, people may rely on a less abstract map that embodies the procedures to be followed to get from one location to another (a route map).

20. Perception and memory are used together to govern navigation. For example, long jumpers begin their run toward the jump board in a stereotyped fashion, without responding to detailed aspects of visual input, but as they approach the board, they modify their steps based on visual feedback. Walking also turns out to be slower and more variable when people are engaged in simultaneous cognitive tasks than when they are not. Whether the source of this interaction is cognition, perception, or muscle control has not been sorted out.

Further Reading

This chapter mentioned classic work by Taub and Berman (1968) which showed that monkeys would be more likely to use a deafferented limb if the other limb was a deafferented limb than if the other limb was not deafferented. It was as if the monkey preferred to use the one limb that had afferent return. A clinical implication of this finding is that patients with difficulty moving a limb might also be led to use that limb if the "good" limb were prevented from moving, for example, by tying it, with the patient's permission, in a sling. For a review of this constraint-induced approach to rehabilitation, see Taub and Uswatt (2006).

The coordination of walking and looking has received some attention (Patla & Vickers, 1997).

A classic study of the visual perception of affordances for stepping on stairs that varied in height was reported by Warren (1984).

For research on mental imagery of walking, see Decety and Jeannerod (1995) and Stevens (2005).

For information about a recently studied problem-solving task for walking, namely, learning to walk on two treadmills at once, one for the left foot and one for the right foot, see Choi and Bastian (2007) and Miall (2007).

For information on the role of audition in walking, particularly for the blind, see Strelow (1985).

Walking on a moving treadway, as occurs at an airport, puts you in a novel state. The relation between your rate of locomotion and the rate of optic flow departs from normal. You quickly adapt to this change and readapt to the normal relation when you step off the treadway. Such adaptation has been studied by Rieser, Pick, Ashmead, and Garing (1995).

Very light touch on a stable surface has a remarkably strong stabilizing effect. Just being able to lightly touch a stable, flat surface greatly reduces the amount of sway that people exhibit, even when their eyes are closed and they are standing on one foot (Jeka & Lackner, 1994).

For a summary of early neuroscience research on the representation of space in the brain, including the discovery of "place cells" in the hippocampus, see O'Keefe and Nadel (1978). For recent work suggesting that place cells fire before animals (rats) go to places corresponding to those places' cells, see Johnson and Redish (2007) and Heyman (2007).

For work on the development of spatial cognition in children, see Newcombe and Huttenlocher (2003).

Advanced statistical techniques have shed light on subtle influences of cognitive states and other variables on walking rate. This work, pioneered by Hausdorff (2007), is also mentioned in Chapter 12.

For videos of wind-driven or string-drawn beach walkers, go to http://www.youtube.com/watch?v=4ZK4V2YUA5U or http://www.strandbeest.com/.

A journal in which walking and related tasks are featured prominently is *Gait and Posture*.

For more coverage of disorders of gait and balance and the treatment of those disorders, see Shumway-Cook and Woollacott (2006).

6

Looking

Blinking	174	**Smooth Pursuit Movements**	194
		Optokinetic Nystagmus	*195*
Accommodation	177	*Vestibular-Oculo-Motor Reflex*	*197*
Pupil Constriction and Dilation	177	**Vergence Movements**	200
General Features of Eye Movements	179	**Eye Movements and Space Constancy**	201
Why Moveable Eyes?	*179*		
Physical Dynamics	*180*		
Activation of the Extra-Ocular Muscles	*182*	**Development and Plasticity of Oculo-Motor Control**	205
Conjugate and Disjunctive Eye Movements	*184*	**Summary**	206
Miniature Eye Movements	*184*		
Saccades	187	**Further Reading**	209
Saccadic Suppression	*191*		
Saccades and Attention	*192*		

To see, you must be able to move your eyes. Eye movement control is one of the most extensively studied topics in human motor control. This is to be expected since vision is arguably the most important sense for humans. Because eye movements are usually unaffected by external, mechanical disturbances, they are also quite faithful to the motor signals that drive them, making them ideal for motor control research.

Looking involves several subsystems. Some rotate the eyeball; others do not. The oculomotor (eye movement) activities in which the eyes do not rotate are blinking, accommodation (changing the focal length of the lens), and pupillary responses (regulating the size of the opening through which light enters the eye). The activities in which the eyes do rotate include saccades (the eye "jumps" that occur in tasks such as reading), pursuit movements (which occur when you visually track a smoothly moving target), and nystagmus (which occurs when your eyes alternate between pursuit movements and saccades—for example, when you look out the window of a moving train). Eye movements of the latter kind are conjugate; they turn the eyes in the same direction. By contrast, vergence movements carry the eyes in opposite directions and so are disjunctive. Vergence movements occur when you shift your gaze between near and far objects or when you visually track an object, such as your fingertip, as it moves toward or away from your face.

In this chapter we will review some of the important features of these oculo-motor activities. We will consider how each activity is triggered and what its main characteristics are. An important question we will also consider is how the activities are coordinated with one another and with movements of the head. The relation between perception and eye movements is another central issue in the analysis of oculo-motor control. It too will see its way into the discussion.

BLINKING

We begin with one of the oculo-motor activities in which the eyeball does not rotate: blinking. Blinking moistens the front surface of the eye or cornea (see Figure 6.1). Blinking also protects the eye against approaching objects. The protective function of blinking is

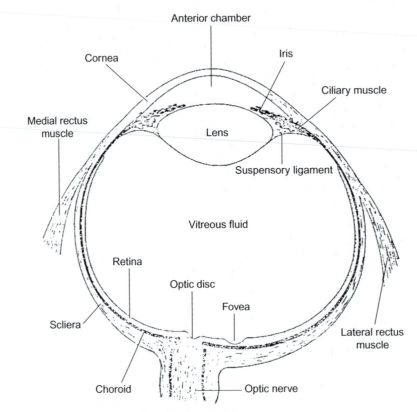

FIGURE 6.1   Cross section of the eye. From Kaufman (1984).

manifested in another way as well. Blinks often occur reflexively when people are exposed to loud, unexpected noises.

A great deal of research has been done on conditioning of the eyeblink. In these experiments, the subject (human or animal) learns to associate an arbitrary stimulus, such as a tone, with a stimulus that automatically elicits a blink, such as a puff of air directed to the open eye. After repeated pairing of the tone (the conditioned stimulus) with the airpuff (the unconditioned stimulus), the subject learns to blink as soon as the tone is presented. Cells in the cerebellum may underlie conditioning of the eyeblink response, at least in rabbits (McCormick & Thompson, 1984). The discovery of these cells has been taken to suggest that some memories may be localized within the mammalian brain.

Acquisition of eyeblink conditioning is not only a low-level process; it can also be learned vicariously. Subjects who watched a videotape of a person in an eyeblink conditioning experiment acted later as if they themselves had been conditioned (Bernal & Berger, 1976). This outcome suggests that responses can be learned without actually being performed—so-called observational learning (Bandura, 1986). In addition, this outcome demonstrates that although blinks can occur automatically or reflexively, they can also be controlled consciously. We can blink at will or blink with one eye (winking). The capacity to control movements automatically on the one hand or deliberately on the other is an important feature of motor control in general. To name just two other motor activities that can be controlled through either method, breathing can go on without attention or with considerable conscious control, as when one inhales for a doctor listening to one's lungs. Similarly, one can deliberately feign a limp, though walking is normally done automatically.

Rates of blinking and the times at which blinks occur indicate one's cognitive state. President Richard Nixon, in his first nationally televised news conference after the Watergate break-in, tried to indicate through his words and tone of voice that his administration had done no wrong. His blinks suggested he knew otherwise. Nixon blinked at a rate of 30 to 40 times a minute. People at ease blink at rates of 10 to 20 times a minute (Vogel, 1989).

That blink rates increase with anxiety has been known since the 1920s, when two investigators secretly counted the blink rates of witnesses in a courtroom. Witnesses under stress blinked at higher rates than witnesses with no cause for worry (Vogel, 1989). More recently, electronic recording techniques have shown that people withhold blinks when taking in vital information—for example, when flying aircrafts in especially perilous circumstances—but they blink more often or for longer durations when they are highly stressed or fatigued. A practical consequence of these observations is that the automatic monitoring of eyeblinks may help provide information about the alertness of individuals involved in activities such as driving cars, flying planes, or monitoring nuclear power plants.

When blinks occur, the eyelids block the view of the external environment. At such times, we do not see the world darken. The darkening is not too quick to be seen, for people can detect the dimming of a light that is shorter than the blink of an eye (about 200 ms). Volkmann, Riggs, and Moore (1980) hypothesized that when an eyeblink is initiated, activity within the central nervous system reduces sensitivity to visual changes. To test this hypothesis, they introduced an optic light fiber through the roof of the mouth and illuminated the fiber at different times relative to the subject's eyeblink. The rationale for the procedure was that some light from the optic fiber would strike the back of the eye and so would be visible as a result of retinal stimulation. It would be harder to make inferences about sensitivity to

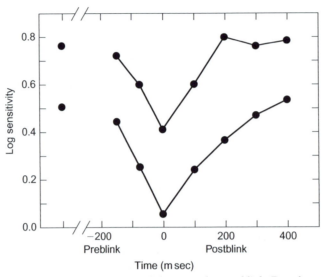

FIGURE 6.2   Reduction in visual sensitivity around the time of an eyeblink. Data from two subjects. Adapted from Volkmann, Riggs, and Moore (1980).

changes in illumination if the light were delivered to the front of the eye and the lids closed for, of course, sensitivity to light would then be reduced. The question Volkmann, Riggs, and Moore sought to answer was whether the light would be less detectable around the time of the blink.

As seen in Figure 6.2, sensitivity to the light decreased during the blink as well as just before and after it. Since the light was not perceived through the eyelids, the change in sensitivity was not due to blockage of the light by the lids. Furthermore, because sensitivity declined before the eyeblink, the change was unlikely to have been caused by peripheral feedback from the lids or the areas around the eyes touched by the lids. Volkmann, Riggs, and Moore (1980) suggested that the drop in visual sensitivity was related to the central generation of the eyeblink command. Their explanation is similar to one given in Chapter 2 for the perceived stability of the visual world during self-induced visual motion: Corollary discharge from a motor center to a perceptual center indicates that a change in stimulation is about to occur, and when the actual change in stimulation arrives, it can be recognized as having stemmed from the movement. In the case of blinking, the center responsible for triggering blinks can tell the perceptual center responsible for monitoring the brightness of the external environment that sudden darkening can be discounted.

As appealing as this idea may be, another possibility must also be taken seriously—namely, that subjects in the study of Volkmann, Riggs, and Moore (1980) sometimes made saccadic eye movements when they blinked, and these eye movements, or the central neural changes associated with them, reduced subjects' visual sensitivity. Saccades occur during blinks (Collewijn, van der Steen, & Steinman, 1985) Because blinks and saccades co-occur, some investigators are not yet convinced that a central suppression mechanism, specifically associated with blinking, needs to be postulated (E. Kowler, personal communication).

ACCOMMODATION

Blinking is one oculo-motor activity that does not, by itself, cause rotation of the eyeball. Accommodation is another. Accommodation is a change in the curvature of the lens of the eye (see Figure 6.1). Accommodation is typically triggered by the sense that an image is out of focus. That sense of blurriness is detected in the visual cortex. Following the detection of blurriness, neural signals are sent from the visual cortex to the third cranial nerve (the oculo-motor nerve), which in turn sends commands to muscles within the eye. These muscles (called ciliary muscles) act on the lens via tiny fibers (zonular fibers). When the ciliary muscles contract, they tug on the zonular fibers, which in turn pull on the lens, stretching it and reducing its curvature. The reduced curvature allows for focusing on distant objects. When the ciliary muscles relax, the lens becomes rounder, and one can focus more easily on nearby objects (Gouras, 1985b). HERE

The lens' ability to regain curvature when the ciliary muscles relax depends on the elastic property of the lens itself. The elasticity of the lens declines with age. Consequently, as people age they are more likely to require glasses. Detailed studies of the histology and biochemistry of the lens and zonular fibers suggest that a number factors cause the age-related decline in lens elasticity (Koretz & Handelman, 1989).

PUPIL CONSTRICTION AND DILATION

When the eye is exposed to bright light, the pupil constricts reflexively, limiting the amount of light that reaches the retina. By contrast, when less light comes to the eye, the pupil dilates reflexively, allowing more light to enter the eye. Pupillary responses are achieved by changing the contraction of the iris (see Figure 6.1). When bright light is directed to just one eye, pupil constriction occurs in the other eye as well. The absence of this consensual reaction in the other eye can be a sign of syphilis (Gouras, 1985b).

Although pupil responses are reflexively controlled, pupil diameter also reflects voluntary states, especially the mental effort expended on a task (Beatty, 1982). Generally, the greater the mental effort, the greater the pupil diameter. For example, when people attempt to memorize strings of aurally presented digits, their pupils enlarge with the presentation of each additional digit (Figure 6.3). Later, when the same people are asked to recall the digits, their pupils first enlarge and then decrease steadily as each digit is recalled (Kahneman & Beatty, 1966).

In a more recent study of the relation between pupil diameter and mental states, Einhauser, Stout, Koch, and Carter (2008) found that pupil dilation changes just before spontaneous perceptual reversals of the Necker cube (Figure 6.4). The Necker cube is the wire frame cube, or its depiction, that seems to spontaneously flip orientation when one views it continuously. First one face seems closest, then the opposite face seems closest, then the first-in-the-front face comes back to the front, and so on. As long as there are insufficient cues to tell how the wire frame is actually oriented, the reversals may continue indefinitely. Einhauser, Stout, Koch, and Carter (2008) discovered that pupil diameter presages these perceived switches.

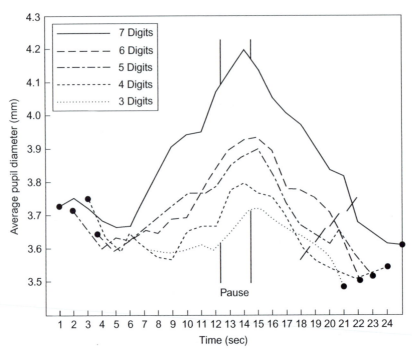

FIGURE 6.3 Changes in the diameter of the pupil during presentation and recall of digit lists containing three to seven digits. Recall begins after the pause. From Kahneman and Beatty (1966).

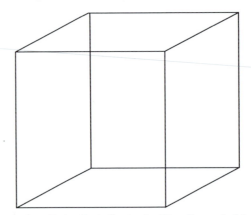

FIGURE 6.4 The Necker cube. From http://upload.wikimedia.org/wikipedia/commons/thumb/e/e7/Necker_cube.svg/400px-Necker_cube.svg.png.

In general, wide pupil diameters are associated with a high degree of interest, whereas narrow pupil diameters are associated with a lower degree of interest. This may explain why candlelight is used in romantic settings. In the dim illumination of candlelight, pupils dilate, conveying the impression that one is interested in one's date. Consistent with this interpretation, people portrayed in photographs are perceived as being more friendly and interesting when their eyes are dilated than when their pupils are constricted (Hess, 1975).

GENERAL FEATURES OF EYE MOVEMENTS

As seen in Figure 6.1, the back of the eyeball has a light-sensitive area called the retina. Near the center of the retina is a small area called the fovea, which is specialized for color perception and fine pattern discrimination. All the eye movement activities to be discussed below bring images of interest onto the fovea. Most eye movements bring or keep images of interest onto the fovea.

Why Moveable Eyes?

Why do our eyes move at all? Why don't we have a very large fovea or even compound eyes like insects (Figure 6.5)? Considering this possibility is more than the stuff of science fiction. It helps explain the role of eye movements in perception.

Tracing nerve projections from different parts of the retina to the visual processing areas of the brain, one finds that much more brain tissue is devoted to the processing of images

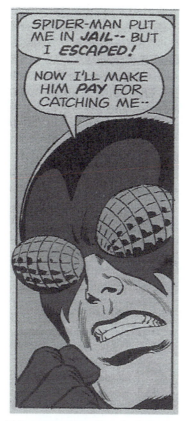

FIGURE 6.5 Eye movements would be unnecessary if we had compound eyes, to those of "Fly Man." From Stan Lee presents: Spidey Super Stories, Electric Company Magazine, June 1986, No. 125, p. 26. Children's Television Workshop.

cast on the fovea than to the processing of images cast on nonfoveal areas. If we had larger foveas, we would need massive enlargements of associated visual processing areas of the brain. Assuming that economizing on brain space is an important evolutionary principle, it was more economical to have minutely foveated, moveable eyes than to have massively foveated, immoveable eyes. This is speculation, of course. To the extent the speculation is correct, one may infer from it that the neural machinery responsible for eye movements is compact and, by implication, that the control of eye movements is achieved in a simple fashion.

Physical Dynamics

The eye rotates in three dimensions: horizontally, vertically, and torsionally (i.e., clockwise or counterclockwise with respect to the depth axis of the eyeball). Three pairs of extra-ocular muscles move the eyeball in these three dimensions (Figure 6.6). One pair, the lateral rectus and medial rectus, is mainly responsible for horizontal movements. Another pair, the superior rectus and inferior rectus, is mainly responsible for vertical movements. A third pair, the inferior oblique and superior oblique, is mainly responsible for torsional movements. Usually, in any given eye movement, the extra-ocular muscles from more than one pair of muscles are active simultaneously. This allows the eye to turn in more than one dimension at a time.

In the 1800s, the Dutch physiologist Franciscus Cornelius Donders (1818–1889) proposed that the position of the eyeball in the eye socket is fixed for any given gaze direction (Figure 6.7). Thus, for any given gaze direction, there is a unique pitch, roll, and yaw of the eyeball in the socket (see Fetter, Misslisch, & Tweed, 1997). This proposed relation has been largely confirmed and has come to be called *Donders' law*.

One can go a step further and ask about the set of eyeball positions associated with different gaze directions. Are the associations between eyeball positions and gaze directions

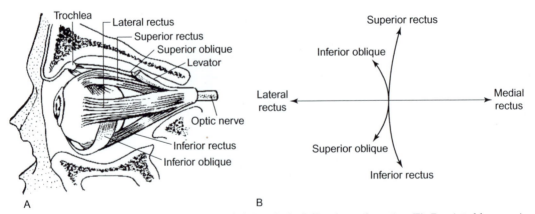

FIGURE 6.6 The extra-ocular muscles (A) and their principal directions of rotation (B). Reprinted by permission of the publisher from Gouras, P. (1985). Oculomotor system. In E. R. Kandel & J. H. Schwartz (Eds.), Principles of neural science (Second Ed.) (pp. 571–583). New York: Elsevier. Copyright © 1985 by Elsevier Science Publishing Co., Inc.

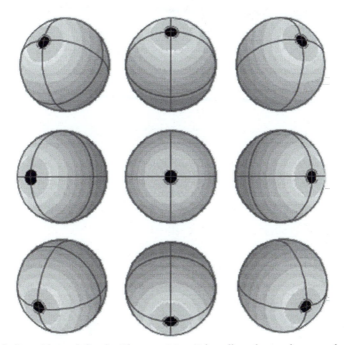

FIGURE 6.7 Eyeball positions, defined with respect to pitch, roll, and yaw, for several gaze directions. The claim that there is a unique eyeball position for each gaze direction is known as Donders' law. Listing's law states that the rotation axes of the eyeball corresponding to all possible gaze directions lie on a single plane. From http://schorlab.berkeley.edu/vilis/whatis.htm.

haphazard or systematic? As one might expect, the relation is systematic. Slight changes in pitch, roll, or yaw yield slight changes in gaze direction. Furthermore, if one plots each gaze direction's pitch, roll, and yaw in a three-dimensional space whose axes are, again, pitch, roll, and yaw, the eyeball position for a given gaze direction can be represented as a point in this 3-space. It turns out that the points in the 3-space for all gaze directions lie on a single plane, called *Listing's plane* (Fetter, Misslisch, & Tweed, 1997). The properties of Listing's plane for each eye provide a way of characterizing oculo-motor abnormalities in the individual for whom such a plane is constructed. One such abnormality is *strabismus*. Here the resting gaze directions of the two eyes are significantly different from parallel.

Donders' law and Listing's plane are thought to have neural rather than mechanical underpinnings. One reason is that in ophthalmic conditions like strabismus, there appears to be nothing wrong with the eye muscles themselves. A second reason is that instantaneous eyeball positions during saccades from one gaze direction to another often bring the eyeball to positions that momentarily depart from Listing's plane. A third reason is that observers' states of mind can affect torsion angles, as shown in a study by Pashler, Ramachandran, and Becker (2006). These investigators asked observers to pay attention to tilted words. The participants' eyeball torsion angles changed as a function of the tilt (Figure 6.8), a result that violates Donders' law.

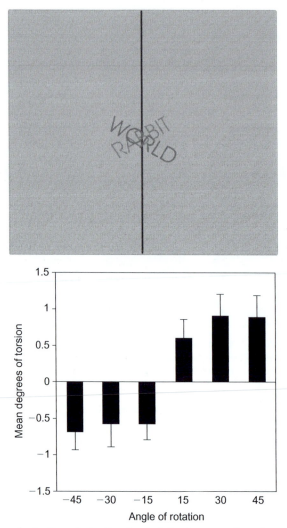

FIGURE 6.8 Tilted words to be selectively attended to (top panel) and mean eyeball torsion angle as a function of angle of word rotation (degrees). From Pashler, H., Ramachandran, V. S., & Becker, M. (2006). *Psychonomic Bulletin & Review*, 13, 954–957. From http://repositories.cdlib.org/cgi/viewcontent.cgi?article = 5988&context = postprints

Activation of the Extra-Ocular Muscles

As seen in Figure 6.6, three pairs of extra-ocular muscles move the eyeball. These muscles are directly innervated by three cranial nerves—the oculo-motor nerve, the trochlear nerve, and the abducens nerve. These nerves emanate from oculo-motor nuclei in the brain stem (Gouras, 1985a). The motor neurons innervating the extra-ocular muscles fire at higher frequencies and over a wider range of frequencies (100–600 impulses/s) than spinal motor neurons (50–100 impulses/s).

Because each oculo-motor neuron has a distinct threshold for continuous firing, additional oculo-motor neurons can be recruited by increasing the activation level of the neuronal pool in which they reside. As more of the neurons are activated, the tension of the extra-ocular muscles increases and the eye's angular deviation from the straight ahead (the eye's eccentricity) increases. Gradually increasing the tension of the extra-ocular muscles appears to be the primary method for generating saccades less than 10–15 degrees (Abrams, Meyer, & Kornblum, 1989; Robinson, 1981). For saccades greater than 10–15 degrees, amplitudes are varied by regulating the time the agonists remain maximally active. Longer periods of activation are associated with larger saccadic excursions (Bahill & Stark, 1979).

These conclusions have been reached by studying peak velocity of the eye as a function of distance covered. The velocity of the eye can be recorded through several techniques, one of which is to mount photodiodes on frames worn by the subject. The photodiodes point toward the eye and detect light reflected from the eye's surface. The amount of light depends on where the eye is pointing, because when the eye rotates, the relative positions of the dark iris and lighter sclera change (see Figure 6.1). Through such recording techniques, which are harmless, it has been found that saccade peak velocities generally increase with saccade amplitudes, reaching a maximum at around 10–15 degrees (Figure 6.9).

This relation has been mathematically reproduced through a model of oculo-motor control that assumes, among other things, that amplitudes of saccades greater than 10–15 degrees are varied by adjusting the durations of commands for maximally activated agonists, whereas amplitudes of saccades less than 10–15 degrees are varied by adjusting durations as well as magnitudes of agonist activation levels (Bahill & Stark, 1979). Holding the eye at the target is achieved by setting the tensions of the agonists and antagonists so they balance out at the target position and by timing the onset of the antagonist activity so it promotes maintenance of the target position at the appropriate times.

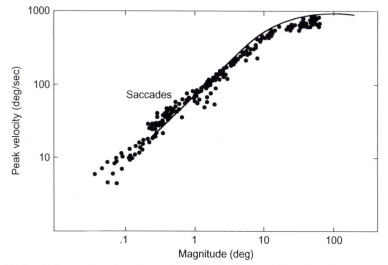

FIGURE 6.9 Peak velocity as a function of saccade amplitude. From Bahill and Stark (1979).

An important feature of this method of control is that it has distinct components—timing control, force control, and mechanical elements such as damping associated with the viscosity of the eye in the socket. Each component can by affected by fatigue or pathology, giving rise to distinct forms of eye movement disturbances. For example, when people are fatigued, they have an increased tendency to display a form of eye movement pattern called glissadic overshoot. Here the eye overshoots a target and then drifts back toward it. Glissadic overshoot can be simulated by assuming that the holding position for the eye is set correctly, but the signal that propels the eye toward the target is set incorrectly.

Even when people are not fatigued, they display variability in the characteristics of their eye movements. The nature of this variability supports the assumption that force and timing are distinct parameters for eye movement control (Abrams, Meyer, & Kornblum, 1989). A similar proposal has been made for hand movements (Keele & Ivry, 1987).

Conjugate and Disjunctive Eye Movements

The two eyes almost always move together. They can move either in the same direction (conjugate movements) or in opposite directions (disjunctive movements). Conjugate movements occur when you visually track an object moving across the visual field or when you select a new object to foveate. Disjunctive movements occur when you visually track an approaching or receding object. Because the eyes can move either in the same direction (conjugate movements) or in opposite directions (disjunctive movements), it follows that any given pair of extra-ocular muscles can play an antagonistic or agonistic role in eye displacement. For example, the medial rectus muscles of the two eyes are antagonists in conjugate movements but agonists in disjunctive movements. Given these two possibilities, the eye movement system must switch between mutual inhibition and mutual excitation of pairs of extra-ocular muscles depending on the oculo-motor task.

Miniature Eye Movements

Let us now consider the subsystems that physically rotate the eye. We begin with miniature eye movements. These are only observable through special recording techniques such as the photodiode recording system discussed above or through careful perceptual experiments such as the one illustrated in Figure 6.10.

There are three types of miniature eye movements (Ciuffreda & Tannen, 1995). As seen in Figure 6.11, one is tremor, which can be thought of as random jitter. The amplitude of tremor is miniscule, less in fact than the diameter of a single visual cone. Tremor frequency is high, around 90 Hz (90 cycles per second). The tremor of one eye is essentially independent of the tremor of the other eye (Carpenter, 1977).

Another class of miniature eye movement is drift. Drifts are slow, covering about 1/60th of a degree of arc per second. Drifts can cover as much as 5/60th of a degree of arc before being terminated (Ditchburn, 1973). One degree of arc is approximately equal to the width of your thumbnail when viewed at arm's length. Drifts bring the fovea toward targets to be looked at and therefore can serve a visual corrective function (Steinman, Haddad, Skavenski, & Wyman, 1973).

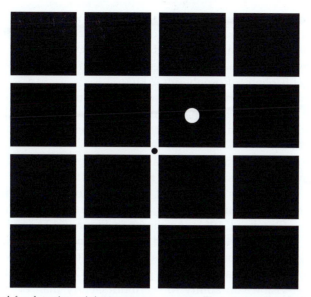

FIGURE 6.10 Method for detecting miniature eye movements. First stare at the black dot in the center of the array for at least 20 seconds. Then stare at the center of the white circle. The afterimage of the array will move with your eye as it undergoes miniature movements. The interactions of the vertical and horizontal contours make the miniature movements apparent. Such interactions are the basis of many illusory effects in "op" art, popular in the 1960's. From Carpenter (1977). Reprinted by permission of Pion Ltd.

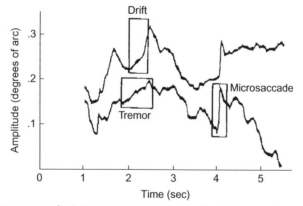

FIGURE 6.11 The three types of miniature eye movements, reflected in simultaneous recordings of the left and right eye (the two curves). Tremor is a series of high-frequency, small-amplitude displacements. Drift is a relatively slow, larger-amplitude displacement. Microsaccades are rapid, relatively large displacements of the two eyes together. From Carpenter (1977). Reprinted by permission of Pion Ltd.

A third class of miniature eye movements is microsaccades. These very small saccades are conjugate (parallel in the two eyes) and may serve a corrective function, bringing the fovea back toward a fixation target from which the eye has drifted, though on occasion they may also take the eye away from the target. Microsaccades differ from drifts and tremors in that they are influenced by volitional factors such as the amount of attention being paid to a task. Thus, after a visual cue is presented, indicating where a visual target is likely to appear, there is an increase in the likelihood of microsaccades in the direction of the cued target (Engbert & Kliegl, 2003; Laubrock, Engbert & Kliegl, 2005, 2007). Analogous tendencies have been observed for the hand when people point to targets, knowing they will soon point to another target (Cohen & Rosenbaum, 2007).

It has been suggested that microsaccades and saccades are members of a single functional category. In support of this suggestion, when peak velocity is plotted against amplitude (Figure 6.9), points for microsaccades and saccades fall equally close to the same best-fitting line (Zuber & Stark, 1965).

When one tries to maintain fixation on a stationary target, the eye often drifts away from the target and then returns to the target via a rapid flick. This behavior serves a useful perceptual function. It ensures that a single set of photoreceptors is not continually stimulated. The consequence of continual stimulation of photoreceptors was revealed in an experiment on retinal stabilization (Pritchard, 1961). As shown in Figure 6.12A, an image was projected onto the retina such that when the eye moved, the image moved with it. Usually when the eye moves, the image of a stationary object shifts across the retina. What would happen, Pritchard wondered, if this retinal shift were prevented? One possibility is that one might enjoy a kind of super-vision—an ability to see more clearly than ever before. In fact, the

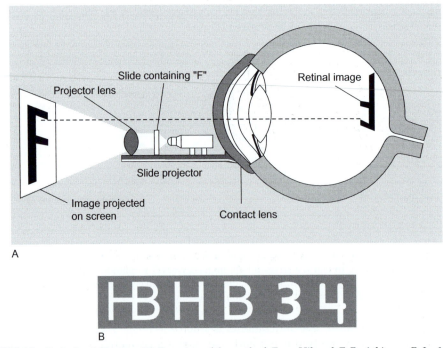

A

B

FIGURE 6.12   Retinal stabilization. (A) Overview of the method. From Hilgard, E. R., Atkinson, R. L., & Atkinson, R. C. (1979). Introduction to psychology. New York: Harcourt Brace Jovanovich, Inc., p. 117. (B) Disintegration of a retinally stabilized image over the course of time (left to right). From Anderson, J. R. (1980). Cognitive psychology and its implications. Copyright © 1980 by W. H. Freeman and Company. Reprinted by permission.

outcome was just the opposite. In a few seconds, participants reported seeing parts of the figure disappear. In the case of a letter, first one stem disappeared, then another, and then another (Figure 6.12B). Ultimately, the letter vanished completely, although when a new letter was projected onto the retina, it could be seen, though it also faded quickly in the same piecemeal fashion. These results show that the miniature movements of the image on the retina serve a useful perceptual function. They keep photoreceptors from fatiguing or adapting (Alpern, 1972; Ditchburn, 1973). Meanwhile, the piecewise perceptual disintegration of visual forms in retinal stabilization studies supports feature-based models of visual perception (Mather, 2006).

Retinal stabilization also occurs outside vision laboratories. For example, it also occurs in severe snow storms. Arctic explorers have reported cases of snow blindness, where they can see nothing, though, ironically, they are surrounded by light. The homogeneity of the visual field produces this effect, a photopic analogue of being on a life raft in the middle of the ocean, with "water water everywhere but not a drop to drink." With light, light everywhere (or light of the same kind), nothing can be seen.

Another perceptual consequence of miniature eye movements is the autokinetic illusion. Stare at a fixed point of light in an otherwise dark room. You will see the point wander over a restricted spatial range. The autokinetic effect is due to oculo-motor activity, for the effect only arises when the eye drifts (Barlow, 1952). The stops, starts, and directions of motion that are visually experienced in the autokinetic effect are directly linked to movements of the eyes (Lehman, 1965).

Some authors have proposed that the autokinetic illusion reflects the operation of a mechanism that compares retinal image displacements with oculo-motor commands or their prior intentions. According to this hypothesis, when retinal image displacements are detected without accompanying registration of oculo-motor commands, the image displacements are ascribed to motion of the target rather than to motion of the eyes (Levy, 1972). This proposal will be considered in more detail later in this chapter, in the section on Eye Movements and Space Constancy.

SACCADES

As already mentioned, saccades are rapid jumps that bring images of points of interest to the fovea. Generally, saccades are voluntary, though they usually do not require conscious intervention. The principal trigger for a saccade is retinal position error—a discrepancy between the projection of a desired point of focus onto the retina and the best place for bringing that point into focus, the fovea. The series of scans that you make when you look at an image is called a saccadic scanpath. Figure 6.13 shows a typical saccadic scanpath from an observer looking at a photograph. The scanpath is nonrandom. In general, observers look at points that are most informative.

The scanpath shown in Figure 6.13 was recorded with a special contact lens to which a lever was attached. The movements of the lever were driven by movements of the eye. By recording the lever movements, it was possible to infer corresponding eye movements (Yarbus, 1967). Other eye-tracking devices make it possible to record the position of the eye

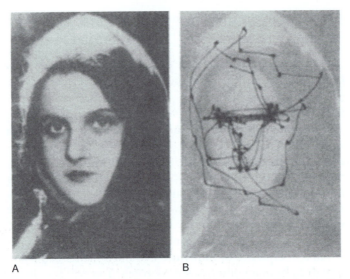

A   B

FIGURE 6.13   Scanpath of the eyes (B) in looking at a picture (A) for 1 minute. From Gouras, P. (1985). Oculomotor system. In E. R. Kandel & J. H. Schwartz (Eds.), Principles of neural science (Second Ed.) (pp. 571–583). New York: Elsevier. Copyright © 1985 by Elsevier Science Publishing Co., Inc. Reprinted by permission of the publisher.

without fixing a sensor to the cornea. For reviews of early eye movement recording techniques, see Ditchburn (1973) and Carpenter (1977). Nowadays it is possible to record eye movements in ways that allow subjects to move freely in the environment (Figure 7.6).

Visual scanpaths and the timing of successive saccades have been studied to reveal the rules governing visual perception and reading. For example, during reading the eyes remain on words that occur with low frequency (e.g., "kiwi") longer than on words that occur with high frequency (e.g., "the"). When readers are presented with words that do not make sense in terms of what they have just read, their eyes dwell for a relatively long time on the odd word. There is also a higher-than-normal likelihood of looking back to an earlier part of a passage being read if one is confused by the text. Findings like these have provided a wealth of information about reading (Rayner & Pollatsek, 2006).

Saccadic patterns have also shed light on altered states of consciousness. Rapid eye movement (REM) sleep is indicative of dreaming. If people are woken up when their eyes saccade beneath their closed eyelids, they are more likely to report dreaming than if they are woken when their eyes are immobile beneath their closed eyelids (Webb, 1973).

Saccades are fast. When a saccade is made, the eyeball can turn at rates of 600 to 700 degrees per second, though peak velocities as high as 830 degrees per second have been reported (Hyde, 1959). Peak velocity increases with saccade amplitude (Fuchs, 1967; Bahill & Stark, 1979), as mentioned earlier (Figure 6.9).

The time to begin a saccade depends on several factors. When subjects simply direct their eyes to a suddenly illuminated point, their saccadic latencies depend on the kind of attentional set they have adopted. If a new target is unexpected, the time to start making a saccade to the target can be 200 ms or longer. If a target is expected, the saccade initiation time can be reduced (Posner, 1978; Vaughan, 1983).

Saccadic latencies can also be reduced if the initial fixation target (the target being looked at initially) is extinguished before another saccadic target is presented (Saslow, 1967). The benefit of extinguishing the initial fixation target may come about because it takes time to disengage attention from the fixated target to make a saccade to the next target. If the initially fixated target is turned off, disengagement of attention can take place before the other target comes on (Fischer & Breitmeyer, 1987).

In the most extreme reduction of saccadic latencies, the latencies actually become negative with respect to stimulus onset—that is, the saccade begins before the target is presented. This occurs when observers fully anticipate targets, as, for example, while looking back and forth between two targets that come on at predictable times and places. Under these conditions, the eye can start saccading to the target even before the target comes on. Thus, saccades reflect predictions (Rashbass, 1961).

A related effect of predictive control is that the time to make the first saccade in a series of saccades increases with the number of saccades to be made, provided the subject knows that the entire series will be required (Inhoff, 1986; Zingale & Kowler, 1987). Similar results have been reported for manual and vocal responses (Henry & Rogers, 1960; Rosenbaum, 1987b; Sternberg, Monsell, Knoll, & Wright, 1978).

Once the process of initiating a saccade is far enough along, it is difficult or impossible to stop it. This demonstration of the point of no return came from a study in which subjects stared at a fixation point that remained on for a while, then was turned off, and then was followed by a target to which subjects were supposed to direct their eyes only if the target remained (Westheimer, 1954). On some trials, after the post-fixation target came on, that target was quickly extinguished and the original fixation point was re-illuminated. The question was whether subjects could withhold their saccades to the target, as they were instructed. It was found that if the delay between illumination of the target and re-illumination of the fixation point was short enough (less than about 200 ms), subjects could usually refrain from making the saccades to the targets. However, if the delay exceeded 200 ms, subjects usually made a saccade to the target even though the target had disappeared. Thus, subjects encountered a point of no return for saccadic initiation. Similar inabilities to stop have been observed for other kinds of responses (Logan & Cowan, 1984).

Although it is impossible to stop a saccade once it has been initiated, it is possible to prepare a saccade while another is under way. This is most clearly demonstrated in the patterns of saccades that people make toward distant targets. For gaze shifts to a target 15 degrees or farther from an initial fixation point, it is not uncommon for two saccades to be made toward the target. The first saccade covers most of the distance but tends to undershoot the required amplitude. The second saccade usually brings the fovea to the target. The important feature of the data from such double-saccade patterns is that the latency of the second saccade (70 ms) is usually much shorter than the latency of the first (200 ms) (Becker & Jurgens, 1979).

Is the second saccade programmed before the first saccade has ended? Evidence bearing on this question comes from studies in which visual targets are moved experimentally after an initial saccade is under way. The first saccade cannot be corrected, but subsequent corrective saccades can begin after the first saccade has been completed, resulting not just in corrective saccades with very short latencies (Becker & Fuchs, 1969), but also, amazingly, in saccades that are curved (van der Stigchel & Theeuwes, 2006; van der Stigchel, Meeter, & Theeuwes, 2006). The implication of this finding is that visual perception is not entirely prevented during saccades and that programming of second saccades can occur while first saccades are under way.

Additional information on this topic comes from studies in which subjects look at a fixation point and then are presented another target to which they are supposed to redirect their gaze (Hallet & Lightstone, 1975). Sometimes, when the saccade to the target is occurring, another target, to which subjects are also supposed to direct their gaze, is presented. The important feature of the second target is that it remains on for only a brief time, sometimes vanishing by the time the first saccade is completed. Nevertheless, subjects can still direct their eyes to the location of the now-invisible second target, provided the timing and spacing of the two targets are "just right." This result indicates that subjects can see the second target during the first saccade and can also remember its location.

Another implication of this result is that the visual system has information about the instantaneous location of the eye when the eye is making a saccade. This implication can be reached because, with the reduced form of stimuli used in the experiment (luminous dots in an otherwise dark environment), the image of the second target on the retina could not have indicated, by itself, where that target was located in the visual field. Because subjects could direct their eyes to the second target location, their visual systems must have registered where the target was physically located. It has been suggested, in fact, that the visual system codes target inputs in terms of spatial rather than retinal locations (e.g., Mays & Sparks, 1980). If the coding were only done with respect to retinal locations, subjects would have made saccades to locations that had the same distance and direction from the line of sight as the target possessed at its time of presentation. The fact that they did not argues for registration of location information per se.

Other studies have provided support for the idea that saccades are directed to target locations per se (Becker & Jurgens, 1979; Mays & Sparks, 1980). In one particularly dramatic experiment (Mays & Sparks, 1980), monkeys made saccades to briefly presented visual targets that were presented at unpredictable locations (see Figure 6.14). Just before

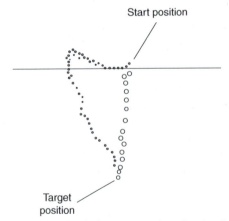

FIGURE 6.14 Position of the eye of a monkey before presentation of a stimulus, while being driven away from the target as a result of electrical stimulation of the superior colliculus, and then back toward the now-absent target (solid points), and position of the eye of the same monkey to the same stimulus location when no collicular stimulation is experimentally administered (empty points). Reproduced from Sparks and Mays (1983).

the monkeys moved their eyes to the stimulus, a small jolt of electricity was delivered to the superior colliculus. The effect of the electricity was to drive the eye to a new position. Nevertheless, after the eye arrived at this new position, it moved directly to the location where the visual target had appeared, even though the target was no longer visible. This result suggests that commands to move the eyes are not given in terms of directions or distances but instead are given in terms of target locations. For further discussion, see Sparks (1996).

Was the command to move to a location given in spatial coordinates or in orbital coordinates? Orbital coordinates specify the orientation of the eyeball in the head. Mays and Sparks (1980) favored the spatial interpretation. Steinman (1986) favored the orbital interpretation. To the best of the author's knowledge, the question of whether saccades are defined with respect to spatial or orbital representations has not yet been resolved. A priori, the orbital view seems preferable because one can easily understand, in biomechanical terms, how an eye movement might be programmed in orbital coordinates. The method would entail setting relative tensions of extra-ocular muscle antagonists. This method would allow for a one-to-one mapping of relative tensions to orbital locations. Programming eye movements in spatial coordinates would be harder, for the spatial coordinates would still have to be translated into appropriate muscle tensions. Given these considerations, it is perhaps not surprising that brain cells have been found that fire predictably before achievement of particular orbital positions (cf. Wise & Desimone, 1988). These cells are located in the supplementary eye fields, rostral to the supplementary motor cortex.

Saccadic Suppression

The studies reviewed above suggest that visual perception can occur during saccades. It may therefore be surprising to learn that other studies have documented a dramatic decline in visual sensitivity when saccades take place. This reduction in visual sensitivity during saccades is called saccadic suppression. Saccadic suppression is similar to the suppression of sensitivity to light during blinks, discussed earlier in this chapter. In general, when saccades occur, we do not see the blurred images that form on our retinas. Laboratory tests have confirmed that the stimulus intensity needed to ensure visual detection is higher when eyes make saccades than when eyes are stationary (see Matin, 1974; Volkmann, 1976, for review).

What causes saccadic suppression? Some investigators have proposed that the phenomenon has peripheral origins. For example, one hypothesis is that saccadic suppression arises from the smeariness of saccadically induced retinal images (MacKay, 1970). Another is that saccadically induced stimuli are masked by stimuli that appear just before and after saccades (Campbell & Wurtz, 1978). It has even been proposed that the physical layers at the back of the eyeball shear against one another when saccades are made and that this shearing reduces the visual resolution that is possible (Richards, 1968).

An alternative class of hypotheses claims that saccadic suppression arises from central interactions between the oculo-motor and visual systems. According to this class of hypotheses, the visual system is informed that commands for saccades have been issued or are about to be issued. The visual system then discounts or suppresses the resulting retinal image displacements. A crucial piece of evidence for this position is that saccadic suppression precedes saccades, albeit by a short time, 30–40 ms (Latour, 1962; Volkmann, Schick, & Riggs, 1969).

Regardless of the exact cause of saccadic suppression, a puzzle remains from the studies reviewed so far. If saccadic suppression is a real phenomenon, how can people respond accurately to visual stimuli that are presented when saccades are under way? One solution to the problem is to note that if sensitivity declines during saccades it does not follow that detection or localization is eliminated. After all, one may be able to determine where a stimulus is located even if it is dimmer than usual. Another less obvious way of solving the puzzle is to note that saccadic suppression may be an artifact of the kinds of responses that are asked for. If subjects are asked to report verbally about the location or presence of a stimulus presented during a saccade, their performance is poor (Matin, 1972), but if they are asked to make nonverbal responses to the stimulus, their performance is quite good. A dramatic demonstration of this phenomenon was offered by Skavenski and Hansen (1978), who asked subjects to strike with a hammer in the dark at briefly illuminated points shown during the subjects' saccades. The subjects protested that they could not see the targets, but when they were encouraged to "go for it" their hammer strikes were accurate. Also see Bridgeman, Kirch, and Sperling (1981) and Hansen and Skavenski, (1985).

The ability of subjects to strike targets shown during saccades, in contrast to their inability to report on the whereabouts of targets shown during saccades, is consistent with the hypothesis that different kinds of visual processing may be handled by different parts of the brain. One part communicates with conscious, verbal centers. The other communicates with centers responsible for perceptual-motor coordination. People may be able to program saccades to targets that are presented while other saccades are under way because the programming-while-executing procedure uses a non-verbal, automatic processing system. By contrast, when people are asked to say where or whether a stimulus has occurred, the method of responding depends on a verbal, less automatic mode of processing. Independent confirmation of the dissociation between these two forms of response has been reported by Weiskrantz, Warrington, Sanders, and Marshall (1974), who described patients with visual cortex lesions. The patients were capable of accurately reaching for targets though they claimed to be unable to see the targets. This syndrome is called *blind sight*.

Saccades and Attention

Because saccades bring the eyes to points of interest, it is reasonable to suppose that they move the eyes to points that attracted attention. Recent work on saccadic control has addressed the question of how attention and eye movements are interrelated. The concept of attention is one of the most alluring concepts in psychology and neuroscience because attention seems to be intimately related to the still more mysterious concept of consciousness (Posner, 1978). If the positions of the eyes show where attention is directed, eye movements may indicate how attention shifts from one place to another or, said more mystically, where one's consciousness is.

Are spatial attention and eye position necessarily linked? A connection between spatial attention and eye position is suggested by the finding, mentioned earlier, that signals informing a subject of the likely whereabouts of a forthcoming stimulus reduce reaction time for saccades to that location (Posner, 1978). The warning signal may be thought of as a prime for spatial attention. Consequently, the reduction of saccadic latencies following a warning signal can be taken to suggest that making a saccade normally depends on a prior shift of attention.

There is evidence that shifts of spatial attention can occur without eye movements. Posner and colleagues conducted studies in which subjects were asked to move their eyes to either primed or non-primed stimulus locations; for a review, see Posner (1978). In control conditions, subjects were asked to make a manual response (release of a lever) as quickly as possible after the presentation of the primed or non-primed stimulus and not to make an associated eye movement. Priming was achieved by presenting a cue that indicated on which side of the fixation point the target stimulus would appear. Generally, the cue was followed by the stimulus it primed, but sometimes a different stimulus was presented. Reaction times were shorter when the presented stimulus was anticipated by the cue. Moreover, the priming effect was essentially the same when subjects moved their hands without moving their eyes or when subjects moved their eyes without moving their hands. Thus, spatial attention could shift without subjects becoming "shifty-eyed" themselves. Shifting attention does not require saccades, though saccades may require prior shifts of attention.

The experimental dissociation of saccades and spatial attention has allowed other investigators to determine where spatial attention and saccades are controlled within the brain. Wurtz, Goldberg, and Robinson (1982) trained monkeys to perform tasks like those used by Posner. While the monkeys performed the tasks, the electrical activity of cells in four areas within their brains were recorded: the superior colliculus, the visual (or striate) cortex, the frontal eye fields, and the posterior parietal lobe (see Chapter 3). The results supported the hypothesis that there is a dissociation of neural activity for eye movements and for attention. As shown in Table 6.1, cells in these four areas responded differently according to these two task demands.

Cells in the superior colliculus and frontal eye fields responded vigorously before saccades were made to primed targets but did not respond above normal resting levels when manual responses were made without accompanying eye movements. Thus, cells in the superior colliculus and frontal eye fields fired in relation to saccadic activity alone.

Cells in the visual cortex fired more whenever visual stimuli were presented than when visual stimuli were not presented. The firing rates of cells in the visual cortex were only slightly higher when saccades were made to primed targets than when saccades were not made to primed targets, and this was true regardless of whether manual responses were performed. Thus, the visual cortex responded to visual targets irrespective of their functional significance or accompanying motor response.

When recordings were made in the posterior parietal cortex, however, firing rates depended on the significance of the target, regardless of the type of response. These cells

TABLE 6.1   Brain Areas and Their Functions Related to Saccades and Visual Attention

Brain area	Conditions yielding enhanced firing rates	Inferred function
Superior colliculus	Saccades but not manual responses to primed targets	Saccadic control
Frontal eye field	Saccades but not manual responses to primed targets	Saccadic control
Visual cortex	Target onsets irrespective of response or significance	Visual processing
Posterior parietal cortex	Saccades or manual responses without eye movements to primed targets only	Attentional control

responded vigorously when a stimulus called for a saccade or a manual detection response but did not respond as vigorously when the same stimuli were presented and no response was required. Likewise, cells in this region responded only minimally when eye movement or manual responses were made without an external visual stimulus. These findings suggest that the posterior parietal lobe is specialized for attention per se (Mountcastle, Lynch, Georgopoulos, Sakata, & Acuna, 1975). Consistent with this interpretation, people with damage to the posterior parietal cortex pay little or no attention to stimuli in the contralateral visual field, though they can see stimuli in that field. This syndrome is known as *spatial neglect*. Spatial neglect can be ameliorated through prism adaptation. If spatial neglect patients wear prisms that shift the visual world to the right, they later show less neglect of the left side of space (Rossetti et al., 1998).

Maintaining fixation rather than moving the eyes can draw upon executive control. An interesting extension of this idea applies to tennis playing. The very best tennis players direct their gaze differently than less skilled players. Careful analysis of high-resolution images of top tennis players and their lesser counterparts shows that the best players keep their gaze where the racquet made contact with the ball after the ball was hit. Less skilled tennis players tend to follow the ball with their eyes (Lafont, 2007). Planning to maintain fixation may confer the advantage of focusing attention more fully on hitting the ball in just the right way.

SMOOTH PURSUIT MOVEMENTS

The preceding section was concerned with saccadic eye movements. Now we pursue smooth pursuit movements. These movements keep the eyes fixated on a target that, typically, moves along smoothly. During smooth pursuit eye movements, the nervous system tries to keep the velocity of the eye the same as the velocity of the target. By contrast, during saccades, the nervous system tries to keep the position of the eye the same as the position of the target. Hence, the main stimulus for smooth pursuit movements is retinal velocity error, whereas the main stimulus for saccades is retinal position error.

The maximum velocity of smooth pursuit movements is around 100 degrees per second, though the eye's tracking ability begins to deteriorates above velocities of 30 degrees per second. The accuracy of tracking with the smooth pursuit system improves if the target being tracked moves predictably. When a smoothly moving target is first selected for tracking, a saccade may be made to it before smooth pursuit begins, for example, if the target is far away from the current fixation point. Corrective saccades also occur if smooth pursuit falters (Carpenter, 1977).

Unlike saccades, smooth pursuit movements usually cannot be initiated at will without an external target. For some time, it was thought that visible targets are necessary to elicit pursuit movements (Alpern, 1972; Robinson, 1968), but this idea was disproved through a clever demonstration: People can make pursuit movements in the dark when tactile stimuli are drawn smoothly across their skin (Lackner & Evanoff, 1977). People can smoothly pursue their own hands in the dark when they move their hands or when their hands are moved passively by someone else (Jordan, 1970). A few people can generate smooth pursuit movements in the absence of any external target (Westheimer & Conover, 1954). It is not unusual for smooth eye movements to occur during REM sleep (Fuchs & Ron, 1968).

The muscles used for smooth movements and saccades are the same, but their mode of operation is different. In saccades, only muscle agonists are used to drive the eye to a new location (Robinson, 1964), but in smooth pursuit movements, agonists and antagonists are both used (Alpern, 1972).

Smooth eye movements and saccades are also controlled through different neural systems. A source of information for this statement is that the two types of eye movement are affected differently by drugs and disease (Alpern, 1972). For example, multiple sclerosis generally affects smooth pursuit movements but leaves saccades unscathed. Direct recording, stimulation, and ablation of various brain regions also suggest that smooth pursuit movements and saccades are controlled by different neural subsystems (Gouras, 1985a).

Despite the differences between saccades and smooth eye movements, both eye movement systems reflect cognitive states. At one time it was thought that smooth eye movements are triggered only by detection of retinal velocity errors—a concept that, if correct, would have made it possible to model smooth eye movements entirely in terms of traditional servo models (Westheimer, 1954). Yet as reviewed above, nonvisual stimuli can also elicit smooth eye movements. That smooth eye movements reflect people's cognitive states has also been demonstrated by recording subjects' eye movements when those subjects look at stationary points, knowing the points will soon move in a particular direction (Kowler & Steinman, 1979). Prior to the motion of the stimulus, the subjects' eyes begin to move smoothly in the expected direction of the stimulus motion (Figure 6.15). Although the velocity of the anticipatory smooth eye movement is slight, its direction correlates with the expected direction of stimulus motion (Kowler & Steinman, 1981). Such results indicate that smooth eye movements, like saccades, provide a "window to the mind." Though saccades and smooth eye movements may be controlled by different brain systems, they both reflect mental states.

Optokinetic Nystagmus

Saccades and smooth pursuit movements can be effectively coordinated, as seen in the phenomenon of optokinetic nystagmus (OKN). OKN can be observed by watching someone's eyes as he or she looks out of a moving train or car. The eyes move in a sawtooth pattern (Figure 6.16), switching between smooth tracking movements (the slow phase) and saccadic jumps (the fast phase). Each smooth movement continues until the tracked object approaches the limit of the visual field, whereupon the eye jumps back to the next object to be followed.

The OKN is often elicited, for clinical purposes, by surrounding a patient with a full-field rotating drum consisting of vertical stripes. This method is useful for diagnosing visual impairments, particularly in patients who are unable or unwilling to report on the clarity of their vision (for example, young children). Because the OKN can only occur if the patient is able to see rotating stripes, the presence of the OKN indicates that the patient can see the stripes even if he or she cannot say so. By varying characteristics of the stripes, such as their width and contrast with the background, one can evaluate the patient's visual capabilities quite well (Collewijn, 1981).

The slow and fast phases of the OKN use typical saccades and smooth pursuit movements, respectively, as shown by the fact that the slow phase of the OKN has the same velocity characteristics as smooth pursuit movements. In the slow phase of the OKN, as in single smooth pursuit movements, the eye tracks most effectively at velocities of 20 to 30 degrees

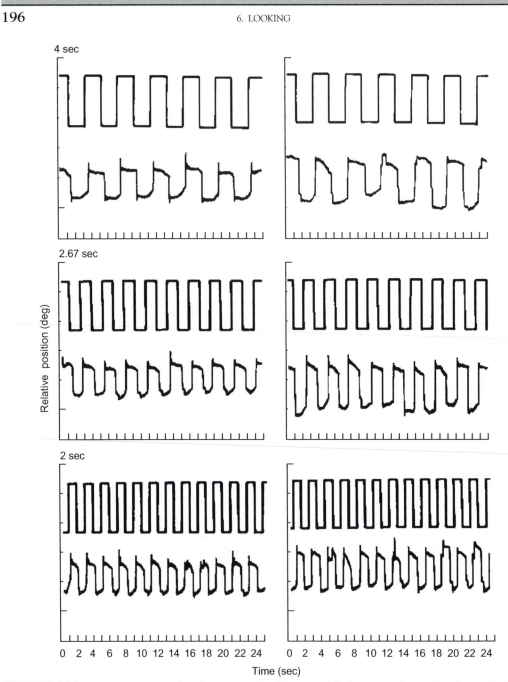

FIGURE 6.15 Anticipatory smooth movements in the direction of forthcoming motion (bottom trace of each panel) when a spot of light moves back and forth horizontally in a stepwise and periodic fashion (upper trace of each panel). The two columns show data from two observers. Each unit on the relative position scale corresponds to 1 degree, with upward points signifying rightward positions. The stimulus moved every 4s (top panels), 2.67s (middle panels), or 2s (bottom panels). From Kowler and Steinman (1979).

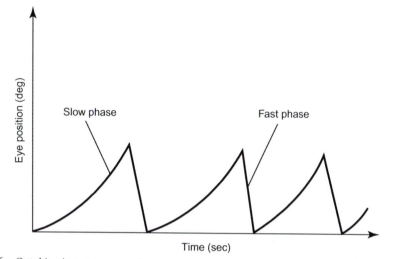

FIGURE 6.16 Optokinetic nystagmus pattern.

per second, and the eye is no longer able to track when velocities approach 100 degrees per second (Carpenter, 1977). The saccades of the OKN (i.e., the fast phase of the OKN) also have the same properties as isolated saccades (Carpenter, 1977). Thus, the OKN can be regarded as a true pattern of alternating saccades and pursuit movements. Because the OKN can be extremely accurate, it is also possible to conclude that exquisite coordination can be achieved between the saccadic and smooth pursuit systems.

Vestibular-Oculo-Motor Reflex

For all the eye movement systems discussed so far, we have conveniently ignored the fact that the head as well as the eyes move. We could ignore head movement because the studies reviewed so far were generally conducted with subjects holding their heads still, often keeping their teeth on bite boards. The studies were conducted in this way for technical reasons. The greatest precision of eye movement recording is possible when the head is still, though with newer recording systems much greater precision is possible even when the head and body can move freely.

The importance of considering movements of the head along with movements of the eyes becomes manifest when you consider what happens when your eyes are fully deviated toward one side or the other. In that circumstance, it is pointless to try to move your eyes to an even more eccentric position. Instead, your must turn your head toward the target and counter-rotate your eyes to keep the gaze fixed on the target. This is where the vestibulo-ocular reflex (VOR) comes in. The VOR is activated when you try to look at a stationary target while turning your head. When the VOR functions properly, the motion of your head is compensated for by counter-motion of your eyes. It turns out that such compensation is virtually perfect under normal circumstances.

How is this possible? The answer is that head movements are sensed by the central component of the vestibular system—the labyrinth of the inner ear (Figure 6.17). The labyrinth

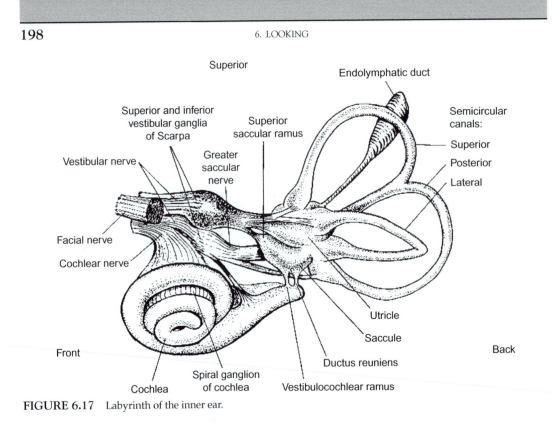

FIGURE 6.17   Labyrinth of the inner ear.

has three semicircular canals oriented at right angles to one other. If a canal undergoes angular acceleration, the fluid within it (the endolymph) changes its rate of flow, pushing against a membrane (the cupula) in one direction or the other depending on the sign of the acceleration (whether the fluid speeds up or slows down). As the cupula is deflected or experiences a pressure differential, tiny hair cells attached to the cupula bend, causing neural signals to be sent to other brain centers and on to the oculo-motor nuclei. From there, efferent commands are delivered to the extra-ocular muscles and the needed eye movement is made (Brown & Deffenbacher, 1979).

The role of the vestibular apparatus in controlling eye movements is apparent in a clinical procedure used to diagnose abnormal dizziness. Tepid water is introduced into the inner ear to stimulate the labyrinths. The result is vestibular-ocular nystagmus, a pattern of alternating smooth and saccadic eye movements similar to that observed in OKN. Detailed characteristics of the nystagmus pattern permit precise diagnoses of the state of the vestibular apparatus (Dell'Osso & Daroff, 1981).

What is the evidence for the claim that the vestibular system underlies normal eye-head coordination? Some of the most important evidence comes from experiments in which monkeys looked straight ahead and then turned the eyes and head toward visual targets presented to the side (Bizzi, 1974). Figure 6.18A shows position-versus-time curves for the eyes and head of a monkey in this situation. The eyes and head began moving at the same time, but because the eyes moved more quickly, they reached the target first. To keep the eyes fixed on the target, the eyes counter-rotated as the head continued to turn.

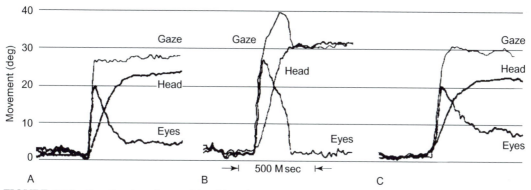

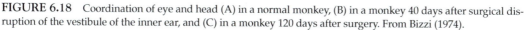

FIGURE 6.18 Coordination of eye and head (A) in a normal monkey, (B) in a monkey 40 days after surgical disruption of the vestibule of the inner ear, and (C) in a monkey 120 days after surgery. From Bizzi (1974).

Figure 6.18B shows what happened when the monkey's vestibular system was surgically disrupted. When the head turned toward the target, the eyes did not counter-rotate. Rather, they moved along with the head and then returned to the target more slowly than usual. This outcome shows that counter-rotation of the eyes during head turning depends on intact functioning of the vestibular system. Even 40 days after vestibular damage, counter-rotation of the eye during head turning was impaired.

What about longer-term adaptation to vestibular damage? After 120 days, some compensation occurred. However, the compensation took a rather different form from normal oculo-motor counter-rotation. As seen in Figure 6.18C, the eye initially undershot the target and then was carried by the head to the target, so a new strategy developed for coordinating the eye and the head when the VOR could not be relied on.

Changes in the coordination of eye and head movements do not occur only as a result of long-term experience. They also can come about quickly if a visual target comes to be expected at a particular location in the periphery. Then the head may actually lead the eye, with the initiation of the eye movement delayed long enough to allow the eye and head to arrive at the target simultaneously (Bizzi, 1974). This strategy eliminates the need for compensatory eye movements and therefore can be relied on when normal vestibular control is impossible.

Long-term learning can occur for the VOR, however, as has been demonstrated with magnifying and minifying lenses. When these types of lenses are placed over the eyes, images on the retina expand or contract, respectively. The lenses also alter the speed at which visual images appear to move when the head turns. Magnifying lenses increase the apparent speed of image displacement, whereas minifying lenses decrease the apparent speed. The consequence of such magnification or minification is that the normal gain of the VOR is initially too small or too large. (Gain is the ratio of effector displacement to stimulus displacement.) When lenses double the image size, the speed of image displacement also doubles, so the optimal gain for the VOR becomes 2.0 rather than the normal 1.0. After a few days of wearing such magnifying lenses in normal illumination, monkeys tested in the dark show gains close to 2.0. Similarly, after minifying lenses are worn, the opposite effect is obtained. After wearing lenses that shrink images to one-quarter their normal size, the gain of the VOR approaches the optimal value of 0.25 (Lisberger, 1988).

These results imply that the VOR adapts to the new relation between eye movement and image displacement. For the gain of the VOR to change, the subject must be exposed to visual input and head rotations simultaneously. Wearing the lens with the head held stationary does not lead to adaptation, nor does moving the head in the dark (Lisberger, 1988). Thus, VOR adaptation in the monkey is achieved by learning new correlations between head rotations and retinal image displacements, much as eye-paw coordination in the kitten is achieved by learning new correlations between walking movements and retinal image displacements (Held, 1965); see Figure 2.16.

What neural mechanism allows for VOR adaptation? One way to find out is to study the times during eye-head counter-rotations when recalibration effects appear. The first response to head turning occurs 14 ms after the head starts to turn and remains unaffected by lens exposure. By 19 ms after the start of head turning, experience-based changes in compensatory eye movements can be detected. Based on the latter result, it has been proposed that there are three components to VOR adaptation: (1) an immediate, unchanging response, (2) a delayed, changing response, and (3) a capacity for introducing changes to subsequent responses based on the outcome of previous eye-head movements. Detailed studies of the neurophysiological underpinnings of the VOR have shown that distinct neural pathways are responsible for these three functions. Thus, even for a response as simple as the VOR, different neural subsystems come into play, each with distinct functional responsibilities. One of these subsystems acts automatically. Another acts rapidly but can be changed through learning. The third tunes the second system based on feedback. Similar three-part schemes for motor learning and control have been identified for other, more complex systems. The fact that all three principles hold for VOR learning highlights the fact that the study of very simple systems can reveal important truths about more complex systems. This, of course, is the article of faith behind the reductionist approach to science and neuroscience in particular (Kandel, 2006). This approach has paid off handsomely in the study of the VOR.

VERGENCE MOVEMENTS

With the exception of some of the miniature eye movements discussed before, all the eye movement activities considered so far keep the lines of sight of the two eyes parallel. Recall that these sorts of eye movements are called conjugate. Parallelism does not characterize all eye movements, however. In vergence eye movements, the lines of sight of the two eyes cross or skew.

There are two kinds of vergence movements. Convergence brings the eyes inward toward the nose as the observer looks at nearer or approaching targets. Divergence brings the eyes out toward the temples as the observer looks at farther or receding targets. When the visual target is very far away, the lines of sight become parallel or nearly parallel.

The main stimulus for vergence movements is retinal disparity (Rashbass, 1981). This is the difference (often very slight) in the retinal projections of a given stimulus on the retinas of the two eyes. Retinal disparity is not the only trigger for vergence, however, as seen in the following demonstration (Alpern, 1957). A target is slowly brought toward one eye while the other eye is blocked. Suddenly, a lens is placed in front of the seeing eye, so that eye's image of the target is blurred. The response of the other, unseeing eye is immediate convergence toward the target. Since there is no retinal disparity in this situation, the trigger for the convergence is accommodation alone.

Because targets at different distances usually require both vergence and accommodation, these two activities usually co-occur. Their joint action is called the accommodation reflex (Gouras, 1985a).

EYE MOVEMENTS AND SPACE CONSTANCY

When the eyes move, the image of the visual world moves across the retina. The same sort of retinal image displacement can also occur if the eyes are held still and objects move before them. How does one determine whether the visual world is stationary and the eyes are moving or the visual world is moving and the eyes are still? There are at least two possible answers, as shown in Figure 6.19.

One is that the visual system receives signals from the oculo-motor centers, indicating how the eyes have been instructed to move. These instructions are then used to guide the interpretation of subsequent visual input. According to this *outflow* model, if an oculo-motor signal is sent to move the eyes 4 degrees to the right, say, a retinal displacement of 4 degrees to the left is predicted. When that retinal displacement occurs, it is interpreted to mean that the visual world remained stationary. If no signal is sent to move the eyes and a 4 degree retinal displacement occurs, the displacement is interpreted to mean that the visual world has moved.

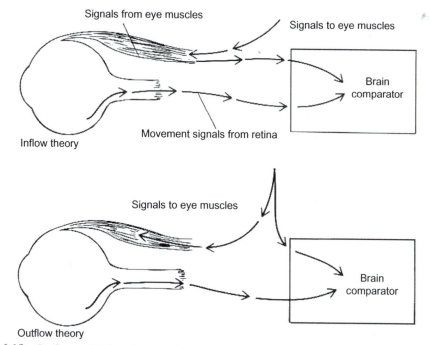

FIGURE 6.19   Outflow and inflow theories of visuo-motor integration. From Gregory (1973).

The alternative to the outflow model is the *inflow* model. Here it is assumed that feedback signals from the eye muscles, rather than commands to the eye muscles or their prior intentions, provide the signals used by the visual system to interpret retinal shifts.

Reliance on feedback from the eye muscles has an advantage over reliance on oculo-motor commands. Because oculo-motor commands may not always be carried out perfectly, the comparison of retinal signals with oculo-motor signals can cause inaccurate interpretations of visual changes. Such errors would be less likely to occur if retinal information were compared with feedback concerning the actual actions of the eye muscles. On the other hand, reliance on outflow has an advantage over reliance on inflow. Efferent information is likely to be available before muscle feedback returns. Thus, a comparator that uses efferent information will generally be faster than one that uses afferent information. From this perspective, the outflow model is preferable to the inflow model.

The debate over inflow and outflow was first posed by the great nineteenth century scientist Hermann von Helmholtz (1821–1894) (see Helmholtz, 1962), whose interest in this topic culminated in his suggestion that perception relies on unconscious inference. Some unconscious inference steps were adumbrated in the preceding paragraph, where the text said, "... if an oculo-motor signal is sent to move the eyes 4 degrees to the right, say, a retinal displacement of 4 degrees to the left is predicted. When that retinal displacement occurs, it is interpreted to mean that the visual world remained stationary." Helmholtz's appreciation of the possibility of unconscious inference in perception actually makes him, rather than Sigmund Freud, the discoverer of the unconscious.

Helmholtz argued that one could decide between outflow and inflow through the following simple demonstration. Close one eye and gently press against the lid of the other eye with your finger. As you repeatedly press your finger against your eye, you will probably see the visual world jump back and forth. This simple observation has a profound implication, though the path to understanding it must be followed carefully.

When you move your eye with your finger, you cause the visual image to move across the retina. Because your eye moved, receptors in the extra-ocular muscles were activated. Therefore, if feedback from the eye muscles were used to interpret retinal displacements, the visual system would not be "fooled into thinking" that the visual world had moved when your finger nudged your eyeball. The fact that you saw the world move suggests that feedback from the eye muscles was not used to discount the retinal displacements. By this line of reasoning, the visual system relies on outflow (efferent commands or their copies) rather than inflow (feedback from the eye muscles) to interpret movement-based retinal displacements (Helmholtz, 1962; Sperry, 1950; von Holst & Mittelstaedt, 1950). In this case, the outflow had to be for the eye muscles per se, because you did use outflow, albeit to your hand, to move your eye.

Now consider another demonstration that leads to the same conclusion. This demonstration was reported by another giant of nineteenth and early twentieth century science, Ernst Mach (1838–1916), the physicist responsible for positivism, the view that all scientific claims must be expressed in terms of observable quantities. Mach observed that when the eyes are prevented from moving by being bunged with putty, one sees the world move when eye movements are tried (Gregory, 1973). The interpretation Mach gave for this phenomenon was similar to the interpretation Helmholtz gave for his demonstration involving eye nudging. When the eyes are commanded to move but do not move, normal feedback from the stretch receptors is presumably absent. The fact that one sees the world shift when the eyes are immobilized suggests that commands to move the eyes, rather than feedback from the eye muscles, allow for the interpretation of retinal displacements associated with eye movements.

To accept this argument, one must accept the assumption that feedback from the stretch receptors when the eyes are commanded to move but cannot move is comparable to the feedback that exists when the eyes are not commanded to move. But suppose feedback from the extra-ocular muscles is in fact somewhat different in these two situations. Then the power of Mach's and Helmholtz's arguments is lost, and the debate between inflow and outflow theory remains unresolved.

A more decisive method for choosing between inflow and outflow theories of space constancy is to physically disrupt the outflow-inflow loop. Pursuing this reasoning, Kornmuller (1930) reported that partial paralysis of the extra-ocular muscles results in the perception of illusory visual motion. Because the eyes presumably did not move or barely moved in this situation, images of external visual stimuli remained fixed on the retina. Since there was little or no feedback from the eye muscles to indicate that the eyes had changed position, the visual centers must have noted that a central signal was issued to move the eyes. These centers then enabled the unconscious inference that the world had moved synchronously with the eyes.

As compelling as this argument may be, it needs to be qualified. Subsequent experiments in which volunteers allowed their eyes to be totally paralyzed did not report seeing illusory motion. The latter experiments were conducted in partial illumination, which may have affected the perceptual judgments that were given. Another concern is that the eye muscles are richly endowed with stretch receptors (see Skavenski, 1972), so it seems odd that the eye muscles cannot provide information about the position or motion of the eye. For a time, it was believed that the receptors of the eye muscles provide no useful information about eye position. This belief stemmed from a report of a person whose eye muscles were physically pulled with a forceps and whose eyelids and eye were anesthetized. The individual could not tell that his eye was being passively rotated (Brindley & Merton, 1960). This subject was probably under duress, however, so his report should be treated skeptically.

A more careful (and humane) study, reported by Skavenski (1972), indicated that proprioceptive information from the extra-ocular muscles may in fact be useful. Skavenski applied a contact lens to the cornea and attached a thread to a stalk projecting from the lens (Figure 6.20). When the thread was pulled, it rotated the eyeball. Subjects in the experiment were responsible for indicating whether they thought their eyes had been moved and in which direction. Though the experiment was conducted in complete darkness, subjects could detect passive motion of the eye and could accurately identify the direction of passive motion. Thus, they had access to proprioceptive information from their eyes. In another experiment, also conducted in darkness, subjects could counter-rotate their eyes to adjust for an external load imposed on the eyeball. The fact that they could do so indicates that they were sensitive to proprioceptive input from their eye muscles (Skavenski, Haddad, & Steinman, 1972).

Adding still more fuel to the conclusion that eye position can be sensed proprioceptively, Wang, Zhang, Cohen, and Goldberg (2007) reported that proprioceptive information about

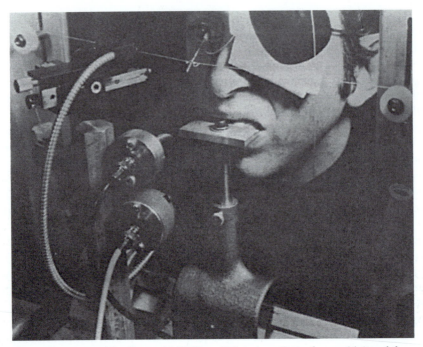

FIGURE 6.20 Apparatus used by Skavenski (1972, p. 224) to investigate the sensitivity of the eye to passive displacement. From Steinman (1986).

eye position is registered in a systematic fashion in the brain. As reported by Wang et al. (2007) and as summarized in a very readable overview of this work (Sommer, 2007), one reason why investigators were long suspicious of the inflow account was that, apart from the checkered career of tests thought to support it, no one had found a region of sensory cortex specifically responsive to extra-ocular muscle stretch. As Sommer noted, Penfield's homunculus had long been known to represent the entire body, but the eyes, mysteriously, were not in view. Wang et al. recorded from a sulcus where they thought eye proprioceptors might have input. That area, Brodman's area 3a, is located near areas of somatosensory cortex that respond to touch on the face, mouth, and lips, but had not been previously investigated. When Wang et al. recorded from this region, they found neural discharge properties closely linked to eye positions. When the eye muscles were paralyzed, the coupling of 3a neural discharge to eye position broke down, suggesting that the 3a activity was not the product of inflow rather than outflow.

A final argument against outflow theory is that in virtually all the studies that have supported it, subjects were exposed to highly restricted visual inputs, typically single points of lights. When several light points could be seen, or when a natural scene was visible, most of the perceptual phenomena that support outflow theory have been eliminated or significantly reduced (Bridgeman, 1983; Matin, Stevens, & Picoult, 1983). For example, a person whose eye muscles were paralyzed saw an isolated visual stimulus drift toward the floor, but the illusion vanished if the room lights were turned on (Matin, Stevens, & Picoult, 1983).

Similarly, as you can confirm for yourself, you may see illusory motion of the illuminated digits of an electronic clock if you make saccades when the room is dark (especially if the clock is off to the side), but there is no such illusion when the room is illuminated. Observations such as these suggest that retinal information alone may provide all the information necessary to distinguish between externally induced motion and internally induced motion. The latter point has been made by advocates of the ecological approach to perception (Gibson, 1979).

DEVELOPMENT AND PLASTICITY OF OCULO-MOTOR CONTROL

One of the most remarkable features of the eye movement system is its capacity for recalibration as a result of experience. We have already considered relevant evidence in connection with the VOR. Recall that in those experiments, after monkeys underwent surgical destruction of the vestibular apparatus, their eyes failed to counter-rotate properly during head turns. With time, however, the amplitude of the initial saccade was adjusted so the eye reached the target and remained on it. Thus, the monkeys could compensate for the altered relation between the movements of their eyes and the movements of their heads.

Such oculo-motor plasticity can be observed without resorting to surgery. Consider what happens when one looks through a lens that shrinks an image. As already discussed, the gain of the VOR can change as a result. For related results, see Berthoz and Melvill Jones (1985) and Collewijn, Martins, and Steinman (1981). Apart from the VOR, wearing a minifying lens causes one's eye movements to have smaller amplitudes than usual. Anticipating this fact, Hoffman and Roffwarg (1983) asked volunteers to wear minifying lenses for 12 days. The researchers found that the amplitudes of the eye movements shortened significantly when the minifying lenses were in place and, briefly, after the minifying lenses were removed. There was also an effect of the lenses during REM sleep, indicating that the recalibration of eye movements was not only based on responses to visual errors.

What of the normal course of development of eye movement control? Most eye movements that humans can make can be made at birth. Ultrasound studies have shown that eye movements occur even prenatally (Birnholz, 1981). By around 16 to 23 gestational weeks, slow eye movements can be seen in ultrasound images, and by around 23 gestational weeks, rapid eye movements are observable. Opening of the eyelids can be detected by around 35 weeks. The fact that these activities develop at different times is consistent with the idea that they are controlled by different neural subsystems.

Although eye movements occur prenatally, they also undergo progressive postnatal development, even past age 5. Kowler and Martins (1983) reported that normal 4- and 5-year-olds did less well at fixating and tracking a target than adults do. There has been controversy about this report (Aslin et al., 1983), but Kowler and Martins' observation raises the interesting possibility that the development of visual acuity in children may be partly determined by factors related to oculo-motor control. To the extent that this hypothesis is correct, it highlights the importance of the interplay between visual perception and its motoric bases; see Coren (1986) for further discussion of this issue.

SUMMARY

1. Looking relies on a number of oculo-motor activities. Some rotate the eyeball. These include saccades (jumps of the eyes from place to place), pursuit movements (the eyes following smoothly moving objects), and nystagmus (alternations between saccades and pursuits), all of which are conjugate movements (the eyes move in the same direction), as well as vergence eye movements, which are disjunctive (the eyes move in different directions). Other oculo-motor activities do not rotate the eyeball: blinking, accommodation, and adjustment of pupil diameter.

2. Blinking protects and moistens the cornea. Blinks can be trained to occur after an unconditioned stimulus such as a tone is associated with a conditioned stimulus such as an airpuff delivered to the eye. The associated learning may be registered in specific brain locations (at least in rabbits). Blinks also depend on high-level cognition, as when one blinks at high rates while lying. Visual sensitivity is attenuated during blinks, presumably due to central programming of the blinks, not just closure of the lids.

3. Another oculo-motor activity that does not result in rotation of the eyeball is accommodation. Accommodation helps focus blurry images. It is triggered by detection of blurriness within the visual cortex and is achieved by contracting and relaxing the ciliary muscles, which are attached to the lens of the eye. Lens elasticity decreases with age.

4. A third oculo-motor activity that does not produce rotation of the eyeball is adjustment of pupil diameter. Like blinking, pupil responses have reflexive and voluntary components. The reflexive component is elicited, under normal conditions, by changes in illumination or by an approaching object. Pupil dilation allows more light into the eye, whereas pupil constriction reduces the amount of light that can enter. Pupil dilation also indexes the mental load invested in a task and changes before spontaneous changes in perception (e.g., reversal of the Necker cube). Pupil dilation is also taken as a social cue about interest in an ongoing task or other person.

5. Regarding activities that rotate the eyeball, it is natural to wonder why the eyeball turns at all. A speculative answer is related to the fact that the foveal projection areas within the brain are massive compared to the nonfoveal projection areas. Moving the eye limits the size of the fovea and the amount of brain tissue associated with it. This argument makes sense if relatively little brain tissue is needed to control eye movements.

6. Eye rotation is achieved with muscles that work in combination to rotate the globe in three dimensions.

7. Donders' law states that a unique eye position (a unique combination of pitch, roll, and yaw) is associated with each gaze direction. Listing's plane contains all the rotation axes for the eye in all its gaze directions.

8. Three pairs of extra-ocular muscles move the eyeball via three cranial nerves whose nuclei are in the brain stem. Saccade amplitudes are increased by firing more motor neurons in these nuclei and by increasing the durations of their firing. Consistent with this model, saccade peak velocities increase with saccade amplitudes, and fatigue causes the eyes to saccade too far and then drift back to targets (glissadic overshoots).

9. Because the two eyes can move in the same direction (conjugate movements) or in opposite directions (disjunctive movements), any given pair of extra-ocular muscles can work as agonists, promoting motion in a common direction, or as antagonists, promoting motions in opposite directions.

10. The smallest eye movements, miniature movements, fall into three classes: drifts, tremors, and microsaccades. Drifts and tremors are mainly involuntary, whereas microsaccades reflect attention and have other features in common with saccades, suggesting that microsaccades and saccades belong to the same functional class.

11. Miniature eye movements refresh photoreceptors, preventing images from disappearing, as occurs when those images are stabilized on the retina. Miniature eye movements also cause the autokinetic illusion, the tendency to see a single, stationary point of light wander about jerkily in a dark surround.

12. Saccades are jumps of the eyes that occur when one reads or inspects a scene. The eye is brought to points of interest.

13. Saccade speeds can be very high. The farther a saccade goes, the higher the peak speed it achieves. Saccades can also be initiated quickly, especially if saccade targets are predictable and the number of to-be-generated saccades is small.

14. It is difficult to withhold a saccade to a target if that target is replaced by another target more than 200 ms later. However, a second saccade can be programmed while a first saccade is underway, revealing not only the capacity for programming of saccades while other saccades are in progress but also sensitivity to visual input during saccades as well as memory for new target positions.

15. How positions of saccade targets are represented is unclear. One possibility is that they are represented in external spatial coordinates. Another possibility is that they are represented in internal orbital coordinates.

16. Despite the accuracy of visual perception during saccades, visual sensitivity during saccades is attenuated. There has been debate about the source of such saccadic suppression. One possibility is that it has central origins. The other possibility is that it has peripheral origins. Both possibilities may be true.

17. Saccadic suppression does not amount to saccadic blindness. Though there is reduced sensitivity to visual input during saccades, consistent with saccadic suppression, targets can be localized even when those targets are not consciously registered, as shown by the fact that people can strike with hammers at stimuli shown during saccades though they claim not to see the stimuli. A related neuropsychological syndrome is blind sight.

18. Attention benefits saccade initiation, though saccades do not have to be directed to targets to which one is attending. Different parts of the brain play different roles in controlling visuo-spatial attention and in controlling saccades, as shown by studies of brain stimulation, brain recording, and neurological disorders such as spatial neglect. Being able to inhibit saccades can be a valuable skill in social and athletic contexts.

19. During smooth pursuit eye movements, the nervous system tries to keep the velocity of the eye the same as the velocity of a target, whereas during saccades, the nervous system tries to keep the position of the eye the same as the position of a target. Smooth pursuit movements occur when one tracks a continuously moving stimulus, though smooth pursuit movements can also be generated at will in some individuals and in response to nonvisual inputs such as moving felt objects.

20. Saccades and smooth pursuit movements are generated with different neural subsystems and are produced through different patterns of activity in the extra-ocular muscles. Antagonists are activated simultaneously in smooth pursuit movements, but are activated asynchronously during saccades. Although saccades and pursuit movements are controlled by different means, they both reveal cognitive states. Expectancies about upcoming target motions can give rise to smooth eye movements in the expected directions.

21. There is effective coordination between saccades and smooth eye movements. One way this is illustrated is in optokinetic nystagmus (OKN), a pattern of eye movements characterized by rapid, regular alternation between quick and slow phases of ocular motility made in response to visual stimuli such as rotating black and white stripes. The properties of the quick phases are the same as the properties of saccades, and the properties of the slow phases are the same as the properties of smooth eye movements.

22. Coordination between the eye and head provides another example of the way different motor systems work together to promote effective vision. The chief way the eye and head are coordinated is through the vestibular-ocular reflex (VOR), which is mediated by the vestibular apparatus, as shown by the fact that stimulation of the labyrinths of the inner ear elicits the VOR and removal of neural inputs from the vestibular apparatus interferes with the eye's ability to counter-rotate as the head turns toward a peripheral target. Following such surgical intervention, alternative strategies can be learned for coordinating the eye and head. Changes can also be made to the VOR following exposure to lenses that magnify or minify images. The temporal dynamics of the VOR following learning suggest levels of control for this very simple response that are strikingly similar to the levels of control for more complex behaviors.

23. Vergence movements allow the eyes to focus on objects at varying distances from the viewer. In contrast to saccades and smooth eye movements, which are conjugate (keeping the lines of sight parallel), vergence movements are disjunctive (allowing the lines of sight of the eyes to cross or skew). The triggers for vergence movements are retinal disparity and detection of blurriness.

24. The analysis of the interaction between vision and eye movements has been pursued in the study of space constancy. The question is how to tell whether retinal displacements are due to motion of external stimuli or to motion of the eyes. Outflow theory states that the brain compares visual input with copies of eye movement commands or their prior intentions. Inflow theory states that the brain compares visual input with proprioceptive feedback from the eye muscles. A third possibility is that visual information alone informs the viewer of the cause of retinal displacement. Evidence has been obtained for all three theories. Outflow theory finds support in observations of external motion when one nudges one's eye with one's finger or when one attempts to move one's eyes but those attempts are unsuccessful. Inflow theory finds support in sensitivity to external tugs on the eyeball administered mechanically and in recent data, indicating tight coupling between eye position and neural discharge properties of cortical area 3a. The hypothesis that visual information alone may be sufficient finds support in the fact that many results consistent with outflow theory or inflow theory depend on participants being in visually impoverished environments.

25. Eye movements occur even before birth. However, eye movements are readily modified by experience and may continue to develop during childhood.

Further Reading

The way the eyes scan a scene differs if one is going to touch objects in the scene or merely search the scene for targets (Epelboim et al., 1997).

A journal in which eye movement control is featured prominently is *Vision Research*.

Donders' law was covered in this chapter. It has been proposed that an analogue of Donders' law may hold for the arm (Gielen, Vrijenhoek, & Flash, 1997; Mitra & Turvey, 2004). In support of this proposal, it has been shown that when people are asked to hold their arms outstretched, with their elbows, wrist, and fingers fully extended but with their shoulders at different angles, the hand angles that are adopted are stereotyped for the various shoulder angles that are produced. On the other hand, much as people's mental states can give rise to violations of Donders' law for the eye (Pashler, Ramachandran, & Becker, 2006), people's mental states can give rise to violation of Donders' law for the arm. Soechting, Buneo, Herrmann, and Flanders (1995) showed that arm torsion for a given pointing direction depends on the previous pointing direction, and Rosenbaum, Vaughan, Jorgensen, Barnes, and Stewart (1993) showed that when people perform series of object manipulations, the postures they adopt anticipate later postures and depart strongly from those predicted by Donder's law (see Rosenbaum, Cohen, Meulenbroek, & Vaughan, 2006, for review).

Bruce Bridgeman of the University of California, Santa Cruz, has made important contributions to the study of visual perception vis-à-vis action. Among his papers is a recent work summarizing his reservations about efference copy theory (Bridgeman, 2007).

This chapter mentioned the special advantage of controlling gaze in tennis (Figure 6.15). For more on gaze control and skill, see Vickers (2007).

For more information about brain mechanisms underlying two-step saccades, see Medendorp, Goltz, and Vilis (2006).

For a review of research concerning microsaccades, see Collewijn and Kowler (2008).

For more about the neural decision mechanisms that guide, control and monitor eye movements, see schall and Boucher (2007). For more information about the work of Jeffrey Schall at Vanderbilt University, see http://psych-s1.psych.vanderbilt.edu/faculty/schalljd/index.php.

OUTLINE

**The Development of Reaching
and Grasping**   214
  Direction   215
  Distance   215
  Orientation   215
  Size   216
  Functional Tuning of Grasps in Infancy 216

Visual Guidance   217
  Vision and Touch   219
  Vision for Action   221
  Eye-Hand Coordination   222

Aiming   225
  Woodworth's Pioneering Study   227

  Fitts' Law   229
  Iterative Corrections Model   230
  Impulse Variability Model   231
  Optimized Initial Impulse Model   232

Equilibrium Point Hypothesis   233

Discrete versus Continuous Movements   237

Intersegmental Coordination   238
  Transport and Grasp Phases   240
  Hand-Space versus Joint-Space Planning 241
  Moving Two Hands at Once   244

Summary   248

Further Reading   249

Much of human culture takes the form it does because of what we do with our hands. We build houses, draw pictures, make bread, play musical instruments, and gesture, all because of the strength, flexibility, and precision of hand movements. Manual performance is so central to human experience that we refer to hand motions when we discuss other topics. We say, "on the one hand and on the other," "I hope this grabs your attention," "These ideas go hand in hand," "an offhand remark," and so on.

Because of the importance of manual control in human experience, several lines of research have grown around it. One is the control of drawing and writing, which will be covered in the next chapter. Another is the control of keyboard performance, which will be covered in the chapter after that. A third is the use of sign language, a topic that has been studied more from the perspective of linguistics and communications than motor control per se, so it is pointed to here but not treated in detail (Emmorey, 2002; Goldin-Meadow, 1999; Goldin-Meadow & Wagner, 2005; Poizner, Klima, & Bellugi, 1987). A fourth is the control of reaching and grasping, which will occupy some of our attention in this chapter, and is the subject of entire books (MacKenzie & Iberall, 1994; Wing, Haggard, & Flanagan, 1996).

Reaching and grasping depend on a blend of initial planning and subsequent correction. The initial planning is based on perception of the objects to be grasped and memory of what the objects afford in the way of grasping. Based on such information, one can decide whether to pick up objects with one hand or two, with a large grip or a small grip force (Gordon, Forssberg, Johansson, & Westling, 1991a,b,c), with all the fingers or only some of the fingers wrapped around the objects (Arbib, Iberall, & Lyons, 1985), and, depending on what will be done with the objects, with one or another placement of the hand on the objects (Fischman, Stodden, & Lehman, 2003; Haggard, 1998; Klatzky & Lederman, 1985; Kleinholdermann, Brenner, Franz, & Smeets, 2007; Marteniuk, MacKenzie, Jeannerod, Athenes, & Dugas, 1987; Rosenbaum, Cohen, Meulenbroek, & Vaughan, 2006); see Figure 7.1.

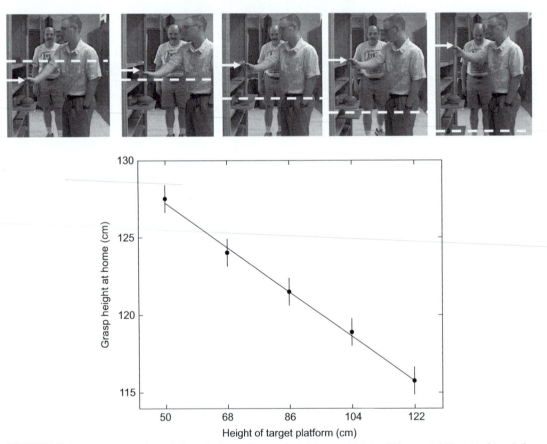

FIGURE 7.1 Grasping an object differently depending on the height to which it will be carried. Top: A subject (who gave permission to have his photo shown here) grasps a plunger on a home platform with different grasp heights (white arrows) before moving the plunger to target platforms at different heights (white dashed lines). The author of this book, also shown here, was responsible for setting up the target platforms. Bottom: Mean grasp heights (± 1 SE) for home-to-target grasps. From Cohen, R. G. & Rosenbaum, D. A. (2004). Where objects are grasped reveals how grasps are planned: Generation and recall of motor plans. Experimental Brain Research, 157, 486–495. With permission.

The chapter is organized as follows. First, we will consider the development of reaching and grasping. The overarching question is at what age different aspects of reaching and grasping tend to come online. In this section, we will be concerned with more than just the extent to which grasps reflect perceptual sensitivity to physical features of objects to be grasped. We will also be concerned with the ability of infants to grasp objects differently depending on what they intend to do with the objects. Identifying the ages at which different abilities are manifested need not be taken to imply a strict stage model of development. Different babies progress at different rates, with some abilities becoming available before others in different individuals (Thelen Corbetta, Kamm, & Spencer, 1993; Thelen, Corbetta, & Spencer, 1996). Thus, describing reaching abilities in a stagewise way is meant to convey a statistical regularity, not a strict stagewise progression.

Next we will look at visual guidance. One of the issues we will consider concerns vision and movement. Given that we rely on vision to help guide our hand movements, one might expect the mappings between vision and movement to be rigid by the time one reaches adulthood. The available evidence suggests otherwise. There is a surprising degree of flexibility in the mappings between the motor system and the visual system. Similarly, there is considerable flexibility in the mappings between vision and touch. Why this is and how it is possible are matters taken up in the section on visual guidance. In this section we will also consider eye-hand coordination and how research on visually guided reaching sheds light on the distinction between two neural systems that have sparked a great deal of excitement in this field of research, the visual "what" system, and the visual "how" system.

The next section will be concerned with aiming. Here we will review work showing that aiming relies on a blend of preprogramming and error correction. A series of models has been developed to characterize this blend. That series of models has taken over a century to unfold. We will review it here in a few pages.

The fourth part of the chapter will be concerned with the equilibrium point hypothesis. The main idea here is that the motor system may have ways of specifying goal positions that eliminate the need for control of the detailed features of the movements to those goal positions.

The fifth part of the chapter will be concerned with a relatively new debate that has sprung up in human motor control: Are movements discrete or continuous? Do we, in other words, move from place to place in steps, or do we move in a smoothly flowing stream?

Sixth and finally, we will look at the coordination of the limb segments involved in reaching and grasping. When we reach for and grasp objects, we do so with our fingers, hands, and arms, and even with our torsos and legs—whatever it takes to impart the forces needed to hold, carry, and manipulate the objects being dealt with. An important principle that has emerged from this area of study is that the limb segments are controlled in a way that reflects sensitivity to their functional interdependence. Recent work on bimanual coupling suggests that this interdependence may stem largely from cognitive factors, not just lower-level aspects of movement execution. This finding highlights the tight links between motor control and mental function. Indeed, the finding that coupling between effectors is largely "in the mind" and not just "in the muscles" shows how cognitive even the most basic voluntary movements are.

Some disclaimers are in order. This chapter will not go into depth for several topics. Differences between the dominant and nondominant hands will not be covered in detail, though the nondominant hand is known to be less efficient in aiming (e.g., in performing series of peg transfers) than is the dominant hand (Annett, Annett, Hudson, & Turner, 1979). More will be said about an exciting new hypothesis concerning differences between the dominant and nondominant hands in the next chapter, Drawing and Writing.

A number of activities deserving of in-depth review will also not be surveyed as copiously as they might be, mostly to keep the length of the chapter manageable. We will not look in detail at the control of throwing (McDonald, van Emmerik, & Newell, 1989), the control of catching (Lacquaniti & Maioli, 1989; McIntyre, Zago, Berthoz, & Lacquaniti, 2001), the control of continuous tracking (Jagacinski & Flach, 2003), adaptation to artificial force fields while interacting with robots (Krakauer, Ghilardi, & Ghez, 1999), or adaptation to Coriolis forces while being immersed in slowly spinning rooms (Lackner & Dizio, 1994). Many of these topics have been covered elsewhere, often in connection with quite technical models of adaptive control (Shadmehr & Wise, 2005).

THE DEVELOPMENT OF REACHING AND GRASPING

By the time a human fetus is around 7.5 weeks of age it has fingers. By around 15 weeks of gestational age it can open and close its hand (Hooker, 1938). By around 24 weeks of age, a prematurely born infant can use its hand in the same way as a full-term baby. It can automatically take hold of an object placed in its palm—a reaction known as the grasp reflex (Twitchell, 1970). The grasp reflex is powerful enough in full-term infants that they can support their own weight (Figure 7.2). This has been taken to suggest that the grasp reflex may have originated with our tree-dwelling forebears. By around 6 months of age, the grasp reflex usually disappears (Touwen, 1971).

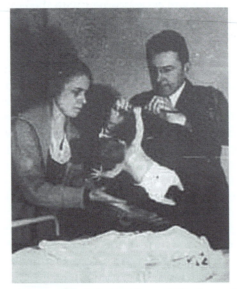

FIGURE 7.2   The grasp reflex. Still photograph from a film made by the psychologist John B. Watson in 1919. Reprinted from Boakes (1984). With permission.

Direction

Infants between the ages of 6 and 11 days can reach with rough accuracy for objects placed in different radial positions—0, 30, or 60 degrees to the right or left (Bower, Broughton, & Moore, 1970). From this result, Bower, Broughton, and Moore concluded that newborns not only have reasonably good control of their reaching movements but can also obtain directional information through vision (also see Bower, 1974).

Other studies have shown that directions of infants' reaches become more precise during the first 4 or 5 months (Hofsten, 1980; Lockman & Ashmead, 1983). By the end of this period, infants are so good at controlling the directions of their reaching and grasping movements that they can direct their hands to future positions of objects in motion, effectively "catching" the objects in midflight (Hofsten, 1980).

Distance

Distance control also improves during the first 4 or 5 months, as has been shown by identifying the distances over which infants are willing or not willing to reach. When an interesting object is out of reach, infants should refrain from reaching for it, but when the same object is within reach, infants should try, or be willing to try, to grasp it. By this logic, if distances that elicit reaches are sharply demarcated from distances that do not elicit reaches and if the boundary between the two kinds of distances approximates the length of the infant's arm, one can conclude that the infant perceives distances veridically and has information about the length of his or her arm.

Based on this logic, Bower (1972) reported that infants as young as 7 to 15 days refrain from reaching for out-of-reach objects, though the distances that elicit reaches are not sharply divided from those that do not. During subsequent development, the boundary between reachable and unreachable distances becomes sharper, until by 5 months of age, infants rarely reach for objects just beyond the maximum extent of the outstretched arm (Field, 1977; Gordon & Yonas, 1976).

Another indication of the quality of distance control is the slowing of the hand as the hand approaches an object to be grasped. By around 5 months of age, infants exhibit significant hand slowing just before contacting to-be-grabbed objects (Hofsten, 1979; White, Castle, & Held, 1964). This suggests that 5-month-old infants are sensitive to the distance and direction of the object to be grasped and of the position of the hand with respect to the object. Whether the slowing is preprogrammed or based on visual feedback is still an open question. An experiment that could resolve the question would be to study the speed with which the hand approaches a target in the dark, given that the target was visible when the hand started reaching for it. It has been established that by 9 months—but not by 5 or 7 months—infants have enough prospective control of their reaching behavior to make successful reaches when the room is darkened upon reach initiation (McCarty & Ashmead, 1999). In the McCarty and Ashmead study, infants were able to complete reaches despite being unable to see the object after reach initiation.

Orientation

As mentioned above, babies exhibit accurate control of the directions and distances of their reaches by around 5 months of age. The control of hand orientation appears to crystallize at a later age. Five-month-old babies orient their hands correctly around a vertically or horizontally oriented bar, but they orient their hands correctly only after physically contacting the bar. Nine-month-old babies, by contrast, orient their hands in anticipation of bar contact based on vision alone (Lockman, Ashmead, & Bushnell, 1984).

Why do babies younger than 9 months not orient their hands correctly before contacting objects to be grabbed? One possibility is that they cannot visually discriminate vertical and horizontal lines. Contrary to this hypothesis, however, even 2-month-olds can make this visual discrimination (Essock & Siqueland, 1981). Furthermore, 5-month-old babies can reorient their hands after physically contacting objects they wish to handle. Apparently, then, babies younger than 9 months lack a fully developed map between visually perceived orientations and corresponding hand orientations.

Size

Another control parameter that appears to be mastered only by 9 months or later is related to the size of the object being grasped. When adults reach for objects of varying size, they vary the distance between the thumb and the other fingers (Jeannerod, 1981). Infants 9 months or older do so as well, but infants younger than 9 months do not (Hofsten & Rönnqvist, 1988). It is doubtful that infants younger than 9 months are unable to visually distinguish large and small objects (Hofsten & Rönnqvist, 1988). Furthermore, infants younger than 9 months are physically able to vary their grip size, for they can spread their fingers farther apart once they have felt a large object (Hofsten & Rönnqvist, 1988). The more likely possibility is that infants younger than 9 months have not yet learned to preprogram grip size on the basis of visual information, just as infants younger than 9 months have not yet learned to preprogram hand orientation on the basis of vision.

Functional Tuning of Grasps in Infancy

Beyond recognizing the physical features of objects to be grasped and directing and shaping grasps accordingly, infants develop the ability to tune their grasps according to the functions they wish to perform. Recent research has shown that the cognitive capabilities linked to anticipatory effects in reaching and grasping appear at a relatively young age.

Claxton, Keen, and McCarty (2003) showed that 10-month-old infants reach more quickly for a ball when engaged in an activity that requires less precision (throwing the ball) than when engaged in activity that requires more precision (fitting the ball into a tube). This outcome is reminiscent of the finding that adults reach more quickly for an object that will be used in a high-precision task than in a low-precision task (Marteniuk, MacKenzie, Jeannerod, Athenes, & Dugas, 1987).

Another series of studies by the group led by Rachel Keen (formerly known as Rachel Clifton) showed that 19- to 24-month-old infants orient their hands appropriately for grasping a spoon, but younger infants (9- to 12-month-olds) do not do so (McCarty, Clifton, & Collard, 1999; McCarty, Clifton, & Collard, 2001). Twelve-month-olds can, however, show improvements in this regard through training (McCarty & Keen, 2005).

These demonstrations show that infants come to see objects more and more accurately and reach for objects in ways that are more accurate relative to how the objects look. The demonstrations also show that infants alter the way they reach for and grasp objects depending on what they plan to do with the objects. Such anticipatory effects have been mentioned before in connection with adult prehension.

Discovering anticipatory changes in physical behavior is of great interest to cognitive psychologists (of which the author is one) because such changes reflect mental representations. Mental representations—thoughts, ideas, reminiscences, predictions, and so on—are likely to underlie tool use, for how else could one explain the purposeful use of a tool to achieve some goal? Discovering anticipatory changes in grasps among infants and monkeys therefore bears on theories of tool development (Johnson-Frey, 2003).

VISUAL GUIDANCE

Reaching for a seen object usually benefits from visual feedback. If one looks at an object to be picked up but keeps one's eyes closed while reaching for it, one's performance typically suffers. Try this for yourself. Assuming your reach turns out to be better with vision than without vision, you will be primed to wonder how visual feedback is used in the control of reaches and grasps.

In approaching this question, it is useful to recognize that visual feedback can be used more and more effectively over the course of development. At around 5 months of age, babies perform about as well when reaching for objects that are seen only briefly as when reaching for objects that are seen continually (Wishart, Bower, & Dunkeld, 1978). After 5 months, reaching benefits more and more from continuous vision until, by around 11 months, the benefit of vision approximates its best level (Figure 7.3).

Learning how to use visual feedback does not end in the first year. Adults can also learn to adjust their reaching behavior based on exposure to new visual conditions. These

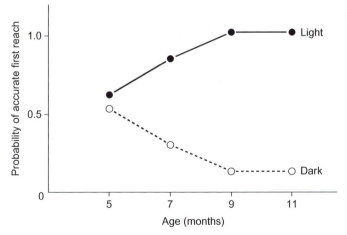

FIGURE 7.3 Accuracy of reaches made in the light (solid points and line) or dark (rings and dashed line) in babies 5–11 months of age. Data from Wishart, J. G., Bower, T. G. R., & Dunkeld, J. (1978). Reaching in the dark. Perception, 7, 507–512. With permission. Adapted from Hay (1984).

conditions can be introduced by having people observe their hand movements through a mirror (which reverses right and left) or by having people observe their hand movements through lenses or prisms that invert, displace, rotate, magnify, or minify (shrink) the image.

One of the first studies of adaptation to visual rearrangement was conducted in the late nineteenth century. The experimenter, George Stratton, wore an inverting lens for 8 days. His purpose was to learn how visual direction is appreciated given that the retinal image of the visual world is normally inverted. Stratton believed that we learn visual directions by associating visual experiences with other forms of sensory feedback, such as proprioceptive input from hand movements. Thus, if the hand is moved to the right, proprioceptive input indicates a rightward movement and allows one to identify the associated visual input as coming from the right rather than the left. Stratton reasoned that if people initially learn visual directions in this way, they should be able to learn new associations between visual and proprioceptive inputs.

Stratton's initial experiences were upsetting:

> If he saw an object off to the right, he would reach for it with his right hand and discover that he should have reached for it with left hand. He could not feed himself very well, could not tie his shoelaces without considerable difficulty, and found himself to be severely disoriented in general. His image of his own body became severely distorted. At times he felt that his head had sunk down between his shoulders, and when he moved his eyes and head the world would slide dizzyingly around [Kaufman, 1984, p. 417].

Gradually he adapted:

> As time went by, Stratton achieved more effective control over his body. He would reach with his left hand when he saw an object on the right. He could accomplish normal tasks like eating and dressing himself. His body image became almost normal, and objects did not appear to move about so much when he changed the positions of eyes and head. He even began to feel as though his left hand was on the right and his right hand was on the left. As long as this new location of his body was vivid, the world appeared to be right side up. Frequently, however, he would experience his own body as upside down in a visually right-side-up world. The visual world became the standard with which he localized his body [Kaufman, 1984, pp. 417–418].

When Stratton removed the inverting lens at the end of the eighth day of the experiment, he frequently made incorrect reaching movements. However, he soon regained his normal perceptual-motor coordination. Because he could adapt to the inverting lens and then read-apt to the normal environment, he showed through his research that perceptual-motor coordination is plastic.

Did Stratton adapt to the inverted lenses by finding a new correlation between vision and proprioception, as he supposed, or did he adapt by finding a new correlation between vision and actively generated motor commands or the intentions giving rise to those intentions?

To test the latter hypothesis, Held (1965) allowed observers to see the reflected image of a square in a horizontal mirror. The observers could move their hands beneath the mirror, but they could not see their hands. The observers' task was to mark the perceived corners of the square with a pencil, but because they could not see where the pencil marks were placed in relation to the square, the only way they could tell where the marks were placed was to compare the seen position of the square with the felt position of the hand. The question was how well observers could perform the task depending on the kind of training they received. One group actively moved their hands while watching their movements through a displacing prism. Another group simply looked at their hands through the displacing prism without making movements. A third group viewed their hands through the displacing prism as their hands were moved passively by the experimenter. After the training session, the three groups returned to the task of marking the corners of the square.

The results were clear. Only the active-movement group exhibited significant adaptation to the prism. The stationary group and the passive movement group did not. Thus, the group that could correlate the altered visual input created by the prisms with their own motor commands (or movement intentions) exhibited more adaptation than the groups that not could not achieve this correlation. Because the subjects in the passive-movement group received approximately the same proprioceptive feedback as the active-movement group, the results argue against Stratton's proposal that we learn to coordinate vision and touch by correlating visual and proprioceptive inputs. Rather, we learn to coordinate vision and touch by correlating visual information with motor commands or their underlying intentions.

Vision and Touch

When one learns new correlations between the way things look and the way things feel, does vision change, does touch change, or both? In the early eighteenth century, the British philosopher George Berkeley argued that touch is more trustworthy than vision because touch puts one in direct contact with the external environment. If Berkeley had been asked to predict what would change in a prism adaptation experiment, he would have said that vision changes but touch does not.

Subsequent experiments have indicated that Berkeley would have been mistaken. If anything, touch changes but vision remains the same. In one relevant experiment, subjects looked through prisms that made a straight rod appear curved (Gibson, 1933). When the subjects were asked to describe how the rod looked and felt, they reported that the rod looked curved and also felt curved. Thus, vision dominated over touch in this experiment. Similar results were obtained when subjects looked through a minifying lens at a cube lying on a cloth (Rock & Harris, 1967). The subjects in this study could reach under the cloth and feel the cube without seeing their hands. When they felt the cube, there was an objective mismatch between its felt and seen size. However, the subjects reported that the cube felt small—as small, in fact, as a physically smaller cube that was viewed normally. Thus, for these subjects, as for the subjects in Gibson's (1933) experiments, vision dominated touch.

What accounts for visual dominance? One possibility is that vision captures attention less effectively than touch does (Posner, Nissen, & Klein, 1976). Tapping someone on the shoulder, for example, is sure to get their attention, but raising one's hand—say, in a classroom—is not guaranteed to summon attention. Vision may dominate over touch, then, because touch has a greater alerting capacity.

Regardless of the exact cause of visual dominance, the phenomenon may have practical benefits. Consider the following curious observation (Tastevin, 1937, reported in Kaufman, 1984). A plaster replica of a person's finger was made to move in step with a subject's moving finger. When the subject saw the replica but not her own finger through a small window, she did not know that the finger she saw was someone else's. In a similar demonstration (Rock & Harris, 1967), a subject was told that she would be able to watch her own hand through a window, but unbeknownst to her, she actually saw the experimenter's hand through a mirror. Provided the experimenter's hand moved in synchrony with the subject's, the subject did not know that the hand being seen was someone else's.

These reports suggest a possible strategy for physical rehabilitation and training. Someone regaining control of a limb might be helped by seeing an image of that limb with greater mobility than it actually has. Giving the patient the impression of limb mobility might provide him or her with the incentive to try moving the limb on his or her own. One could also imagine a more draconian approach, where the movement one sees is *less* than the movement generated, in which case the patient might be persuaded to try harder to move.

An approach that builds on such visual changes has been taken with robotic aids to movement. Here, patients with limited mobility, typically after stroke, have been assisted in their movements toward specific targets. The idea is to get patients to move more and more independently by building on their returning movement abilities (Volpe et al., 2008).

The approach has also been pursued in a manner that relies solely on vision. The method entails showing amputees mirror images of their extant limbs (Figure 7.4). A mirror is placed so the image of the amputee's remaining limb appears where the amputated limb would be if it still existed. In some patients, witnessing the image of the remaining limb helps "unlock" the patient's phantom limb (Ramachandran & Rogers-Ramachandran, 1996). For example, one patient whose phantom hand had been in a clenched, painful position for years felt the phantom hand's fingers unfurl after experiencing the mirror treatment, and the pain associated with the phantom hand abated. This method has received quite a bit of popular press. The promise of the approach was extolled in the Science section of the *New York Times* (Angier, 2008).

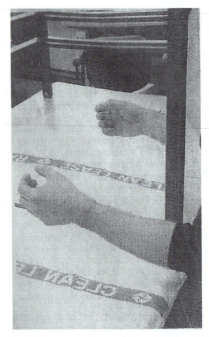

FIGURE 7.4 The one remaining hand of an amputee and the reflection of that hand in a mirror. From Angier, N. (2008). Reflections on the simple mirror. The Global Edition of The New York Times, Thursday, July 24, 2008, p. 10.

Vision for Action

No less intriguing than the effects described above are effects related to changes in perception accompanying reaching and grasping. From a conventional view of perception, one might expect perception to be the same if one were looking at a scene for the sake of recognizing objects or for the sake of acting. On the other hand, the hypothesis that there are two visual systems, one for recognition (the "what" system") and one for action (the "how" system), would allow perception to differ in these two contexts; see Figure 2.13. A number of studies have supported the two visual system hypothesis. The tack taken in these studies has been to ask whether visual illusions that arise in non-action, recognition contexts, disappear in action contexts.

An influential study done along these lines (Aglioti, DeSouza, & Goodale, 1995) relied on the fact that a circle of fixed size tends to look smaller when surrounded by large circles than when surrounded by small circles (Figure 7.5). What would happen, Aglioti, DeSouza, and Goodale asked, if instead of merely looking at the standard circle, participants reached for it? The researchers had participants reach for a poker chip surrounded by large or small disks. The participants wore infra-red emitting diodes on their index finger and thumb so the distance between the index finger and thumb could be recorded with a motion tracking

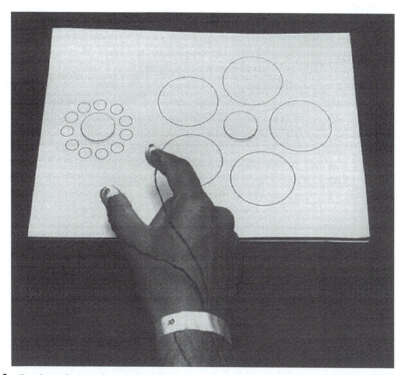

FIGURE 7.5   Reaching for a poker chip of fixed size surrounded either by small or large disks. From http://www.current-biology.com/content/article/fulltext?uid = PIIS0960982295001333&origin = SD.   Original   source: Aglioti, S., DeSouza, J. F., & Goodale, M. A. (1995). Size-contrast illusions deceive the eye but not the hand. Current Biology, 5, 679–685. With permission.

system as participants reached for the poker chip. The result was that the maximum separation between the index finger and thumb during the reach was unaffected by the size of the disks around the poker chip even though the consciously perceived size of the poker chip depended on the surrounding disks. The absence of a size contrast effect for the fingers was not due to participants seeing their fingers and correcting the separation seen between them.

The results of Aglioti, DeSouza, and Goodale (1995) are consistent with the two visual system hypothesis. That said, it should be acknowledged that these results and others obtained in this tradition have generated as much heat as light. Questions have been raised about what such results actually mean theoretically (e.g., Glover, 2002) and doubts have been expressed about methodological features of the studies and the inferences the results allow (Franz, 2001; Smeets & Brenner, 2006).

Eye-Hand Coordination

Continuing this overview of research on the visual guidance of reaching and grasping, it is natural to ask about eye-hand coordination. A number of studies have shown that when people move the hand as quickly as possible from one location to another, the eyes generally make saccades to the target location shortly before the hand. Lags between the eye and hand movements typically range from 60 to 100 ms (Angel, Alston & Garland, 1970; Prablanc, Echallier & Jeannerod, 1979). Neural signals driving the eyes and hand may be delivered simultaneously, as shown by the fact that arm-muscle EMGs begin at virtually the same time as the first sign of eye movements (Biguer, Jeannerod, & Prablanc, 1982, 1985). These results suggest that the eyes and hand comprise a "pointing synergy" whose neural commands may be generated simultaneously (Jeannerod, 1988). Consistent with this hypothesis, eye movement latencies and arm movement latencies are usually positively correlated. Trial-by-trial correlations between times to start moving the eyes and times to start moving the hand can be as high as +0.8 (Herman, Herman & Maulucci, 1981).

Because the eyes can generally travel to a target more quickly than the hand, the eye generally reaches the target before the hand (Abrams, Meyer, & Kornblum, 1990; Gribble, Everling, Ford, & Mattar, 2002; Herman, Herman, & Maulucci, 1981; Reina & Schwartz, 2003). Given that the eye then dwells on the target, what is the advantage of initiating eye and hand movements together? The benefit may derive from the ability of the oculo-motor system and manual-control system to share spatial information. The eye can "point" to the target and the hand can then move to the target, drawing on information about where the gaze is directed in space. The ability to move the eyes to a target aids hand movements, even when the target cannot be seen after the eyes have carried out the saccade (Abrams, Meyer, & Kornblum, 1990). The latter result indicates that the hand has access to spatial information about where the eye is pointing.

Additional evidence for the coupling of the eye and hand comes from studies in which the eye tracks the hand during slow, ongoing hand movements. The hand can be tracked by the eyes even when the hand cannot be seen (Gauthier, Vercher, Mussa-Ivaldi, & Marchetti, 1988). A moving image projected from one's own hand can be tracked more accurately than the projection of someone else's hand, even when the person whose eye movements are monitored does not know which hand is the source of the image displacement (Steinbach & Held, 1968). Perhaps most remarkably, the maximum velocity of smooth pursuit eye movements—about 40 degrees per second in the case of a conventional visual target (Westheimer, 1954)—is more than doubled (to 80 to 100 degrees per second) when the visual target is moved by the subject him- or herself (Gauthier, Vercher, Mussa-Ivaldi, & Marchetti, 1988).

What mechanism allows for such tight coupling between the eyes and hands in tracking one's own hand movements? Presumably, when one voluntarily moves one's hand, one can predict where the hand-driven stimulus will be. Prediction enables the oculo-motor system to anticipate the position of the moving stimulus. Tracking a conventionally driven external stimulus, by contrast, does not derive such anticipatory benefits.

Anticipation is so sophisticated that when the eye tracks the hand, if the hand causes a target to reverse direction, the eye can track the target virtually perfectly, with no measurable delay, at the reversal point (Gauthier et al., 1988). It is difficult to imagine how such near-perfect tracking could be based on a mode of control not involving some form of prediction.

As tightly coupled as the eye and hand may be, the eye and hand should also be free of one another in some circumstances. It would be unappealing to be forced to visually track one's hand movements, for example. Young babies and children with severe cerebral palsy cannot achieve such de-coupling. If the hand happens to fall into view, visual attention is captured, and the eyes are "dragged along" by sight of the hand (Gauthier et al., 1988). In the course of normal development, such coupling can be broken if necessary and the hands can perform one task while the eyes are directed elsewhere. The importance of this observation is that eye-hand synergies are task-dependent. Such task dependency is also evident in the discovery that the way the eyes scan an array of targets differs depending on whether the observer is merely looking at the targets or is preparing to tap the targets with the finger (Epelboim et al., 1997).

Beyond these fundamental observations, some creative studies of eye-hand coordination have allowed for inferences about naturalistic performance, the relation between performing actions and watching others perform those actions, and the understanding of language.

Regarding naturalistic performance, Hayhoe and Ballard (2005) described work that took advantage of the fact that eye movement recording technology has become more portable in recent years than it was before. Whereas in the past, a researcher interested in eye movements had to have a subject sit still in a head mount or even on a bite block, eye movements can now be recorded with the subject moving freely (Figure 7.6). With this new type of apparatus, it is possible to record where people look as they engage in everyday activities like stacking blocks or making peanut butter and jelly sandwiches (Hayhoe & Ballard, 2005).

Regarding the second of the topics referred to above, namely, the relation between performing and watching others perform actions, Flanagan and Johansson (2003) found that people generated similar scanpaths when they stacked blocks or watched someone else stack the same blocks. Subjects looked at critical points where they themselves would grasp blocks for stacking, and they looked at those same critical points when they watched someone else do the "heavy lifting." This outcome suggests a tight connection between one's own plans for action and one's appreciation of others' action plans.

Regarding the third of the topics mentioned above, the understanding of language, psycholinguists have relied on eye-hand coordination to investigate speech perception.

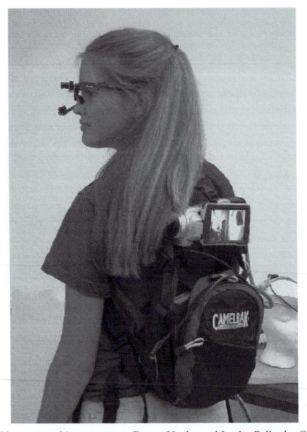

FIGURE 7.6 Portable eye-tracking system. From Hayhoe, M. & Ballard, C. (2005). Reaching in natural behavior. Trends in Cognitive Sciences, 9, 188–194. With permission. From http://www. sciencedirect.com/science?_ob = ArticleURL&_udi = B6VH9-4FM9MR7-1&_user = 209810&_rdoc = 1&_ fmt = &_orig = search&_sort = d&view = c&_acct = C000014439&_version = 1&_urlVersion = 0&_userid = 2098 10&md5 = b9b045735ab772ace5b0edd6947afa28.

Behind this work is the idea is that if subjects need to reach for one of two objects named in an experimental trial, subjects' eye movements over the scene may reveal how the subjects process the heard name of the object. If there are two objects, one a piece of candy and the other a candle, for example, the subjects may only look at the object to be named after the distinguishing syllable is heard: the "y" of candy or the "le" of candle. By contrast, if there are two objects, one a piece of candy and the other a pickle, subjects may look at the object to be named earlier, at the moment of the first distinguishing phoneme. All that is needed to distinguish "pickle" from "candy" is the first phoneme. If people can distinguish words immediately after their distinguishing phonemes are heard, they should be able to move their eyes to the candy more quickly when the alternative is a pickle than when the alternative is a candle. This is just what has been found (Allopenna, Magnuson, & Tanenhaus, 1998; Tanenhaus, Spivey Knowlton, & Eberhard, 1995).

AIMING

Much of the research on the control of hand movements has been concerned with the task of moving the hand from one position to another, generally as quickly and as accurately as possible. How people correct their errors has been a topic of long-standing interest.

In approaching this problem, it is useful to remember that errors arise when initial movements are incorrect. From this perspective, it is useful to note some of the errors reflect biases in the way movements are made.

Figure 7.7 shows data from a study that revealed an important feature of such biases. In this study (Gordon & Ghez, 1994), participants moved one hand from a home position to each of a number of targets. Some of the targets were near the home position and others were farther away. Participants were told that they did not have to correct their movements if the movements ended off target. Under this instruction, the distribution of endpoints for the movements could be taken to reflect the biases of the movement system.

As seen in Figure 7.7, the endpoint distributions were elliptical: The endpoints were more widely spread along the line connecting the start point to the target point than along the line perpendicular to the line connecting the start point to the target point. This result implies that participants were better at getting the direction of movement right than at getting the amplitude of movement right. From this outcome, one would expect amplitude corrections to be more strongly needed than direction corrections.

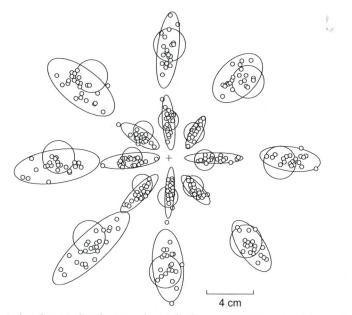

4 cm

FIGURE 7.7 Elliptical end-point distributions obtained when participants moved from a home position (+) to each of a number of targets (circles) but did not have to correct the movements they made. From Gordon, J., & Ghez, C. (1994). Accuracy of planar reaching movements: I. Independence of direction and extent variability. Experimental Brain Research, 99, 97–111. With permission. From http://www.ncbi.nlm.nih.gov/pubmed/7925800.

Amplitude errors are of two main kinds. One is going farther than required. The other is going shorter than required. Going farther is more time consuming than going shorter. It takes longer to turn back than to go farther (Vince & Welford, 1967). This outcome makes sense in terms of mechanical inertia. It may also explain why participants take longer to resolve direction uncertainty than extent uncertainty when preparing to move to targets with different directions and extents (Rosenbaum, 1980). They may pay more attention to getting direction right before movements begin than to getting amplitudes right before movements begin because direction errors are harder to correct than are amplitude errors.

Figure 7.8 shows another important finding from Gordon and Ghez (1994). This figure shows speed profiles for the movements in their task. As seen in Figure 7.8, the speed profiles are bell-shaped, with the bell shapes being larger for movements to far targets than for movements to near targets. This outcome suggests that from the start of the movements, participants moved at rates that scaled with the distance to be covered. The movements were ready in their entirety before being executed, or at least their principal features were

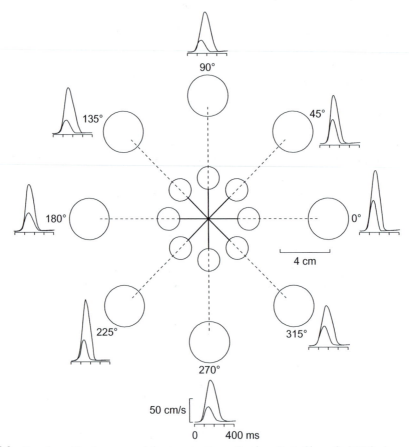

FIGURE 7.8 Speed profiles to near and far targets. From Gordon, J., & Ghez, C. (1994). Accuracy of planar reaching movements: I. Independence of direction and extent variability. Experimental Brain Research, 99, 97–111. With permission. Experimental Brain Research. From http://www.ncbi.nlm.nih.gov/pubmed/7925800.

ready in advance, such as their lengths and directions. Before they started to move, the participants knew, at some level, just how they would do so.

This outcome helps explain why one sometimes has the uncanny feeling, while making a movement, that the movement is doomed to fail. Similarly and more positively, it helps explain why one may sense that a movement will be successful (Gray, Beilock, & Carr, 2007). A report of such a feeling was reported in the sports news while the author was working on this second edition of *Human Motor Control*. On the evening of April 7, 2008, the University of Kansas beat the University of Memphis for the NCAA national basketball championship. With just 2.1 seconds left in regular play and with Kansas behind Memphis by 3 points, Mario Chalmers hit a 3-pointer. The two teams went into overtime and Kansas went on to beat Memphis 75–68. In the author's local newspaper, the *Centre Daily Times*, this quote from Mario Chalmers appeared the next morning: "I had a good look at it. . . . When it left my hands it felt like it was good, and it just went in."

Woodworth's Pioneering Study

We turn now to error correction itself. How well can people aim for targets? Pioneering work on aiming was done by Woodworth (1899) for his doctoral dissertation at Columbia University. Woodworth was impressed by the speed and accuracy with which construction workers hammered nails. He wondered how these workers could achieve the speed and accuracy they did. To answer this question, he set up an experiment in which people moved a stylus back and forth through a slit, reversing the direction of the movements at two visually marked locations. Woodworth recorded subjects' movements by allowing the pencil to draw a line on a paper roll that turned beneath the work surface. (Computers and other electronic data-recording devices were not yet available.) Subjects were asked to make the back-and-forth movements at different rates specified by a metronome. In one set of conditions, subjects made the movements with their eyes open. In another set of conditions, they made the movements with their eyes closed.

Woodworth's results are shown in Figure 7.9. The dependent measure was mean absolute error, defined as the mean absolute value of the distance between the point where the pencil reversed direction and where it should have reversed direction (the target). The independent measure was the mean movement velocity. As seen in Figure 7.9, when subjects had their eyes closed, their mean absolute error remained more or less constant as velocity increased. When subjects had their eyes open, their mean absolute error decreased as velocity decreased.

Woodworth accounted for these results by saying that in the eyes-closed condition subjects' movements were entirely preprogrammed, being guided by what he called the *initial impulse*. By contrast, in the eyes-open condition, the subjects' movements were preprogrammed but could be corrected with visual feedback, or what Woodworth called *current control*. Woodworth hypothesized that the first part of an aiming movement is achieved through initial impulse control and the later parts are achieved with current control. He based this hypothesis on observations of participants making large, quick, target-directed movements followed by smaller, slower, target-capturing movements.

By Woodworth's way of thinking, if a movement is made in too short a time for current control to be possible, the movements should be just as error-prone if visual feedback is

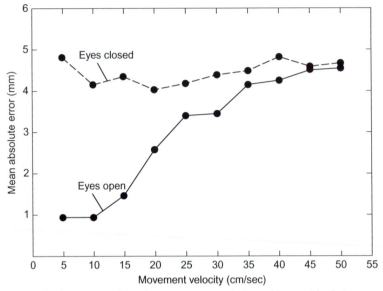

FIGURE 7.9 Mean absolute error of hand movements made by subjects with their eyes open or closed. Data from Woodworth (1899). Adapted from Woodworth, R. S. (1899). The accuracy of voluntary movement. Psychological Review, 3, 1–119. With permission.

present or not. Conversely, if a movement is made in enough time for current control to be possible, the movements should more accurate if visual feedback is present than if not. Seeing where along the required velocity axis there is a transition from no benefit of visual feedback to some benefit of visual feedback lets one estimate the critical velocity for using visual feedback. Because a single distance was used in Woodworth's experiment, the critical velocity could be translated to a critical time (since velocity equals distance divided by time). Woodworth estimated the critical time for visual feedback to be a fifth of a second.

Later research largely confirmed Woodworth's estimate. It did so based on the following logic. Suppose it takes t ms to process visual feedback. Movements that take longer than t ms should then be impaired if visual feedback is suddenly withdrawn, but movements that take less than t ms should be carried out equally well regardless of whether visual feedback is available or not. This reasoning allowed Keele and Posner (1968) to estimate t. They trained subjects to move a stylus from a home position to a target position in different amounts of time: 150 ms, 250 ms, 350 ms, or 450 ms, +10% for each target time. In a block of trials, the subject repeatedly tried to make the movement within the target time, but on some trials the room lights went off unpredictably as soon as the movement began. Aiming accuracy was affected by the presence or absence of visual feedback only when movements took about 200 ms or more. From this outcome, Keele and Posner (1968) concluded that it takes about 200 ms to use vision to correct aiming movements. Subsequent research has suggested that visually based corrections may take less time than Keele and Posner (1968) proposed (Carlton, 1981; Zelaznik, Hawkins, & Kisselburgh, 1983). Nonetheless, it is safe to say that the time for the visual feedback loop is between 100 ms and 200 ms.

Fitts' Law

The idea that aiming movements have an initial, ballistic phase followed by a feedback-based homing-in phase has been pursued with a number of methods. One is to have subjects move a stylus back and forth between two targets as quickly as possible, where the distance between the targets and the widths of the targets varies (Fitts, 1954). The time to bring the stylus from one target to another increases with the distance between the targets. It also increases as the targets become narrower. This relation was summarized by Fitts (1954) as follows:

$$MT = a + b \log_2(2A/W),$$
(7.1)

where MT denotes movement time, A denotes the amplitude (or distance) between the centers of the targets, W denotes the width of the target, and a and b are empirical constants. The term $\log_2(2A/W)$ is called the index of difficulty, or ID.

Equation 7.1 says that MT increases linearly with ID, a claim that has been confirmed experimentally (Figure 7.10). In fact, Equation 7.1 has been found to do such a good job predicting movement times for so many aiming tasks that it has come to been called Fitts' law (Keele, 1968). Fitts' law is one of the few laws in psychology.

Other tasks where Equation 7.1 applies include discrete ("one-shot") aiming movements (Fitts & Peterson, 1964), transferring pegs over a distance to be inserted into a hole (Annet,

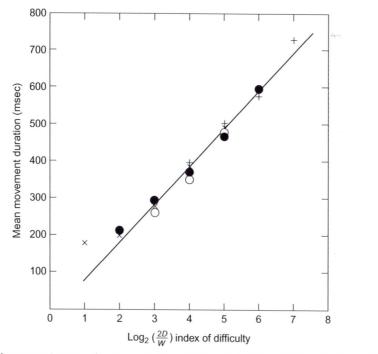

FIGURE 7.10 Movement time as a function of index of difficulty in Fitts' (1954) study. From Meyer, Smith, Kornblum, Abrams, and Wright (1990).

Golby, & Kay, 1958), moving a joystick or turning a handle to move a cursor on a screen (Jagacinski, Repperger, Moran, Ward, & Glass, 1980; Meyer, Smith, & Wright, 1982), throwing darts at a target (Kerr & Langolf, 1977), carrying out aiming movements under water (Kerr, 1973), and manipulating objects under a microscope (Langolf, Chaffin, & Foulke, 1976).

Some mathematical variants of Fitts' law have been proposed (Beamish, Bhatti, Mackenzie, & Wu, 2006; Kvalseth, 1980; Plamondon & Alimi, 1997), but the main idea behind Fitts' law has never been questioned, namely, that the farther one has to go and the tighter the accuracy constraints of the target, the longer the movement takes, provided one tries to go as quickly as possible.

Fitts' law or variants of Fitts' law (Elliott, Helsen, & Chua, 2001) have also been pursued by considering other related tasks, including moving around obstacles (Jax, Rosenbaum, & Vaughan, 2007) and moving through restricted pathways (Accot & Zhai, 2001). People can engage in motor imagery in accordance with Fitts' law (Decety & Jeannerod, 1995; Sirigu et al., 1996) and can see actions as possible or impossible depending on whether those actions are consistent with Fitts' law (Grosjean, Knoblich, & Shiffrar, 2007). Fitts' law can also be violated when extraneous targets are present in the workspace (Adam, Mol, Pratt, & Fischer, 2006), and decisions about optimal movement choices, as defined by Fitts' law, can be made in some tasks (Augustyn & Rosenbaum, 2006), but not others (Young, Chau, & Pratt, 2008).

Iterative Corrections Model

How can one explain the main relation suggested by Fitts' law? One idea, embodied in the *iterative corrections* model of Crossman and Goodeve (1963/1983; Keele, 1968), is that Fitts' law is mainly attributable to current control. According to this model, an aiming movement consists of a series of discrete submovements, each of which is triggered by feedback that the target has yet to be attained. By hypothesis, each submove takes the hand (or a handheld stylus) a fixed proportion of the distance to the target. For example, if the hand is 20 cm from the center of the target and each submove takes the hand 50% closer to the center of the target, then the first submove brings the hand 10 cm from the target center, the second submove brings the hand 5 cm from the target center, the third submove brings the hand 2.5 cm from the target center, and so on. As the width of the target decreases, the hand falls within the target later in the series of submoves. Similarly, as the distance of the target increases (for a given target width), the first submove for which the hand falls within the target is also delayed. Qualitatively, then, the model accounts for the relationships implied by Fitts' law. Quantitatively, the model predicts a linear increase of total movement time with index of difficulty (Fitts' law), provided one assumes that each correction takes a constant amount of time (Keele, 1968).

The iterative corrections model has been supported by detailed analyses of movement trajectories. Discrete submoves of the sort assumed in the model have been recorded (Annett, Golby, & Kay, 1958; Carlton, 1981; Crossman & Goodeve, 1963/1983; Jagacinski et al., 1980; Langolf, Chaffin, & Foulke, 1976; Woodworth, 1899). A representative example is shown in Figure 7.11.

Further research has shown, however, that the iterative corrections model is a bit off target. When discrete submoves are present, they appear as distinct peaks in the function relating velocity to time, yet one does not always see these distinct velocity peaks (Langolf et al., 1976). In addition, when distinct submovements are detectable, they do not have constant

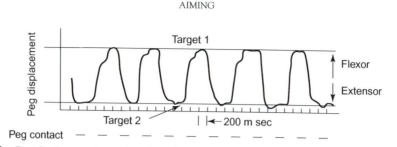

FIGURE 7.11   Peg displacement as a function of time in an aiming task performed under a microscope. The "plateaus" prior to the targets reflect momentary slowing of the hand. Data from Langolf, G. D., Chaffin, D. B., & Foulke, J. A. (1976). An investigation of Fitts' Law using a wide range of movement amplitudes. Journal of Motor Behavior, 8, 113–128. With permission. Adapted from Smyth, M. M. (1984). Memory for movements. In M. M. Smyth & A. M. Wing (Eds.), The psychology of human movement (pp. 83–117). London: Academic Press. With permission.

durations (Jagacinski et al., 1980; Langolf et al., 1976), nor do they travel constant proportions of the distance remaining to the target (Jagacinski et al., 1980). These problems have led investigators to seek an alternative to the iterative corrections model.

Impulse Variability Model

One alternative says that Fitts' law represents the initial impulse phase of movement rather than the current control phase (Schmidt, Zelaznik, Hawkins, Frank, & Quinn, 1979). The experiments that led to this model differed from the kinds of experiments that Fitts (1954) conducted. Whereas Fitts had his participants get to a defined target area in as little time as possible, Schmidt et al. had their subjects get to a target within a prescribed amount of time, trying to minimize the spatial variability of the movement endpoints. Specifically, subjects in the experiments of Schmidt et al. were supposed to move within 200 ms, a time that was unlikely to permit much current control. The targets were between 10 and 30 cm from the home position. A single movement was made in each trial. The measure of interest was the spatial variability of the movement endpoints.

Schmidt et al. observed that the standard deviation of the endpoints, denoted W_e, increased with the distance, D, to be covered and decreased with the duration, T, of the movement:

$$W_e = k(D/T),\qquad(7.2)$$

which can be rearranged as

$$T = k(D/W_e).\qquad(7.3)$$

This relation between time, distance, and effective target width is similar to Fitts' law.

What property of the motor system could give rise to this relation? Schmidt et al. proposed that rapid arm movements are achieved by, in effect, flinging the arm toward a target. The flinging is achieved with a neuro-motor impulse delivered to the arm muscles. The impulse causes the muscles to exert a burst of force for the first half of the movement time. During the second half of the movement time, the limb coasts (moves passively) toward the target.

A further assumption is that there is variability in the forces driving the arm toward the target as well as variability in the time during which the forces are produced. The standard deviation of the force is assumed to be proportional to the amount of force, and the standard deviation of the time during which impulses are delivered is assumed to be proportional to the time during which the impulses are delivered. Thus, if more force is used to cover a larger distance, more force variability results, and if more time is spent propelling the limb toward the target, more time variability results as well. Because time and force can be independently controlled in the model, the participant's challenge is to find the time and force that minimize the variability of both factors. According to Schmidt et al., Fitts' law represents the solution to this problem.

The impulse variability model has much to recommend it, at least as a model of rapid movements. It recognizes the inherent variability of neuro-motor processes, and it represents this variability in simple terms.

Schmidt et al. tested their assumptions about force and time variability by having subjects make isometric movements, producing different magnitudes of force for varying amounts of times. As predicted by the model, standard deviation of force was proportional to the force produced, and standard deviation of time was proportional to the time spent moving.

As encouraging as these results were for the impulse variability model, the model cannot account for all the effects observed in rapid aiming tasks. Submoves based on feedback are often observed, as noted in the last section, yet the impulse variability model makes no provision for feedback-based correction. Furthermore, questions have been raised about the model's assumptions concerning force and time variability (Newell & Carlton, 1988). Finally, some questions were raised about the way Schmidt et al. derived Fitts' law from their underlying assumptions, although Fitts' law can be derived in a less controversial manner if the assumptions are refined (Meyer, Smith, & Wright, 1982).

Optimized Initial Impulse Model

So far, we have considered two ways of explaining Fitts' law. One, the iterative corrections model, explains Fitts' law solely in terms of current control. The other, the impulse variability model, explains Fitts' law solely in terms of initial impulse. Neither model fully accounts for the data on manual aiming, so one is left hoping for a better model. Such a model was proposed by Meyer, Abrams, Kornblum, Wright, and Smith (1988). Their *optimized initial impulse* model is a hybrid of the iterative corrections model and the impulse variability model.

The starting point for the optimized initial impulse model is shown in Figure 7.12. By hypothesis, the subject makes a first movement toward the target. If the movement lands within the target, the task is completed, but if the movement lands outside the target, another movement is necessary. The second movement can either land within the target or not. If the second movement does not reach the target, another movement must be made, and so forth. The subject's task is to reach the target as quickly as possible, so ideally s/he should make just one, high-velocity movement directly to the target. The problem is that, according to the model, the spatial accuracy of movements is imperfect. The standard deviation, S_i, of the endpoint of any movement i is assumed to increase with the distance, D_i, covered by that movement and to decrease with its duration, T_i, that is,

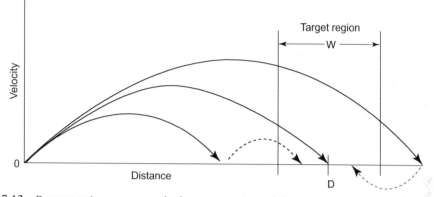

FIGURE 7.12 Representative sequences of submovements toward the target region assumed in the optimized initial impulse model of Meyer, Abrams, Kornblum, Wright, and Smith (1988). From Meyer et al. (1988). Optimality in human motor performance: Ideal control of rapid aimed movements. Psychological Review, 95, 340–370. Copyright © 1988 by the American Psychological Association. Adapted by permission.

$$S_i = k(D_i / T_i),$$ (7.4)

where k is a constant. The subject therefore faces a dilemma. To get to the target as quickly as possible, s/he could make a movement with a long distance (large D) and short time (small T), but this would result in a large standard deviation (S in Equation 7.4) and a low probability of hitting the target. Alternatively, the subject could make a movement with a long duration (T in Equation 7.4) and s/he could make a series of short movements (small values of D) and be sure of hitting the target, but the total movement time would be very long. The best thing to do, then, is to find the balance of D's and T's that minimizes the total movement time. According to Meyer et al. (1988), Fitts' law represents such an optimal balance.

The optimized initial impulse model is interesting not just because it does a good job of accounting for data from aiming studies, but also because it implies that even when people engage in a task as mundane as bringing the hand to a target, they employ sophisticated strategies to optimize performance. This conclusion reinforces the point that has been made repeatedly in this book and that is arguably the most important general principle of all of motor control research, namely, that even simple motor tasks that appear on first glance to be computationally trivial are far from it.

EQUILIBRIUM POINT HYPOTHESIS

In the research reviewed above, subjects were instructed to move very quickly. Not all aiming movements are performed this way, however. When movements are performed at slower rates, are they controlled through heavy reliance on feedback? An experiment reported by Polit and Bizzi (1978) provided surprising feedback on this question.

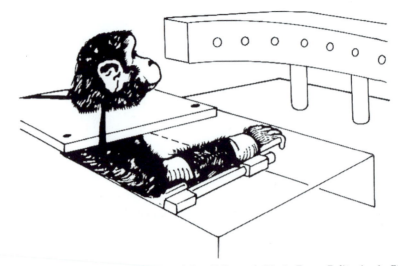

FIGURE 7.13 Experimental arrangement used by Polit and Bizzi. From Polit, A. & Bizzi, E. (1979). Characteristics of motor programs underlying arm movements in monkeys. Journal of Neurophysiology, 42, 183–194. Reprinted by permission of the American Physiological Society.

Polit and Bizzi (1978) investigated monkeys' pointing responses to target lights (Figure 7.13). On any given trial, one of the lights was turned on and the monkey was supposed to point to the illuminated light, holding its arm there for 1 second to receive a sip of juice. The monkey could not see its arm, so it received no visual feedback about the position of its arm relative to the light. The position of the arm was recorded with a splint attached to a vertical axle. The axle rotated when the monkey's arm moved, and the angular position of the axle was recorded. The axle could also be turned with a torque motor. When the torque motor came on, it caused the monkey's arm to be displaced. The torque motor was turned on unpredictably from trial to trial but usually came on after the target light was illuminated and before the monkey moved its arm.

The question Polit and Bizzi (1978) sought to answer was what would happen to the accuracy of pointing when the arm was displaced. For monkeys with normal proprioceptive feedback, pointing accuracy was high, consistent with the notion that when the monkey felt its arm being displaced, it introduced appropriate compensatory responses. However, an additional aspect of the experiment suggested that feedback was not the only source of information that monkeys relied on. After the initial phase of the experiment (described above), the dorsal roots of the monkey's spinal cord were severed. These fibers supply sensory feedback to the central nervous system (see Chapter 3). Thus, cutting the dorsal roots prevented the monkey from feeling anything below the neck, as confirmed in behavioral and physiological tests. Given this state of affairs, one would expect the monkey to be unable to compensate for the perturbation. Yet it could do so. When the monkey was again supposed to point to the target lights, it could do so accurately, even after the perturbation was applied.

How can this surprising result be explained? Polit and Bizzi (1978) appealed to the notion that muscles act like springs (Asatryan & Feldman, 1965; Crossman & Goodeve, 1963/1983). To appreciate the analogy, consider the following experiment, which you can set up yourself.

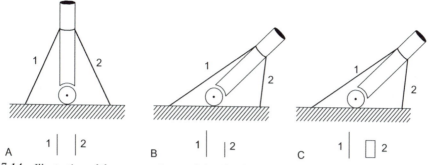

FIGURE 7.14   Illustration of the mass-spring model with a hinged cylinder and two rubber bands. (A) Resting lengths and stiffnesses of the rubber bands are equal. (B) Resting length of rubber band 1 is less than the resting length of rubber band 2 but the stiffnesses are equal. (C) Resting lengths of the rubber bands are equal but the stiffness of rubber band 2 is greater than the stiffness of rubber band 1 (indicated by the thicknesses of the bands in the rest position).

Take two identical rubber bands and attach one to one side of a hinged board and the other to the other side of the board, as shown in Figure 7.14. Orient the board parallel to the ground so the forces provided by the rubber bands are orthogonal to (perpendicular to) the force of gravity. Now pull the board to one side and release it. It will swing back and forth for a while and then come to rest at approximately 90 degrees. Next, try releasing the board from different starting positions. It will return to the same final position. This demonstrates that a spring system can achieve the same final position regardless of its starting position—a property known as *equifinality*. If the primate arm were controlled like the simple spring system of Figure 7.14, it too would be able to arrive at the same final position regardless of the position from which it starts, and it could do so even without feedback.

Unlike the board in Figure 7.14, a biological arm can get to different final positions. Can a simple spring system achieve different final positions? There are two ways it can. You can demonstrate one of these methods with a hinged board and two rubber bands of different length but the same stiffness. (You can make two such rubber bands by cutting one rubber band into two pieces of unequal length). Attach the two rubber bands to either side of the hinged board and again try releasing the board from different starting positions. Again the board will always end up at the same final position, but this time the final position will not be at 90 degrees. Instead, it will be in the direction of the shorter rubber band (see Figure 7.14B). In general, the board will end at the position where the opposing forces of the two rubber bands balance out, at the equilibrium position. If the left rubber band has a shorter resting length than the right rubber band, the board will end up pointing to the left. If the right rubber band has a shorter resting length than the left rubber band, the board will end up pointing to the right. The greater the discrepancy between the resting lengths of the two rubber bands, the more extreme the board's final position will be. This follows from the fact that, for ideal springs, the tension exerted by a spring is proportional to the distance it is stretched from its resting position, a principle known as Hooke's law. Because it is possible to obtain different equilibrium positions by changing the resting lengths of opposing springs, the biological motor system might achieve different limb positions by altering the resting lengths of the opposing muscles acting on the limb (Berkenblit, Feldman, & Fucson, 1986).

Another way to achieve different final positions with a simple spring system is to vary the stiffnesses of the springs (see Figure 7.14C). You can observe this effect by using two rubber bands of equal length but different stiffnesses. Use three identical rubber bands and place two on one side of the board for this purpose. Displace the board and let it swing freely. It will end up in the direction of the stiffer rubber band. In general, the stiffer the rubber band on one side relative to the other, the farther away from 90 degrees the board's final position will be. This outcome suggests that another way for a biological motor system to vary a limb's final position is to vary the stiffnesses of the limb's opposing muscles (Polit & Bizzi, 1978, 1979).

Why might it be advantageous for the motor system to treat muscles as springs? The main reason is that regulating muscle resting length or muscle stiffness is a simple way of directing a limb from one position to another. If the limb naturally behaves as an equilibrium point system, it is sensible for the motor system to treat it as such. If the motor system could not exploit the spring-like nature of muscle, it might be necessary to specify the entire trajectory of the limb, which could be onerous. Treating the limb as a equilibrium point system affords the possibility of significantly reducing the computational demands of trajectory planning.

Assuming that the study reported by Polit and Bizzi (1978, 1979) demonstrates reliance on an equilibrium point strategy for monkey limb control, what evidence is there that the equilibrium point model applies to human performance? One source of information is an experiment in which human patients who lacked sensory feedback from their fingers moved a finger from one position to another without being able to see their finger move (Kelso & Holt, 1980). After performing this task, the patients were asked to reproduce the movement they had just performed, passing the finger either over the same distance or to the same location as in the first task. Location reproduction should be possible, according to the equilibrium point model, even if the position of the finger cannot be sensed and even if the finger is passively displaced while moving toward the target. Distance reproduction, however, should be difficult, particularly if the finger is perturbed by an external force. The results supported the equilibrium point model. Although the patients could not feel their finger, they could bring the finger from one location to another, even when the finger was momentarily displaced by a torque motor. When the same patients were asked to cover the same distance as in the first task, their performance was significantly worse than when they were asked to reach the same location. This result suggests that subjects were not simply clever about finding ways of compensating for their handicaps.

Because the study of human patients by Kelso and Holt (1980) is like the study of monkeys by Polit and Bizzi (1978, 1979), one might think that the equilibrium point model can only be demonstrated with feedback-deprived subjects who must compensate for unexpected limb displacements. The model's success is more widespread, however. When a person with normal proprioception is asked to use the forearm to drag a load over a horizontal surface to a target, if the load is suddenly released and the subject does not attempt to compensate, the resulting hand trajectories are as predicted by the mass-spring model (Asatryan & Feldman, 1965). Furthermore, a computer simulation of the equilibrium point model (Cooke, 1980) predicts a characteristic of rapid aimed hand movements that has been obtained in several studies—a bell-shaped speed profile, with the peak of the curve near the midpoint of the displacement (Abend, Bizzi, & Morasso, 1982; Cooke, 1980).

There has been debate about the equilibrium point hypothesis, however. One point of contention is whether muscle resting lengths or stiffnesses are regulated to bring limbs to new positions. Bizzi and colleagues favored the stiffness regulation view, and in support of this hypothesis, they argued that even in the absence of afferent feedback it is possible to identify cells in the spinal cord (of the frog) that when stimulated drive the leg to well-defined positions (Bizzi, Mussa-Ivaldi, & Giszter, 1991).

Feldman and colleagues favored the resting length view, arguing that a well-established mechanism can be used for regulating muscle resting length. That mechanism is changing the threshold for the muscle stretch reflex (Feldman & Latash, 2005). Feldman and colleagues contended that the results obtained by Bizzi et al. are compatible with this interpretation. A demonstration you can try for yourself to perhaps convince you that Feldman and colleagues are correct is to squeeze on an object—a can of soda, say—and then pull the object out from between your squeezing fingers. Your fingers will quickly come to rest at a position within the now-absent object. This position corresponds to the resting lengths your muscles adopted while you held the can.

Others have argued that neither the stiffness view nor the resting length view is correct. Kawato and colleagues questioned the equilibrium point hypothesis altogether, based on research indicating that participants have much finer control of limb trajectories than might be expected if the equilibrium point hypothesis were correct (Gomi & Kawato, 1996). Burdet, Osu, Franklin, Milner, and Kawato (2001) argued that it is not as difficult to learn to control limb trajectories as advocates of the equilibrium point hypothesis assert. Burdet et al. showed that even in the face of highly unstable dynamics (forces and torques acting on the limb), people could learn to make adaptive movements. Thus, the subjects of Burdet et al. could do quite well on a task that, according to proponents of the equilibrium point hypothesis, should be impossible or at least very difficult.

DISCRETE VERSUS CONTINUOUS MOVEMENTS

Implicit in the foregoing discussion of the equilibrium point hypothesis is the assumption that movements are discrete: A movement is made to an endpoint, then the next movement is made to its endpoint, and so on. According to the equilibrium point hypothesis, if casual observation suggests that someone is moving in a smoothly flowing fashion, the underlying control is actually discrete, such that one starts before another ends. So are reaching movements fundamentally discrete or fundamentally continuous? Are they discrete with overlap that makes them appear continuous, or are they continuous with stops that make them appear discrete?

Again, as might be imagined, this has been a topic of debate in the motor control community. Evidence has been offered for the view that continuous-appearing movements may in fact arise from cascading discrete movements. Much of this evidence has relied on demonstrations that complex movement sequences with apparently seamless transitions can in fact be decomposed into overlapping submovements. Work on the optimized initial impulse model took this tack (Meyer et al., 1990), as did studies of infant reaching movements (Berthier, 1996) and corrective movements by human adults (Henis & Flash, 1995).

Henis and Flash (1995) asked what would happen when participants try to bring the hand to one target but then had to bring the hand to some other target that suddenly appeared. In their experiment, Henis and Flash had participants make horizontal planar arm movements with the preferred hand, displacing a stylus from a start location to a target location. In the control trials, a single target location appeared and participants were supposed to make direct movements to that target. In the experimental trials, the first target was extinguished and a different target appeared at either of two equally likely locations. Henis and Flash found that the observed kinematics of the hand could best be explained with a discrete cascade model. According to the model, two independent movements simply add together if a second target appears. One movement corresponds to the initially planned displacement from the start position (A) to the first target (B). The second movement corresponds to the displacement from the first target (B) to the second target (C). How the movements add— where in the movement from A to B the movement from B to C is added—depends on the timing of the second target relative to the motion of the hand away from the home position. An interesting feature of this model was that it avoided an appeal to the idea that participants aborted the first movement if a second target appeared. Rather, the second movement was simply added to the first and the first movement was allowed to run its course. This strategy is always guaranteed to work, provided the two movements are carried out correctly, because the two movements comprise two vectors that, when added, are guaranteed to bring the hand from its start position to the necessary end position.

Henis and Flash's model is noteworthy because it illustrates how seemingly continuous kinematics can arise from discrete control. Yet it does not follow that all continuous kinematics arise this way. In an influential study that pushed things in the other direction, Guiard (1993) asked whether the back-and-forth movements observed in the Fitts' reciprocal aiming task are in fact discrete. Guiard studied the kinematics of the hand in back-and-forth aiming tasks with varying indices of difficulty (IDs). Guiard found, as shown in Figure 7.15 (bottom panel), that when ID was high (a difficult aiming task), the function relating acceleration to displacement was essentially a straight line, or more properly, a series of points that ascended and descended along a line that was approximately straight. However, as ID decreased (aiming became easier), the function relating acceleration to displacement contained loops in the vicinity of each target. Guiard (1993) took these results to suggest that the normal way of moving is to move continuously rather than in a discrete point-to-point fashion.

Others have chimed in in favor of Guiard's all-is-continuous view (Mottet & Bootsma, 1999; Schöner, 1990). Others have argued that there are, in fact, two distinct modes of controlling movements—the discrete way and the continuous way (Buchanen, Park, & Shea, 2006; Hogan & Sternad, 2007; van Mourik & Beek, 2004). Investigators are still sorting out the issue.

INTERSEGMENTAL COORDINATION

In the last section we considered the question of whether motions of the hand, treated as a single point, are part of one continuous stream or discrete displacements chained together. How, we asked, are series of movements coordinated?

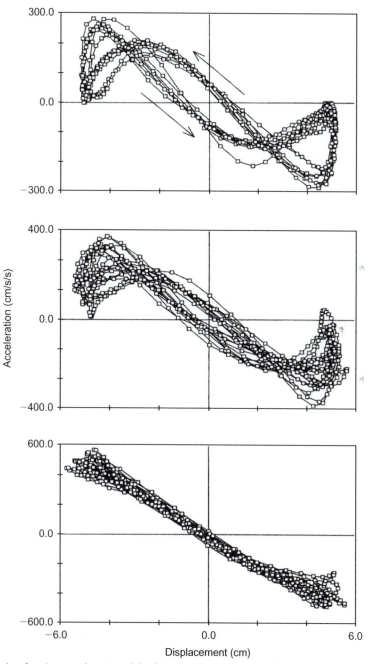

FIGURE 7.15 Acceleration as a function of displacement for back-and-forth aiming movements with a low (top panel), medium (middle panel), and high (bottom panel) index of difficulty. From Guiard, Y. (1993). On Fitts's and Hooke's laws: Simple harmonic movement in upper-limb cyclical aiming. Acta Psychological, 82, 139–159(1993). With permission.

We turn now to coordination of a somewhat different kind, coordination of different limb segments acting simultaneously. The limb segments to be considered are the hand, fingers, wrist, elbow, and shoulder. Because most people have two hands, the question of coordination naturally also extends to the analysis of two-hand motions. However, it is important to remember that while coordination can be studied in terms of the effectors that are usually involved in reaching and grasping, coordination need not be studied only in those terms. One might grasp an object with one's mouth, for example, which is not at all unusual if one is a bird, dog, or baby. Whatever principles apply to coordination of the canonical effectors for reaching and grasping—the fingers, hand, wrist, elbow, and shoulder—those principles might also apply to the coordination of other effectors. A general theory of coordination ought to accommodate coordination of any effectors, even effectors that extend to tools.

Transport and Grasp Phases

Reaching for an object and taking hold of it appear to take place in two distinct phases—a transport phase and a grasp phase. During the transport phase, the hand is carried toward the object. During the grasp phase, the fingers are wrapped around the object. These two phases appear to be controlled by different areas of the brain. Damage to the pyramidal tract (see Chapter 3) results in impairments of fine finger control, including impairments in grasping objects. Damage to the extra-pyramidal tract results in impairments of gross arm movements, including damage to hand transports prior to object manipulation (Kuypers, 1973). Developmentally, the pyramidal tract also matures after the extra-pyramidal tract (Lawrence & Hopkins, 1972), which may explain why fine finger control is possible only after gross arm movements come to be controlled relatively skillfully. Behavioral studies also support the hypothesis that the transport phase and grasp phase are governed separately. Changing the size of an object to be grasped does not affect the rate at which the arm is moved but does affect the maximum separation between the thumb and index finger as the hand approaches the to-be-grasped object (Jeannerod, 1981, 1984).

There is some dependency between the grasp and transport phases, however. The maximum separation between the thumb and index finger when the hand is brought toward an object depends on the speed with which the grasp must be completed. Thus, when subjects try to reach for objects quickly, they spread their fingers farther apart than when they try to reach for the same objects at a leisurely pace (Wing, Turton, & Fraser, 1986). Greater finger widening increases the likelihood of capturing the object when the hand travels at high speed.

Another kind of dependency between transport and grasp concerns the timing of the opening and closing of the hand and the speed with which the hand is transported. As reported by Jeannerod (1981, 1984), the distance between the thumb and index finger is usually greatest when the hand begins the final, slow-approach phase of the movement (see Figure 7.16). Even individuals with prosthetic hands exhibit this effect (Fraser & Wing, 1981). The coincidence of maximal finger widening and the start of the slow-approach phase may reflect a tendency to time-lock related behavioral events. Having the events occur simultaneously reduces the number of degrees of freedom that must be independently controlled by the motor system. Models have been developed for such timing in reaching and grasping

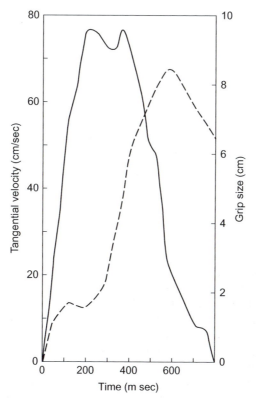

FIGURE 7.16 Tangential velocity of the hand (solid line) and grip size (dashed line) as a function of time. From Jeannerod, M. (1984). The timing of natural prehension movement. Journal of Motor Behavior, 26, 3, 235–254. With permission.

performance (Meulenbroek, Rosenbaum, Jansen, Vaughan, & Vogt, 2001; Rosenbaum, Meulenbroek, Vaughan, & Jansen, 2001; Smeets & Brenner, 2002).

Hand-Space versus Joint-Space Planning

As the hand moves to pick up an object, the angles of the shoulder and elbow joints usually change. Muscle torques are applied at these joints to cause the arm to move. The muscle torques are selected on the basis of a chosen path for the hand to follow through extrapersonal space.

In robotics, determining how the endpoint of a system of hinged levers is displaced when certain torques are applied to the levers is called the *forward dynamics* problem. The *inverse dynamics* problem is the problem of determining the torques that should be applied to the levers given that the endpoint of the levers is supposed to traverse some path. The inverse dynamics problem is the one that is usually required in motor control. One reason why it is interesting to ask how the joint angles of the arm change during aiming movements is to learn how the motor system solves the inverse dynamics problem.

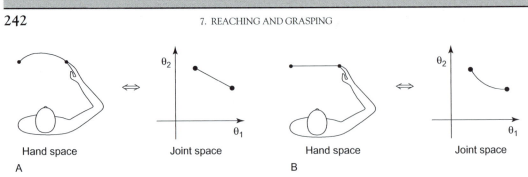

FIGURE 7.17   Trajectories expected if hand movements are planned in joint space (A) or in hand space (B). From Hollerbach, J. M. & Atkeson, C. G. (1986). Characterization of joint-interpolated arm movements. In H. Heuer & C. Fromm (Ed.), Generation and modulation of action patterns (pp. 41–54). Berlin: Springer-Verlag. With permission.

Suppose the inverse dynamics problem is so hard for the motor system that it effectively sidesteps it. Suppose that instead of selecting a direct path for the hand to follow on its way to a target, the motor system actually selects a set of muscle torques and then, perhaps after some trial and error in the planning process, allows the hand to get to the target through a path that may be straight or may just as well be curved. If this strategy were used, one would expect considerable simplicity in the pattern of joint angles that occur during aimed hand movements but considerable complexity in the patterns of associated hand paths. By contrast, if the motor system had no difficulty with the inverse dynamics problem, and so could select direct hand paths and then find the muscle torques that would produce them, one would expect simple hand paths but complex joint angle patterns. The question, then, is whether the motor system plans movements with respect to *joint* space, which uses the intrinsic coordinates of the body, or *hand* space, which uses the extrinsic coordinates of the external surroundings.

Figure 7.17 illustrates possible consequences of joint-space or hand-space planning. If planning is based on the extrinsic coordinates of hand space, the hand would be expected to move in a straight line. Conversely, if planning used the intrinsic coordinates of joint space, then joint angles, or the function relating joint angles to time, would be expected to follow a straight line. Note that only one of these outcomes is possible. If the hand moves in a straight line, the joint angles cannot do so, and if the joint angles move in a straight line, the hand cannot do so.

Data bearing on this distinction were collected by Morasso (1981). He recorded hand trajectories on a two-dimensional surface when people pointed to targets. He found that subjects' hands tended to move in straight lines, but their joints went through complex angular changes. Even when subjects were told to draw curved lines, detailed analyses of their hand trajectories suggested that they actually generated series of straight-line segments (Abend, Bizzi, & Morasso, 1982). These results suggest that the nervous system can in fact plan hand movements in extrinsic coordinates. Once it has done so, it determines the muscles torques that should act on the joints.

Not all investigators are convinced that planning is achieved in hand space, however. Hollerbach, Moore, and Atkeson (1986) proposed a way of directly controlling the joints that can yield straight-line hand trajectories. Their method simply entailed varying the onset times for the motions of the joints, allowing all the joints to stop together at the end of the movement. This method can yield approximately straight hand paths given appropriate onset delays

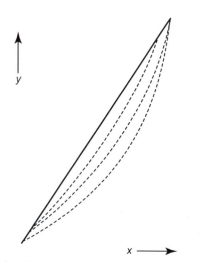

FIGURE 7.18 Motion of the hand in the x and y dimensions when the onsets of elbow and shoulder motion are staggered to varying degrees. From Hollerbach, J. M., Moore, S. P., & Atkeson, C. G. (1987). Workspace effect in arm movement kinematics derived by joint interpolation. In G. N. Gantchev, B. Dimitrov, & P. Gatev (Eds.), Motor Control (pp. 197–208). Plenum. With permission.

(see Figure 7.18). Moreover, consistent with the staggered-time proposal of Hollerbach, Moore, and Atkeson, the motions of the joints of the arm actually appear to be timed so all the joints do in fact reach their final positions simultaneously (Kaminski & Gentile, 1986).

Another source of evidence that there may be joint-based planning is the observation that during the performance of simple pointing movements, invariant relations can be observed among the joints. Soechting and Lacquaniti (1981) studied how people perform the simple act of pointing to a target. Initially, the subjects stood with their arms hanging freely at their sides. When they felt ready to do so, they pointed to the target, located on a vertical surface directly in front of them. Soechting and Lacquaniti found that the peak angular velocities of the elbow and shoulder joints were reached at the same time. In addition, the ratio of the peak velocities of the two joints equaled the ratio of the radial distances that the joints covered. Such regular relations would not be expected if the planning system did not take the joints into account.

A similar result was reported by Kots and Syrovegnin (1966), who recorded the angular positions of the wrist and elbow during the two tasks shown in Figure 2.4. In one task, which can be called the *congruent articulation* task, subjects attempted to flex the wrist while flexing the elbow or they attempted to extend the wrist while extending the elbow. In the other task, which can be called the *incongruent articulation* task, subjects attempted to flex the wrist while extending the elbow or flex the elbow while extending the wrist. Kots and Syrovegnin (1966) found that in the congruent articulation task, the beginnings and ends of the joint motions occurred nearly simultaneously. However, in the incongruent articulation task, the motions of the joints were not well synchronized. Apparently, the elbow and wrist joints were controlled via some sort of coordinative structure (Turvey, 1977) or synergy (Latash, 2008b). Such a structure can help reduce the number of degrees of freedom that must be individually controlled (Bernstein, 1967). One would not expect such simplify-ing structures if arm motions could simply be controlled by directing the hand to move in straight lines in external space.

Moving Two Hands at Once

Do coordinative structures also apply to the coordination of the joints of one arm? Consider the child's game of rubbing the stomach and patting the head. Because this osten-sibly simple task is actually quite difficult—it is hard to keep the shape of one hand's move-ment from infiltrating the other's—one may suppose that there are coordinative structures for the two arms as well.

A number of investigators have sought to provide detailed descriptions of the interactions between the two arms. As noted in Chapter 2, the German physiologist Erich von Holst (see von Holst, 1973) recorded the activities of the two arms of human subjects as the subjects oscillated their arms at different relative frequencies: 1:1, 1:2, 2:3, and so forth. Only at rela-tive frequencies of 1:1 and 1:2 could the two arms move in a stable fashion over repeated oscillations.

Interactions between the two arms also arise when people point to two targets at once. Kelso and colleagues (Kelso, Putnam, & Goodman, 1983; Kelso, Southard, & Goodman, 1979) took advantage of the fact that the time to move the hand to a target depends on the target's index of difficulty, or ID, as discussed earlier in connection with Fitts' law. Kelso and co-workers asked what would happen if each hand had to move to a target with a dif-ferent ID. If each hand could be controlled independently, then each hand's movement time should have only depended on the ID of the target to which it moved. In fact, the movement times of the two hands tended to be approximately equal, even when the IDs of the two targets differed. Specifically, the hand that had an easier targeting task (a lower ID) slowed down so its movement time matched the other hand's. Because subjects were not instructed to synchronize the movements of their two hands, their tendency to do so derived from the operation of some mechanism governing two-hand movements.

What is the nature of this mechanism? One possibility is that each arm is controlled with one or more oscillators, and the oscillators for the two arms are functionally coupled (Haken & Kelso, 1985). This hypothesis is attractive because coupled oscillators are likely to underlie locomotion (see Chapter 5) and the arms were used for walking earlier in evolu-tion. Evidence has been obtained for oscillator control of arm movements in studies where subjects first let one arm dangle freely, then press the arm against a rigid surface, and then dangle the arm freely again (Craske & Craske, 1986). When the arm hangs freely before being pressed against the wall, it displays some oscillation, as would be expected from the fact that the arm, when suspended from the shoulder, can be viewed as a pendulum (Fenn, 1938). More importantly, when the arm dangles freely after being pressed against the wall, it oscillates in the plane of the applied pressure. Craske and Craske (1986) suggested that oscillators responsible for the initial direction of motion become fatigued or adapt during strenuous arm-pressing. Later, when those oscillators are unable to contribute as much as they normally do, the observed direction of oscillation changes. Try this exercise yourself if you wish.

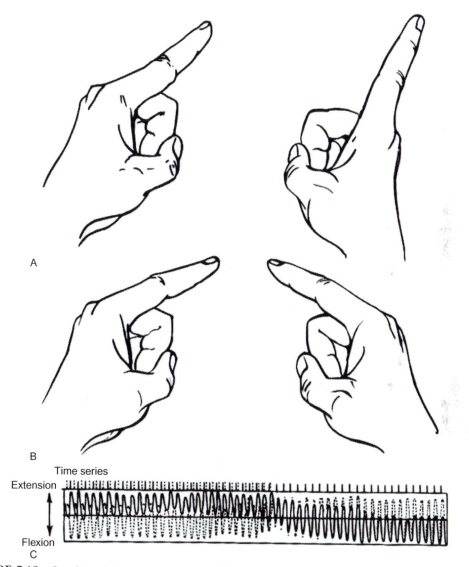

FIGURE 7.19 Coupling of the two index fingers. (A) At low frequency, the two fingers can stay in anti-phase (one finger extending while the other flexes). (B) At high frequency, only an in-phase relation can be maintained (both fingers flex or extend). (C) Time series showing the transition from anti-phase to in-phase relation as oscillation frequency increases. Positions of right finger appear as a solid line. Positions of left finger appear as a dotted line. From Haken, H., Kelso, J. A. S., & Bunz, H. (1985). A theoretical model of phase transitions in human hand movements. Biological Cybernetics, 51, 347–356. With permission.

Another observation that accords with the oscillator hypothesis is another you can make yourself. Position your two index fingers as in Figure 7.19 so your left index finger flexes and you right index finger extends. Now allow the fingers to reverse position, so the right index finger flexes and the left index finger extends. Alternate between these two positions, slowly at first, but then at higher and higher rates. Keep going faster and faster until your fingers move as quickly as possible. What you may notice is that your fingers switch from an anti-phase pattern, where one finger flexes while the other finger extends, to an in-phase pattern, where both fingers flex together or extend together. The switch only occurs from anti-phase to in-phase patterns. If you start at a slow rate with the fingers in-phase, speeding up does not cause a switch to anti-phase coupling. This phenomenon has been investigated in detail by Haken, Kelso, and Bunz (1985), who modeled the switch in terms of nonlinear, coupled oscillators.

Regardless of whether coupling between the hands is due to nonlinear coupled oscillators or some other mechanism, a question that has intrigued motor control researchers concerns the locus of the interactions. Is it in the neuro-muscular periphery—for example, in the spinal cord—or is it in higher centers? These alternatives are not mutually exclusive.

Several sources of evidence indicate that the locus of bimanual coupling is in higher rather than lower levels of motor control. One source of evidence concerns split-brain patients. Research with such patients has shown that they can achieve greater spatial independence between the hands than normal individuals can (Franz, Eliassen, Ivry, & Gazzaniga, 1996). This outcome would not be expected if bimanual coupling resided in the spinal cord because in split-brain patients it is the corpus callosum, the bridge between the two cortical hemispheres, that is severed surgically (to relieve the spread of severe epileptic seizures).

Another source of evidence for a higher rather than a lower level of control as the source of bimanual coupling comes from Franz, Zelaznik, Swinnen, and Walter (2001), who asked participants to move their two hands in synchrony in the frontal plane so the two hands behaved in different ways (Figure 7.20). In one condition, the two hands reached their *zeniths* at the same time (top-top). In another condition, the two hands reached their *nadirs* at the same time (bottom-bottom). In another pair of conditions one hand reached its zenith while the other hand reached its nadir (top-bottom or bottom-top).

One of these four conditions was dramatically harder than the others. In the bottom-top condition, when the arcs drawn by the two hands came together rather than going apart, participants basically "fell apart." Their movements became chaotic. Because there was no obvious biomechanical reason for this breakdown, and because the participants commented

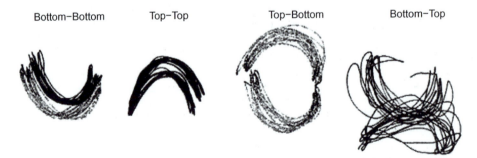

FIGURE 7.20 Motions of the two hands in the four conditions studied by Franz, Zelaznik, Swinnen, and Walter (2001). From Franz, E. A., Zelaznik, H. N., Swinnen, S., & Walter, C. (2001). Spatial conceptual influences on the coordination of bimanual actions: When a dual task becomes a single task. Journal of Motor Behavior, 33, 103–112. With permission.

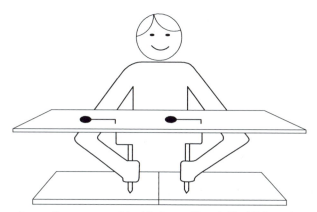

FIGURE 7.21   The crank-gear-flag setup used by Mechsner, Kerzel, Knoblich, and Prinz (2001) and two target configurations. From Mechsner, F., Kerzel, D., Knoblich, G. & Prinz, W. (2001). Perceptual basis of bimanual coordination. Nature, 414, 69–73. With permission.

on how hard it was to conceptualize the movements in this particular condition, Franz, Zelaznik, Swinnen, and Walter ascribed the participants' difficulty in the bottom-top condition to a conceptual failure rather than to a failure of movement execution per se.

If conceptual failures make some bimanual actions difficult, conceptual advantages might make other bimanual actions easy. Support for this possibility came from Mechsner, Kerzel, Knoblich, and Prinz (2001). In one of their experiments, they had participants turn cranks beneath a table (Figure 7.21). Rotation of the cranks caused two flags to turn above the table surface, and the flags were observed by the participants as they turned the cranks. The especially clever feature of the setup was that the cranks were linked to the flags through gears. This made it possible for the required ratios of the two hands' motions to be whatever the experimenters wanted for a given flag phase lag. For example, to have the two flags come together in the middle of the workspace at the same time—what can be called a zero-degree phase lag—the crank handles could be turned with the same phase lag or some other phase lag depending on the gears installed at the time. Through this methodology, Mechsner et al. showed that it was not the physical turning of the cranks that predicted the ease or difficulty of performance but rather the simplicity of the perceptual display that participants had before them. For example, even if it took a frequency ratio of 4:3 to make the two flags reach the center of the workspace at the same time, participants had no trouble generating that frequency ratio. Normally, however, they found it difficult to do so.

Other studies have similarly shown that it is the difficulty of perception or conception that accounts for bimanual coupling in humans. Diedrichsen, Hazeltine, Kennerley, and Ivry (2000) and Kunde and Weigelt (2005) showed that the cognitive representations of goals to be achieved with the two hands accounted more fully for difficulties of bimanual coordination than did the sheer physical demands of coordination. Similarly, Rosenbaum, Dawson, and Challis (2006) showed that when participants made two-hand movements by haptically tracking two moving objects—letting each hand stay in contact with a moving object through gentle touch—the participants could move their two hands essentially independently with no training. Haptic tracking was chosen as an experimental preparation by this group of investigators because it was thought that haptic tracking might bypass the intentional system responsible for macroscopic movement planning (establishing the general shape and timing of the movements to be performed). Finding that the two hands could move independently via haptic tracking, along with the other lines of work reviewed here, suggest that cognitive factors play a major role in interlimb coordination (see also Lee, Blandin, & Proteau, 1996; Oliveira & Ivry, 2008).

SUMMARY

1. Hand movements occur *in utero*. Later, by 5 months of age postpartum, infants can reliably control the direction and distance of reaches and grasps. By around 9 months, they can reliably control the orientation and size of their reaches and grasps. By around 10 months of age, they can adjust their movement speed depending on task demands. Later still, they can grasp objects differently depending on what they intend to do with the objects.
2. The use of visual feedback is susceptible to experience. As shown in the late nineteenth century, people can adapt to inverting lenses. Adaptation to such visual distortion is achieved by correlating changes of visual input with actively generated movements.
3. Vision dominates touch. Relevant illusions may have practical benefits in physical therapy.
4. Vision for action may use a different neural subsystem than vision for recognition of objects.
5. The eye and hand are tightly coupled in visually guided manual aiming tasks. Studies of eye-hand coordination have shed light on language processing and other functions.
6. When aiming for targets, amplitude errors tend to be larger than direction errors. However, speed profiles tend to scale with the distance to be covered.
7. Manual aiming for a target is often achieved in two phases, an initial ballistic phase and a secondary homing-in phase. The time for vision to be used in aiming is between 100 ms and 200 ms.
8. One domain where feedback processing has been studied in detail is manual aiming. In the so-called Fitts' task, the subject moves the hand to a spatial target, usually as quickly as possible. Fitts (1954) introduced a formula for the time needed to reach a target depending on the distance of the target from the starting position and the target's diameter: The time to reach a target increases with the distance of the target from the start position and decreases with the target's width. Because Fitts' formula does an excellent job of accounting for movement time data from a wide range of tasks, it has been called Fitts' law.
9. Several explanations have been offered for Fitts' law. The iterative corrections model says that the law mainly reflects corrections for movement errors. The impulse variability model says that the law mainly reflects the initial impulse that drives the limb toward the target. The optimized initial impulse model, which is the most successful model to date, says that both factors are important.
10. According to the equilibrium point hypothesis, a way to move a limb from one position to another is to take advantage of the spring-like properties of muscle. There are two

ways to exploit these spring-like properties—change the resting lengths of the muscle or change the stiffness of one muscle relative to the other. Several studies suggest that one or the other of these methods may be used. Treating muscles as springs may be economical from a computational standpoint. However, challenges have been raised to the equilibrium point hypothesis.

11. Another question is whether positioning movements are discrete or continuous. Data have been marshaled on both sides.

12. During reaching and grasping, two distinct phases of movement can be identified—the transport phase, during which the hand is brought toward the object, and the grasp phase, during which the fingers enclose the object. The transport and grasp phases may be controlled by different brain areas, and their underlying control mechanisms appear to develop at different rates. Some dependencies exist between the two phases.

13. Although it is convenient when studying reaching and grasping to view the hand as a single moving point, the hand is only one part of a complex set of joints. The hand often follows a straight path when people point to objects, an outcome that has been taken to suggest that movements are planned in the extrinsic coordinates of hand (or extra-personal) space rather than in the intrinsic coordinates of joint (or intra-personal) space. The fact that people exhibit straight-line hand trajectories suggests that the motor system does not compromise hand trajectories when it solves the inverse dynamics problem—the problem of determining the muscle torques that bring an end effector (such as the hand) through a desired trajectory. However, regularities in the relations of joint positions during aiming movements suggest that there may be some joint-based planning.

14. Simultaneous flexion of the wrist and elbow is easier than flexion of the wrist and extension of the elbow, or extension of the wrist and flexion of the elbow. The greater ease with which people can simultaneously flex (or extend) the wrist and elbow suggests that there are coordinative structures for the two joints. Such coordinative structures can reduce the number of degrees of freedom to be independently managed by the manual control system.

15. Coordinative structures also characterize interactions between the two arms and hands. For example, there is a tendency for the two hands to begin and end aiming movements simultaneously. Similarly, when the left and right index fingers flex and extend simultaneously, as the oscillation frequency increases, there is a tendency for the fingers only to flex together and only to extend together. Coupling between the hands appears to be centrally based rather than peripherally based.

Further Reading

Aiming movements can be perturbed by extraneous visual stimuli. See Tipper et al. (1992, 1997), Welsh and Elliott (2004), Welsh and Pratt (2008), and Finkbeiner, Song, and Nakayama (2008).

The latter study pertained to psycholinguistic influences on reaching. For other studies on this topic, see Glover, Rosenbaum, Graham, and Dixon (2004), Spivey (2007), and van der Wel et al. (2009).

Shapes of hand paths for manual positioning tasks carry over from one task to the next. See Jax and Rosenbaum (2007) and van der Wel, Fleckenstein, Jax, and Rosenbaum (2007) for data concerning such hand-path priming, as these authors called it.

Prism adaptation research has progressed, thanks in part to the work of Redding and Wallace (1997, 2008).

Coupling of grasping and fore-aft motion of the forearm has been demonstrated by Flanagan and colleagues (Flanagan, Tresilian, & Wing, 1993).

Complementing studies of unimanual grasps on objects to be moved are studies of bimanual grasps on objects to be moved (Hughes & Franz, 2007).

Researchers have studied reaching and grasping in virtual reality (Zahariev & MacKenzie, 2007) and in surgery, including surgical contexts where visual feedback magnifies the workspace or reveals tissue that is not directly visible, as in endooscopic procedures (Zheng, Verjee, Lomax, & MacKenzie, 2005). A leading investigator in this area is Christine MacKenzie of Simon Fraser University (http://www.sfu.ca/hmsl/mackenzie/).

The analysis of aiming in two spatial dimensions (aiming within a plane) has been generalized to aiming in three dimensions (aiming in open space). See MacKenzie, Marteniuk, and Dugas (1987) and Hansen, Elliott, and Khan (2008).

Sabes and Jordan (1997) suggested that people reach around obstacles in ways that take into account resistance to unexpected perturbations.

Work has been done on socially mediated reaching and grasping. See Mason and MacKenzie (2005) for a study of grip forces in passing objects from one person to another. Mottet, Guiard, Ferrand, and Bootsma (2001) studied two-person performance of the Fitts aiming task.

Shadmehr and Wise (2005) provided a mathematically in-depth treatment of reaching, grasping, and related topics.

An integrated treatment of hand function can be found in Jones and Lederman (2006).

A monograph on cognition and tool use was authored by Baber (2003).

Using a handheld tool benefits from wielding the tool. Wielding—holding an object and shaking or rotating it—provides useful information about the object's physical properties. See Carello and Turvey (2004).

This chapter covered the development of reaching in infancy. Reaching has also been studied in the elderly. See Pratt, Chasteen, and Abrams (1994) and Liao, Jagacinski, and Greenberg (1997).

For a superb review of research on aiming, see Elliott, Helsen, and Chua (2001).

O U T L I N E

Drawing	254	*Reaction Time Evidence for*		
Planning of Strokes	254	*Allograph Selection*	265	
The Isogony Principle	257	*Writing Size, Relative Timing,*		
Two-Thirds Power Law	258	*and Absolute Timing*	266	
Drawing Smoothly	262	*Context Effects*	268	
		Writing and Handedness	270	
Control of Writing	263			
Error Analyses	263	**The Dynamic Dominance Hypothesis**	272	
Dysgraphia	263	**Summary**	273	
Reaction Time Evidence for				
Grapheme Selection	265	**Further Reading**	275	

One of the primary functions of human motor control is to allow for communication with others. The activities we have considered so far—walking, looking, reaching and grasping— only incidentally allow for such communication. By contrast, the activities considered here, drawing and writing, mainly provide for the expression of thoughts to others. Based on this observation, it is natural to consider a theoretical perspective for analyzing drawing and writing. The perspective relies on the assumption that communicative acts generally represent the culmination of several internal stages. First, one has an idea to be expressed. Then this idea is represented in some abstract form, in the "language of thought." The abstract message is then translated into drawn or written segments that allow for expression of the idea. Those segments come to be realized via a series of motor commands. Feedback about progress in each of these stages can be used to move forward.

If such a model captures what occurs in the control of drawing and writing, one should find evidence for the stages in the initiation of drawing and writing acts. This hypothesis has motivated much of the research on drawing and writing and is the basis around which this chapter is organized.

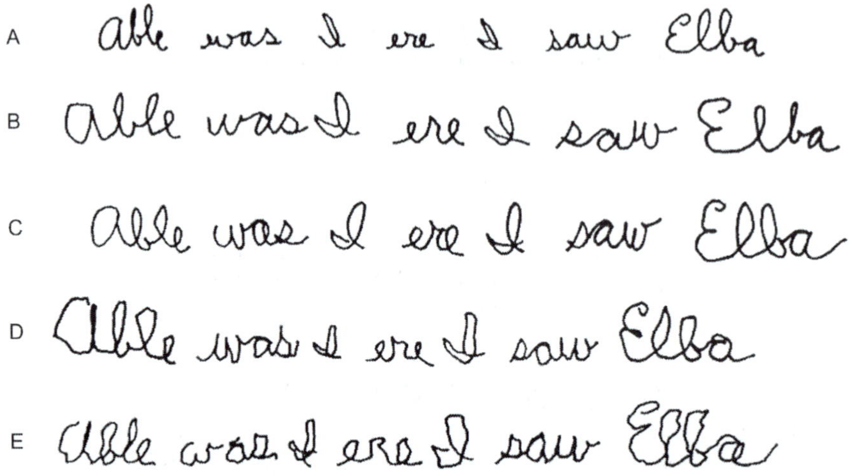

FIGURE 8.1   Handwriting achieved through different means: (A) with the right (dominant) hand; (B) with the right arm but with the wrist immobilized; (C) with the left hand; (D) with the pen gripped between the teeth; (E) with the pen attached to the foot. Reprinted from Raibert, M. H. (1977). Motor control and learning by the state-space model. Technical Report AI-TR-439, Artificial Intelligence Laboratory, MIT. With permission.

Before we turn to the full review of work on drawing and writing, it is worth mentioning a general finding that corroborates the stage model suggested above. As shown in Figure 8.1, people can write with a consistent style even when using different effectors—in this case, writing with the right hand or left hand, the right foot or left foot, or the mouth (with a pen held between the writer's teeth). These examples are reminiscent of the illustrations of motor equivalence described in Chapter 2, where we saw that there are alternative means of getting the same job done with different effectors.

Less dramatic evidence but of no less concern to researchers in human motor control, writing style is also preserved when one scrawls across a blackboard or writes with minis-cule script on a bank check. A person's signature, for example, is still unmistakably his or hers in both of these contexts. So too is one's drawing style.

A dramatic way of illustrating the preservation of writing style while writing over different expanses is to write your name in large letters on a blackboard and then to project your signature on that surface with a transparency machine, having written your name in a small area such as a narrow box on a plastic sheet. The two signatures will probably overlap nearly perfectly. By contrast, two signatures of the same name produced by you and another person will not. Professor Arnold Thomassen of Radboud University (formerly the University of Nijmegen) came up with this clever demonstration.

These observations highlight the capacity for motor equivalence, emphasized in Chapter 2. The observations suggest that different production mechanisms—corresponding, say, to different limbs—provide alternative means of realizing the same high-level graphic representation. Said another way, the control of writing, and presumably the control of drawing, too, is at least partly hierarchical: The same abstract idea, and the same spatio-temporal segments, are expressed by different implementation systems such as the fingers in the case of writing a check or the entire arm in the case of scrawling a message across a blackboard.

Perhaps the most intriguing question in the study of the control of drawing and writing is how the motor system solves the problem of expressing the same high-level intentions in different ways. One answer to this question is to propose planning constraints that the output mechanisms obey. Such constraints help limit the range of behavioral options that are considered.

One planning constraint that may help in this regard is people's tendency to move in straight or nearly straight lines as they connect points on a plane (Morasso, 1981). As discussed earlier in this book, it has been suggested that this tendency reflects a planning constraint for minimizing jerk, the third time derivative of position (Flash & Hogan, 1985; Hogan, 1984). Later in this chapter, we will see that this constraint also accounts for other aspects of people's drawing and writing behavior.

In addition to the question of how writing and drawing styles are preserved in widely different contexts, another central question in this area of study is why people's graphic outputs are so distinctive. The individuality of writing style is so reliable that signatures are used for identification purposes. It has been suggested that writing styles indicate personality traits. For example, writing analysts (graphologists) who subscribe to Freudian theory have suggested that the way one forms lower loops in letters such as "g" and "p" reflects the state of the unconscious id (the part of the psyche related to sexual urges, according to Freud). The overall slant and size of handwritten letters also supposedly reflect extraversion or self-esteem (Hughes, 1966). Graphology is taken so seriously in some countries that it has been used in hiring decisions. However, the validity of graphology is doubtful (Fischman, 1987).

Without personality as a basis for explaining differences in writing style, we are left with the question of why one person's writing differs so dramatically from another's. To the best of the author's knowledge, there has been little scientific research on this question. It would be worth trying to pull apart the relative contributions of nature (genes) and nurture (experience) to the properties of handwriting because both factors are likely to play a role.

In this connection, the author will share an anecdote, though because it is an anecdote, it should be taken only as a goad to future research, not a statement of established findings. Once, upon looking through envelopes delivered to his home, the author glanced upon an envelope he was sure was from his mother. After he looked at it again, the author saw that it actually came from the author's second cousin on his mother's side, someone whose writing he had never seen. It turns out that this second cousin grew up several decades after the author's mother did and in a different country—he in the United States, she in Germany, from where she emigrated in 1939. Did this writing resemblance bespeak genetic biases in the subtleties of letter formation? Perhaps. As will be seen in the final chapter of this book, an ever-growing body of evidence points to strong genetic contributions to behavioral tendencies.

There is one more general question about drawing and writing that is worth mentioning here to help prime you for what's to come. As everyone knows, most people prefer to write and draw with one hand rather than the other, and for most people the hand they prefer to write with is the right. What accounts for this preference? Relevant work will be summarized in the final part of this chapter.

DRAWING

Because the capacity to draw precedes the capacity to write, we will begin with a discussion of drawing. First, we will consider the high-level control of drawing. Then we will turn to the execution of drawing strokes.

Planning of Strokes

Much of the research that has been done on drawing has been concerned with the planning of drawing behavior, especially in young children. Children's drawings become progressively more refined over the course of development (Goodnow, 1977). Presumably this is because children become more and more sophisticated in their motor planning and control, as well as their perceptual and attentional capabilities (Figure 8.2).

Because children can draw before they can write, it has been suggested that early drawing behavior may provide clues about young children's cognitive abilities. For example, it has been proposed that drawing may be governed by high-level rules of the sort underlying language processing (Goodnow & Levine, 1973; van Sommers, 1984). Consequently, some investigators have proposed that the development of drawing may parallel the development of language.

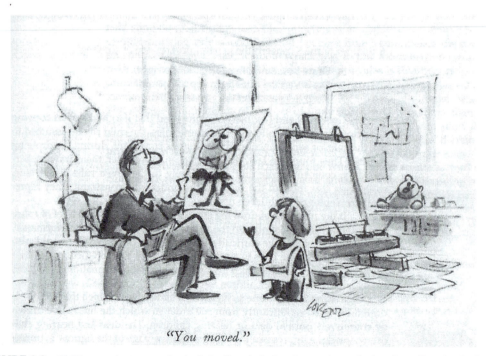

"You moved."

FIGURE 8.2   Children are just as creative in defending their drawings as in producing them. Drawing by Lorenz © 1987 The New Yorker Magazine, Inc.

Goodnow and Levine (1973) pursued this possibility in a seminal article called "The grammar of action: Sequence and syntax in children's copying." The authors recorded the drawing paths that children followed when copying simple two-dimensional shapes such as squares and triangles. Based on their observations, the authors proposed that children rely on rules for sequencing drawing strokes. Two rules pertain to the starting point:

1. Start at the leftmost point.
2. Start at the topmost point.

Two other rules pertain to the starting strokes:

3. Start with a vertical line.
4. Given a figure with an apex such as a diamond or a triangle, start at the top and descend the left oblique.

A final set of rules concerns the general progression of copying:

5. Draw horizontal lines from left to right.
6. Draw vertical lines from top to bottom.
7. Keep the pencil on the paper at all times.

Goodnow and Levine (1973) proposed that if a child's overt copying behavior follows these rules, the child can be assumed to use the rules, or some functionally analogous constraints, in his or her copying. Goodnow and Levine found that as children grow older, their drawing performance conforms more and more closely to the seven rules listed above.

If the planning of drawing strokes does indeed rely on rules for drawing and if those rules are similar to the rules underlying linguistic performance, then children who have difficulty sequencing spoken words should have trouble drawing lines in a rule-governed fashion. This prediction was confirmed in a study of children with profound sentence-forming difficulties (agrammatic aphasia). The children in the study (Cromer, 1983) were asked to copy figures such as the one in Figure 8.3. The order in which the lines were drawn by these children deviated significantly from the order in which the lines were drawn by deaf or normal children. Deaf and normal children copied the figures in a way that took advantage of the figures' symmetric organization. The deaf and normal children mostly started at the top of the figure, drawing a left and right branch, proceeding down a level, and so forth. The agrammatic aphasic children drew in a more haphazard fashion, often starting at the bottom of the figure and drawing all the way to the top before filling in the

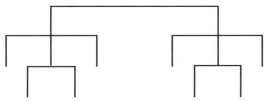

FIGURE 8.3 Stick figure to be copied by the children in Cromer's (1983) study. From Cromer, R. F. (1983). Hierarchical planning disability in the drawings and constructions of a special group of severely aphasic children. Brain and Cognition, 2, 144–164. With permission.

mirror-image line within that subsection. The failure of the agrammatic aphasic children to capitalize on the hierarchical organization of the figure suggests that the ability to sequence behavior may depend on a central, amodal rule system (Keele, 1987).

Apart from the fact that postulating sequencing rules may help explain observed behavior, what is the rationale for the rules? How do the rules help?

The rules may simplify planning. For example, the availability of a simple left-to-right drawing rule—Goodnow and Levine's rule 5—eliminates the need for decision-making about which way to proceed when attempting to draw a horizontal line. Rules may also reduce the number of distinct motor programs that must be maintained in memory. Suppose there were no rules for drawing and one had distinct programs for squares of different sizes. The storage requirements of this set of programs would be much greater than if there were a single program that could be modified to allow for the production of squares of any size (Schmidt, 1975). Rules therefore allow for flexibility of performance while reducing memory storage costs.

If rules are useful for drawing, one would expect adults as well as children to rely on them. Investigations of adult copying and drawing behavior bear out this expectation. In an intensive study of the stroke paths used by adults while copying two-dimensional shapes, van Sommers (1984) found that similar drawing paths were followed by different individuals, consistent with the view that those individuals subscribed, implicitly, to the same rules. The following statement captures some of the regularities van Sommers observed:

> Take a pencil and quickly draw the sun the way it is typically illustrated in children's books—straight rays coming out of a simple circle. . . . If you are right-handed you very likely began at the top of the circle and drew in a counterclockwise direction. Then you probably put the first ray on at the top, starting at its upper end and drawing downwards towards the circle. The next ray was drawn to its right and as you progressed clockwise around the disk, you changed from drawing inwards to drawing outwards (usually after one or two strokes) and then reverted to inward strokes at about nine o'clock
>
> [van Sommers, 1986, p. 62].

What is the source of rules for drawing? A reasonable first hypothesis is that they come from pressure to satisfy biomechanical constraints. People choose to draw so the writing surface can be held down while the pen is in motion, for example. They also try to avoid extreme joint angles, perhaps explaining why they change the direction of ray drawing as a function of ray orientation in the example just given. Research by Ruud Meulenbroek and his colleagues at Radboud University bears this out (Meulenbroek, Rosenbaum, Thomassen, & Schomaker, 1993; Meulenbroek & Thomassen, 1991).

Mechanical or biomechanical factors are not the only determinants of drawing strategies, however. van Sommers (1984) found that people's drawings were also sensitive to the verbal labels given to shapes being copied. For example, if the pattern shown in Figure 8.4 was identified as a cocktail glass, it was drawn with different stroke patterns then if it was identified as a man holding a telescope. When the shape was described as a cocktail glass, the glass was usually drawn first and the cherry was added later. When it was described as a man holding a telescope, the head was usually drawn first, the stem and feet were drawn second, and the arms were drawn third. Because the meanings attached to the patterns affected the way the patterns were drawn, van Sommers (1984) concluded that semantic or perceptual factors influence drawing plans. This outcome suggests that rules for copying are deployed after meanings or representational goals are defined. Drawing, therefore, may be a top-down process, which accords with the view that drawing is hierarchically controlled.

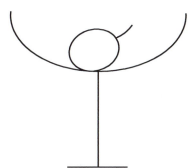

FIGURE 8.4 A figure that could be described as a man with a telescope or a cocktail glass with a cherry. The stroke patterns used to copy the figure depended on the description. Adapted from Van Sommers, P. (1986). How the mind draws. Psychology Today, May, 62–66. With permission.

The Isogony Principle

No matter how the sequencing of drawing strokes is planned, the sequence must be realized physically. One way to study the execution of drawing strokes is to allow people to draw very simple patterns over and over again. In one such study (Lacquaniti, Terzuolo, & Viviani, 1983), subjects were asked trace figure eights (see Figure 8.5A). The trajectory of the pen was recorded with a graphics tablet—a device that records the x-y coordinates of the pen tip periodically (e.g., every 10 ms). Figure 8.5C depicts the most important result from the study. The ordinate represents the angle of pen movement relative to an arbitrary reference frame; the abscissa represents time (see Figure 8.5B). As seen in Figure 8.5C, the absolute value of the average angular velocity in the top and bottom loops was nearly constant. (Angular velocity is the change in angle per unit time. Average absolute angular velocity is the arithmetic mean, over time, of the rectified change in angle per unit time; for rectified changes, all negative changes are made positive.)

Looking again at Figure 8.5, we see that the total angle of the top loop to be drawn was 360 degrees and the total angle of the bottom loop to be drawn was also 360 degrees. Because each loop was drawn with the same constant angular velocity, the total time to draw each loop was the same. Lacquaniti, Terzuolo, and Viviani (1983) summarized this finding in one statement: *Equal angles are described in equal times.* They called this the *isogeny* principle.

The success of the isogeny principle for drawing figure eights is surprising in view of the fact that another control principle could have also operated. A priori, the time to draw each loop could have depended on its arc length, in which case the time to complete the top loop would have been shorter than the time to complete the bottom loop.

What does the isogeny principle tell us about the control of drawing? It suggests two features of drawing control. One is that a complex, continuous curve such as a figure eight is segmented into components, each of which is drawn as a distinct unit or stroke. Research on handwriting, to be summarized later in this chapter, suggests that letters are indeed written by concatenating individual segments, which makes sense from the point of view of dealing with limits on how much one can plan in advance (see Chapter 4). Successful models of

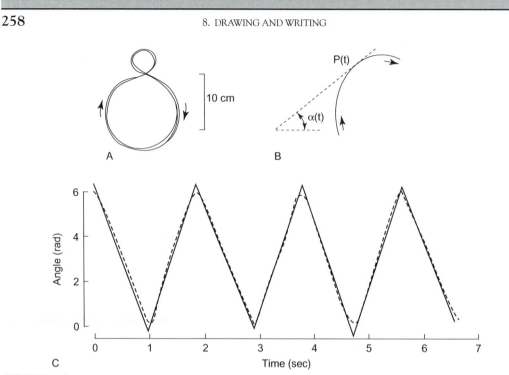

FIGURE 8.5 (A) A figure eight drawn continuously. (B) Method used to define the angle of the pen movement at each point in time (the angle was defined as the tangent to the trajectory formed with respect to a reference line). (C) Angle of pen movement as a function of time. From Lacquaniti, F., Terzuolo, C., Viviani, P. (1983). The law relating the kinematic and figural aspects of drawing movements. Acta Psychologica, 54, 115–130. With permission.

writing have incorporated this stroke-based approach (Bullock, Grossberg, & Mannes, 1993; Edelman & Flash, 1987; Meulenbroek, Rosenbaum, Thomassen, Loukopoulos, & Vaughan, 1996; Rhodes, Bullock, Verwey, Averbeck, & Page, 2004).

The second implication of the isogeny principle is that a primary control feature in the execution of drawing is *timing*. When people draw, or at least when they draw figure eights, they try to complete each segment in a set amount of time.

Two-Thirds Power Law

Lacquaniti, Terzuolo, and Viviani (1983, 1984) observed another important regularity in drawing behavior. They observed this regularity in scribbling behavior, a sample of which is shown in Figure 8.6A. The angular velocity of the pen while drawing the scribble (Figure 8.6B) varied irregularly as a function of time. On first blush, these data look like chaos. But when the pen's angular velocity was plotted as a function of the curvature of the line being drawn, an orderly pattern emerged (Figure 8.6C). The relation could be captured by the equation

$$A(t) = kC(t)^{2/3},$$ (8.1)

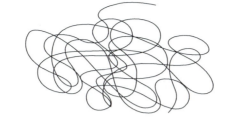

A

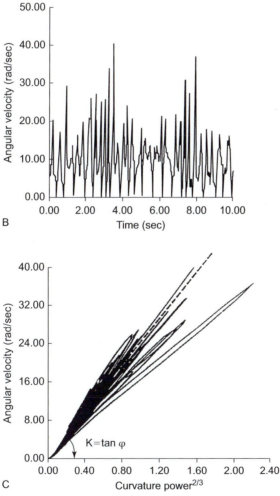

B

C

FIGURE 8.6 (A) A scribble produced by one subject in the study of Lacquaniti, Terzuolo, and Viviani (1984). (B) Angular velocity of the pen as a function of time. (C) Angular velocity as a function of curvature raised to the two-thirds power; each segment applies to a distinct segment of the trajectory. From Lacquaniti, F., Terzuolo, C., Viviani, P. (1984). Global metric properties and preparatory processes in drawing movements. In S. Kornblum & J. Requin (Eds.), Preparatory states and processes (pp. 357–370)., Hillsdale, N.J.: Lawrence Erlbaum Associates. With permission.

where $A(t)$ denotes angular velocity at time t, k is an empirical constant, and $C(t)$ is curvature at time t. Lacquaniti, Terzuolo, and Viviani called this the *two-thirds power law*.

To understand what the two-thirds power law means, it helps to review the meaning of its terms. First, regarding $C(t)$, which stands for the curvature of the arc being drawn at time t, one can think of the curvature of an arc at a moment in time t in terms of the curvature of three points, A, B, and C, in a plane. By the time, t, that point C has been reached, one has drawn the arc ABC. The curvature of ABC can be found by identifying another point—call it X—that is equidistant from A, B, and C. The smaller the distance from X to A, B, and C, the higher the curvature of ABC. Conversely, the larger the distance from X to A, B, and C, the lower the curvature of ABC. As the distance from X to A, B, and C approaches infinity, the curvature of ABC approaches 0 and ABC is nearly perfectly straight.

Knowing these things, you can hopefully appreciate what the two-thirds power law says about drawing. The law say that as an arc becomes more curved, the pen's angular velocity increases. However, the angular velocity does not increase *linearly* with curvature. Rather, it increases in a curvilinear fashion such that $C(t)$ increases at a lower and lower rate as $C(t)$ increases more and more, as reflected in the fact that the (positive) exponent is less than 1.

If angular velocity increases with curvature, albeit at a diminishing rate, how can this result be squared with the isogeny principle, which says that equal angles are described in equal times? How, for example, can the high-curvature arc at the top of a figure eight be drawn in the same amount of time as the lower-curvature arc at the bottom of the same figure eight? If the angular velocity is higher for the high-curvature arc, isogeny requires that something else must counteract the effect of curvature.

Inspection of Equation 8.1 provides the needed solution. In it is the term k, a constant of proportionality fitted to the data, as is the 2/3 exponent. It turns out that isogeny is achieved if k increases with arc *length*. Thus, for arcs of different lengths inscribed on circles of different curvature (Figure 8.7), k is larger for wide arcs than for narrow arcs. Said another way and in specific reference to Figure 8.7, the three points shown in each of the four circles

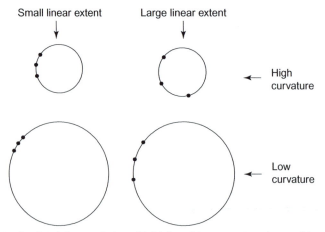

FIGURE 8.7 Triplets of points lying on circles with high and low curvature (top and bottom row, respectively) and separated by small and large linear extents (left and right columns, respectively). Each of the three points along each of the four circles would be reached at the same times according to the isogeny principle.

depicted in this figure would be occupied at the same times if pens were moving around their respective circles in ways that respected the two-thirds power law, provided that three things were true: (1) k increased identically with arc length; (2) the pens started at the same angular points around the circles; and (3) the pens went in the same direction (both counterclockwise or both clockwise).

So does k increase with arc length in a way that ensures isogeny? To find out, Lacquaniti, Terzuolo, and Viviani (1983, 1984) studied the production of spirals. They focused on spirals because the arms of a spiral have varying length. As the pen approaches the center of a spiral, the arms of the spiral become shorter and shorter (see Figure 8.8A).

Figure 8.8B shows that during the drawing of spirals, the pen's angular velocity increased linearly with curvature raised to the 2/3 power, replicating what was observed for scribbles. In addition, distinct angular velocity lines were evident for the distinct arcs of the spiral, with the slopes of the lines varying according to the length of the loop being drawn. Thus, a single control parameter, corresponding to k, varied with the linear extent of the arc being drawn in a manner that made it possible for equal angles to be drawn in equal times.

The fact that such arc length scaling occurs for individual line segments suggests that the drawing of spirals is achieved by segmenting the spiral into series of strokes. Somehow, while drawing, the person who is drawing sets the gain of the manual control system according to the length of the forthcoming arc. This conclusion bears on the issue discussed

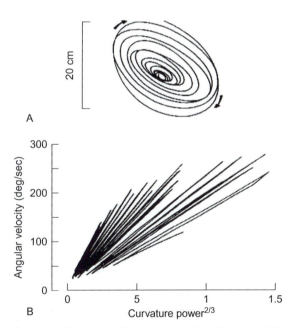

FIGURE 8.8 (A) A spiral produced by one subject in the study of Lacquaniti, Terzuolo, and Viviani (1984). (B) A plot of angular velocity as a function of curvature raised to the 2/3 power. The slope of the angular velocity function depends on the linear extent of the arm of the spiral. From Lacquaniti, F., Terzuolo, C., Viviani, P. (1984). Global metric properties and preparatory processes in drawing movements. In S. Kornblum & J. Requin (Eds.), Preparatory states and processes (pp. 357–370)., Hillsdale, N.J.: Lawrence Erlbaum Associates. With permission.

in Chapter 7 in the section on discrete versus continuous movements. The success of the two-thirds power law can be taken to support the hypothesis that movements are discrete.

What underlying mechanisms account for the two-thirds power law? Lacquaniti, Terzuolo, and Viviani (1984) suggested that the relation may result from the coupling of two independent oscillators. If the output of the oscillators is sinusoidal, the phase relations and relative amplitudes of the sinusoids can be modulated to produce curves of varying length and curvature. Simulations have shown that coupled-oscillator systems can indeed generate a wide range of graphic outputs (Hollerbach, 1981), making this proposal attractive. Another appealing feature of the coupled-oscillator hypothesis is that oscillators are biologically realistic.

Drawing Smoothly

Despite the apparent success of the two-thirds power law, some investigators have not been convinced by it. Wann, Nimmo-Smith, and Wing (1988) noted that significant departures from the 2/3 exponent have been observed in some studies of drawing and handwriting (Thomassen & Teulings, 1985). On the other hand, Wann, Nimmo-Smith, and Wing did not question the fact that angular velocity is generally a power function of curvature, that is, that angular velocity is equal to curvature raised to some power.

Wann, Nimmo-Smith, and Wing (1988) did take issue with the explanation of the power law in terms of (sinusoidal) oscillations. They said that while sinusoids are mathematically appealing, real motor systems rarely behave in such an ideal sinusoidal fashion (Saltzman & Kelso, 1987). Furthermore, according to Wann, Nimmo-Smith, and Wing, while sinusoids are mathematically convenient, it is hard to see why they would have been favored in natural selection.

A more biologically plausible explanation of the power law, according to Wann, Nimmo-Smith, and Wing (1988), is that writers and drawers attempt to generate graphic behavior as smoothly as possible. This goal is consistent with the minimum jerk model of Hogan (1984) and Flash and Hogan (1985). Recall that the minimum jerk model says that movement trajectories are planned so as to minimize the mean-squared value of the third time derivative of position. Writing smoothly appears to be a goal in graphic production as shown, for example, by the fact that children write more smoothly as their writing improves (Wann, 1987). Wann, Nimmo-Smith, and Wing (1988) showed that the minimum jerk model could also give rise to a power law of the kind endorsed by Lacquaniti, Terzuolo, and Viviani (1983, 1984).

With the oscillator model and the minimum jerk model as possible explanations of the two-thirds power law, how should one choose between them? A reason to prefer the minimum jerk model is that it may also account for people's tendency to draw straight lines when connecting two points (Flash & Hogan, 1985). The ability of the minimum jerk model to account for both results could be taken to suggest that jerk minimization, or some constraint related to smoothness of performance, may be a general determinant of drawing and writing behaviors. On the other hand, oscillators are also known to underlie basic motor acts such as walking, making it hard to say which group of investigators is correct. Perhaps both are. Oscillatory movements are certainly smooth, and even time-varying patterns that are not perfectly cyclic can be composed with oscillations that are.

CONTROL OF WRITING

Because writing and drawing are physically similar behaviors, it is reasonable to expect that they are controlled in similar ways. In this section we look at evidence indicating that handwriting, like drawing, is controlled hierarchically.

Error Analyses

An influential source of support for hierarchical control of handwriting comes from slips of the pen. Ellis (1979) compiled a corpus of such slips by recording his own writing errors over a period of 18 months (see Table 8.1). Sometimes Ellis substituted one word for another (example 1) or substituted one letter for another (example 2). On other occasions, he repeated a letter too many times (example 3) or replaced one letter with another, capitalizing the intruding letter if the replaced letter should have been capitalized (example 4). On still other occasions, he made errors involving single writing strokes (example 5).

To account for these results, Ellis proposed that writing is initiated in four stages whose outputs are (1) words, (2) graphemes, (3) allographs, and (4) graphs. Words (stage 1) are the entities selected in the first stage of the programming process. Errors in this stage lead to lexical errors (production of the wrong word). Graphemes (stage 2) are the letters of the alphabet. Mistakes in grapheme selection account for errors of the sort shown in examples 2 and 3. Allographs (stage 3) are a grapheme's categorical variations—for example, the upper- and lowercase form of a letter. An allograph stage is suggested by errors like the one in example 4. Graphs, or strokes, are selected at the lowest level of the hierarchy (stage 5). Errors of graph selection lead to mistakes like the one in example 5.

Dysgraphia

The slips of the pen described above were occasional errors made by a neurologically normal individual. Another source of support for hierarchical control of handwriting comes from

TABLE 8.1   Examples of Writing Errors*

Example	Error	Description
1	*low* — *two*	Lexical error
2	*lapse from* — *lapse time*	Letter substitution
3	*looks* — *brooks*	Letter repetition
4	*cognitive* — *Kr...*	Letter substitution and case change
5	*Wednesday* — *Wednesday*	Extra stroke

*Data from Ellis (1979).

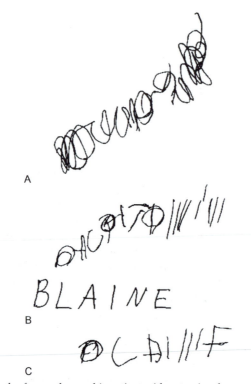

A

B

C

FIGURE 8.9   Writing samples from a dysgraphic patient with extensive damage to the right frontal and parietal lobes 1 month after stroke. (A) The man's signature. (B) His printed name. (C) A copied name, with the model above the copy. From Margolin, D. I., & Wing, A. M. (1983). Agraphia and micrographia: Clinical manifestations of motor programming and performance disorders. Acta Psychologica, 54, 263–283. With permission.

neurological patients. Some neurological patients have difficulty writing, though their motor control, perception, and spelling are otherwise intact. Their syndrome is known as *dysgraphia* (Roeltgin, 1985). Dysgraphia occurs rarely without other neurological impairments. However, the forms it takes comport with the hierarchical model. Particular aspects of handwriting corresponding to particular levels of the writing hierarchy are disrupted in dysgraphia.

A dysgraphic patient was described by Margolin and Wing (1983). This man suffered damage to the right frontal and parietal lobes (see Chapter 3). He could not write words on command, but he could copy words with a modicum of skill (see Figure 8.9). Based on a detailed analysis of the patient's writing and drawing, Margolin and Wing concluded that this individual had difficulty producing writing strokes. The patient's writing difficulty was not due to perceptual deficits, for he could copy reasonably well, and the errors he made were qualitatively different from those exhibited by normal individuals subjected to altered visual feedback (Smith, McCrary, & Smith, 1960). Because the patient did not have difficulty retrieving words, graphemes, or allographs (the first three stages in Ellis' model), his symptoms were consistent with the hypothesis that he had a problem with graphs per se. For this to be the case, it appears that there is a mechanism for generating writing strokes that is separate from the mechanisms governing generation of words, graphemes, and allographs.

Rounding out this story, other dysgraphic patients exhibit writing deficits limited to words, graphemes, or allographs (Roeltgin, 1985). Miceli, Silveri, and Caramazza (1985) described a patient who made frequent spelling errors while writing, though his writing strokes were essentially normal and the words he selected, though spelled incorrectly, were appropriate. Because this patient could accurately copy text, his deficit was apparently localized at the grapheme selection stage (Margolin, 1984).

Reaction Time Evidence for Grapheme Selection

Another way to test the hypothesis that there are distinct stages in the control of handwriting is to measure writing reaction times. Using this technique, Teulings, Thomassen, and van Galen (1983) obtained convergent evidence for the grapheme selection stage. These authors displayed a single handwritten letter on a screen and then presented another letter, either to the left or right of it. The subject's task was to copy the completed letter pair as soon as possible after the pair was completed by addition of the second letter to the first. The result was that the time to start writing was shorter when the two letters matched than when they did not match. This outcome corroborates the hypothesis that subjects could access pre-formed letter-production programs (graphemes) before starting to write. Apparently, less planning was needed when a single letter-production program could be executed twice in a row than when two letters had to be prepared. That conclusion would only hold if letters (graphemes) were relevant units for the preparation process.

There are other ways to account for the matching-letter advantage obtained by Teulings, Thomassen, and van Galen (1983). One is that matching letters could be visually coded more easily than non-matching letters. Teulings, Thomassen, and van Galen argued against this view based on data from studies of letter perception. They also argued against another possible explanation of their result—namely, that subjects benefited from identical letter pairs because the letters in the pairs used common strokes. According to this interpretation, subjects initiated matching letter pairs more quickly than non-matching letter pairs because fewer strokes had to be specified in the former case than in the latter. Other experiments by Teulings, Thomassen, and van Galen led these researchers to conclude that sharing strokes did not reduce reaction times.

Reaction Time Evidence for Allograph Selection

The writing reaction time study just summarized provided evidence for the grapheme selection stage (stage 2 in Ellis' model). Another reaction-time study of writing behavior provided evidence for the allograph selection stage (stage 3 in Ellis' model). Stelmach and Teulings (1983) informed subjects that they would be required to write one of two letter strings but that one of the letter strings would be much more likely than the other. The question was how the time to start writing the ultimately required letter string depended on its relation to the other possible string. Making one of the letter strings very likely encouraged subjects to prepare to write it. Writing the other string required a switch from the initially readied program to the ultimately required program.

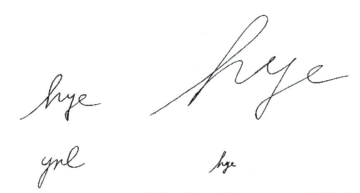

FIGURE 8.10 Letter pairs similar to those copied by subjects in the experiment of Stelmach and Teulings (1983). From Stelmach, G. E. & Teulings, H-L. (1983). Response characteristics of prepared and restructured handwriting. Acta Psychologica, 54, 51–67. With permission. (A) Two strings with different letter shapes. (B) Two strings with different letter sizes.

Stelmach and Teulings (1983) applied their priming paradigm to two choice contexts (see Figure 8.10). In one, the response alternatives were letter strings that required different letter shapes—the lowercase strings *hye* and *ynl*. When the improbable member of this pair was performed (for example, *ynl* when *hye* was likely), the time to start writing was 128 ms longer than when the probable member was performed. In the other choice condition, the response alternatives differed with respect to size; the alternatives were a large and small rendition of the letter string *hye*. In this choice condition, when the improbable response was called for (for example, the small rendition of *hye* when the large rendition was primed), the reaction time cost was only 63 ms, about half the cost in the shape difference condition. Stelmach and Teulings (1983) suggested that the reaction time cost was smaller for the different-size condition than for the different-shape condition because letter size could be specified after letter shape was established, whereas letter shape required shape and then size specification. This is what Ellis' model predicted. His model asserted that allograph selection follows grapheme selection.

Writing Size, Relative Timing, and Absolute Timing

Let us now consider in more detail how writing size is governed. Some authors have proposed that writing size may be controlled by modulating a single control parameter that allows one's writing to stretch or contract as if it were produced on a rubber sheet. We encountered this proposal earlier in this chapter when we saw that in the production of spirals, the angular velocity of the pen is proportional to the linear extent of the loop being drawn (Lacquaniti, Terzuolo, & Viviani, 1983, 1984). A possible mechanism for this and related effects (to be described below) is that an internal clock paces writing performance, with the clock's speed influencing the size of the strokes being created. According to this hypothesis, writing size depends on writing rate. The principle is called *rate scaling*.

A test of the rate-scaling hypothesis was provided by Wing (1978). He measured writing times as subjects altered the overall size of their writing. As the letters grew, the time to produce them grew as well, as predicted by the rate-scaling hypothesis.

Another, more exotic, study also lent support to the rate-scaling view. Here, subjects were asked to breathe nitrous oxide in oxygen while copying short prose passages (Legge, Steinberg, & Summerfield, 1964). As the concentration of nitrous oxide increased, the height of the produced letters also increased. Nitrous oxide is a central nervous system depressant. When its concentration is increased, reactions slow. Increasing concentrations of nitrous oxide may have led to increases in writing size because the neural processes underlying writing performance became more sluggish.

Another exotic study involved hypnosis. Zimbardo, Marshall, and Maslach (1971) told hypnotized individuals "to allow the present to expand and the past and future to become distanced and insignificant." One of the behavioral changes that was observed in individuals affected by these instructions was that their handwriting expanded.

If global rate scaling underlies variation in the overall size of written characters, does it also underlie the minute variations in letter size that occur when one writes within a given size window? For example, if you sign your name repeatedly on a narrow strip of paper and particular letters happen to change size as you repeat your signature, are these size variations due to changes in writing rate?

Viviani and Terzuolo (1980) proposed that changes in writing rate do in fact cause spontaneous changes in writing size. They were led to this position by an observation reproduced in Figure 8.11. Each curve in this figure corresponds to the tangential velocity of a pen used by one person while writing the letter *a*. (Tangential velocity is the slope of the line joining two points in a space of *n* dimensions; in this case, *n* equals 2.) Although the sizes of the strokes varied, when the tangential velocity profiles were arranged from top to bottom according to the total duration of writing the letter (shortest duration at the top, slowest duration at the bottom), Viviani and Terzuolo could fit straight lines through the reversal points (the points where the sign of the velocity changed from positive to negative, or vice versa). The fact that straight lines could be fit to these points means that the ratios of successive stroke durations within the letter were approximately constant, even though the absolute durations of the strokes varied. Apparently, changes in the sizes of the letter were associated with variations in the absolute times of the letter's strokes, though the relative times of the strokes were approximately constant. See Gentner (1987) and Heuer (1988) for discussions of this statistical approach.

The distinction between relative and absolute timing may help explain individual differences in writing style—an issue raised at the beginning of this chapter. Consider the curves in Figure 8.12. These curves, like the ones shown in Figure 8.11, display a pen's tangential velocity profile as a function of time during production of the letter *a*. Each curve in Figure 8.12 comes from a different writer. The *a*'s produced by the writers look different, but the relative times of the strokes are approximately constant. This result suggests that the identity of a letter—what makes an *a* an *a*, for example—may be defined by its relative timing pattern, not to mention its major spatial features. Differences in absolute timing, on the other hand, may explain why one person's writing looks different from another's.

The data just described were obtained by two investigators (Vredenbregt & Koster, 1971) who also built a writing machine that could produce letters with different forms (Figure 8.13). The machine had two pairs of motors. One pair produced vertical movements; the other produced horizontal movements. To produce different letters and different forms of the same letter, the timing of the motors (when they came on and off) was varied, but no other control

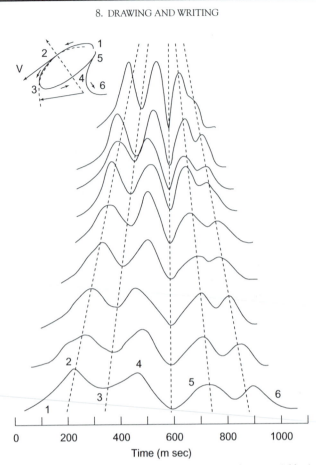

FIGURE 8.11   Tangential velocity profiles of the letter *a* when it was drawn quickly (top) and more and more slowly (bottom). From Viviani, P., & Terzuolo, C. (1980). Space-time invariance in learned motor skills. In G. E. Stelmach & J. Requin (Eds.), Tutorials in motor behavior (pp. 525–533). Amsterdam: North-Holland. With permission.

parameters were manipulated. The mechanical inertia and viscosity of the system allowed smooth lines to be produced even though the motors were abruptly activated and deactivated. The device could produce shape variations similar to those produced by different writers. The letter shape variations were produced by changing the absolute timing of individual strokes. The identities of letters were preserved by maintaining the relative timing of the directional reversals of the moving pen. This writing machine was so successful that it inspired others to design artificial writing systems based on similar principles (Denier van der Gon & Thuring, 1965; Edelman & Flash, 1987; Hollerbach, 1981; Plamondon & Lamarche, 1986).

Context Effects

One aspect of handwriting that is missing from Vredenbregt and Koster's (1971) model is sensitivity to context. The shape and timing of a letter depend on what letter precedes it

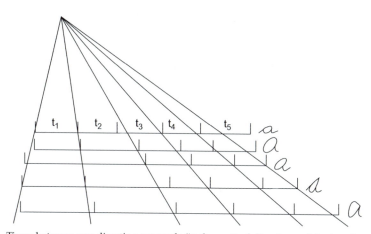

FIGURE 8.12 Times between pen direction-reversals (in the vertical direction only) when five subjects wrote the letter *a*. Each row is for a different subject. Each completed letter is shown on the right side. From Vredenbregt, J. & Koster, W. G. (1971) Analysis and synthesis of handwriting. Philips Technical Review, 32, 73–78. With permission.

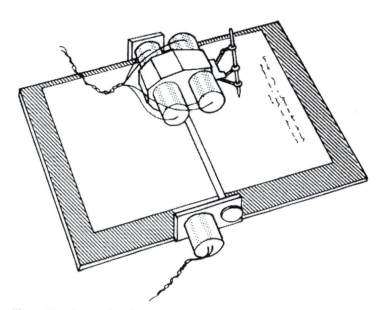

FIGURE 8.13 The writing device of Vredenbregt and Koster (1971).

(Greer & Green, 1983; Wing, Nimmo-Smith, & Eldridge, 1983) and on what letter follows it (Teulings, Thomassen, & van Galen, 1983). For example, Greer and Green (1983) found that when people produced the same letter repeatedly (as in cursive versions of *ee* and *ll*) they could write more quickly than when they alternated between different letters (such as cursive versions of *el* or *le*). Greer and Green (1983) proposed that when the same letter is produced over and over again, a single timing and force program can be used repeatedly, but when different letters are produced in alternation, the program elements change.

Presumably, it takes time to make the needed programming changes, and this slows performance (Rosenbaum, Weber, Hazelett, & Hindorff, 1986; Rosenbaum, Cohen, Jax, van der Wel, & Weiss, 2007).

Greer and Green's (1983) work suggests that there are limits on the extent to which global rate scaling can be used in handwriting (Gentner, 1987). Nevertheless, the demonstration of context effects by these investigators is consistent with the hierarchical model advocated here because hierarchical models predict that the way a response is produced depends on its relation to earlier and later responses.

Writing and Handedness

One of the most striking features of handwriting is that it is most often performed with the right hand. One way to develop an explanation for this fact is to note that the left hemisphere, which is the hemisphere that is primarily responsible for control of the right hand, is generally specialized for language. Because handwriting is a linguistic activity, the right hand might be specialized for writing because it is controlled by the "linguistic" hemisphere.

If this reasoning is correct, then for most people the same hemisphere should control language and handwriting. In fact, it does appear that most individuals whose language is centered in the left hemisphere write with the right hand, and most individuals whose language is centered in the right hemisphere write with the left hand (Levy, 1982).

There are some individuals for whom this generalization may not apply, however. Levy and Reid (1976) proposed that people who write with the hand in an inverted position— that is, with the hand held above the line and the pen pointed down toward the bottom of the page (see Figure 8.14)—may have language and manual control centered in different

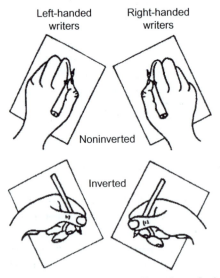

FIGURE 8.14 Inverted and normal handwriting postures. From Levy, J., & Reid, M. L. (1976). Variations in writing posture and cerebral organization. Science, 194, 337–339. With permission.

hemispheres. These individuals are sometimes called hookers, by reference to the hooked appearance of their hand. Their method of writing contrasts with the more usual method in which the hand is held below the line, with the pen pointing up toward the top of the page. Hooking is rare in right-handed writers, but occurs fairly often in left-handers. About 50% of left-handed American writers write with a hooked posture (Smith & Moscovitch, 1979).

To evaluate the hypothesis that hookers have language and writing in different cerebral hemispheres, Levy and Reid (1976) tested right- and left-handed writers who were either hookers or not in tasks designed to reveal whether the left or right hemisphere is specialized for language. In the experiment, a numeral and a nonsense syllable were flashed on a screen, with the horizontal positions of the stimuli randomized from trial to trial. The question was which stimulus would be reported. Levy and Reid (1976) assumed that the nonsense syllable would be reported with higher probability than the numeral if it was projected to the hemisphere specialized for language function. By appealing to the known anatomy of the visual system, they also assumed that if the nonsense syllable was reported with high probability when it appeared on the right side of the display, the subject's left hemisphere was specialized for language, but if the nonsense syllable was reported with high probability when it appeared on the left side of the display, the subject's right hemisphere was specialized for language.

The result was that for hookers, the nonsense syllable was reported with higher probability when it appeared on the side of the screen opposite the writing hand, but for non-hookers, the nonsense syllable was reported with higher probability when it appeared on the same side of screen as the writing hand. This result suggested that for hooked writers, verbal function is localized in the hemisphere ipsilateral to (on the same side as) the preferred writing hand, whereas for non-hooked writers, verbal function is localized in the hemisphere contralateral to (opposite) the preferred writing hand. This outcome accords with Levy and Reid's (1976) hypothesis that in hookers writing and language are controlled by different hemispheres, whereas in non-hookers writing and language are controlled by the same hemisphere.

As intriguing as this outcome is, it was questioned by Moscovitch and Smith (1979), who suggested that hookers may process visual information differently from non-hookers. In Moscovitch and Smith's (1979) study, hookers and non-hookers were asked to respond with either the left or right hand to an auditory, visual, or tactile stimulus. In each block of trials, the identity of the stimulus and the identity of the response were revealed ahead of time, and the subject's task was simply to respond as quickly as possible after detecting the stimulus. Moscovitch and Smith (1979) found that hookers responded more quickly to visual stimuli presented opposite the responding hand than to visual stimuli presented on the same side as the responding hand. This result accords with Levy and Reid's (1976) view that for hookers, each hand is controlled by the ipsilateral rather than by the contralateral hemisphere. Also consistent with Levy and Reid's (1976) view, non-hookers in Moscovitch and Smith's (1979) study were quicker to respond to visual stimuli presented in the visual field on the same side as the responding hand. This result accords with Levy and Reid's proposal because it suggests that in non-hookers, each hand is controlled by the contralateral hemisphere rather than the ipsilateral hemisphere. The problematic results for Levy and Reid (1976) concerned detection of auditory and tactile stimuli. For these stimuli, Moscovitch and Smith (1979) found that hookers and non-hookers responded most quickly when the stimuli were presented on the same side as the responding hand. This is what would be expected if each hand were primarily controlled by the contralateral hemisphere in both types of writers. The latter result flies in the face, and quite squarely between the eyes, of Levy and Reid's (1976) hypothesis.

How can Moscovitch and Smith's results be explained? Perhaps the simplest explanation is that hookers and non-hookers code visual stimuli in different ways. This hypothesis helps explain why laterality tests with a strong visual component are effective at distinguishing hooked and non-hooked left-handed writers (Smith & Moscovitch, 1979). It also fits with the result that electrophysiological measures reveal laterality differences in the occipital lobe (a center for visual processing), but not in other brain areas (Herron, Galin, Johnstone, & Ornstein, 1979).

THE DYNAMIC DOMINANCE HYPOTHESIS

It would still be desirable to know why most people write or draw with the right hand. Analytically, this question can be broken into two. One is, Why is one hand preferred over the other? The other is, Why does the preferred hand happen to be the right?

No one, to the author's knowledge, has provided a satisfying answer to the second question. However, a promising lead has been made to answering the first question. That lead came from Robert Sainburg (2002), a colleague of the author's at Penn State University.

According to Sainburg (2002), one hand may be specialized for *movement* while the other hand may be specialized for *position*. More specifically, one hand may be especially good at forming trajectories and for dealing with, and exploiting, dynamics (force- and torque-related changes). The other hand, by contrast, may be adept at keeping things steady at desired locations, perhaps via expertise in impedance control (see Chapter 3).

This *dynamic dominance* hypothesis is more attractive than some other hypotheses that amount to little more than just-so stories about why one hand is more dexterous than the other. An attraction of the dynamic dominance hypothesis is that, considering the evolutionary past of Homo sapiens, it makes sense to believe that our forebears benefited from having a hand that was good at holding a tree branch while the other hand was good at feeding. Our ancestors may likewise have been aided by having a hand that was good at holding a bone while the other hand was good at picking meat from it, or by having a hand that effectively secured a baby to one's breast while the other hand gathered food or pointed the way for others. Being able to draw especially well with one hand might have been a by-product of these adaptations, although it is conceivable that having well-drawn maps may have helped our ancestors remember where they could find desirable things like food and water or undesirable things like vicious beasts and hidden crevices.

To subscribe to the dynamic dominance hypothesis, one must buy into the idea that the development of special abilities for one hand results in diminution of other abilities for the same hand. One must also subscribe to the idea that there is reciprocity between the two hands: If one hand gets good at dynamics and not so good at position control (statics), the hand will get good at statics and not so good at dynamics.

It would help to have evidence for the dynamic dominance hypothesis so its claims about handedness can be checked and so the other, far-reaching implications suggested above can be either endorsed or repudiated depending on how the data turn out. It turns out that Sainburg and his colleagues have obtained data that are quite persuasive for the dynamic dominance hypothesis (for a review, see Sainburg, 2005).

One such finding was the observation that the reliability of adopted positions was higher for the non-dominant arm than for the dominant arm. Wang and Sainburg (2007) found that, for the dominant arm, performance was more accurate when reaching from one fixed starting position to multiple targets than when reaching from multiple starting positions to one fixed target. For the non-dominant arm, the pattern of results was the opposite. Another finding, obtained in other studies by Sainburg and his colleagues (Duff & Sainburg, 2007; Sainburg, 2002, 2005) was that the dominant arm was better able to compensate for imposed loads than the non-dominant arm was. This pair of results—the first showing superiority of the non-dominant arm for position retention and the second showing superiority of the dominant arm for dynamics adaptability—argues against any simple-minded hypothesis about the dominant arm simply being "smarter" than the non-dominant arm. Each arm, or each arm's hemisphere (the left hemisphere for the right arm and the right hemisphere for the left arm), has its own specialization. The implication for hand preference in drawing and writing is that drawing and writing benefit from skill at movement more than skill at maintaining single positions. From this perspective, it makes sense that in most people the right hand is preferred over the left for drawing and writing (Oldfield, 1971).

SUMMARY

1. Writing and drawing may be controlled through a series of stages—from ideas to graphic segments to motor commands.
2. A demonstration of the validity of the stage model is the preservation of writing styles across different means of writing—for example, when writing with different parts of the body or when writing over differently sized spaces such as a blackboard or a bank check. Some questions for research on drawing and writing are why individuals write with different styles and why, for most people, writing and drawing are easier with the right hand than the left.
3. To draw, one must determine the order in which drawing strokes are made. Research on drawing in children and adults suggests that rules may be called upon during the planning of drawing behavior. The rules may ensure mechanical efficiency, but other factors—notably the semantic interpretation of the figure to be drawn—may also affect the order in which strokes are produced. Semantic biases in drawing provide additional support for the view that drawing, and graphic behavior in general, is largely a top-down process.
4. A way to study the execution of drawing strokes is to record the kinematics of the pen during simple, repetitive drawing tasks such as scribbling, drawing figure eights, or

drawing spirals. Research on such elementary drawing tasks has suggested the isogony principle, which asserts that equal angles are covered in equal times. The isogony principle implies that figures are segmented into manageable pieces by the graphic production system and that an effort is made to produce segments, or sets of segments, in equal amounts of time.

5. Another control principle that has emerged from studies of drawing is the two-thirds power law. According to this principle, angular velocity increases with curvature and also with arc length.

6. A possible explanation of the two-thirds power law is based on the coupling of oscillators. Another possible explanation is based on the assumption that it is desirable to move as smoothly as possible. It may be that two-thirds power law is based on both factors.

7. Another way to study the control of handwriting is to classify the kinds of errors that writers make. Based on one such classification scheme, four stages may be identified for the generation of handwriting. The outputs of these stages are (a) words, (b) graphemes or letters, (c) allographs or letter forms, such as upper- and lowercase versions of the same letter, and (d) graphs or strokes.

8. People with the neurological disorder known as dysgraphia display errors consistent with the hierarchical stage model. Some dysgraphic patients have difficulty producing well-formed writing strokes, though their spelling and word choices are appropriate. Others produce well-formed writing strokes but have difficulty spelling (in writing only), though their word choices are legitimate.

9. Reaction time studies with normal individuals lend further support to the hierarchical model of writing. Facilitation of reaction times in various task conditions suggests that people can selectively ready grapheme-level (letter-level) programs.

10. Other reaction time results suggest that people can also selectively ready allograph-level programs (programs for the same letter appearing in different forms).

11. Writing size may be controlled by altering writing speed. Although absolute times of writing strokes may increase as writing size increases and may distinguish writing styles by different individuals, relative times of strokes within letters or words remain remarkably invariant over size changes or writers and so help define particular letters. Writing machines designed on the basis of these observations produce letters that simulate personal writing styles.

12. A property of writing that must be captured in a complete theory of handwriting is the presence of context effects. The speed with which one letter is written depends on which other letters have just been written or are about to be written. Context effects suggest hierarchical control because they suggest that information about forthcoming written responses is available when earlier written responses are produced.

13. In most people, the hand used for handwriting (the right hand) is controlled by the brain hemisphere specialized for language (the left hemisphere). It has been proposed that this principle may not hold for people who write with a hooked hand posture. However, this proposal has been supplanted by the hypothesis that "hookers" and "non-hookers" may process visual or spatial information differently.

14. The dynamic dominance hypothesis says that the left hemisphere is specialized for movement control (dynamics) while the right hemisphere is specialized for position

control (statics). In support of this hypothesis, it has been found that returns to start positions are more reliable for the non-dominant arm than for the dominant arm, while adaptation to force fields is better for the dominant arm than for the non-dominant arm.

Further Reading

For a study of limb contributions to drawing, see Meulenbroek, Rosenbaum, Thomassen, and Schomaker (1993).
For evidence that visual recognition of writing relies on embodied cognition, see Parkinson and Khurana (2007).
Why can't most people draw what they see? See Cohen and Bennett (1997).
What can we learn about drawings by the blind? See Kennedy (1983) and Kennedy and Juricevic (2006).
Computer technology has been used to distinguish forgeries from authentic paintings by established masters like Vincent Van Gogh. Statistical properties of brush strokes provide a clue, as reported by two Penn State University professors, James Wang of Information Sciences (http://wang.ist.psu.edu/cgi-bin/zwang/pub/show_publication.cgi?sort=4) and Jia Li of Statistics (http://www.stat.psu.edu/~jiali/).
Handwriting recognition by computers is a topic that has received extensive coverage in two journals: *IEEE Transactions on Pattern Analysis and Machine Intelligence*, and *Pattern Recognition*.
Dysgraphia is one of many neuropsychological disorders. The journal *Neuropsychology* focuses on such disorders, as does the journal *Neuropsychologia*. Textbooks on neuropsychology are available as well (e.g., Zillner, 2008).

Reaction Time	279	*Event Timing*	297	
Simple Reaction Time	279	*Amodality of Timing*	299	
Choice Reaction Time	280	*Integration of Serial Order and Timing*	300	
Stimulus-Response Compatibility	282	*Adjusting the Rate of Production*		
Ideo-Motor Accounts of Stimulus-		*for Entire Sequences*	301	
Response Compatibility	284	**Typing**	303	
The SNARC Effect	285	*Historical Issues*	304	
The Simon Effect	286	*Units of Typing Control*	306	
The Stroop Effect	286	*Typing Errors*	307	
Response-Response Compatibility	287	*Timing of Keystrokes in Typewriting*	307	
Simultaneous and Sequential		*Rumelhart and Norman's*		
Finger Presses	288	*Model of Typewriting*	312	
Simultaneous Keystrokes	288	**Piano Playing**	314	
Sequences of Keypresses	289			
Learning Keyboard Sequences	293	**Summary**	317	
Control of Rhythm and Timing	294	**Further Reading**	321	
Hierarchical Time Keepers	296			

On June 28, 2004, the Associated Press reported that a new record had been set for text messaging. Kimberly Yeo, a 23-year-old woman in Singapore, managed to text message the following passage in just 43.24 seconds: "The razor-toothed piranhas of the genera Serrasalmus and Pygocentrus are the most ferocious freshwater fish in the world. In reality they seldom attack a human." The message was entered by Ms. Yeo using her thumbs only. The message had 160 characters, including spaces. Given the number of characters and the time needed to enter them, Ms. Yeo managed to enter the characters at the impressive rate of 3.7 characters per second, or about 270 ms per character. Not bad for someone who, at the time, was all thumbs!

In case you are so impressed with this speed of text messaging that you feel tempted to dispose of your computer keyboard and rely on your cell phone to type your next novel, be mindful that typists, who have the luxury of using all their fingers, can produce 60 or even 90 words a minute. With an average of 5 characters per word and one space between words, a rate of 90 words a minute amounts to 450 keystrokes a minute, or one keystroke every 133 ms. That is about twice as fast as the record-setting rate for all-thumbs text messaging.

Pianists can produce keystrokes at even higher rates, particularly when they play chords. If a pianist plays three notes per chord with each hand at a rate of three chords per second per hand, the pianist's keystroke rate is 18 keystrokes per second, or more than one keystroke every 56 ms.

How are such high rates of keyboard performance achieved? The rapidity of text messaging with the two thumbs may be ascribed to quick reaction times, for reaction times, which are recorded when people respond to external signals, tend to be between 250 and 300 ms, although the actual value depends on the nature of the reaction time task and the nature of the performer, as described later in this chapter. High speeds of typing and piano playing cannot be ascribed solely to rapid responding to sensory signals, however, for the times are too short. High rates of keyboard performance must be ascribed instead to internal plans that guide production of the series of keystrokes (Lashley, 1951). Understanding the nature of these plans and how they are executed is the central aim of basic research on keyboarding. Understanding how keyboarding can be made easier is the central aim of applied research in this area.

The organization of the chapter is as follows. First, we will consider performance in reaction time tasks. These tasks, though elementary, provide windows into the mechanisms by which stimulus-response associations are realized. Data from reaction time tasks constrain models of more complex keyboard sequencings. For example, the fact that reaction times for individual keypresses are longer than times between keystrokes in rapid typing and piano playing indicates that rapid keyboard sequences must be based on plans. As will be seen in this chapter, reaction time research has proven helpful in resolving other, more general, questions about human perception and performance.

The second part of the chapter concerns performance in tasks requiring sequences of button presses. Such tasks have enabled researchers to develop detailed models of the memory representations underlying sequential behavior. One of these models assumes that manual response sequences are hierarchically controlled. Another assumes that there are internal timing mechanisms for motor production that may also serve perception. The basis for these claims will be examined here.

The next section of the chapter will be concerned with typewriting. An important principle from typewriting research is that typists type quickly by moving their fingers and hands in an overlapping fashion, without each keystroke awaiting completion of the keystroke before it. Another insight from typing research is that features of individual keystrokes play a role in keystroke planning, namely, which hand and which finger are used for individual strokes. The most detailed model of typing was developed in the early 1980's by Rumelhart and Norman (1982). It remains a standard against which future models can be measured. Owing to the success of Rumelhart and Norman's model, and owing to its deeper theoretical importance about human motor control generally, it is reviewed in some depth here.

The coda of the chapter concerns piano playing. Much of the work in this area reinforces principles covered in the preceding sections, but two new ideas are presented. One is that variations in force can be used to communicate musical phrasing. The other is that speeding up and slowing down can express musical emotion. Such changes in tempo become routinized with practice and turn out to be less spontaneous than one might expect. Because such timing changes become highly stereotyped over repeated performances of a piece of music, they become an integral part of the piece's memory representation.

REACTION TIME

The speed with which one reacts to a signal—one's reaction time (RT)—is a widely used measure of performance. When there is just one possible signal and response in a block of trials, the dependent measure is the *simple* RT. When there is more than one possible signal and response in a block of trials, the dependent measure is the *choice* RT. Choice RTs are usually longer than simple RTs.

Many factors affect simple and choice RT: the state of the participant, the nature of the stimulus, the nature of the response, and the relations among these factors. The literature on RT is massive, so no attempt will be made here to review all of it. For summaries of classic work, see Keele (1986), Luce (1986), Meyer, Osman, Irwin, and Yantis (1988), Welford (1980), Woodworth (1938), and Woodworth and Schlosberg (1954). Some findings that are important for our concerns are reviewed below.

Simple Reaction Time

A number of factors affect simple RT. People who are younger or more alert generally have shorter simple RTs than people who are older or less alert (Woodworth & Schlosberg, 1954). People practiced at a reaction time task generally produce shorter simple RTs than people who are unpracticed (Woodworth & Schlosberg, 1954). If a person is sure about when a signal will occur, his or her simple RT is usually shorter than if s/he is uncertain about the signal's arrival time (Klemmer, 1957). If the time of the signal is completely certain, responses can be made to coincide with the signal, yielding RTs close to 0 ms. If the participant anticipates the signal, s/he may be able to respond before the signal appears, yielding negative RTs. Experimenters often admonish subjects not to produce negative RTs. Beyond this, they also introduce "catch trials" in which no reaction signal appears. In such trials, the subject is supposed to refrain from responding. Because participants in RT experiments are so apt to anticipate when signals will appear, it is reasonable to suppose that the participants have an internal time-keeping ability, perhaps made possible by one or more internal "clocks." We will explore this issue later in this chapter.

The strength of the reaction signal affects simple RT. People are generally faster to respond to bright lights than to dim lights, particularly when the intensity of the signal is uncertain (Teichner & Krebs, 1972). Similarly, people are generally faster to respond to loud sounds than to soft sounds; again, this effect is more pronounced when the sounds' times are unpredictable.

The type of response also affects the simple RT. Effectors of large mass generally have longer simple RTs than effectors of small mass. For example, the finger, forearm, and upper arm have simple RTs of 156, 166, and 173 ms, respectively (Anson, 1982). These RT differences are mainly attributable to mechanical factors, as shown by the fact that the simple RTs of electromyographic activity in these three effectors (the times when significant EMG activity can be observed after reactions signals) are the same (Anson, 1982).

Some response factors that one might expect to influence simple RT do not. There is hardly any difference between the simple RTs of the dominant and non-dominant hand, and there is hardly any difference between the simple RTs for the different fingers (Woodworth, 1938).

Choice Reaction Time

As mentioned above, choice RTs are generally longer than simple RTs. On the other hand, if the probability of a choice stimulus is high enough, the corresponding choice RT can approximate a simple RT. This outcome follows from the fact that simple and choice RT occupy a probability continuum. In a simple RT task, the probability of a response reaches the maximum probability of 1. If the probability of response in a choice RT task approaches 1, the corresponding choice RT approximates the simple RT for that same stimulus-response pair.

Why do choice RTs decrease (get faster) for likely stimuli? Is the effect due to a change in stimulus processing, a change in response processing, or both? This question has been addressed by mapping more than one stimulus to a response (Bertelson, 1965); see Figure 9.1. Bertelson reasoned that if subjects respond more quickly to a stimulus because of preparation to make a particular response, their choice RTs should be reduced by repeated testing of that response regardless of which stimulus was assigned to it. On the other hand, if subjects respond more quickly to repeated presentation of a stimulus because of their perceptual set for that stimulus, their choice RTs should be reduced only by repeated presentation of that stimulus.

The results indicate that response preparation contributes to the reduction of choice RTs. In Bertelson's (1965) experiment, two stimuli, SA and SB, were assigned to the same response. When stimulus SA was presented repeatedly, choice RTs decreased. When stimulus SA was replaced with stimulus SB, there was some elevation of choice RTs, but the elevation was much smaller than when stimulus SA was replaced by a stimulus that called for a different

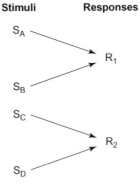

FIGURE 9.1 Mapping of stimuli to responses in Bertelson's (1965) study. From Bertelson, P. (1965). Serial choice reaction-time as a function of response versus signal-and-response repetition. Nature, 205, 217–218. With permission.

response—SC or SD. Thus, response preparation helped reduce choice RTs, but perceptual set also contributed to the choice RT decline. Other experiments have led to the same conclusion; see Keele (1986).

As the number of possible stimulus-response pairs in a choice RT experiment increases, the choice reaction time also increases. Figure 9.2 shows the results of such an experiment, where in each trial one of n lights was turned on and the subject's task was to press the key beneath it. Choice RTs increased linearly with the logarithm to the base 2 of the number of stimulus-response alternatives. (The logarithm of a number is the exponent to which some base is raised to yield that number. The logarithm of 8 to the base 2 is 3 because $2^3 = 8$, the logarithm of 16 to the base 2 is 4 because $2^4 = 16$, and so on.) The linear increase of choice RT with the logarithm to the base 2 of the number of stimulus-response alternatives is known as the Hick-Hyman law. It was discovered by Hick (1952) and by Hyman (1953) and is one of the most famous relations in RT research and one of the few laws of psychology.

In the Hick-Hyman law, it is assumed that decision making can be characterized by the number of binary digits, or "bits," that uniquely define a particular response. In effect, the subject is assumed to play 20 questions to determine which response should be made when

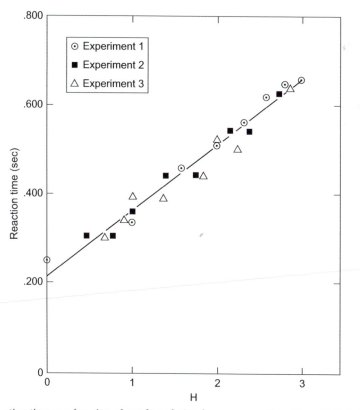

FIGURE 9.2 Reaction time as a function of number of stimulus-response alternatives, H. Data from three experiments and best fitting straight line between reaction time and H. From Posner, M. I. (1967). Characteristics of visual and kinesthetic memory codes. Journal of Experimental Psychology, 75, 103–107. With permission.

a stimulus has appeared. The number of bits (or "questions") for n equally likely stimulus-response alternatives is $\log_2 n$. According to the Hick-Hyman law, bits are set (binary decisions are made) at a rate approximating the slope of the best-fitting straight-line function relating choice RT to $\log_2 n$. For the data shown in Figure 9.2, the rate is about 150 ms per bit. Another way of saying this, and another way of expressing the Hick-Hyman law, is to say that choice RTs increase by an equal amount—for example, by 150 ms—with each doubling of the number of stimulus-response alternatives.

Characterizing decision making as a series of binary decisions was consistent with an influential theory of communication developed in the late 1940's, called *information theory* (Shannon & Weaver, 1949). The theory's application to human information processing received a boost through the success of the Hick-Hyman law. Information theory is commonly used today in the way we refer to computer memory capacity. If your computer's hard drive can store 8 gigabytes, it can hold 8 billion 8-bit strings of 1's and 0's. A convention in computer science is to refer to 8 bits as a "byte." A million bytes is a megabyte, a billion bytes is a gigabyte, and a trillion bytes is a terabyte.

Despite the usefulness of information theory in technology, the application of information theory to psychology received a setback in the 1950's when it was shown that the amount of information that can be held in human short-term memory depends not on how many bits the information has (roughly, the number of questions required to uniquely identify it), but rather on how many meaningful units or "chunks" it contains (Miller, 1956). It was not possible in 1956, nor has it been possible since, to measure meaningfulness in terms of information theory. Developing an objective measure of meaningfulness has remained a challenge of cognitive science. Ironically, one of the most succinct quantitative measures of meaning, or at least meaningfulness, was offered by B. F. Skinner, who said that the meaningfulness of a stimulus is defined by the number of associations it has. Skinner's contribution here is ironic because he was a behaviorist—indeed the foremost behaviorist of his time.

Stimulus-Response Compatibility

Another blow to information theory, or at least the Hick-Hyman law, came from studies of stimulus-response (S-R) compatibility. In a classic experiment demonstrating the power of S-R computability, Leonard (1959) asked subjects to rest their fingers on small vibrators. Whenever a vibrator came on, the subject was supposed to press the finger resting on it. Leonard found that as the number of possible vibrators increased, there was virtually no increase in choice RT. Thus, choice RTs did not consistently increase with the number of stimulus-response alternatives.

What accounted for this lack of an uncertainty effect? Leonard (1959) found that choice RTs did obey the usual uncertainty effect when his subjects were asked not to respond with the stimulated finger but instead were asked to respond with *another* finger assigned to the vibrator that came on. Based on the *absence* of an uncertainty effect when subjects pressed fingers that received vibration, coupled with the *presence* of an uncertainty effect when subjects pressed fingers that did not receive vibration, Leonard concluded that when the responding and stimulated finger were the same, there was a highly effective, or compatible, mapping between stimulus and response. Conversely, when the finger to be pressed did not directly contact the vibrator, the stimulus-response mapping was less compatible, and a more deliberate, time-consuming process was required, akin to the one implied by the Hick-Hyman law. Strictly speaking, Leonard's data did not disprove the Hick-Hyman law. Rather, his data showed that the slope of the function relating choice RT to uncertainty can go to zero. This outcome limited the generality of the Hick-Hyman law.

Stimulus-response (S-R) compatibility is an important factor in virtually all kinds of RT tasks, including button pressing (Craft & Simon, 1970; Inhoff, Rosenbaum, Gordon, & Campbell, 1984), handwriting (Greenwald, 1970), speaking (Gordon & Meyer, 1987a, b; Rosenbaum, Gordon, Stillings, & Feinstein, 1987), and aiming for targets (Fitts & Deininger, 1954). S-R compatibility has also been used to shed light on the codes used for movement initiation. A classic study on this topic was reported by Wallace (1971), who asked how quickly subjects could respond to a visual signal appearing on the left or on the right when the associated response was made with the left hand or right and when the hands were either crossed or uncrossed (Figure 9.3). Wallace found that S-R compatibility was principally defined by the spatial relation between the stimulus and response, not by the anatomical identity of the hand making the response. Thus, subjects were faster to respond on the same side of the body midline as the signal, regardless of whether the hand making the response was the anatomical left or right hand. This outcome suggests that S-R compatibility is defined primarily by the mappings between stimulus and response *locations*.

This outcome is similar to Tolman's (1948) classic finding for spatial navigation, which was described in the chapter on walking (Chapter 5). Recall that Tolman discovered that maze locations tend to be learned in terms of spatial layouts, not in terms of movements. This was the basis for his famous "cognitive maps." Wallace's (1971) study, as well as an analogous study that appeared at around the same time (Brebner, Shephard, & Cairney, 1972), showed that the same cognitive map principle applies to more elementary stimulus-response mappings. From this pair of outcomes—one concerning navigation through the environment and one concerning button presses—we see that common principles can be found for seemingly disparate aspects of human motor control.

Another study, focusing on the fundamentals of conditioning, led to the same conclusion. Wickens (1938; reviewed by Gallistel, 1980) had subjects hold their hands palm-side down on a device that transmitted an electrical shock to the fingertip. The shock was regularly preceded by a tone. After a few exposures to the tone-shock pair, subjects learned to withdraw the finger from the shocker as soon as the tone was presented but before the shock came on. To make the withdrawal response, subjects extended the finger.

Wickens (1938) next asked his subjects to turned their hands over, leaving the palm up. Would they *extend* the finger, which is the response they had made before in terms of muscle activity, or would they *flex* the finger, which is the response they had made before in terms of spatial displacement, bringing the finger away from the shock? The answer was that they flexed the finger, the response that was muscularly opposite the earlier response but spatially congruent with the response made before. This behavior was adaptive for avoiding the shock.

The latter result reinforces the conclusion from the other studies considered above. Again, we see that learned responses are often defined with respect to spatial features, not muscle features. Obtaining this result across a wide range of tasks—choice RT tasks, navigation tasks, and instrumental conditioning tasks—shows how different lines of evidence from various sources can point to the same general principles.

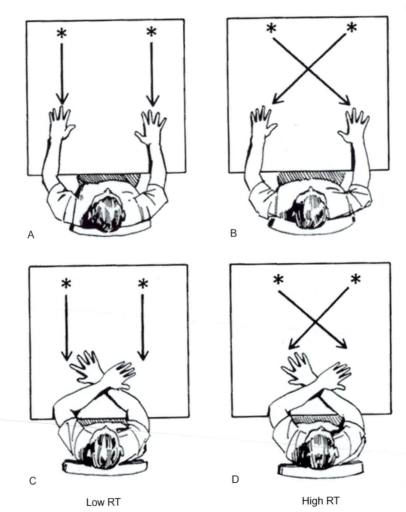

Low RT   High RT

FIGURE 9.3   Four stimulus-response arrangements in Wallace's (1971) experiment. (A) Compatible mappings between stimulus locations and button locations, and also between stimulus locations and effector (hand) locations; (B) Incompatible mappings between stimulus locations and button locations, and also between stimulus locations and effector (hand) locations; (C) Compatible mappings between stimulus locations and button locations but not between stimulus locations and effector locations; (D) Compatible mappings between stimulus locations and effector locations but not between stimulus locations and button locations. Choice reaction times were shorter in conditions (A) and (C) than in conditions (B) and (D).

Ideo-Motor Accounts of Stimulus-Response Compatibility

What accounts for the fact that some stimulus-response mappings are compatible, as indexed by the brevity of their choice RTs, whereas other stimulus-response mappings are incompatible, as indexed by the greater length of their choice RTs? We have seen that spatial factors often predict compatibility. However, that fact does not imply the mechanism underlying the phenomenon.

One hypothesis about the mechanism is that the time to respond to a stimulus simply depends on the number of times that the S-R pair has been experienced. On this account, the distinction between compatible and incompatible stimulus-response associations amounts to a distinction between often-made and seldom-made responses to particular stimuli. Consistent with this view, the more often a response is made to a stimulus, the shorter the RT, as already mentioned.

Still, there might be something more to S-R compatibility than sheer probability of stimulus-response association. An idea of what that something more might be is that the basis for S-R compatibility effects is *ideo-motor* activity. This term was broached in earlier chapters, where we saw that some investigators have appealed to the idea that a prerequisite for voluntary action is an internal representation of the perceptual changes that the voluntary action produces. Having such an internal representation can instigate the action itself, according to ideo-motor theory. In fact, in its strongest form, the theory says that having the internal representation of a desired percept automatically triggers the act that makes that percept possible.

Such a hypothesis provides a ready account of S-R compatibility. Compatible S-R associations are ones for which summoning stimuli strongly resemble the stimuli their response will produce; those resulting stimuli are called *reafferent* stimuli. Incompatible S-R associations, by contrast, are ones for which summoning stimuli do not strongly resemble reafferent stimuli. Data consistent with the ideo-motor perspective have been reported in a number of studies; for a review, see Hommel, Musseler, Aschersleben, & Prinz (2001). To cite one illustrative study, published after the review by Hommel et al., Brass, Bekkering, and Prinz (2001) asked participants to initiate finger movements in response to finger movements produced by a model that the experimental participants viewed on a video monitor. If the required movements went in the same direction as the observed movements, the choice RTs were shorter than if the required movements went in the opposite direction. This outcome fits with ideo-motor theory because the theory says that seeing a movement that is similar to the movement to be made should facilitate the movement's generation. Conversely, seeing a movement that is dissimilar from the movement to be made should interfere with the movement's generation.

The SNARC Effect

One should not infer from the foregoing discussion that ideo-motor theory is the only way to explain S-R compatibility effects. S-R compatibility effects can also be explained by saying that stimuli and responses share abstract representations or a common code (Hommel, Musseler, Aschersleben, & Prinz, 2001). An example is the SNARC effect (Dehaene, 1997), which arises when people press a button on the left to indicate that a number is even or press a button on the right to indicate that a number is odd. The effect, described empirically and in its canonical form, is that left button responses have short RTs for small numbers and long RTs for large numbers. The opposite outcome is obtained for right button responses. This outcome has been explained by saying that numbers are mentally represented along a mental line that runs continuously from left to right, with small numbers to the left and large numbers to the right. The acronym SNARC refers to spatial number analogue representation compatibility. SNARC-y data are also obtained when the left button press is used to indicate that numbers are odd rather than even or, in other conditions, that numbers are even rather than odd. It doesn't matter much whether the left button press signals oddness or evenness. What does matter—what fulfills the SNARC effect—is that the number triggering a left response is small and the number triggering a right response is large. Those mappings yield short RTs. The opposite mappings yield long RTs.

The Simon Effect

Nothing in the instructions to subjects in SNARC effect experiments requires them to code numbers as leftward or rightward. Yet they code the numbers that way, albeit unconsciously. The fact that the SNARC effect concerns an incidental feature of stimuli and responses adds to its intrigue.

Other studies of S-R compatibility have turned up similar incidental effects. A famous effect of this kind is the Simon effect (Simon, 1990). In typical experiments in which the Simon effect is observed, participants are asked to press a button on the left if a stimulus is of one color—for example, green—or to press a button on the right if a stimulus is of another color—for example, red. Even though the side where the stimulus appears is logically irrelevant to the task, left button presses have shorter RTs to responses made to stimuli on the left than to stimuli on the right, and right button presses have shorter choice RTs for stimuli on the right than for stimuli on the left. This outcome echoes the result concerning S-R compatibility discussed earlier in this chapter, where it was found that left-side responses have shorter choice RTs to left-side stimuli than to right-side stimuli, and vice versa for right-side responses (Brebner, Shephard, & Cairney, 1972; Wallace, 1971). In the latter studies, however, stimulus side was the defining feature of the stimulus, the feature that explicitly defined the required response. By contrast, in studies showing the Simon effect, stimulus side is a purely incidental feature of the stimulus. The existence of the Simon effect shows that incidental features can yield S-R compatibility, just as explicit features can.

The Stroop Effect

Another example of a task in which incidental features of stimuli and responses produce marked effects is one in which participants are asked to name the color of the ink in which words are presented regardless of what the word is. If participants could comply with this instruction and ignore all information that is strictly irrelevant to the decision, it would not matter whether the word whose ink color is to be classified matches the name of the ink color. It should take no longer to say "green" to the word "RED" printed in green ink than to say "green" to the word "GREEN" printed in green ink, for example.

The actual outcome is different. As discovered by Stroop (1935), people take much longer to say "green" when the word "RED" is shown in green ink than when the word "GREEN" is shown in green ink. The reason can be traced to *response competition*. Seeing the word "GREEN" automatically activates the "green" response, but that response is incompatible with saying "red" in response to red ink. With two possible responses—"green" and "red"—fighting it out, so to speak, extra time is needed to sort out the fray. Executive control processes come online to select the response that befits the instructions, and this takes extra time.

The *Stroop* effect is one of the most reliable and robust phenomena of RT research; for a review, see MacLeod (1991). Apropos this chapter's emphasis on keyboarding, the Stroop effect has been demonstrated in experiments in which participants type rather than say color words aloud (Logan & Zbrodoff, 1998). As might be expected, to obtain the Stroop experiment in typing contexts, the participants must be very skilled typists, for otherwise they would not have the automatic tendency to type the words they are reading. Based on this idea, the Stroop effect provides a measure of the automaticity of responses to stimuli, whether in keyboarding or other performance domains.

Response-Response Compatibility

In the Stroop effect, the response that happens to be called up by the word that is shown to the participant interferes with the response that is called up by the word's ink. In other tasks, such interference between possible responses is also suggested. Changes to choice RTs due to relations between or among possible responses, whether called for implicitly or explicitly, are known as *response-response* (R-R) compatibility effects.

One of the first reports of the R-R compatibility effect came from an experiment (Kornblum, 1965) in which subjects performed in two different choice RT conditions. In one, they chose between a button press with the *index* finger of the right hand and a button press with the *middle* finger of the right hand. In the other, they again chose between a button press with the index finger of the right hand and a button press with the middle finger of the *left* hand. The signals were the same in the two conditions, yet the choice RT for the common right index finger was shorter when the alternative response was the left middle finger than when the alternative response was the right middle finger. Thus, the choice RT for the same response to the same signal was affected by the identity of the other possible response.

What accounts for this result? Kornblum (1965) suggested that there is more competition or inhibition between fingers of the same hand than between fingers of different hands. The index finger and middle finger of the same hand are linked mechanically, whereas the index finger of one hand and the middle finger of the other hand are more mechanically independent. You can demonstrate this difference for yourself by trying to hold your right index finger rigid while oscillating either your right middle finger or your left middle finger. It is nearly impossible to keep your index finger still while wiggling the middle finger of the same hand, but it is easy to keep your index finger still while oscillating the middle finger of the other hand. The greater independence between the fingers of the two hands makes it easier to prepare to respond with one of those fingers.

Further support for this account of R-R compatibility came from an experiment in which participants were encouraged to get ready to respond with a right index finger response and on most trials were asked to respond with that finger. However, on other trials they were called upon to respond with another possible finger—either the right middle finger or the left middle finger (Rosenbaum & Kornblum, 1982). The time to switch to the less prepared response was longer when it was made with the right middle finger than when it was made with the left middle finger, consistent with the hypothesis that while the right index finger response was prepared, participants found it easier to maintain a secondary state of readiness for the other-hand response.

SIMULTANEOUS AND SEQUENTIAL FINGER PRESSES

In the studies reviewed so far, subjects pressed a button with one finger when a signal was presented. Because the aim of this chapter is to shed light on the control of extended sequences of keypresses, it is also important to consider laboratory tasks in which subjects perform more than one keypress per trial. Two tasks are relevant in this connection. In one, subjects press two or more keys simultaneously; that is, they produce chords. In the other, they produce series of keypresses, either in response to external signals indicating which key is to be pressed or in response to their own memories.

Simultaneous Keystrokes

There has been surprisingly little research on chord production, although simultaneous keypressing is indispensable in a wide variety of practical domains. Pianists play chords, of course, and so do courtroom stenographers, who use chord typewriters to transcribe oral testimony. The most efficient way to type Japanese characters is to press several keys at once (Yamada, 1983).

Rabbitt, Vyas, and Fearnley (1975) asked how quickly people could make chord responses on a laboratory keyboard, where the combination of keystrokes at any time was designated by combinations of lights above the keys. Rabbitt et al. found that the choice RT to produce a chord increased with the number of keystrokes within it. In addition, choice RTs were shorter for responses that used homologous fingers of the two hands (e.g., the two index fingers or the two middle fingers) than for responses that used non-homologous fingers of the two hands (e.g., the left index finger and the right middle finger). Choice RTs also depended on the relation between the number of keystrokes in successive chords. As the number of chord keystrokes increased, the choice RT for the subsequent chord also increased. This result may have been due to the time demands of monitoring response accuracy, for Rabbitt et al. also found that the time to detect errors in a chord increased with the chord's complexity.

Another study of chord performance addressed the question of how well people could learn to produce different chords in response to different letters (Gopher, Karis, & Koenig, 1985). There were three different rules for assigning letters to chords in this study (Figure 9.4). In one, the keys pressed with the two hands were spatially congruent, so if a letter was assigned to the two left keys for the left hand, the subject was also supposed to depress the two left keys for the right hand. This meant that different fingers of the two hands had to be pressed simultaneously. In another arrangement, the keys pressed with the two hands were manually congruent, so all two-hand chords used homologous fingers. A third arrangement combined spatial congruity and manual symmetry. This was achieved by vertically tilting the keyboards for the left and right hands (see Figure 9.4) so homologous fingers were used to press keys that were also spatially congruent. In all three conditions, subjects were shown letters and were asked to produce the corresponding chords as quickly and as accurately as possible. The question was what arrangement of keys and what assignment of letters to keys would be learned most easily. Gopher et al. found that subjects performed at the best level in the combined arrangement, subjects performed at the

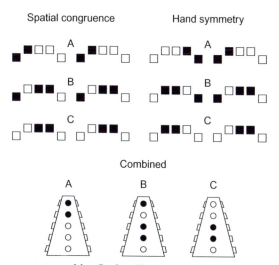

FIGURE 9.4   Chord arrangements used by Gopher, Karis, and Koenig (1985). From Gopher, D., Karis, D., & Koenig, W. (1985). The representation of movement schemas in long-term memory: Lessons from the acquisition of a transcription skill. Acta Psychologica, 60, 105–1134. With permission.

intermediate level in the spatial congruity arrangement, and subjects performed at the worst level in the hand symmetry arrangement.

What caused this outcome? We can first evaluate the possibility that the superiority of the combined arrangement was due to the vertical posture of the hands, which was unique for the combined-arrangement condition. When subjects from the combined-arrangement group were later asked to perform with their hands in the flat orientation, they still did very well. Moreover, when a new group of subjects was taught to adopt the same stimulus-response mapping rule as the combined group but with their hands held flat, they also performed well. Thus, vertical hand postures alone did not ensure efficient chord typing. More likely is that the combined arrangement was especially effective because it allowed subjects to alternate between spatial and anatomical coding strategies. This interpretation implies that the way subjects mentally represent stimulus-response mappings plays a significant role in performance (Proctor & Reeve, 1989).

Sequences of Keypresses

Let us now consider the production of sequences of keystrokes. We will begin with studies in which successive keypresses are called for by signals that are typically presented shortly after the last response, without an intervening warning signal—the so-called serial choice RT. After that discussion, we will turn to studies in which successive keystrokes are produced from memory.

Rabbitt and Vyas (1970) performed a serial choice RT experiment in which subjects were asked to press one key at a time with the index and middle fingers of the left and right hands following the appearance of one of four digits on a screen. Subjects were fastest when they pressed a finger of one hand after a response was made with the homologous finger of the other hand, they were somewhat slower when the finger to be pressed was on the same hand as the immediately preceding response but used a different finger (for example, left index finger after left middle finger), and they were slowest when the finger to be pressed used a different hand and was non-homologous to the finger used in the immediately preceding response (for example, left index finger after right middle finger).

One way to interpret this pattern of results is that when subjects used one hand after the other, they could prepare one response while the preceding response was being completed. By contrast, when successive responses were made with one hand, the preparation of one response could not begin until the previous response was completed. This is essentially the same explanation as the one given earlier for the findings regarding R-R compatibility. The same idea will prove useful again when we consider typewriting, later in this chapter.

The advantage of performing successive responses with homologous fingers suggests that the neural representations of homologous fingers are linked in some way and that the activation of one neural representation primes the other. Recall that this hypothesis was supported in the chord study just reviewed (Rabbitt, Vyas, & Fearnley, 1975), where it was found that people were faster to perform two-hand homologous finger combinations than when they were to perform two-hand non-homologous finger combinations. As will be seen in the section on typewriting, aspects of typewriting behavior also support the hypothesis that there are functional linkages between homologous fingers.

In Rabbitt and Vyas' (1970) serial choice RT study, the sequence of signals from trial to trial was random. In other studies, investigators examined performance when the train of signals was structured. This work has shown that people are adept at taking advantage of structure when it is available. When signals follow a predictable pattern, people can respond to the signals more quickly and accurately than when the signals are unpredictable (Restle, 1970). For example, it is easy to learn sequences such as 123, 234, 345, 456, . . . , but it is hard to learn random sequences such as 143, 256, 265, . . . (Restle, 1970; Simon & Kotovsky, 1972). Sequences of the former kind are well described by rules, and may be compactly represented by computer programs, such as the following program written in MATLAB:

```
for  i = 1:5
        for j = 1:3
                y(i, j) = i + (j-1);
        end
end

y
```

The output from this program is

```
y =
1  2  3
2  3  4
3  4  5
4  5  6
5  6  7
```

The high rapidity and accuracy of the rule-governed sequence suggests that the internal representation for the sequence is more than just a linear sequence of event-to-event associations. Instead, rules defining relations among the events (as well as relations among the relations) form part of the sequence's memory representation. This is not to say that linear associations are never used. They may be used when a rule-based description has not been discovered or when the sequence is very short (Keele & Summers, 1976).

When the memory representation for a sequence is rule-based, it is hierarchical. This is true because rules defining relations among the basic elements of a sequence presuppose superordinate relations between or among those elements (Jones, 1981).

If sequences can be represented hierarchically, are they executed in a way that depends on that hierarchical organization? Data suggesting they are were reported by Collard and Povel (1982). Their participants performed two different finger-tapping sequences with the right index finger (I), right middle finger (M), and right ring finger (R). One sequence was IMRRMI. The other sequence was MRRMII. Both sequences were performed over and over again as quickly as possible. Notice that the latter sequence is the same as the former sequence, just shifted over by one finger. Collard and Povel found that the times between finger presses had a characteristic profile which followed the *number* of the finger press in the sequence, not the *finger* used to make each press. The first press in the sequence had the longest latency, the second press in the sequence had the second-longest latency, and the third press in the sequence had the shortest latency.

A similar finding was reported by Rosenbaum, Kenny, and Derr (1983), who asked subjects to perform short keyboard sequences from memory. One such sequence was IiIiMmMm, where I and i denote keypresses made with the right and left index fingers, respectively, and M and m denote keypresses made with the right and left middle fingers, respectively. Subjects were instructed to perform the sequence over and over again as quickly and accurately as possible until they were told to stop (after the series was completed for the sixth time).

The profile of mean inter-response times for each response in the sequence was similar to the one reported by Collard and Povel (1982). As shown in Figure 9.5, the speed with which each response was performed depended on its serial position in the sequence. Responses 1 and 5 had the longest latencies, responses 3 and 7 had intermediate latencies, and responses 2, 4, 6, and 8 had the shortest latencies. The errors followed a similar pattern.

To account for these results, Rosenbaum, Kenny, and Derr (1983), like Collard and Povel (1982), developed a model whose main claim was that motor programs are not only structured hierarchically but also are executed in a way that depends directly on that hierarchical structure. According to the model, motor programs are structured in nested fashion and are "unpacked" during their execution. The process can be likened to accessing files in a file cabinet. To access a file, you need to open the appropriate drawer, then locate the correct folder, and then find the right sheet of paper within that folder. If the next sheet of paper that you need is in the same folder, you can access it relatively quickly, but if it is in a different folder of the same drawer, you need more time to access it, and if it is in a different folder in a different drawer, the time you need is longer still. Time is not the only dependent variable that changes with "file distance." The opportunity for making an error in accessing the proper file also increases with the number of compartments that must be accessed.

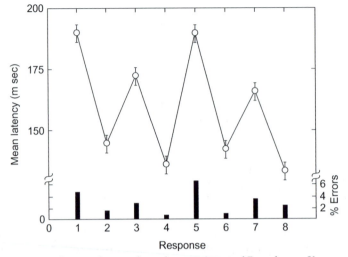

FIGURE 9.5 Inter-response times and errors from the experiment of Rosenbaum, Kenny, and Derr (1983). The times and errors associated with response 1 are restricted to productions of response 1 after response 8, in the second through sixth cycles of the sequence. From Rosenbaum, D. A., Kenny, S., & Derr, M. A. (1983). Hierarchical control of rapid movement sequences. Journal of Experimental Psychology: Human Perception and Performance, 9, 86–102. Copyright © 1983 by the American Psychological Association. Reprinted with permission.

Graphically, this process can be depicted as a *tree-traversal* process (see Figure 9.6). The picture allows you to count the number of nodes between successive responses to see whether that number predicts the delay between successive output events (retrieving a sheet of paper or pressing a key). The model provides a good account of the latency data in the experiment.

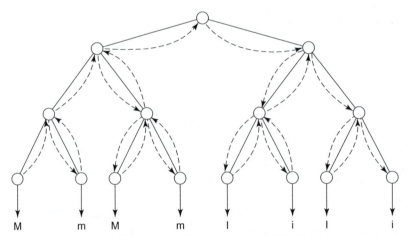

FIGURE 9.6 Tree-traversal model of Rosenbaum, Kenny, and Derr (1983). M, m, I, and i denote keypresses with the left and right middle fingers and left and right index fingers, respectively. From Rosenbaum, D. A., Kenny, S., & Derr, M. A. (1983). Hierarchical control of rapid movement sequences. Journal of Experimental Psychology: Human Perception and Performance, 9, 86–102. Copyright © 1983 by the American Psychological Association. Reprinted with permission.

Latencies increased with the number of nodes to be traversed between successive keypresses. In addition, the number of errors increased with the number of nodes to be traversed. The types of errors that were made could also be accounted for with the tree-traversal model.

This model of performance implies that the program for a sequence of keyboard responses is structured hierarchically and is also executed hierarchically. The success of the model implies that motor programs are not simply linear strings of instructions. If they were, the errors and latencies from the study described above would have been uniform or chaotic across serial positions.

Another model that can be rejected by the data we are focusing on assumes that motor programs are hierarchically organized but are executed linearly. Such a model predicts a flat latency curve, which is not what was found. It appears then, that subjects in the experiments of Rosenbaum, Kenny, and Derr (1983) and Collard and Povel (1982) relied on a tree-traversal process to produce their responses. The fact that they apparently did so suggests that the memory system responsible for storing low-level motor commands cannot hold a large number of commands at once. Instead, the memory system for motor commands has very limited storage capacity, much like the sensory buffers that hold incoming visual (Sperling, 1960) or auditory information (Darwin, Turvey, & Crowder, 1972). Despite this limited capacity, the motor system can generate movements very quickly. The way it does so, according to the tree-traversal scheme, is to traverse branches of the relevant memory tree at very rapid rates.

The picture that emerges—a limited capacity for holding motor commands coupled with a system capable of rapid unpacking of information at higher levels—is reminiscent of the picture that has emerged from studies of perceptual processing. There too it has been found that despite limited capacities for maintaining sensory information in a format that can be held for very long, there is rapid access to higher-level memory representations aroused by those sensory inputs (Potter, Kroll, & Harris, 1980). Discovering that perception and action work in this common way complements the view that common codes underlie perception and action (Hommel et al., 2001). Not only are the codes the same. The associated processes are similar as well.

Learning Keyboard Sequences

How do people learn keyboard sequences such as those described above? Researchers concerned with this question have focused on three main issues. One is how and whether hierarchical representations are formed. The second is whether the learning of keyboard sequences requires conscious awareness. The third is what information is actually remembered.

The main way these issues have been pursued has been to use serial RT tasks. In the simplest version, signals are associated with keypresses and the same S-R associations are maintained throughout learning. In addition, the series of signals and associated responses is either structured or random. It has been found that structured sequences are learned more quickly than random sequences. Moreover, for this learning to occur, participants do not have to be consciously aware of the sequence. Participants' RTs diminish though they claim they have no awareness of which stimulus-response pair will be tested after a given stimulus-response pair has been tested (Nissen & Bullemer, 1987).

In a more complex version of the task, the requirements change after some amount of training. By introducing such changes, investigators can ask what has been learned. If what has been learned is a set of associations between signals and response locations, then shifting the fingers used to press keys at those locations should have no effect on performance. Subjects should be able to respond just as quickly as when the same fingers were used at those locations. By contrast, if what has been learned is a set of associations between signals and finger movements, shifting the fingers should hurt performance.

To a first approximation, the data support the notion that what is learned are associations between signals and response locations, not associations between signals and finger movements. This outcome agrees with the results reviewed earlier concerning cognitive maps (Tolman, 1948) and S-R compatibility (Brebner, Shephard, & Cairney, 1972; Wallace, 1971).

Control of Rhythm and Timing

So far we have considered how people control the serial order of responses that are supposed to be produced as quickly as possible. Now we turn to the question, How do people control delays between successive keypresses? In a typical experiment concerned with this question, people are asked to tap a key at a rate specified by a metronome. The metronome goes off soon after the person starts tapping. A computer records the times between the taps the person produces.

Among the results that have been obtained with this procedure are two that are noteworthy for present purposes (Wing & Kristofferson, 1973). First, times between successive keypresses are negatively correlated. That is, if one inter-response interval is long, the next one tends to be short, and vice versa. The second important finding is that the variances of inter-response intervals grows with the means of the intervals. (The variance of a set of inter-response intervals is the sum of the squared differences between each inter-response interval and the arithmetic mean of the entire set, all divided by the number of intervals in the set. The arithmetic mean of a set of inter-response intervals is the sum of the intervals divided by their number.)

Wing and Kristofferson (1973) developed a model to account for these results. The model has two components (see Figure 9.7). One is a clock. The other is a motor delay between clock events and subsequent overt responses.

Wing and Kristofferson's model predicts that successive response intervals should be negatively correlated. To see why, consider what happens if the motor delay for a response happens to be longer than normal. Because that response defines the end of one interval and the start of the next, the longer-than-usual motor delay results in a shorter-than-usual subsequent interval. Similarly, if the motor delay for a response happens to be shorter than usual, the shorter-than-usual motor delay results in a longer-than-usual subsequent interval. Thus, variations in motor delays yield negatively correlated successive inter-response intervals or, as they are also called, negative lag-1 auto-correlations. The latter term refers to correlations between variables of the same type within a set (hence "auto") computed for variables that follows in immediate succession (with lag 1).

Negative lag-1 auto-correlations have been observed in tapping studies. In fact, they were reported as long ago as 1886 (see Wing, 1980), when they were attributed to the operation of a feedback correction mechanism in which the performer in effect said to him- or herself,

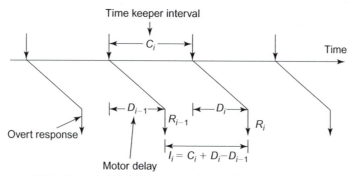

FIGURE 9.7 Wing and Kristofferson's (1973) timing model. According to the model, there is a motor delay D_{i-1} between the trigger for response $i-1$ and its execution, just as there is a motor delay D_i between the trigger for response i and its execution. The observed interval between response i and response $i + 1$ is $C + D_{i+1} - D_i$, where a timekeeper delay, C_i, is used to control the delay between the triggers for the two responses. The observed interval between the two responses is I_i.

"That last interval was longer than usual so I'll make the next interval shorter than usual," or vice versa. Wing and Kristofferson showed that such a mechanism need not be invoked. Spontaneous variation in motor delays without explicit feedback correction could give rise to negatively correlated successive inter-response intervals, all else being equal.

Wing and Kristofferson also showed in the context of their model that the variability of inter-response intervals should increase with the size of the interval produced. This prediction arises from the fact that a neural clock "pulsing" away at a variable rate will give rise to more and more variability as it pulses more and more. Figure 9.8 shows data consistent with this prediction. These data were obtained in an experiment in which subjects tried to tap a finger repeatedly and as evenly as possible at a rate specified by a metronome. As the inter-tap interval increased, the variance of the intertap interval also increased.

Perhaps the most intriguing aspect of Wing and Kristofferson's model is that it allows for the derivation of independent estimates of the variance of motor delays and the variance of clock delays. The method for doing so relies on mathematics that need not be rehearsed here; for a review, see Wing and Beek (2002). Figure 9.8 shows that the estimates of clock variance and motor delay variance behave as expected from Wing and Kristofferson's model. As the inter-response interval increases, the clock variance increases, but the motor delay variance remains approximately constant. This result is consistent with the hypothesis that motor delays and clock delays are independent.

Further support for the independence of motor delays and clock delays was obtained in a patient with Parkinson's disease, where the disease was restricted to one brain hemisphere (Wing, Keele, & Margolin, 1984). The patient in question showed increased clock variance when using the hand contralateral to the diseased hemisphere but normal clock variance when using the hand contralateral to the normal hemisphere. Neither hand showed unusual motor delay variance. Dissociating clock delay variance and motor delay variance in a neurological patient suggests that the two mechanisms are distinct, as assumed in the Wing and Kristofferson model.

One difficulty of the Wing and Kristofferson model is that analyzing data to test the model's assumptions entails buying into those assumptions. This is because the method for estimating

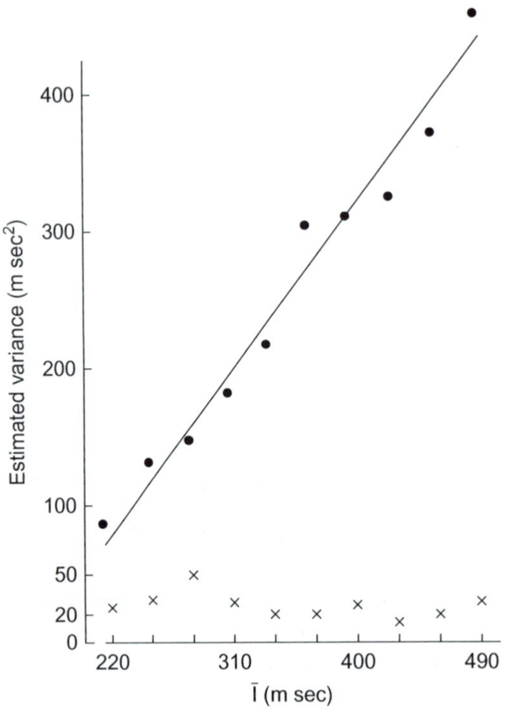

FIGURE 9.8   Estimated time keeper variance (dots) and motor delay variance (crosses) as a function of mean inter-response interval. Adapted from Wing, A. M. (1980). The long and short of timing in response sequences. In G. E. Stelmach & J. Requin (Eds.), Tutorials in motor behavior (pp. 469–486). Amsterdam: North-Holland. With permission.

clock variance and motor delay variance assumes that these two mechanisms exist and are independent. Another assumption that is required to test the model is *stationarity*, the tendency of a system's underlying parameters to remain fixed or, if they vary, to vary about fixed means rather than drifting in some consistent fashion. Contrary to the stationarity assumption, tapping rates sometimes increase or decrease, in which case statistical tools are needed to detrend the data, that is, to take out the observed drift (Collier & Ogden, 2004). Interestingly, the drift that is observed rarely persists forever. Instead, it generally "comes to rest" on or around a preferred tapping rate. When such changes in tapping rate are observed, the asymptotic rates can be ascribed to drift toward resonance, the oscillation frequency of a mechanical system with the largest ratio of oscillation amplitude to input energy (Yu, Russell, & Sternad, 2003).

Hierarchical Time Keepers

Wing and Kristofferson's (1973) model is linear. The only practical way to increase the time between responses is to add more clock pulses. A possible drawback of this system is that in rhythmic performance it might be difficult to "keep the beat." That is, because there are no higher-level units controlling groups of responses, the delay between the first note in one measure and the first note in the next measure could be just as variable as the sum

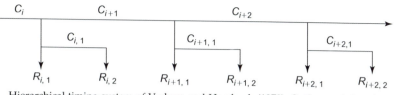

FIGURE 9.9   Hierarchical timing system of Vorberg and Hambuch (1978). C_i, C_{i+1}, and C_{i+2} denote clock delays for the ith, $i+1$th, $i+2$th . . . measure; $C_{i,1}$, $C_{i+1,1}$, and $C_{i+2,1}$ denote lower-order clock delays for the first interval within each measure; and responses are denoted with letter R's.

of the delays between the successive notes within a measure. From a musical standpoint, it would be desirable if the beat were steady even if the notes within the measures happened to speed up or slow down. Listening to a good drummer makes the point clear. The drummer's foot keeps pounding the bass drum at a relatively constant rate though his or her drumsticks may strike the other drums at rates that fluctuate depending on the difficulty of the sequence being performed or on subtle "bends" the drummer adds to the rhythm.

Pounding a bass drum while other events are occurring exemplifies a model of timing and rhythm control developed by Vorberg and Hambuch (1978, 1984) and shown in Figure 9.9. The model says that internal timers specify delays between the lead notes of each measure in parallel with the delays between notes within each measure. The key feature of the model is that it is hierarchical.

How can such a hierarchical model be tested? As mentioned above, if the start of each measure is timed relative to the trigger of the immediately preceding response, as in the Wing and Kristofferson (1973) model, the variance of the delays between successive downbeats should equal the sum of the variances of the delays between the notes lying between the downbeats. On the other hand, if the start of each measure is timed relative to the start of the preceding measure, as in Vorberg and Hambuch's (1978, 1984) model, the variance of the delay between downbeats should be smaller than the sum of the variances of the notes between the downbeats.

The prediction of the hierarchical model was tested and confirmed in a study of piano playing (Shaffer, 1984a, b). Using a specially equipped piano that allowed for electronic recording of individual keystrokes, Shaffer found, in performances of works by Bach, Beethoven, and Chopin, that the variances of delays from one bar to the next were less than the sum of the variances of the individual notes between the bars.

Vorberg and Hambuch (1984) also tested their model and found support for it in sequences with unequal intervals. Sequences with equal intervals appeared to be timed linearly: Downbeats did not confer any special reduction in timing variance. From these and related results, it appears that performers have at their disposal different methods of controlling timing depending on the complexity of the sequences being produced (Jagacinski, Marshburn, Klapp, & Jones, 1988; Rosenbaum, 2002; Summers et al., 1993; Peper, Beek, & Wieringen, 1995).

Event Timing

Another way hierarchical control of timing may be expressed is in terms of critical events for timing. Critical events are represented at a high level, whereas movements made

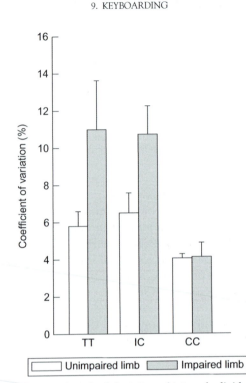

FIGURE 9.10 Coefficient of variation (standard deviation of intervals divided by corresponding mean intervals) for tapping (TT), intermittent circle drawing (IC), and continuous circle drawing (CC) in the hand controlled by the damaged cerebellum (impaired limb) and in the hand controlled by the undamaged cerebellum (unimpaired limb). Data from Spencer, R. M. C., Zelaznik, H. N., Diedrichsen, J., & Ivry, R. B. (2003). Disrupted timing of discontinuous but not continuous movements by cerebellar lesions. Science, 300, 1437–1439. With permission. Image from http://www.sciencemag.org/cgi/content/full/300/5624/1437.

between those critical events are represented at a lower level. By analogy to a travel itinerary, cities to which one travels are generally represented at a higher level than the means of getting to those cities. Arrivals at the cities are the critical events. Travels between the cities are the means to those critical ends.

Spencer, Zelaznik, Diedrichsen, and Ivry (2003) provided evidence for such a distinction in the neural control of timing. Focusing on patients with unilateral damage to the cerebellum, they showed that in such patients there is disrupted timing of discontinuous movements but not of continuous movements (Figure 9.10). When such patients tried to tap at a regular pace, their tapping times showed higher variability when performed with the hand controlled by the damaged portion of the cerebellum than when performed by the hand controlled by the undamaged portion of the cerebellum. When the same patients drew circles with pauses at the tops of the circles' paths, their drawing times also showed higher variability when drawn with the hand controlled by the damaged portion of the cerebellum than when drawn by the hand controlled by the undamaged portion of the cerebellum. Remarkably, however, when the same patients drew circles *continuously*, they showed no differences between timing variability of the two hands.

This outcome suggests that there is an important functional difference between continuous timing and discontinuous timing. The cerebellum, according to Spencer, Zelaznik, Diedrichsen, and Ivry (2003), plays a special role in the timing of critical events. By analogy to planning a trip between cities, the cerebellum seems to cares about the major events—arrivals at cities, so to speak—while other brain regions care more about the continuous motions that connect those key points.

Amodality of Timing

Because many responses must be timed with reference to external events—hitting an approaching baseball, playing a note in time with a conductor's downbeat, reaching out and shaking another person's hand—it is plausible that the mechanisms used for timing movements are also used for timing perceptual events. Several lines of evidence suggest that this is the case.

The late Steven Keele and his colleagues (Keele, 1987; Keele & Ivry, 1987; Keele, Pokorny, Corcos, & Ivry, 1985) asked people to make regular tapping responses with the finger or foot. Over subjects, the variance of inter-response intervals correlated significantly between the finger and foot. Thus, a person with low variability in finger tapping was also likely to have low variability in foot tapping. The individuals in this study also varied in their ability to judge brief intervals between auditory events. Most importantly, individuals who were good at perceptual timing were also good at motor timing. The correlation between tapping and perceptual judgment was about the same as the correlation between tapping with the finger and tapping with the foot, just as one would expect if one thought that timing is controlled with a mechanism that is amodal (i.e., not specifically tied to a particular modality).

In evaluating this result, it is important to consider a possible artifact. It may be that some people are simply more conscientious than others, or have less "neural noise" than others. If this were the case, one would expect people who are good at timing to be good at controlling muscle forces, another task that probably benefits from care or steadiness. Keele, Ivry, and Pokorny (1987) found, however, that accuracy of controlling muscle forces was not correlated with precision of timing control, though the force control achieved with the finger was correlated with the force control achieved with the forearm or foot. From the fact that force accuracy was not correlated with timing accuracy, it appears that the significant correlations between motor timing and perceptual timing observed by Keele, Pokorny, Corcos, and Ivry (1985) were not artifacts. Instead, timing and force may be governed independently, perhaps by different parts of the brain (Keele & Ivry, 1987). Recall that independent control of force and timing was postulated for eye movements in Chapter 6.

A second line of evidence for the hypothesis that timing is not tied to a particular modality, and so is amodal, is that people have equal difficulty controlling rhythmic responses with one hand while performing an opposing rhythm with the other hand or while perceptually monitoring an opposing external rhythm. Recall from Chapters 1 and 6 that people find it difficult to perform cyclical movements with one hand without influence from the other hand. Tapping 3 against 4 is very difficult, for example (Peters, 1977). Likewise, it is difficult to tap one rhythm and orally produce another incompatible rhythm (Klapp, 1979). Finally, tapping one rhythmic sequence while listening to a sequence of tones with another rhythmic structure leads to disruptions in ongoing performance (Klapp, Hill, Tyler, Martin, Jagacinski, & Jones,

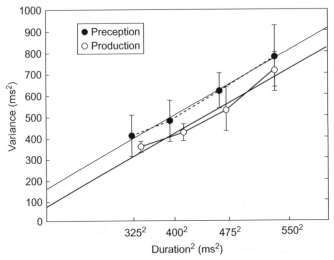

FIGURE 9.11   Estimated duration variance as a function of mean duration squared in perception and production. From Ivry, R. B. & Hazeltine, R. E. (1995). Perception and production of temporal intervals across a range of durations: Evidence for a common timing mechanism. Journal of Experimental Psychology: Human Perception and Performance, 21, 3–18. With permission.

1985). The fact that rhythmic interference extends across output modalities (manual and oral) and between hearing and tapping suggests that the locus of the interference is not tied to a single input channel or output channel. The same suggestion can be made on the basis of the fact that difficulties in generating polyrhythms are of roughly equal magnitude if one generates the polyrhythm with fingers of two hands or fingers of one hand (Semjen & Ivry, 2001).

A third source of evidence for the amodality of timing came from a study by Ivry and Hazeltine (1995). These investigators had participants produce or judge time intervals. When the authors plotted the standard deviation of the produced intervals against the means of the intervals (Figure 9.11), the slope of the best-fitting straight line was very similar to the slope of the best-fitting straight line obtained by plotting the standard deviation of estimated time intervals, based on perceptual judgments, as a function of interval means. This outcome led Ivry and Hazeltine to conclude that timing is amodal. According to these authors, there is no need to posit a timing system for production separate and apart from a timing system for perception. The same conclusion was reached in an earlier study using other methods (Rosenbaum & Patashnik, 1980), where it was found that the time to prepare for the production of a time interval is similar to the time to prepare for the perception of that same time interval.

Integration of Serial Order and Timing

So far, we have considered the timing and serial ordering of keystrokes as if they were two separate control problems. In practice they are not. If the timing of responses is specified, their serial order is determined (Rosenbaum, 1985). Said another way, once you know that the time between event A and event B is +5s, then you know that A precedes B, provided the sign has been defined that way. Thus, once the timing of two events is specified, their serial order is also known. This fact suggests that serial order and timing may not require separate control mechanisms. The studies described next support the hypothesis that they do not.

A representative study was conducted by Summers (1975). He trained subjects to press nine keys in a specific order and with a specific timing pattern indicated by flashing lights. The durations of the lights indicated the durations to be produced. For one group of subjects, the first light stayed on for 500 ms, the second light stayed on for 500 ms, the third light stayed on for 100 ms, and then this same "500-500-100" pattern was repeated two more times. For another group of subjects, the first light stayed on for 500 ms, the second light stayed on for 100 ms (rather than 500 ms), the third light stayed on for 100 ms, and then this cycle was repeated twice more. The important feature of the experiment was that only the rhythms differed in the two conditions. The fingers making the responses and the locations where the responses were made were the same.

After performing the same sequence for nearly 500 trials over two sessions, the subjects in both groups were asked to perform the original sequence as quickly as possible but without regard to the original timing pattern. The subjects succeeded at producing the sequences at a higher rate than before, but they could not escape the original rhythm. This finding suggests that the timing of each finger sequence became an integral part of the memory representation for the sequence. With additional practice, the original timing pattern disappeared (Keele & Summers, 1976).

Adjusting the Rate of Production for Entire Sequences

If the timing of a sequence of keyboard responses becomes integrally related to the serial order of the sequence, then finding such an integral relationship suggests that the timing of the sequence was learned along with its serial order. Pursuing this line of thinking, Terzuolo and Viviani (1980) provided one of the most intriguing and, as it turns out, controversial findings in human motor control. Terzuolo and Viviani explored the possibility that adjustments in the overall rate of production for a response sequence may be achieved by modulating the rate at which a clock triggers all the responses within the sequence. Suppose you have learned to produce a sequence of four button presses so the delay between the first response and second is 500 ms, the delay between the second response and third is 250 ms, and the delay between the third response and fourth is 100 ms. An efficient way to slow the entire sequence is to slow a clock that triggers all the responses. For example, to slow the sequence by 20%, you could change the value of a multiplicative rate parameter, r, from 1 to 1.2. Thus if the timing of the sequence was represented (symbolically) as $r(500, 250, 100)$, changing r from 1 to 1.2 would cause the inter-response intervals to take on the values 600, 300, and 120 ms. Alternatively, if r were changed from 1 to 1.5 to produce a 50% slowdown, the inter-response intervals would be 750, 375, and 150 ms. Plotting the inter-response intervals for $r = 1.0, 1.2$, and 1.5, the resulting pattern would be a fan (see Figure 9.12A). Another way to plot the data would be to turn the data sideways, placing the successive responses of a sequence produced at a particular rate on a time line (see Figure 9.12B). The result would be a fan oriented vertically rather than horizontally.

Terzuolo and Viviani (1980) presented typewriting data that supported the hypothesis that timing can be controlled with a multiplicative rate parameter (Figure 9.13). The data

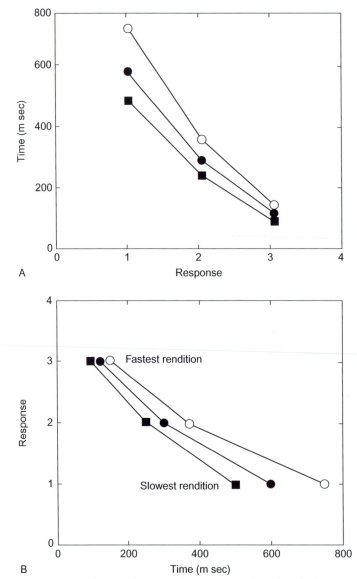

FIGURE 9.12 (A) Inter-response time as a function of response number when the basic time sequence has been scaled by a multiplicative rate parameter, r, with three different values: $r = 1.50$ (empty circles); $r = 1.20$ (filled circles); $r = 1.00$ (filled squares). (B) Same data turned sideways.

came from different renditions of the word "enclosed," produced at different speeds by one typist. As seen in Figure 9.13, the vertical fan effect was apparent, and straight lines could be fit to the individual keystrokes, as predicted by the multiplicative rate model. Viviani and Terzuolo obtained similar results for handwriting (see Chapter 8), which they took to suggest that this method of controlling response rates is general.

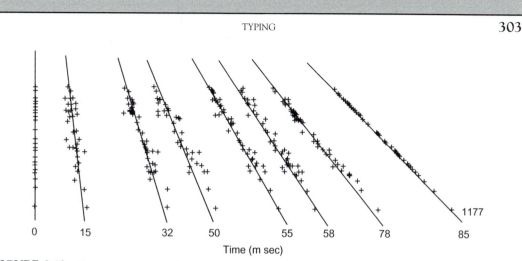

FIGURE 9.13 Fan representation of the word "enclosed." From Viviani, P., & Terzuolo, C. (1980). Space-time invariance in learned motor skills. In G. E. Stelmach & J. Requin (Eds.), Tutorials in motor behavior (pp. 525–533). Amsterdam: North-Holland. With permission.

Terzuolo and Viviani's (1980) model is compelling and their graph is visually striking. However, in a detailed review of the literature on the multiplicative rate hypothesis, Gentner (1987) came to the conclusion that the evidence favoring the hypothesis is tenuous. Gentner proposed a more stringent test of the multiplicative rate hypothesis than the one developed by Terzuolo and Viviani. Gentner reasoned that if the hypothesis is correct, then when a word is typed at different rates, the time to type any given letter in the word after the immediately preceding letter should be a constant proportion of the word's total duration. To understand this prediction, consider the hypothetical response sequence described earlier in this section. Recall that the sequence had inter-response times of 500, 250, and 100 ms at the fastest speed, inter-response times of 600, 300, and 120 ms at the intermediate speed, and inter-response times of 750, 375, and 150 ms at the slowest speed. The total durations for these renditions were therefore 850 ms, 1020 ms, and 1275 ms. If we consider any of the responses in the sequence—say the last response—its latency is a constant proportion of the total sequence duration: $100/850 = 120/1020 = 150/1275 = 0.1176$. Constancy of this kind is therefore diagnostic of multiplicative rate modulation.

When Gentner (1987) tested this prediction, he found it to be wanting, so he concluded that the multiplicative rate hypothesis is incorrect. A question remaining from Gentner's analysis is whether his statistical test was too stringent. A difficulty with his test is that it is valid only if one assumes that all responses have the same motor delay (Heuer, 1988). Relaxing this assumption makes the multiplicative rate hypothesis more credible.

TYPING

Let us now consider typing in more detail, having just mentioned one of the studies that used it. First, we will consider some of the historical issues surrounding typing research. Then we will discuss typing errors and what they reveal about the units of typing control.

Next, we will focus on keystroke timing. The final part of this section will review an influential theory of typing control developed by Rumelhart and Norman (1982).

Historical Issues

Keyboards are so common today that it is hard to imagine that society ever functioned without them. In fact, the typewriter as we know it did not come into wide use until the 1800's. The first practical typewriter was developed in Milwaukee in the mid-1800's and was manufactured by a company that then specialized in gun making, E. Remington and Sons. Typewriters soon were used by professional authors. The first complete typewritten manuscript was *Tom Sawyer*, by Mark Twain (Cooper, 1983).

The most common arrangement of keys on the keyboard was developed by the entrepreneur who promoted the typewriter in the United States, Christopher Sholes. His *Qwerty* keyboard was named after the positions of the top left keys (see Figure 9.14A). Rumor has it that Sholes chose the Qwerty arrangement to make it hard to use. By placing common letter pairs far apart, Sholes allegedly attempted to discourage typists from jamming the keys by

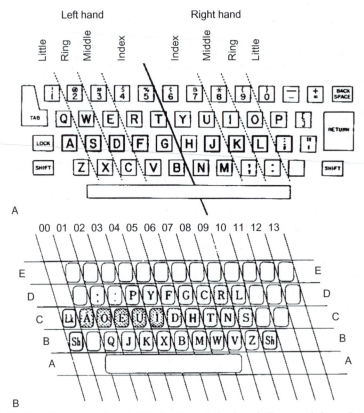

FIGURE 9.14 (A) The Qwerty keyboard. (B) The Dvorak keyboard. Reprinted from Cooper, W. E. (1983). Introduction. In W. E. Cooper (Ed.), Cognitive aspects of skilled typewriting (pp. 1–38). New York: Springer-Verlag. With permission.

typing too quickly. The story is most likely false because large spaces between keys do not slow performance. Furthermore, the Qwerty arrangement was made possible before widespread adoption of rapid touch typing (Gentner & Norman, 1984).

Other keyboard designs have since been developed, and some of them permit higher typing speeds than the Qwerty. The best known example is the Dvorak keyboard (Figure 9.14B), designed at the University of Washington in the 1930's. The switch to Dvorak was hampered by economic considerations. It was difficult to induce already skilled typists to relearn old typing habits, and it was hard to pry typewriter companies from their established manufacturing designs, though in the long run their profit margins might have improved if they had done so (David, 1985).

Whether typing is faster with ten fingers or two, as in the "hunt-and-peck" method, was hotly debated in the early years of the typewriter. Resolution of the debate came in a highly publicized speed-typing contest held in Cincinnati in 1888 between two men claiming to be the world's fastest typist. The winner typed with ten fingers and memorized the layout of the keyboard beforehand, enabling him to keep his eyes on the page he was copying. In the wake of his victory, touch typing came to be accepted as the preferred method for office personnel.

One of the first questions asked in the scientific study of typewriting performance was where the eyes are in relation to the hand. What characters do typists look at while typing? There has been remarkably little research on this topic, and most of it was done in the 1930's and 40's (Butsch, 1932; Fuller, 1943). This work indicated that the eye typically leads the hand by about four to eight letters—a lag commonly referred to as the *eye-hand span*. The eye-hand span is considerably shorter than the eye-voice span—the lag between where one looks and what one reads aloud. The eye-voice span is about 12 to 24 characters.

Delays between successive visual fixations are longer in typing than in reading, and locations of fixations appear less related to word boundaries when one types than when one reads (Cooper, 1983). Butsch (1932) summarized the role of eye movements in typing by saying that the typist "reads only rapidly enough to supply the copy to the hand as it is needed" (p. 113). As would be expected from this claim, typists often report that they have little or no comprehension of what they type, at least in copy typing situations. Highly proficient typists can engage in conversations while typing, and they suffer little or no reduction in typing speed or accuracy (Shaffer, 1975).

What one transcribes has effects on the speed with which one types. Transcribing words arranged in a haphazard order does not slow performance compared to transcribing words that are ordered normally. Nonwords are typed significantly more slowly than words, however (Fendrick, 1937).

One way the importance of words over nonwords has been demonstrated is to vary the amount of preview that typists have of the material they copy. As seen in Figure 9.15, normal prose can be typed at its maximum rate when eight or more characters are visible in advance. The maximum rate for prose is approximately the same as the rate attained with fully previewed, random word streams. By contrast, random letter strings, like random words, benefit from preview, but random letter strings do not benefit as much from preview as do random words. Even when eight characters of a nonword can be seen in advance, the mean typing rate is slower than when the eight characters form a word (Shaffer, 1973).

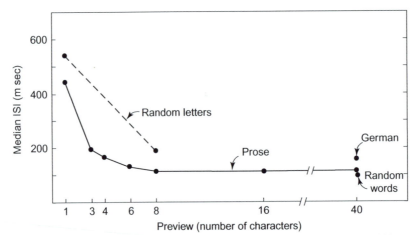

FIGURE 9.15   Median interstroke interval (ISI) when a variable number of characters could be previewed and where different kinds of material were to be typed. From Shaffer Shaffer, L. H. (1973). Latency mechanisms in transcription. In S. Kornblum (Ed.), Attention and performance IV. New York: Academic Press. With permission.

These effects of preview accord with Butsch's hypothesis that there is a "supply line" between the eye and the hand. In terms of information-processing models of performance, the results shown in Figure 9.15 suggest that perceptual information is held in a buffer until it can be accessed or decoded by a system that ultimately produces keystrokes (Cooper, 1983; Logan, 1983). Another implication of the preview results is that typists produce keystrokes in units no longer than a word. If the units were longer than a word, word order would be expected to have an effect on typing speed.

Units of Typing Control

Because words are typed more quickly than nonwords, words have special status as production units for typing. It does not follow, however, that words are the smallest units for typing. Because words are made of letter strings, it is possible that letters, or transitions between letters, might be even more basic production elements, that is, elements that are explicitly or individually controlled by the motor system. One source of evidence that there are production elements smaller than the word is that typists can stop typing upon hearing a tone equally well if they are within a word or between words (Logan, 1982). If words were the most basic production elements, it would impossible to stop them in midstream.

Typists also stop within words when they spontaneously detect errors. Long (1976) asked typists to stop and correct errors as soon as they detected any errors. In the vast majority of cases, typing ceased as soon as an error was committed. Similarly, Rabbitt (1978) asked typists to stop typing without bothering to correct the mistake afterward as soon as they detected a mistake. They succeeded in stopping on 95% of the occasions when an error was made.

Some errors appear to be detected even before they are made. Incorrect keystrokes are made less forcefully than correct keystrokes (Rabbitt, 1978), and incorrect keystrokes have longer latencies than correct keystrokes (Shaffer, 1975). Because incorrect keystrokes are produced differently from correct keystrokes, information about the accuracy of the keystrokes is available before the errors are made.

Typing Errors

What is known about the nature of the errors made during typing? Lessenberry (1928) compiled 60,000 typing errors and counted the number of times that a given letter was typed when that or another letter was apparently intended. Lessenberry found that the majority of errors consisted of hitting the key that was horizontally adjacent to the intended letter (for example, typing miatake instead of mistake), the next most frequent error was hitting the key vertically adjacent to the key that should have been struck (for example, typing mixtake instead of mistake), and the third most common mistake was substituting the finger of one hand for the like-named finger of the other hand—so-called homologous finger substitutions (for example, typing d instead of k with the middle finger).

Lessenberry (1928) suggested that hitting keys horizontally or vertically adjacent to the correct key was due to misaiming: The correct finger simply went too far to the left, too far to the right, too high, or too low. Subsequent film analyses revealed that this explanation was off target. Grudin (1983) found that when the wrong key was typed, it was almost always struck by the correct finger. Thus, in an error such as miatake, the a was typed with the little finger, not with the ring finger. Thus, the error was not one of misdirecting the correctly chosen finger, as Lessenberry (1928) supposed, but instead consisted of selecting the incorrect key but using the correct finger for that key. This observation suggests that keys and fingers are identified separately. Keys may be identified on the basis of their remembered spatial locations, but the fingers associated with those locations are apparently selected separately, in a distinct stage of processing, presumably after the key's location has been picked.

Homologous finger substitutions, which are the third most common error recorded by Lessenberry (1928), add further weight to the hypothesis that fingers are explicitly identified during keystroke selection. The substitution of one finger for its twin suggests that decisions are made to use a particular type of finger but incorrect decisions may be made about the hand to which the finger belongs. For example, in substituting k for d, which are both struck with the middle finger, the decision to use the middle finger is apparently dissociated from the decision to use the left hand or right.

Error analyses suggest that there is yet another "low-level" keystroke feature that may play a role in typewriting control. Grudin (1983) and Munhall and Ostry (1983) observed that b and n are sometimes substituted for one another, but b and u rarely are. b and n both have down and "inward" movement components (when the hands are brought in from the home row of the keyboard), but b and u are achieved with movements of opposite direction. If movement direction were not specified explicitly, one would not expect b-n confusions to be more prevalent than b-u confusions.

Timing of Keystrokes in Typewriting

As stated at the beginning of this chapter, skilled typists can type at impressive speeds, and as mentioned in the last section, typing speeds are higher for words than for nonwords.

In general, the higher the frequency of a word, the more quickly it can be typed (Fendrick, 1937; Gentner, Larochelle, & Grudin, 1988; Shaffer, 1973; West & Sabban, 1982). The frequency with which one letter follows another within a word—its digraph frequency—also affects typing speed. The higher the digraph frequency, the shorter the time between the first letter and second (Gentner, Larochelle, & Grudin, 1989; Terzuolo & Viviani, 1980).

Times between keystrokes also depend on the relation between the finger and hand making the keystrokes. Transitions between keystrokes made by different hands are faster than transitions between keystrokes made by different fingers of the same hand, and transitions between different fingers of the same hand are faster than transitions between repeated keystrokes made by the same finger (Coover, 1923). The basis for this effect is mechanical. Films of typists' hands show that the hands and fingers move continually, not waiting for previous keystrokes to be completed (see Figures 9.16 and 9.17). Each finger moves toward its target, subject only to mechanical interference by previous keystrokes (Gentner, Grudin, & Conway, 1980; Larochelle, 1983; Olsen & Murray, 1976). This outcome helps explain why the text-messaging speed of 3.7 keystrokes per second, mentioned at the start of this chapter, is impressive but does not hold a candle to the speeds of even less-than-world-record typing.

Can other keystroke timing effects also be explained mechanically? For example, are word frequency and digraph frequency effects due to mechanical factors? The alternative hypothesis is that these effects derive from central limitations, such as the speed with which typists can access lexical memory, the part of memory where word representations are functionally housed.

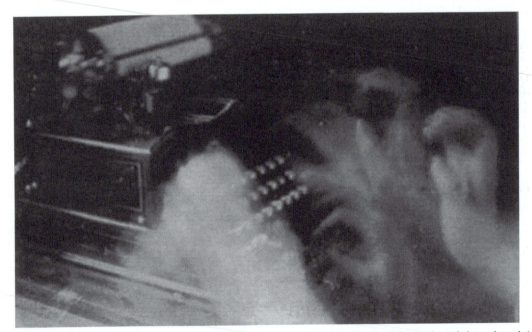

FIGURE 9.16　Touch typing as recorded through stroboscopic photography. From http://people.brunel.ac.uk/bst/3no2/Papers/Steve%20Dixon.htm.

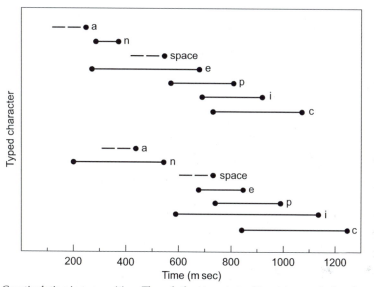

FIGURE 9.17 Coarticulation in typewriting. Though the i in epic is ultimately typed after the e and p, it is initiated before either letter. Similarly, the first time epic is typed, the e is initiated before the n in the preceding word (an). The data were obtained from film records. From Gentner, D. R., Grudin, J., & Conway, E. (1980). Finger movements in transcription typing. La Jolla, CA: University of California, San Diego, Center for Human Information Processing, (Technical Report 8001). With permission.

One approach to this problem has been to study keystroke timing when subjects become highly prepared to produce brief bursts of keystrokes. As one author put it, ". . . the inability to take advantage of a preparation interval seems to indicate that the programming of typing movements is intimately linked to their execution" (Ostry, 1983, p. 225). By this line of reasoning, if mechanical factors account for the fact that cross-hand transitions are faster than within-hand transitions, then even when typists can prepare keystrokes in advance, the cross-hand benefit should be seen.

A study by Sternberg, Monsell, Knoll, and Wright (1978) confirmed this prediction. These investigators asked skilled typists to produce letter strings from memory following the appearance of a reaction signal. On each trial, a letter string appeared and then a series of warning tones sounded to enable subjects to become highly prepared to respond. On 85% of the trials, the reaction signal was presented at the end of the series of warning tones and the subject was supposed to produce the sequence as quickly as possible. On the remaining 15% of the trials, no reaction signal was presented and the subject was supposed to withhold the response. These catch trials were included to discourage subjects from anticipating.

As seen in Figure 9.18A, the time for the first keypress increased with the number of keystrokes to be typed. The rate of increase for the latency function was higher for keystroke sequences requiring strict hand alternation than for keystroke sequences requiring only one hand. Meanwhile, sequence durations (Figure 9.18B) increased with sequence length, as one would expect, but more interestingly, the rate of production (the time per keystroke) *decreased* as sequence length increased, as seen in the greater steepness of the function as the number

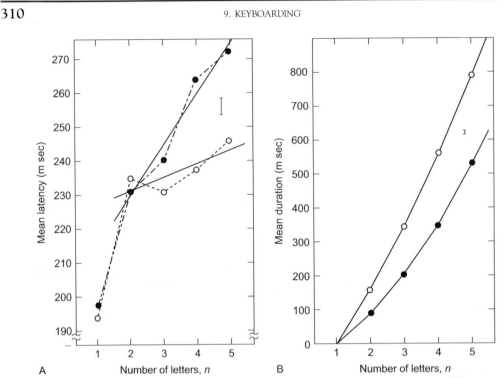

FIGURE 9.18   (A) Mean latency to produce the first keystroke in a sequence of n keystrokes following a reaction signal. Linear functions fitted to the data for $n \geq 2$. (B) Mean durations of complete sequences. Sequences completed with alternating hands are shown with filled dots. Sequences completed with one hand are shown with empty dots. From Sternberg, S., Monsell, S., Knoll, R. L., & Wright, C. E. (1978). The latency and duration of rapid movement sequences: Comparisons of speech and typewriting. In G. E. Stelmach (Ed.), Information processing in motor control and learning (pp. 117–152). New York: Academic Press. With permission.

of letters, n, increased. Meanwhile, keystroke rates were again higher for two-hand sequences than for one-hand sequences. A final result, not shown in Figure 9.18, is that keystroke times for words were indistinguishable from keystroke times for random letter strings.

Consider these data in light of the criteria given earlier for mechanical sources of performance effects. First, the difference between within-hand and between-hand timing was apparently due to motor execution, since this difference was obtained even under a state of high preparation. At the very least, the data do not force rejection of the mechanical account. Second, the difference between words and nonwords was apparently not due to execution, since this difference vanished when subjects could become highly prepared to type one letter string at a time.

Gentner, Larochelle, and Grudin (1989) offered additional criteria for distinguishing between mechanical and central sources of timing effects in typewriting. They focused on digraph and word frequency effects, seeking to determine why high-frequency words are typed more quickly than low-frequency words, and why high-frequency digraphs are typed more quickly than low-frequency digraphs.

First, it is possible to reject the hypothesis that high-frequency words are simply faster than low-frequency words because they are made up of high-frequency digraphs. The correlation between the frequencies of words and the frequencies of their constituent digraphs is surprisingly modest (Gentner, Larochelle, & Grudin, 1989).

Gentner, Larochelle, and Grudin (1989) reasoned that if the source of the digraph frequency effect is central rather than peripheral, then if a digraph is frequent in one language but infrequent in another, the speed of typing the digraph should be different in the two languages. On the other hand, if the source of the digraph frequency effect is peripheral rather than central, then, since the mechanics of the hands are the same for speakers of the two languages, the speed of typing the digraph should be the same for both groups.

Using Dutch and American typists, Gentner et al. (1989) obtained evidence for a mechanical basis of the digraph frequency effect. They found that the difficulty of producing digraphs did not depend on the frequency of the digraphs within the two languages. The difficulty of producing whole words did, however, depend on the words' frequency within the typist's language. Based on these results, Gentner et al. concluded that digraph frequency effects are peripherally, or mechanically, based whereas word frequency effects are centrally based. Recall that the same conclusion about word frequency effects was reached in connection with the findings of Sternberg et al. (1978), who found that word frequency effects disappeared under conditions of maximal single-word preparation.

Gentner et al. (1989) offered another reason why word and digraph frequency effects have different origins. As seen in Figure 9.19, these authors found that words that were initially typed slowly were typed more and more quickly as the words were repeated. By contrast, digraphs that were typed slowly at first continued to be typed slowly no matter how often they were repeated. The fact that digraphs did not improve with practice suggests that the factor limiting their performance was in the periphery, where practice presumably has little short-term effect on performance speed.

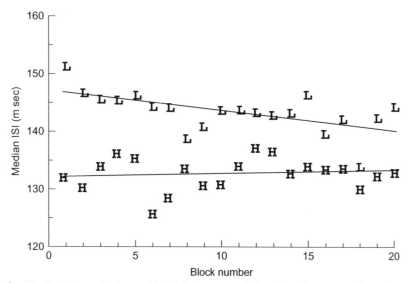

FIGURE 9.19 Median interstroke interval for high-frequency (H) and low-frequency (L) words as a function of practice. From Gentner, D. R., Larochelle, S., & Grudin, J. (1988). Lexical, sublexical, and peripheral effects in skilled typewriting. Cognitive Psychology, 20, 524–548. With permission.

Rumelhart and Norman's Model of Typewriting

The foregoing discussion has shown that there are a number of robust phenomena in typewriting research. It would be gratifying if all of the phenomena could be accounted for with one unified theory. The most comprehensive theory that has been developed was proposed by Rumelhart and Norman (1982). The theory deserves careful attention not only because of its usefulness for the analysis of typewriting but also because of its historical importance for cognitive science at large. Rumelhart and Norman's model was a precursor of connectionist models of memory and performance (Rumelhart and McClelland, 1986). A connectionist model consists of units, often represented as points or "nodes," joined by links. Information is stored in the network by virtue of the connections among its units. In general, the only kind of activity in a connectionist network is activation or inhibition.

In Rumelhart and Norman's (1982) typing model (see Figure 9.20) distinct nodes exist for each key of the keyboard. Each node is the site for associating a particular finger with a particular key. Thus, the node for the letter "v" associates the left index finger with the "v" key. When a decision is made to type a word such as very, the v, e, r, and y nodes are activated, along with the connections among them. The connections define the serial order of the letters. The v node inhibits the nodes for e, r, and y; the node for e inhibits the nodes for r and y; and the node for r inhibits the node for y. When a node is activated, its keystroke is initiated, but once the keystroke has been initiated, its own node is inhibited. At first, the only node that is uninhibited is v, so the v keystroke can be initiated. A short time

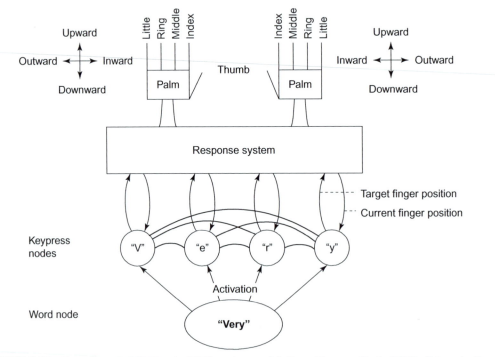

FIGURE 9.20   Rumelhart and Norman's (1982) typing model. From Norman, D. A. (1981). Categorization of action slips. Psychological Review, 88, 1–15. With permission.

later, the v node is inhibited and so it stops inhibiting the other nodes. As a result, one node is now uninhibited—the one for e—and so the e keystroke begins. Shortly thereafter, the e node is inhibited, so it stops inhibiting the nodes for r and y. Consequently, the r node is released from inhibition, so it is initiated, and finally its self-inhibition allows the y keystroke to begin. This method of controlling serial order is, in essence, the one proposed by Estes (1972) as discussed in Chapter 4; see Figure 4.4.

In Rumelhart and Norman's (1982) model, nodes are self-inhibited as soon as their corresponding keystrokes are initiated, but they can also be self-inhibited before their corresponding keystrokes are completed. Because the self-inhibition of a node can occur while its keystroke is still in progress, subsequent keystrokes can begin while preceding keystrokes are under way. This provides a way of explaining the simultaneous activity of hands and fingers during typewriting.

Another important feature of Rumelhart and Norman's (1982) model is that many of the timing relations between keystrokes arise entirely from the mechanical coupling of the hands and fingers; they are not explicitly controlled by the network. If a keystroke is initiated while another keystroke is under way, its trajectory is influenced by the earlier stroke. Specifically, each keystroke proceeds more and more directly to its target the less it is mechanically coupled to the hand or finger still performing an earlier keystroke. If the keystroke being performed uses the identical finger to the keystroke before it, it undergoes a significant detour; if it uses a different finger of the same hand, it undergoes less of a detour; and if it uses the other hand, it undergoes even less of a detour. Thus, the model relies on mechanical interactions to account for the within-hand and between-hand timing effects observed in typewriting. Note that this reliance on physical properties of the system being modeled is what we have seen in other domains of human motor control, such as the analysis of walking, where important advances have been made by relying on preflexes as well as reflexes (see Chapter 5).

Another important feature of Rumelhart and Norman's (1982) model is that it deliberately lacks a mechanism for timing, though it does have a mechanism for serial ordering (the inhibitory connections from early response nodes to late response nodes). At first blush, the absence of a timing mechanism is appealing, for generally one wants to have the most parsimonious model possible. Nevertheless, it may be that a timing mechanism is necessary. For example, Grudin (cited in Gentner & Norman, 1984) observed that transposition errors preserve the timing of correct keystroke orders. When typists typed thme instead of them, for example, the m was typed at the time that e usually occurs. A priori, one might expect e and m to be typed in the wrong order because the initiation of m happened to come a bit too early relative to the initiation of e. If that were the case, m and e would often be typed almost simultaneously, though by chance there would be a few instances in which m happened to come first. Grudin observed instead that the delays between m and e were usually as long as the delays between e and m. This surprising phenomenon suggests that timing may be independently represented in the plan for keystrokes, contrary to what Rumelhart and Norman (1982) assumed.

Another timing-related problem with Rumelhart and Norman's model is that it appears to make some wrong predictions about variations in overall typing rate. The only way to vary typing rates within the model is to change inhibition levels among letter nodes. When this is done, however, the simulated timing changes do not agree with those observed in real typists (Gentner, 1987, p. 272). Whether this difficulty can be repaired without an explicit timing mechanism remains to be seen.

Yet another assumption in Rumelhart and Norman's model accounts for some obtained results but not others. Rumelhart and Norman allowed for nodes called type nodes but not nodes called token nodes. (These two terms are used in domains that have nothing to do with typewriting.) A type node is a unit for any of a set of particular instances, any one of which would be represented by a token node. Rumelhart and Norman allowed type nodes (for example, the o type) but not token nodes (for example, o1 and o2). Thus, these authors assumed that there could be only one node per key. To account for the fact that some words use the same letter twice in a row, Rumelhart and Norman assumed that there must be a "doubling operator." Consistent with that assumption, they found that typists often double the wrong letter of a word with a repeated letter (for example, llok instead of look). The price paid for the exclusion of tokens, however, was that sequences with repeating, displaced elements had to be broken into two subsequences. For example, ABCA had to be broken into two subsequences, one containing the first A and the other containing the second A. A prediction arising from this state of affairs is that the typing of the first segment would be unaffected by characteristics of the second segment, and vice versa, since the two segments were assumed to be separate. Yet coarticulation effects are widespread in typing and extend across subsequences containing the same letter (Shaffer, 1975a). Hence, this feature of Rumelhart and Norman's model needs to be revised. So too may the fact that, in its current form, the model does not acknowledge a lexical level of representation. Thus, it fails to predict that words should be typed more quickly than nonwords. The model also lacks a level of representation below the keystroke, and so it does not predict homologous substitutions, homologous direction errors, and finger misidentification errors (reviewed above).

In spite of these shortcomings, Rumelhart and Norman's model is the most comprehensive and detailed model of typewriting currently available. It represents an important advance in the modeling of human motor control. The author's intent in leveling criticisms against the model is to inspire others to improve upon it.

PIANO PLAYING

In typing, one's job is to produce printed output as quickly and accurately as possible. The timing of one's keystrokes and the forces one applies to the keys are not usually available for public scrutiny. In piano playing and other forms of musical keyboard performance, however, the times and forces of one's keystrokes must be controlled to shape the rhythm, phrasing, and expressiveness of the piece being played. How are these aspects of keyboarding controlled?

A study by Sloboda (1983) provides useful information on this issue. He showed pianists two scores. The notes in the two scores were the same but the positions of the notes with respect to the bar lines were different. Consequently, only the phrasing differed (see Figure 9.21). The pianists were asked to play the pieces for a listener. Because the notes were the same, any differences in phrasing had to be communicated through the timing or forces of the pianist's keystrokes. To study these features of performance, Sloboda used a piano—the

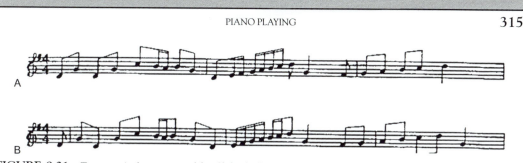

FIGURE 9.21 Two musical scores used by Sloboda (1983). The notes are the same, but their positions in the measures differ. From Sloboda, J. A. (1983). The communication of musical metre in piano performance. Quarterly Journal of Experimental Psychology, 35A, 377–396. With permission.

same one used by Shaffer (1984a, b)—fitted with optical sensors. Two sensors were dedicated to each hammer. One detected movement of the hammer near its resting position, making it possible to record when the hammer left the home position and returned to it. The other sensor detected movement of the hammer near the string, making it possible to record when the hammer approached the string and returned from it. The time between departure from the resting position and striking of the string was used to estimate how hard the hammer struck the string, and therefore how loud the note was. Loudness was assumed to be inversely related to the hammer's travel time.

Figure 9.22 (top panel) shows the loudness profile for the 18 notes in the two sequences. Although the profiles were produced by the same pianist, they differed systematically. The peaks of the loudness functions were displaced by one note, as were the bars for the two scores. The times between the notes, however, were nearly identical (see Figure 9.22, bottom panel).

Several implications can be drawn from these results. First, pianists can communicate musical meter by modulating keystrokes forces. Second, changes in the forces of keystrokes can be achieved without observable timing changes. Pianists can independently vary keystroke times and forces, allowing for a wider range of expression than if force and time were dependent. This result is reminiscent of the finding, reviewed earlier in this chapter, that force control and timing control are only weakly correlated (Keele, Ivry, & Pokorny, 1987). Third, when distinct timing profiles are observed for rapid series of keystrokes, they need not be attributed to force modulation alone. This makes it safe to attribute timing variations to the manifestation of internal control processes.

The fourth implication of Sloboda's (1983) timing data stems from the fact that his data show a remarkable periodicity, stretching over an eight-note span (see Figure 9.22, bottom panel). Similar patterns were observed by Shaffer (1984b), who found that the timing of keystrokes for a Chopin etude had a period of four bars, with peaks in the interstroke function apparent at the start of each four-bar section (corresponding to the major phrases of the piece). Patterns like these are similar to the ones reported by Povel and Collard (1982) and by Rosenbaum, Kenny, and Derr (1983), discussed earlier in this chapter (see Figure 9.5). As in the latter studies, the regular pattern of peaks and troughs in piano keystroke timing can be taken to reflect hierarchical control of successive keystrokes and groups of keystrokes (Shaffer, 1984b).

One last comment about piano music concerns the opportunity it affords for the study of free timing changes (rubatos). In Chopin's music, for example, the expressiveness of the piece depends on the pianist's judicious departure from a strict tempo. The rhythm must

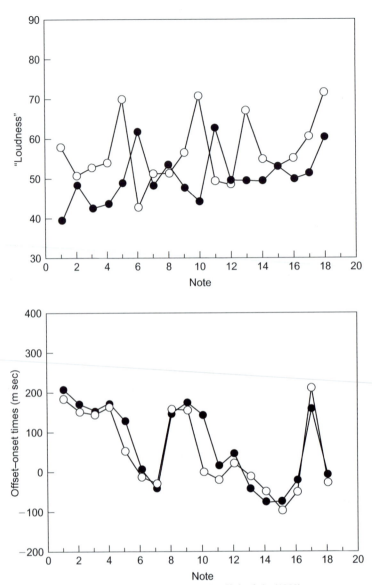

FIGURE 9.22 Top: "Loudness" values for the 18 notes in Sloboda's (1983) two sequences. Loudness was defined as the reciprocal of the time between when the hammer departed from its resting position and when it struck the string. Bottom: Times between release of one note and onset of the next for the same 18 notes. The data come from one pianist. From Sloboda, J. A. (1983). The communication of musical metre in piano performance. Quarterly Journal of Experimental Psychology, 35A, 377–396. With permission.

"bend" to reflect ebbs and flows of emotion. Little is known about the control of rubato, although it has been established that the rubato pattern for a piece becomes highly stereotyped with practice (Seashore, 1938; Shaffer, 1984a, b). For more recent work on this topic, see Repp (1999, 2005).

Shaffer (1984a, b) suggested that rubato timing variations are controlled at a lower level than the musical meter (the "beat"). Controlling meter at a higher level allows it to remain fixed or to drift on its own, rather than being at the mercy of local timing changes. Recall the earlier comment about the drummer keeping the beat with his or her foot.

There are many other interesting questions that can be addressed about piano playing, as well as the playing of other keyboard instruments. One is how pianists select fingering patterns, especially when they sight-read. Improvisation at the keyboard is another worthwhile, though difficult, topic that warrants more investigation. Jazz pianists invent new keyboard patterns while playing. Recording the timing and intensity of their keystrokes might shed light on the process of musical invention. Preliminary studies of brain activity during improvisation at the keyboard hold promise for shedding new light on the creative processes underlying musical and other forms of expression (Bengtsson, Csikszentmihalyi, & Ullen, 2007; Berkowitz & Ansari, 2008; Limb & Braun, 2008).

Another new line of work concerns piano playing with others rather than alone. Pianists playing in ensembles, like musicians playing other instruments in groups, are capable of remarkable sensitivity to the timing of performance by others, as shown not only by when they hit the keys but also in the way they sway with the other performers (Keller, 2008).

SUMMARY

1. Although people can text message at fairly high rates, they can type on keyboards at even higher rates and can play musical chords at higher rates still. Because times between keystrokes can be shorter than reaction times to external signals, rapid sequences of keystrokes are likely to be based on central plans.
2. Studies of reaction time provide useful information about the preparation of motor responses as well as the organization of the information processing system as a whole. When subjects know in advance what signal will be presented and what response will have to be performed when a signal appears, the time of their response relative to the signal is the simple RT. Simple RTs depend on the subject's practice, alertness, and age, as well as the strength of the signal and, to a small extent, the type of response being performed. Mechanical inertia accounts for differences in simple RTs for large and small effectors.
3. When there are several possible stimuli and responses, the times to respond are choice RTs, which are usually longer than simple RTs. Choice RTs depend on response preparation as well as stimulus expectancy.
4. Choice RTs increase linearly with $\log_2$ of the number of possible stimulus-response pairings in an experiment. This relation is known as the Hick-Hyman law, a law that is consistent with *information* theory, where information is measured in terms of binary digits or "bits"—roughly the number of yes-no decisions needed to uniquely identify a signal from a set of possible signals. Information theory is used in computer science, as in referring to a hard drive that has 5 gigabytes (5 trillion 8-bit storage capacity). However, information theory was dealt a blow by the discovery that the capacity of human short-term memory is defined by the number of meaningful elements or "chunks," not by the number of bits.

5. Another blow to information theory came from the discovery of stimulus-response compatibility effects for choice RT. Here, choice RTs depend on how "natural" the mappings are between stimuli and responses. "Naturalness" is not a well-defined concept in information theory. Choice RTs depend on the number of S-R alternatives when S-R compatibility is low but do not depend on the number of S-R alternatives, or depend only slightly on the number of S-R alternatives, when S-R compatibility is high. In choice RT tasks where manual responses are made to visual stimuli at different spatial positions, S-R compatibility is defined by the relations between stimuli and response *locations*, not by the relations between stimuli and the *hands* used to make the responses. The special role of learned relations between stimuli and response locations has also been found in studies of spatial memory, as well as in studies of instrumental conditioning.

6. Although choice RT decreases with the number of times an S-R pair is tested, S-R compatibility can also be ascribed to ideo-motor processes. Here, the more a reaction signal resembles the reafferent stimulus of the summoned response (the stimulus that will be produced by that response), the shorter the choice RT tends to be.

7. S-R compatibility effects are also elicited in making judgments about numbers, such as whether the numbers are odd or even. The *SNARC* effect is the tendency of left button responses to have short RTs for small numbers and the tendency of right button presses to have short RTs for large numbers. The SNARC effect has been taken to suggest that numbers are mentally represented in analogue form, with small numbers to the left and large numbers to the right. Hence, there is spatial-numerical analogue response compatibility (SNARC).

8. In the Simon effect, left button presses have shorter RTs to responses made to stimuli on the left than to stimuli on the right, and right button presses have shorter choice RTs for stimuli on the right than to stimuli on the left, even when the side where the stimulus appears is strictly irrelevant to the task, for example, when the color of the stimulus defines the necessary response. The Simon effect shows that *implicit* S-R relations can give rise to S-R compatibility effects.

9. In the Stroop effect, people have difficulty naming the color of a word when the word's color mismatches the word's name. Thus, it takes longer to say "green" when the word "RED" is shown in green ink than when the word "GREEN" is shown in green ink. This effect is due to automatic activation of the response from the printed word as well as the time-consuming process of resolving the ensuing response competition.

10. Choice RTs reflect response-response compatibility—relations between or among possible responses. For example, when there are two possible responses that can be made with different hands, choice RTs are generally shorter than when the two possible responses are made with the same hand.

11. Choice RTs for chord responses increase with the number of responses in the chord to be produced as well as the number of responses in the chord just performed. There is a benefit to producing chords using homologous fingers of the two hands (for instance, using the left and right index fingers). Learning to produce chords associated with distinct stimuli is facilitated when the chords use homologous fingers and when the constituent responses are spatially congruent to one another.

12. In serial choice RT tasks, each stimulus calls for a response following a preceding response. Serial choice RTs are shortest when successive responses are made with

homologous fingers of the two hands. Thus, the homologous finger advantage found for chord production tasks is also found for serial choice RT tasks.

13. Sequences of finger patterns are facilitated when the sequences are organized hierarchically. Data on latencies and errors made in producing rapid keystroke sequences from memory suggest that such sequences are executed via a tree-traversal process, that is, a process that involves translating units into successively smaller units.

14. The success of tree-traversal models suggests parallels between the way information is taken into the perceptual system and how it is emitted via the motor system. Limited-capacity storage buffers appear to be used in both systems. The limited capacity of these storage buffers is compensated for by rapid access to high-level codes.

15. Serial RT tasks have been used to study the learning of S-R sequences. People can learn S-R sequences without conscious awareness, and they can learn associations between stimulus locations and response locations more easily than between stimulus locations and response effectors (fingers for those locations).

16. When people vary delays between successive finger taps, they may rely on a system, proposed by Wing and Kristofferson (1973), in which responses are triggered at time intervals controlled by an internal time keeper or clock. According to the model, time-keeper variability is independent of motor delay variability.

17. When it is necessary to "keep the beat" while other, more rapidly changing notes are being produced, it is desirable to rely on hierarchical time keepers that control delays between musical measures independently of lower-level time keepers that control delays between notes within measures. Consistent with this desideratum, it has been found that variances of times between musical bars can be smaller than the sums of the variances of times between individual notes within measures.

18. The cerebellum may control critical events for timing. The evidence for this is that patients with unilateral cerebellar damage tap with more temporal variability when using the hand controlled by the damaged part of the cerebellum than when using the hand controlled by the undamaged part of the cerebellum. Likewise, they draw circles with pauses with more temporal variability when using the hand controlled by the damaged part of the cerebellum than when using the hand controlled by the undamaged part of the cerebellum. However, they draw circles *continuously* with equal variability when using the two hands.

19. Time keepers serve perception as well as motor control, and so can be said to be *amodal*. Evidence for amodality of timing comes from several sources. People who are good at motor timing are also good at perceptual timing. Rhythmic performance suffers when conflicting rhythms must be produced in disparate motor subsystems or when a rhythm must be produced while a conflicting rhythm is visually monitored. The time to prepare for the production of a time interval is similar to the time to prepare for the perception of that same time interval. Timing variability is similar for time production and for time perception.

20. The timing of a keyboard sequence can become integrally related to the memory for the serial order of that sequence. After a sequence has been performed repeatedly with a particular timing pattern, it is difficult to perform the sequence more quickly without a vestige of the original timing pattern.

21. Adjusting the overall rate of performance for a sequence of responses, keyboard or otherwise, may be achieved by altering the rate at which the individual responses are triggered. This may be done by adjusting a multiplicative rate parameter for the entire sequence. The evidence for this method is controversial.

22. Keyboards became popular in the nineteenth century, as did the "Qwerty" keyboard and the "touch typing" method. The benefits of touch typing were not immediately obvious, but became incontrovertible later on. Typing benefits from an eye-hand span of about four to eight letters. Typists do better when typing words than when typing nonwords, but type randomly ordered words as quickly as sentences, suggesting that words, but not phrases, are production units for typewriting.

23. Although words may be production units for typing, words are not produced as indivisible units. Typists can stop typing within words upon hearing a stop tone or upon detecting an error. The fact that typists can stop typing within words implies that individual keystrokes may also be production units for typing.

24. Keystrokes are the not the "atoms" of keyboarding, however. Still lower-level units are implied by typing errors. Typists sometimes make mistakes in key locations, finger types (index, middle, ring, or little), hands used, and directions of motion of keystrokes. Because all these features need to be specified to define individual keystrokes, the keystroke itself need not be viewed as the most fundamental unit of keyboard control.

25. Some aspects of the timing of keystrokes are attributable to mechanical interactions between the hands and fingers. Times between successive keystrokes made by the two hands are shorter than times between successive keystrokes made by different fingers of the same hand, and times between successive keystrokes made by different fingers of the same hand are shorter than times between successive keystrokes made by one finger. Film analyses indicate that such timing differences are due to differences in the opportunity for one finger to move toward its target while the previous keystroke is being performed. Simultaneous movement is easiest when the preceding keystroke is made by the opposite hand and is hardest when the preceding keystroke is made by the identical finger.

26. A model of typewriting control, developed by Rumelhart and Norman (1982), relies on mechanical interactions to account for observed timing effects. The model assumes that there are nodes in memory that allow for associations between fingers and keys. Inhibitory connections between the nodes provide for the serial order of keystrokes. Rumelhart and Norman's model is a *connectionist* model of memory and performance.

27. Piano playing has rhythmic and expressive elements not typically found in typewriting. Pianists can convey different metrical organizations of the same notes by varying the times and forces of their keystrokes. The timing of piano sequences appears to be well remembered, for subtle timing variations associated with rubato (expressive slowing and speeding) become routinized with practice. Rubato may become an integral part of the memory representation for a keyboard sequence. Timing of non-musical finger-tapping sequences has also been found to be an integral part of the memory representation for those sequences.

Further Reading

Recent work on isometric force production by multiple fingers has turned up interesting findings concerning dependencies between the digits. The total force that can be generated by several fingers on one hand is less than the sum of the forces that can be generated by each of the fingers alone. For a review, see Zatsiorsky and Latash (2008).

A researcher who has done a great deal of valuable research on piano playing is Caroline Palmer, of McGill University. Just a few of her publications are Palmer and Pfordresher (2003), Palmer (2005), and Pfordresher, Palmer, and Jungers (2007). Her website is http://www.mcgill.ca/spl/palmer/.

Another leading researcher in this area is Bruno Repp, who was cited here. His website is http://www.haskins.yale.edu/staff/repp.html. Repp has studied synchronization in great detail. For a review of his and others' research on this topic see Repp (2005). Repp and Knoblich (2004) showed that pianists can discriminate between their own and others' recordings of the same pieces of music. The authors took this outcome to support the hypothesis that common codes are brought to bear in perception and action.

As one would expect given the large number of people who take piano lessons at one point or another in their lives, there is a large literature on piano pedagogy. Much of this work has been developed separately from the scientific literature on the control of keyboarding. An interesting website that focuses on playing just the most essential notes in a piece as it is being learned is http://alfanopianostudio.com/INCORP_2.html. A personal memoir about learning to play the piano has been written by Noah Adams (1996) of National Public Radio.

Keyboarding sometimes gives rise to overuse syndromes such as focal dystonia, an undesirable muscular contraction or twisting of the hands or arms. For a useful portal to work on focal dystonia and other overuse syndromes in pianists, see http://www.balancedpianist.com/pianoinjury.htm. Carpal tunnel syndrome is an overuse syndrome well known to chronic keyboard and computer mouse users. The world-wide web offers many leads to work on this topic.

For an interesting finding concerning the role of embodied cognition in the perception of text among typists, see Beilock and Holt (2007). These authors found that typists preferred letter pairs that are easy to type over letter pairs that are hard to type, though the typists had no idea why they had this preference.

For applied work on keyboarding, see the journal *Human Factors*, which often has articles on this and related topics. A fine textbook on human factors is Proctor and Van Zandt (1994).

Jeff Miller of the University of Otago in New Zealand (http://psy.otago.ac.nz/staff/miller.html) has done pioneering work on the time course of information processing using reaction times and brain waves. Some of his publications are Miller and Low (2001), Miller and Navon (2002), and Miller, Ulrich, and Rinkenauer (1999).

For an in-depth study of the many steps leading up to a piano recital, see Chaffin (2002) and Chaffin and Imreh (2002).

For more information about learning of serial RT tasks, see Bird and Heyes (2005), Bird, Osman, Saggerson, and Heyes (2005), Rhodes, Bullock, Verwey, Averbeck, and Page (2004), Witt, Ashe, and Willingham (2008), Willingham (1998), and Willingham, Wells, Farrell, and Stemwedel (2000).

For recent research on the question of whether timing is integrally represented in keyboard sequences, see Shin (2008).

For work on the development of timing abilities, see McAuley, Jones, Holub, Johnston, and Miller (2006).

A comprehensive book on timing is one edited by Grondin (2008).

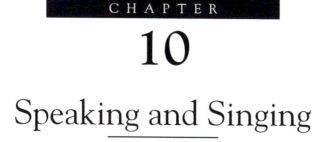

The Issues	324	A Mechanism for Relative Positioning	341	
Overview of the Chapter	326	A Parallel Distributed Processing System for Coarticulation	343	
The Vocal Tract and Articulatory Dynamics	328	**High-Level Control of Speech**	346	
The Respiratory System	328	Word Games	346	
Laryngeal Mechanisms	329	Laboratory Studies of Speaking Speed	347	
Articulatory Mechanisms	331	Speech Errors	349	
The Pharynx	332	**Brain Mechanisms Underlying Speech**	353	
Vowels	332			
Consonants	333	**Bird Song**	354	
Variability	335	**Motor Resonance**	357	
The Motor Theory of Speech Perception	336	**Summary**	359	
The Target Hypothesis	337	**Further Reading**	362	
Relative Positions and Acoustic Targets	339			

   Like the other activities discussed in this book, speaking and singing have special properties. Two are most critical for present purposes. First, their most important output is auditory rather than visual or proprioceptive. Second, they are usually carried out for purposes of communication.

   Because of the centrality of communication for human affairs and because of the uniqueness of human language, the control of speech has been studied in detail by investigators from a large number of disciplines—psychology, physiology, linguistics, engineering, and speech pathology, among others. The control of singing has received somewhat less attention than the control of speech because, at least for humans, singing is not the primary means of verbal communication. Singing will be covered here in less detail than speech, not just because less research has been done on it, but also because most, though certainly not all, of the important principles of vocal control can be documented by considering speech alone.

THE ISSUES

How should we approach the control of speech and singing? To begin, it is useful to say what vocal outputs consist of. Some of the sounds we produce—coughing, burping, and sneezing—have vegetative or survival value. Because they are nonlinguistic, they will not be analyzed in this chapter.

When we speak, we produce words. These consist of *phonemes* (roughly, vowels and consonants), which allow for meaning distinctions in a language. /l/ and /r/ are phonemes in English, as shown by the fact that "lip" and "rip" have different meanings. In Mandarin Chinese, however, word meanings are never distinguished by /l/ or /r/. Thus, /l/ and /r/ are not phonemes in Mandarin Chinese. On the other hand, speakers of Mandarin Chinese distinguish between [l] and [r]. They say [l] only at word beginnings and [r] only at word endings. [l] and [r] are therefore said to be two *phones* of Mandarin Chinese. Phones are sound categories that can but do not necessarily convey meaning. In English, [l] and [r] are distinct phones that also happen to be phonemes. In Mandarin Chinese, [l] and [r] are phones that happen not to be phonemes. Notice that phonemes are denoted here with slashes (/ /) while phones are denoted with brackets ([ ]).

English, like Mandarin Chinese, has phones that are not phonemes. Place your hand in front of your mouth while saying "pit" or "spit." You should feel a burst of air following the p in "pit" but not in "spit." This indicates that the two p sounds are produced differently. The difference reflects a subtle rule of English that until now you probably knew only unconsciously: p in the initial position of a word is aspirated (it is accompanied by a breath of air), but p in a non-initial word position is unaspirated. The fact that we distinguish between aspirated and unaspirated p's even though aspiration does not distinguish word meanings implies that aspirated and unaspirated p's are phones in English but not phonemes. Linguists refer to the sound elements distinguishing phones as *phonetic features*. Aspiration is a phonetic feature of English.

Distinct phones in a language that are not distinct phonemes are called *allophones*. [p] in spit and [p] in pit are English allophones. In Hindi, a language mainly spoken in India, aspiration affects meaning, so aspirated and unaspirated p's are not allophones in this language.

When we speak, we also vary intonation and stress. In English, intonation and stress help convey meanings about entire phrases. Saying in a matter-of-fact way, "OK, I'll pay you $500 to fix my car," means something different from exclaiming in anger, "OK, I'll pay you $500 to fix my car!" The meanings of the individual words are the same, but the meanings of the sentences differ. Intonation and stress provide cues to the listener about sentence-level or phrase-level meaning. In other languages—so-called tone languages—intonation affects individual word meaning as well as phrase and sentence meaning. Mandarin Chinese is a tone language. Some phonemes in this language are differentiated by pitch alone. In English, meanings of individual vowels and consonants are not typically distinguished just by pitch, though they can be.

Another aspect of speech that must be controlled by the speaker and correspondingly used by the listener is timing. You can speak at different rates, but you do not uniformly speed up or slow down your vocal output the way a record player does when it is run at different speeds (33, 45, or 78 rotations per minute). Instead, as you speak more quickly, you reduce the durations of vowels more than the durations of consonants. You also take various shortcuts, omitting all but the most critical elements needed to ensure intelligibility. Finally, when you speak quickly, you tend to flatten the intonation profiles of your speech, as you can confirm by reading this sentence as quickly as possible or by recalling very fast-talking advertisements on TV or radio.

Maximum speech rates are about 200 words per minute (Goldman-Eisler, 1968. Because words in English have an average of seven phonemes, speakers of English can speak at rates of about 1,400 phonemes per minute. It has been estimated that it takes 1/10 of a second to produce a single phoneme. Using the latter figure, it follows that we should be able to produce no more than 10 phonemes a second, or 600 phonemes per minute. How do we manage, then, to speak at more than twice that rate?

The answer is that phonemes are not produced one after the other in a strictly serial fashion. Rather, the vocal apparatus makes use of parallel activity, much as the hands do in the simultaneous movements of the fingers in typing (Figure 9.16). X-ray movies of the tongue, jaw, and other parts of the vocal tract, made by temporarily attaching tiny metal pellets to the speaker's articulators, have shown that the articulators move in several directions at once. You can observe the capacity for parallel articulation by looking into a mirror and watching your lips as you say, rather deliberately, "construe." Notice that your lips become rounded even before you say "str" (Kozhevnikov & Chistovich, 1965; Daniloff & Moll, 1968). Anticipatory lip rounding illustrates *coarticulation*—the tendency for different articulatory objectives to be met simultaneously, generally through parallel articulatory activity. Another example of coarticulation occurs in the word "boo." When you say this word emphatically, your lips round before you produce the b. Anticipatory lip rounding is not always necessary for saying b, however, as you can see by saying "bed." No anticipatory lip rounding occurs for this word. Anticipatory lip rounding only occurs in anticipation of vowels for which the lips need to be rounded.

As the preceding discussion indicates, there are many aspects of vocal output that must be controlled by the speaker (or singer). A successful theory of vocal control must explain how such control is achieved. In addition, a theory of vocal control must explain why some sounds or sound combinations are part of our linguistic repertoire and others are not. Some sounds are physically impossible to make—no one can shout as loud as a jet plane, for example—but other sounds are physically possible but rarely if ever uttered, at least in normal speech contexts. For instance, among the thousands of languages in the world, none appears to use, as part of everyday speech, brief "snoring" sounds (Ohala, 1983). Such sounds can of course be made, as bedmates can attest. The absence of snoring sounds in natural language cannot be attributed to a universal concern for etiquette, for the sounds made by speakers in some languages are considered rude by some speakers of other languages. Not all Americans, for example, are enamored of gutterals—the "ch" sound so common in Dutch, Hebrew, and other languages. A more likely reason for the absence of certain sounds in virtually all languages is that the production of these sounds in ongoing speech would violate principles of biomechanical efficiency (Lindblom, 1983; Ohala, 1983). Yet another possibility is that inclusion of these sounds would violate deep-seated grammatical rules, perhaps common to all people (Chomsky, 1975). According to the latter view, computational factors constrain the sound combinations that comprise natural languages.

As we consider the requirements of a theory of speech production, we must also take account of the fact that speech can be produced in the presence of physical changes to the vocal apparatus. A familiar example is talking with a pipe in one's mouth. The fact that people can speak intelligibly while holding pipes between their teeth suggests that their speech production systems are tuned to the proprioceptive feedback they receive. Experiments bear this out (Lindblom, 1983).

A final issue that must be dealt with in the analysis of speaking and singing concerns the interplay between vocal output and hearing. One important question is how we distinguish among heard speech sounds. The problem is nontrivial, as suggested by the fact that we mainly communicate with computers via keyboards, though we mostly communicate with one another in everyday life via speech. Artificial speech recognition is a difficult technical problem.

A related problem is how we regulate our ongoing vocal output as we hear ourselves speak and sing. How do we control the loudness of our voices, for example? A method that has been used to investigate the role of auditory feedback in speaking is to delay the auditory feedback that a speaker or singer receives from his or her own voice. In the case of singing, delayed auditory feedback affects the frequency and amplitude of vibrato. Vibrato is the intentional wavering of the voice used by singers to produce rich-sounding notes. (Musicians also produce vibrato on their instruments, of course.) Changes in vocal vibrato appear with feedback delays as short as 100 ms. This result has been taken to suggest that singers respond to auditory feedback as often as 10 times a second (Deutsch & Clarkson, 1959). A comparable result comes from delayed auditory feedback studies of speech. When auditory feedback from speech is postponed by 100 ms or more, speaking can be seriously disrupted, with the resulting speech pattern resembling stuttering (Lee, 1950). Based on this result, it has been suggested that one cause of stuttering may be a kind of perennial mismatch between expected and actual auditory feedback delays (Costello, 1985).

If one has learned to speak with the benefit of hearing but one becomes deaf, it is possible to continue to speak normally for weeks or even months. Beyond this time, however, the quality of speech usually deteriorates. Manipulating the amount of time that people can receive auditory feedback while learning to talk is not ethically acceptable, of course, so much of the research on this topic has been done with birds, a species that communicates through vocalization. Some exciting discoveries have been made through work on the neural control of bird song. We will look at research in that area in the last part of the chapter.

OVERVIEW OF THE CHAPTER

The chapter will be organized as follows. First, we will consider the vocal tract and articulatory dynamics. Here we will look at the anatomy of the vocal tract and the mechanics of the air flow that creates sounds within it. Then we will turn to some of the problems that the articulatory system must solve to produce recognizable speech sounds. Key among these is the achievement of desired articulatory configurations. Because the articulators rarely occupy a single, fixed position before a given speech sound is produced, the problem of achieving desired articulatory configurations is one of the fundamental problems to be solved by the speech controller. It happens that the speech perception system is remarkably forgiving of variations in the speech signal. Listeners usually do not notice small, artificial deletions in the speech signal when those deletions are replaced by noise of approximately equal amplitude—a phenomenon known as *phonemic restoration* (Warren & Warren, 1970). Similarly, when people repeat what they hear as soon as they hear it—a task called *shadowing*—they instantly correct errors in the input (Marlsen-Wilson & Tyler, 1980). These phenomena indicate that people extract meaning from speech signals despite major variations in the signal itself. This capability relieves the speech production system from having to "worry too much" about producing perfectly accurate sounds.

The next issue that will be discussed will be the relation between speech and hearing. Here we will review two influential theories of speech perception. One is primarily concerned with how we perceive speech. It claims that we recognize speech sounds by recruiting knowledge about how speech sounds are produced (Liberman, Cooper, Shankweiler, & Studdert-Kennedy, 1967). The other theory is primarily concerned with how we produce speech. It claims that the programming of speech uses perceptual representations of likely auditory consequences (Guenther, Hampson, & Johnson, 1998; Ladefoged, DeClerk, Lindau, & Papcun, 1972; MacNeilage, 1980). A variant of the latter theory holds that invariant relative positions of the articulators define target states toward which the articulators move.

The next section reviews a theory of coarticulation that makes use of a network of interconnected, neuron-like units (Jordan, 1986a, b). Network models are receiving more and more attention because of their apparent similarity to the brain.

Another model of this kind has also been found to account for phenomena related to the planning of sentences and their constituents (Dell, 1986). The phenomena being modeled are "slips of the tongue." Traditionally, such speech errors have been explained by assuming that information passes in a single direction from high to low levels in the language production system (Fromkin,1973; Garrett, 1975; Levelt, 1989; Shattuck-Hufnagle, 1979). The network model described later in this chapter also allows information to pass from low levels to high levels.

Another topic to which we will turn is the brain's control of speech and song. Because much of our current knowledge of speech derives from analyses of speech disorders following brain injury, it is useful to look for correspondences between the types of language disorders produced by damage to different parts of the brain and the speech errors that occur when the brain is intact.

The penultimate part of the chapter will be concerned with the control of bird song. As suggested above, neuroscience has made significant strides in this line of investigation.

The final part of the chapter will be concerned with motor resonance—the tendency of perceptual input to arouse physical action tendencies that in turn affect the way perceptual input is interpreted. Speech is one area where this idea has been documented.

Two topics will not be treated here in as much detail as might be expected—the acquisition of speech and the diagnosis and treatment of speech disorders. The major points of basic research on the motor control of speaking and singing can be covered without delving into these topics, each of which requires a considerable amount of space to be dealt with adequately. References to work in these area will be given in the Further Reading section.

THE VOCAL TRACT AND ARTICULATORY DYNAMICS

To speak and sing, air must be pushed through the vocal tract. The resonance of the column of air in the tract gives rise to sound. To produce specific, desired sounds, the speech system must achieve fairly precise control of the shape of the vocal tract. It does so by modulating the behavior of three subsystems (see Figure 10.1): the *respiratory* subsystem, the *laryngeal* subsystem, and the *articulatory* subsystem. Figure 10.2 presents a schematic diagram of these components.

The Respiratory System

The respiratory section includes the lungs and associated muscle groups. Two major muscle groups promote inhalation (breathing in). One of these major muscle groups is the diaphragm, which lies at the base of the rib cage. Another major muscle group is the external

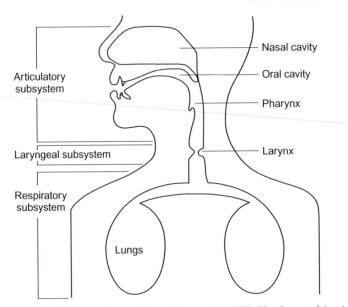

FIGURE 10.1 Cross section of the vocal tract. From Harvey, N. (1985). Vocal control in singing: A cognitive approach. In P. Howell, I. Cross, & R. West (Ed.), Musical structure and cognition. (p. 289). London: Academic Press. With permission.

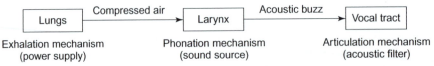

FIGURE 10.2 Schematic diagram of the vocal system. From Harvey, N. (1985). Vocal control in singing: A cognitive approach. In P. Howell, I. Cross, & R. West (Ed.), Musical structure and cognition. (p. 289). London: Academic Press. With permission.

intercostals. This group of muscles lifts and expands the rib cage, allowing for exhalation (breathing out). The internal intercostals pull down on the rib cage and push air out of the lungs. The internal intercostals are the most important respiratory muscles for normal speech and singing, for they are the muscles that propel air out through the mouth and nose. In general, the greater the pressure of the escaping air, the louder one's voice.

Breathing is very different when one is vocalizing or silent. During silence, inhalation and exhalation proceed at a more-or-less even rate, but during vocalization there is a short period of inhalation followed by a longer period of exhalation. In singing, it is sometimes necessary to take a deep breath in a short amount of time to allow for a sustained period of singing with few interruptions. Studies of the control of inhalation during singing indicate that singers, or at least professional singers, regulate the amount of air they inhale and the speed with which they do so depending on the length and loudness of the phrase they are about to sing (Harvey, 1985).

The timing of respiratory muscle activity during the inhalation-exhalation cycle of speech has also been studied (MacNeilage & Ladefoged, 1976). After the lungs have filled with air, the rib cage recoils elastically from a state of complete or near-complete expansion. During this period, the external intercostals, which promote inhalation, remain active until receptors within these muscles indicate that the lungs have been fully filled. After the elastic recoil process has continued and the lung volume has decreased to a critical value (which, by the way, is well above complete emptying of the lung), the external intercostals shut off based on feedback from stretch receptors within them. This event signals the internal intercostals to contract, which allows for active exhalation and production of the next utterance. Because the internal intercostals do not contract until the lungs have also begun to contract, they take advantage of the inertia of lung contraction—an example of exploitation of physical mechanics similar to what we have seen in other activities.

As air is expelled from the lungs, the activity of the internal intercostals increases. When the volume of the lungs reaches a critically low value, other muscles come into play to ensure that exhalation continues. Finally, when the lung volume reaches a base level, the next inhalation begins.

The foregoing description illustrates sustained activity in the respiratory muscles. There is also transient activity. The internal intercostals produce clearly demarcated pulses. These pulses were once hypothesized to occur at, and indeed define, syllable beginnings (Stetson, 1951). However, subsequent work revealed that syllables need not be accompanied by transient activity of the internal intercostals (Ladefoged, 1967).

Laryngeal Mechanisms

As seen in Figure 10.1, the area of the branching structure that feeds air to the lungs (the trachea) contains the larynx. This structure serves four main functions. First, it regulates the characteristic pitch of the voice. Second, it modulates aspiration. Third, it permits whispering. Fourth, it creates the buzzing sound known as voicing.

The role of voicing can be appreciated by placing your index finger and thumb on your Adam's apple while making two sounds: a prolonged "f" and a prolonged "v." When you say "v" you can feel your vocal cords vibrate, but when you say "f" you cannot feel your vocal cords vibrate. This is because "f" and "v" are distinguished by the presence or absence

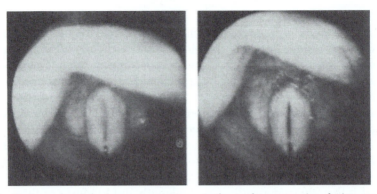

FIGURE 10.3 Photographs of the larynx in positions similar to those occurring during production of (left) voiced and (right) unvoiced consonants. From Sawashima, M. & Hirose, H. (1983). Laryngeal gestures in speech production. In P. F. MacNeilage (Ed.), The production of speech (pp. 11–38). New York: Springer-Verlag. With permission.

of vocal cord vibration or voicing. "v" is a voiced consonant, whereas "f" is a voiceless consonant.

Voicing is controlled by adjusting the distance between the vocal cords, which are two folds that lie across the roof of the larynx. Figure 10.3 shows a picture of the vocal cords, taken with a special optic fiber camera system. During production of voiced consonants such as "v" and "b," the distance between the vocal cords is small, but during production of unvoiced consonants such as "f" and "p," the distance increases to the point where air flowing between the cords does not cause vocal cord vibration. The muscles involved in separating the vocal folds have been analyzed in some detail despite the formidable technical difficulties of doing so (MacNeilage & Ladefoged, 1975; MacNeilage, 1983).

The shape of the larynx accounts in part for the fact that some people have better singing voices than others (Sundberg, 1977). People with exceptionally fine singing voices can lower their larynxes more than people with unexceptional singing voices. The enlarged cavity that accompanies larynx lowering allows for an extra formant—that is, an extra concentration of energy in part of the auditory frequency range. This extra formant—sometimes called the "singer's formant"—allows the voice to be projected more effectively than usual. As a result, a fine opera singer can be heard over an orchestra without a microphone. Someone unable to produce the extra formant would have to scream or rely on artificial amplification to be heard in such places.

It has been known at least since the time of Leonardo da Vinci that the vocal cords control pitch as well as voicing (Peschel & Peschel, 1987). da Vinci studied cadavers and concluded that the mass of the vocal cords affects vocal pitch. As the vocal cords enlarge, they vibrate at a lower frequency. During puberty in males, the release of male sex hormone (testosterone) causes enlargement of the vocal cords, causing the voice to drop. To prevent this from happening, boys at various times in history have been castrated (Peschel & Peschel, 1987; see Figure 10.4).

If changing the mass of the vocal cords were the only way to change pitch, it would be impossible to change pitch rapidly. To produce rapid pitch changes, the speech production system regulates the frequency of vocal cord vibration, principally by changing the stiffness

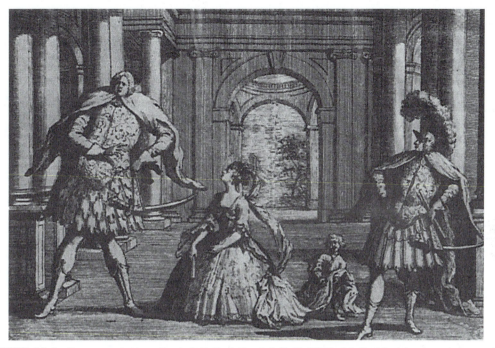

FIGURE 10.4   Two castrati. From Peschel, E. R. & Peschel, R. E. (1987). Medical insights into the castrati in opera. Amercian Scientist, 75, 578–583. With permission.

of the vocal cords. To understand how this is achieved and why it has the desired effect, try the following simple experiment. Imitate the sound of a power lawn mower as it speeds up or slows down. To produce the sound of a slow-running lawn mower, let your lips flap back and forth passively while you force air through your mouth. Now gradually increase the stiffness of your lips to produce the higher-pitched sound of the mower "in high gear." Notice that your lips vibrate at a higher rate than they did before, allowing a higher-pitched sound to emerge. This is essentially what happens to your vocal cords when you produce sounds of varying pitch. The cords stiffen to vibrate at higher rates so higher-pitched sounds are produced, and they relax to allow for vibration at lower rates so lower-pitched sounds are produced. The vibration itself is passive, driven by air pushed from the lungs and by counteracting physical forces, a phenomenon known as the Bernoulli effect.

Articulatory Mechanisms

So far, we have considered how speakers and singers adjust the amplitude, frequency, voicing, and degree of aspiration of their vocal output. We have not yet considered how the other distinctions in speech come about. How do speakers distinguish between l's and m's, for example, or between g's and j's? In general, how do speakers produce the full range of consonants and vowels they do? It turns out that they rely not just on mechanisms at the level of the larynx and below, but also on mechanisms at the level of the larynx and above.

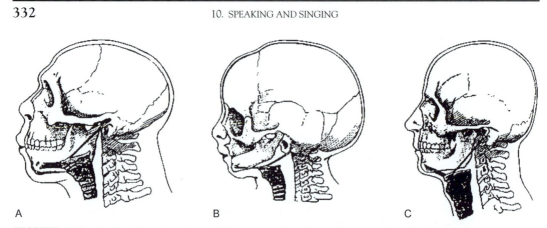

FIGURE 10.5   Skulls of the Neanderthal (A), human infant (B), and human adult (C). From Miller, G. A. (1981). Language and speech. New York: Freeman. San Francisco. With permission.

These include the pharynx (the cavity lying between the larynx and the mouth or oral cavity), the mouth, jaws, and lips, the nasal tract, and the velum (a movable flap connecting the nasal tract and oral cavity) (see Figure 10.1).

The Pharynx

The shape of the pharynx constrains the vowels that can be made. Because adult humans have long necks, low larynxes, and large mobile throats (see Figure 10.5), their pharynxes possess resonance properties suitable for production of certain vowels, such as [a], [i], and [u]. The resonance of a body is the frequency at which it vibrates with the greatest amplitude for each unit of energy supplied . The throats of human infants and of apes do not have these characteristics, however. Human infants and apes have short necks, relatively high larynxes, and small immobile throats, making it impossible for them to say [a], [i], and [u]. Based on this observation, an intriguing hypothesis was proposed about the evolutionary origins of human language (Lieberman, 1984). According to this hypothesis, the Neanderthal ape, a pre-human species that lived about 35,000 years ago, was unable to say [a], [i], and [u], because its throat was more like that of modern apes and human infants than like that of modern human adults. If this hypothesis is correct, it would imply that the full range of human speech sounds developed recently in evolution (within the past 35,000 years) and so may have arisen through a genetic mutation, as some have speculated (Chomsky, 1975).

Not all researchers are convinced that speech as we know it only emerged this recently. Alternative interpretations of the fossil evidence as well as other archaeological samples have led others to argue that our human forebears spoke much as we do as long as 2 million years ago (Bower, 1989).

Vowels

An effective way to understand how articulatory mechanisms allow for the production of different classes of speech sounds is to consider the classes one by one. This is the approach taken in this section and in the next. We first consider vowels.

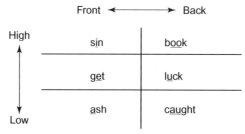

Front ◄————► Back

High

	sin	book
	get	luck
	ash	caught

Low

FIGURE 10.6   Locations of the tongue body in production of so-called lax vowels—vowels produced with the root of the tongue retracted. Tense vowels, by contrast, have the tongue root advanced, as in "teen" or "boot." From Akmajian, A., Demers, R. A., & Harnish, R. W. (1979). Linguistics: An introduction. Cambridge, MA: MIT Press. With permission.

All vowels are voiced. Only consonants can be unvoiced. Vowels differ on several articulatory dimensions (see Figure 10.6). One is the position of the tongue body—either high or low in the mouth and either toward the front of the mouth or toward the back. To produce the vowel in "sin," for example, the tongue body is placed high in the mouth and toward the front. Consequently this vowel is categorized as high-front. To produce the vowel in "book," the tongue body is placed high in the mouth and toward the back. Consequently, this vowel is categorized as high-back. The vowel in "get" requires placement of the tongue body low in the mouth and toward the front. Hence, this is a low-front vowel. The vowel in "luck" requires placement of the tongue body low in the mouth and toward the back. As a result, this is a low-back vowel. There is also a vowel that requires an extremely low front tongue placement (the "a" in ash), and there is a vowel that requires an extremely low back tongue placement (the "augh" in caught).

Consonants

The production of consonants, like the production of vowels, depends on where the tongue is placed. Consonants are also affected by the positions and activities of the lips, jaw, and velum.

Linguists have categorized consonants according to their manner and place of articulation. Manner of articulation refers to the way the air stream is constricted by the articulators—for example, whether the air is momentarily stopped by closure of the lips. Place of articulation refers to the location where the constriction occurs. Tables 10.1 and 10.2 list several manners and places of articulation.

A number of points should be kept in mind as you study Tables 10.1 and 10.2. First, the tables do not list all the consonants of English. It would be educational and entertaining for you to synthesize other possible consonants by combining the features shown in Tables 10.1 and 10.2. An example of such a synthesized consonant is the sound associated with the letters ng, as in "song"; this is a velar/nasal.

Second, the entries in Tables 10.1 and 10.2 are for American English. Other languages use many of the same places and manners of articulation as in American English, but some other languages or dialects also use other places and manners of articulation. For example,

TABLE 10.1   Manners of Articulation

Type	Example	Description
Stops	*pug*	Total interruption of air flow by lips, tongue, velum, or glottis
Constrictives	*forth*	Narrowing of air stream by lip or tongue
Nasals	*mine*	Nasal passage opened by lowering velum
Liquids	*reel*	Tongue tip near alveolar ridge
Glides	*wet*	Narrowing of air stream by lips with voicing and velum open
Affricates	cru*tch*	Stop followed by constrictions

TABLE 10.2   Places of Articulation

Type	Example	Description
Bilabials	*m, b*	Lips brought together
Labiodentals	*f, v*	Lower lip brought into contact with teeth
Dentals	*then*	Tongue tip brought into contact with teeth
Alveolars	*d, s*	Tongue tip brought into contact with alveolar ridge
Palatals	*rich*	Tongue body brought into contact with hard palate
Velars	*kid*	Tongue body brought close to soft palate
Glottals	bu*tt*on	Brief closure of the vocal cords

French has uvulars, as in the r of "rouge," where the uvula, the little appendage hanging from the soft palate of the roof of the mouth, is touched or approached by the back of the tongue.

Knowing that the examples in Tables 10.1 and 10.2 refer to American English should help you interpret the examples correctly. The t's in "button," for example, are reduced to glottal stops in American English, but in formal British English are pronounced as hard t's. Hard t's are produced by touching the tongue to the alveolar ridge, the protrusion behind the teeth, which you can feel with the tip of your tongue.

A final comment about Tables 10.1 and 10.2 is that, for ease of communication, this text does not use the special symbols used in the field of phonetics to represent speech sounds precisely. These symbols can be found in a number of sources, such as Akmajian, Demers, and Harnish (1979) and Halle and Clements (1983).

Whereas Tables 10.1 and 10.2 introduce different types of articulatory features and consonants that possess them, it is also possible to construct tables that show, for any given consonant, the articulatory features it possesses. Similarly organized tables can be drawn up for vowels. Representing consonants and vowels in this way was a major achievement of the approach taken by Chomsky and Halle (1968) in what has come to be called the "standard theory" of phonology. According to the standard theory, each phoneme is coded according to its distinctive features.

Table 10.3 presents part of a distinctive-feature matrix for a few consonants in American English. Note that the entries in the table are pluses and minuses, reflecting the fact that articulatory features are assumed in the theory simply to be present (+) or absent (−). For

TABLE 10.3 Binary Values of Selected Phonetic Features for a Few English Consonants

| | Consonants | | | | | | | |
Feature	p	b	m	t	d	n	k	g
Nasal	−	−	+	−	−	+	−	−
Stop	+	+	+	+	+	+	+	+
Affricate	−	−	−	−	−	−	−	−
Sibilant	−	−	−	−	−	−	−	−
Glottal	−	−	−	−	−	−	−	−
Labial	+	+	+	−	−	−	−	−
Interdental	−	−	−	−	−	−	−	−

example, a consonant is assumed to be either nasal or not—that is, produced with the velum closed or open. When the velum is open, air can pass through the nasal cavity. Similarly, a consonant is assumed to be a stop or not—that is, it is produced with or without complete constriction of the air stream. A consonant is an affricate or not, that is, it is produced with or without a temporary stop of the air stream, released into a constrictive state. Likewise, a consonant either is or is not a sibilant, that is, it either has or does not have a hissing sound. A consonant also is a labial or not, that is, it is made or not made through lip closure. Likewise, a consonant is or is not an interdental, that is, it is made or not made by pushing the tongue against the teeth, yielding a slight hissing sound. And finally, a consonant either is or is not glottal, that is, it is made or not made by briefly stopping the air flow with the vocal cords.

Implicitly, the standard theory of phonology suggests a way that distinct speech sounds might be produced: The articulators might be brought to specific positions to ensure that particular articulatory features are present or absent. In ongoing speech, a series of such articulatory positions would be achieved to ensure that the appropriate sequence of articulatory feature vectors is produced.

As straightforward as this idea may seem, it runs into a problem. Articulatory positions exhibit tremendous variation. Actual speech is not as neat and tidy as the standard theory would suggest, raising questions about how useful the theory may be in practice. The next section covers the nature of variability in speech production.

VARIABILITY

One source of evidence for the variability of speech comes from analyses of the acoustic properties of speech sounds. Such analyses have relied extensively on the sound spectrograph, a device that converts sound to visible traces (see Figure 10.7). When sound spectrograms were first produced, they revealed something disconcerting. We hear distinct phonemes—for example, a "b" as a "b" regardless of whether it occurs in "bag" or in "big"—but sound spectrograms reveal little in common between the energy profiles of these two initial consonants. If we hear b's as b's but the two b's have little in common acoustically, what is the source of that perceptual invariance?

H–U—M–AN M—O——TO–R CON—TR——O—L

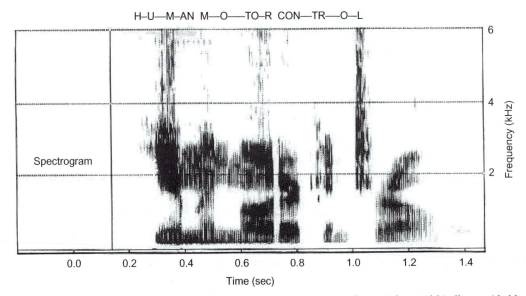

FIGURE 10.7 A sound spectrogram of the phrase "human motor control" as spoken and kindly provided by Professor Neil Stillings, Hampshire College, Amherst, Massachusetts.

The Motor Theory of Speech Perception

In the 1960's a group of researchers at Haskins Laboratories, then in New York City and now in New Haven, Connecticut, suggested that we hear certain speech sounds as the same because, in effect, we invoke the commands needed to produce them. On this view, acoustic invariance arises from articulatory invariance. This idea is known as the *motor theory* of speech perception (Liberman, Cooper, Shankweiler, & Studdert-Kennedy, 1967).

The motor theory has precedent. Part of the legacy of behaviorism was the belief that the activity called thinking is actually a subtle form of movement. To test this hypothesis, electromyographic (EMG) recordings of the muscles of the mouth and throat were made while subjects engaged in various sorts of cognitive activity. The experiments showed that subtle movements do indeed occur in the vocal apparatus. When people think, they may engage in subvocal speech (Sokolov, 1972.

Recently, this fact was put to practical use. It was realized that amplifying subvocal speech could be useful in noisy environments where instructions must be given but are hard to hear, in public places where conversations may be annoying or distracting to others, or in covert operations where overt speech may be dangerous. It was realized that these problems could be averted by attaching painless electrodes to speakers' throats to pick up subvocal electromyographic activity. Amplifying the EMG signals and turning the signals into sound for the intended listener make it possible for remote listeners to hear what the speaker is saying, albeit after computer algorithms responsible for converting the EMG signals into acoustic signals are suitably "trained" and the speaker learns how to make suitable vocal movements without speaking out loud.

Even if subvocal speech can be picked up when people try to generate it or when they are told simply to "think," it does not follow that subvocal speech is necessary for thought. In fact, other studies have shown that it is not. One study relied on a heroic subject who allowed himself to undergo complete, temporary paralysis while being presented with new information to be recalled later. After recovering from the paralysis, he could recall what was presented to him. This result indicates that he could form new memories without overt motor involvement (Smith, Brown, Toman, & Goodman, 1947).

What do these findings imply about the motor theory of speech perception? Plainly they rule out any form of the theory that says speech perception requires overt muscle activity. For the theory to be taken seriously, therefore, it must be taken to mean that when speech is heard, it evokes tendencies for speaking, if not speech itself.

If the motor theory is interpreted this way, how can it be tested? According to the theory, the speech motor commands for any given consonant or vowel should be the same even if the sounds that are emitted depend on the context in which the consonant or vowel occurs. One way to test this hypothesis is to measure the electrical activity of the speech musculature when particular phonemes are produced. If the motor theory is correct, the electrical activity associated with particular phonemes should be the same. Initial studies, conducted in the late 1960's, provided encouraging support for this prediction, but as more data were collected, it became clear that the hoped-for invariances would not emerge. For example, MacNeilage and DeClerk (1969) found that the electromyographic patterns of 36 consonant-vowel-consonant syllables differed considerably depending on the identity of the phonemes that came before or after. This result as well as others showed that variability was more the rule than the exception in speech production (MacNeilage, 1970). Motor theory was therefore dealt a blow by this research.

If we do not produce invariant motor commands and our speech motor activity is highly variable, how do we reliably get out the speech sounds we do? One solution—if it can be called that—is simply to say that the speech production system is inherently noisy. One noted speech scientist proposed such a view:

> Imagine a row of Easter eggs carried along a moving belt; the eggs are of various sizes, and variously colored, but not boiled. At a certain point, the belt carries the row of eggs between the two rollers of a wringer, which quite effectively smash them and rub them more or less into each other. The flow of eggs before the wringer represents the series of impulses from the phoneme source. The mess that emerges from the wringer represents the output of the speech transmitter [Hockett, 1955, p. 210].

This is not a very satisfying model. Speech may be difficult to analyze, but if it lacked underlying regularity, human communication would be even less reliable than it is.

The Target Hypothesis

In 1970, Peter MacNeilage offered a theory to explain how the speech production system might reliably generate speech sounds (MacNeilage, 1970). He proposed that feedback from the articulators is used, via γ motor neurons (see Chapter 3), to bring the articulators to specific target positions. Because the articulators can be in different positions before a target position must be reached, the commands used to move the articulators need not be invariant.

Recall from Chapter 3 that the gamma system allows muscles to contract until they reach desired lengths. If an entire group of muscles must move to a target position, the gamma system can be used to bring each muscle to the position it must reach. Thus, MacNeilage's (1970) target hypothesis provides a physiologically plausible mechanism for achieving target positions. An advantage of the theory is that, in principle, it provides a way for the articulators to respond to physical disturbances or variations.

MacNeilage (1970) offered several kinds of evidence for this idea. One was that a patient with normal hearing and normal motor control but virtually no somesthetic feedback was unable to produce intelligible speech (MacNeilage, Rootes, & Chase, 1967). This outcome was consistent with the assumption that sensory feedback plays a role in speech production, as required for the gamma system to work. Similarly, experimental manipulations that temporarily disrupt oral feedback impair the quality of speech (Scott & Ringel, 1971).

Another result that fits with the target hypothesis is that people with normal feedback are adept at compensating for disturbances within the vocal apparatus. We have already considered pipe smokers in this connection. They can speak intelligibly with a pipe between their teeth. MacNeilage (1970) noted that whenever one speaks with clenched teeth, the necessary tongue and lip movements are dramatically different from their normal pattern. Yet speakers can speak intelligibly in this state, suggesting that they can make effective use of oral feedback and alter the ensuing motor commands based on the feedback they receive. If speech were produced with fixed efferent commands, such compensation would be impossible.

A final result that MacNeilage adduced in support of his theory concerned the stability of articulatory targets despite variability in articulatory starting positions. MacNeilage, Krones, and Hanson (1969) found that with repetitions of an utterance, there was much less variation in final jaw positions than in initial jaw positions. Such consistency could reflect updating of jaw position information with feedback.

A related finding, reported by Kozhevnikov and Chistovich (1965), was that the maximum velocity of the lower lip as it approached the upper lip in producing /p/, /b/, or /m/ increased with the amount of lip opening for an immediately preceding vowel. Again, this result fits with the view that the speech production system strives for final target positions.

As encouraging as these results were for MacNeilage's (1970) target hypothesis, further results found it to be off target. One difficulty was that the muscle lengths required to produce intelligible speech when the teeth are clenched are in fact different from the muscle lengths that are normally required (Lindblom & Sondberg, 1971). Because the gamma system regulates muscle length, it alone cannot produce the effective compensations achieved by pipe smokers.

A related result came from a study in which a block was sometimes placed between the lips of speakers who were asked to produce consonants that required lip closure (Smith & Lee, 1971). The target hypothesis predicted an increase in lip muscle activity with the block in place because the gamma loop would cause the muscles to work harder than usual to get to the target position. What was seen, however, was a *reduction* in lip muscle activity, not an *increase*.

A final challenge to the target hypothesis was that quite different articulatory configurations can be used to produce vowels with similar acoustic characteristics (Nooteboom, 1970). If reliance on the gamma system were the means of achieving desired articulatory targets, such wide variations would not be expected.

Relative Positions and Acoustic Targets

In the face of so much contradictory evidence for the spatial target theory, the theory could not be accepted. Faced with this discouraging state of affairs, some investigators stepped back and asked, "What is speech for?" Considering this basic question helped them arrive at a more accurate theory of how speech is controlled.

The reason we speak is, of course, to communicate with others, to transmit recognizable acoustic waveforms to listeners. Recognizing this point, several authors, including MacNeilage (1980), came to the view that commands for speech may be specifically designed to achieve desired *acoustic* targets rather than desired *spatial* targets (Guenther, Hampson, & Johnson, 1998; Ladefoged, DeClerk, Lindau, & Papcun, 1972; Nooteboom, 1970). Subsequent work helped indicate how acoustically based targets might be achieved. The central insight in this more recent research is that proper acoustic results can be realized when the articulators achieve proper *relative* positions. The *absolute* positions of the articulators are less important (Abbs, 1986; Abbs, Gracco, & Cole, 1984; Turvey, 1977, 1990).

A study that supported this view was concerned with the positions of the upper and lower lips when speakers repeatedly produced a simple utterance such as [apa]. As seen in Figure 10.8, the positions of the lips were inversely related: When the upper lip happened to be higher than usual, the lower lip was lower, and when the upper lip happened to be lower than usual, the lower lip was higher. From this observation, it appeared that the speech production system controls the relative positions of the upper and lower lips, not their absolute positions. From an acoustic point of view, when one wants to say [p], what is needed is to bring the lips together, so it is the relation between the lips that matter, not their exact locations.

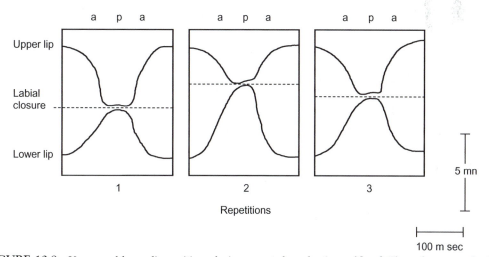

FIGURE 10.8 Upper and lower lip positions during repeated productions of [apa]. These data were obtained while the speaker clenched his teeth on a stationary bite bar that immobilized the jaw. From Abbs, J. H. (1986). Invariance and variability in speech production: A distinction between linguistic intent and its neuromotor implementation. In J. S. Perkell & D. H. Klatt (Eds.), Invariance and variability in speech processes (pp, 202–219). Hillsdale, NJ: Erlbaum. With permission.

Several additional points should be made in connection with the relative-position hypothesis. First, although we have noted the importance of relative spatial positions, other variables also seem to be represented as coordinated articulatory goals. For example, the relative velocities of the upper and lower lip may be coordinated as well. Relative lip velocities have been found to co-vary in the production of sounds for which proper relative velocities are important (Hasegawa, McCutcheon, Wolf, & Fletcher, 1976).

Second, the achievement of proper relative positions among articulators seems to be computed very rapidly, enabling the system to compensate almost immediately for perturbations within the speech apparatus (Lindblom & Sundberg, 1971). For example, Abbs, Gracco, and Cole (1984) found that within 20–30 ms of the sudden application of a downward load on the lower lip, there was a greater than usual descent of the upper lip, provided the utterance being produced demanded bilabial closure (see Figure 10.9). Compensations for unexpected disruptions are widespread in the vocal system. They occur in naive subjects, even if subjects are told not to compensate and even if the disruptions are introduced after movement has begun. They also occur in remote articulatory sites if the compensation is adaptive for the current acoustic target (Kelso, Vatikiotis-Bateson, Tuller, & Fowler, 1984).

A third comment about the relative-position hypothesis is that it reflects a general tendency of the motor system to achieve motor equivalence—"the capacity of a motor system to achieve the same end product with considerable variation in the individual components that contribute to them" (Hughes & Abbs, 1976, p. 199). Speaking and singing demand this capacity as much as any other motor activity. Apart from speaking with a pipe in one's mouth, people can speak while eating, while enduring extra weight on their chests, with lesions in areas of the spinal cord that cause paralysis in some respiratory muscles, and following the loss of teeth or the addition of orthodontic braces (Abbs, 1986).

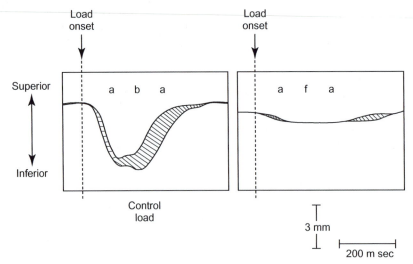

FIGURE 10.9   Responses of the upper lip to unexpected downward loads applied to the lower lip. The upper lip descends more than normally during production of [aba], which requires bilabial closure, but not during production of [afa], which does not. From Abbs, J. H. (1986). Invariance and variability in speech production: A distinction between linguistic intent and its neuromotor implementation. In J. S. Perkell & D. H. Klatt (Eds.), Invariance and variability in speech processes (pp, 202–219). Hillsdale, NJ: Erlbaum. With permission.

It is interesting that one of the main sources of evidence for motor equivalence in speech production—the finding that the lips tend to reach correct relative positions when one lip is pulled down suddenly (see above)—has been replicated for the fingers. In a pinching task, where one finger was unexpectedly pulled back as the other finger approached it, the response of the other finger was to cover a greater distance than usual, as needed to achieve finger contact (Abbs, Gracco, & Cole, 1984). Here again, the motor system manages to achieve a functionally defined goal (bringing the fingers together) despite sudden impediments.

Another context in which this principle is seen to operate is in the arm. Reflex compensations at the elbow following perturbation of the whole arm are consistent with the goal of maintaining desired joint torques rather than of maintaining any intrinsic muscle parameters such as muscle length or tension (Lacquaniti & Soechting, 1984).

A Mechanism for Relative Positioning

What mechanism might achieve this sort of motor equivalence? Figure 10.10A shows a simple pulley system that serves as a metaphor for the two lips. The weights on either end of the pulley represent the upper and lower lips. Because the weights are connected, when one of them is pulled in one direction the other moves in the opposite direction. This has the effect of keeping an imaginary point, $p = u + l$, at a fixed vertical position between the two weights; here u is the vertical position of the weight corresponding to the upper lip, and l is the vertical position of the weight corresponding to the lower lip.

To achieve such a relation between the upper and lower lips, one can use mutual inhibition between their respective motor neuron pools. The inhibitory connection is only potentiated if the acoustic target requires achievement of a particular relative position—for example, if the speaker wants to produce a bilabial stop. A simple way for the inhibitory connection to work is for each lip to inhibit the other by an amount that is positively related to its distance from a resting position, assumed here to be where the lips are comfortably apart. Thus, as the lower lip reaches a higher position, it exerts a greater inhibitory effect on the upper lip. Similarly, as the upper lip reaches a lower position, it exerts a greater inhibitory effect on the lower lip. If the lower lip cannot go as high as it usually does—for example, if the lower jaw is suddenly pulled downward—it inhibits the upper lip less than usual, and so the upper lip can descend toward the lower lip more quickly than usual.

This scheme has been implemented in a computer program in which the lips (or representations of the lips) begin apart, and activation is provided to each lip in each time step until the lips meet, whereupon they return to their original position, halving the distance back to the original position in each time step. Prior to the meeting of the lips, each lip's position is simply the sum of the activation coming to it, plus its position in the previous time step, minus a proportion of the position of the other lip in the previous time step; the latter term corresponds to the inhibitory connection. If the lower lip gets stuck—that is, if it is not allowed to rise above some height before contacting the upper lip—the upper lip descends more rapidly than when the lower lip is allowed to cover its normal range (see Figure 10.11). Hence the upper lip appears to compensate for the perturbation applied to the lower lip, even though no active correction occurs. Happily, the lips meet at the same time regardless of whether they both move normally or one lip cannot move beyond a set position.

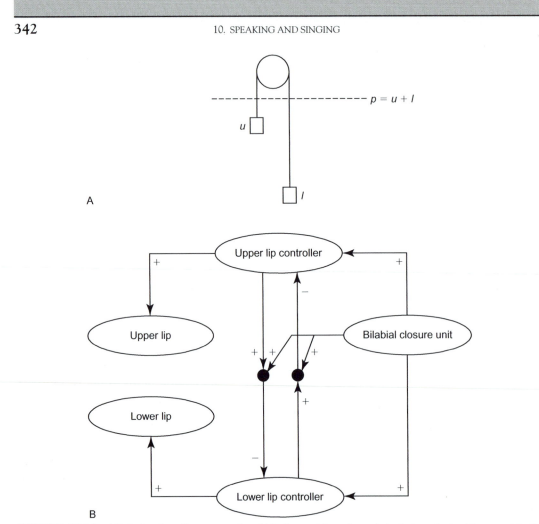

FIGURE 10.10   (A) A simple pulley system in which the position of a point p is invariant with respect to the positions of the upper weight u and lower weight l. (B) A circuit that can achieve similar invariance for the upper and lower lips. When the bilabial closure unit is turned on, it activates the upper and lower lip controllers as well as intermediate units (dark circles). Each intermediate unit is also activated by one of the lip controllers and has an inhibitory effect on the controller for the opposing lip. The inhibitory effect only occurs when the bilabial closure unit is on.

The simplicity of this model suggests that it may comprise a reasonable approximation of the biological mechanism used for relative positioning of the upper and lower lips. Note that the physiological channel for mutual inhibition is not, and need not be, explicitly specified in the model. The inhibition can be mediated by peripheral feedback or by centrally issued efferent commands. An important feature of the model is that it relies on a form of interaction that is seen at low levels of the motor system, for example, in reciprocal inhibition between muscle antagonists (see Chapter 3). Based on this observation, it is reasonable to suppose that even in achieving high-level goals like producing speech, the nervous system uses tried-and-true functional mechanisms.

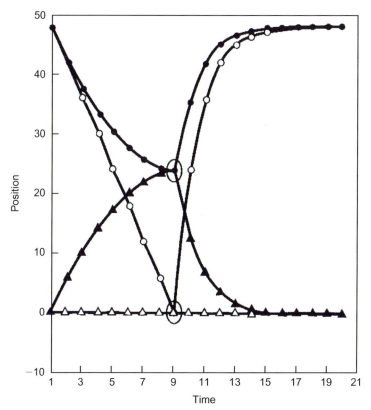

FIGURE 10.11 Theoretical results of the bilabial coordination network. When the lower lip (solid triangles) can ascend normally, the upper lip (filled dots) descends gradually. However, when the lower lip is prevented from ascending (empty triangles), the upper lip descends more rapidly (empty dots). The lips meet at the same time in both instances (ovals).

A Parallel Distributed Processing System for Coarticulation

The circuit shown in Figure 10.10B is one example of a class of models that is gaining considerable attention in cognitive science and neuroscience. Because all behavior derives from the workings of the nervous system, behavioral scientists have become increasingly interested in the neural circuits that allow for behavior. Not all such work requires "wet" physiology, however. The formidable complexity of the brain also invites the design of *possible* circuits, where evaluation of the effectiveness of the circuit is done analytically or through computer simulation, as in the model just described. In this section, we consider another such model (Jordan, 1986a, b), which was designed to account for three of the most basic phenomena of the production of speech: resistance to perturbations, parallel activity (exhibited in coarticulation), and serial ordering.

Coarticulation has already been mentioned in this chapter, where it was illustrated by referring to the tendency of the lips to round before lip rounding is absolutely necessary.

Another example is pre-nasalization—opening the velum in anticipation of a nasal consonant (see Tables 10.1 and 10.3). An example of pre-nasalization is opening the velum before
producing the nasal /n/ in "freon"; the velum opens even before the first syllable of this
word (Moll & Daniloff, 1971). Anticipatory velar opening only occurs in languages for
which nasalization carries no meaning. In English, opening the velum during pronunciation of "freo-" has no effect on the meaning of these phonemes, but in French it does, and
in French, velar opening does not occur much in advance of /n/. Coarticulation is therefore
language-dependent. By implication, it is not simply a result of the physical dynamics of the
speech apparatus or of other low-level aspects of speech control.

The neural network model developed by Jordan can account for these effects. It is made
up of units connected in such a way that their pattern of activation allows units linked to
muscles (output units) to bring about particular, desired actions. The starting point for
Jordan's analysis is the assumption that any action can be described as an n-dimensional
vector. The dimensions are simply independent characteristics of the action. In the case of
speech, the dimensions can be phonetic features, such as those shown in Tables 10.1, 10.2,
and 10.3: nasalized, affricate, sibilant, and so forth.

Suppose speech actions can be described in terms of three dimensions, a, b, c. Then a
series of three successive speech actions can be represented as

$$
\begin{vmatrix} a_1 \\ b_1 \\ c_1 \end{vmatrix} \begin{vmatrix} a_2 \\ b_2 \\ c_2 \end{vmatrix} \begin{vmatrix} a_3 \\ b_3 \\ c_3 \end{vmatrix}
$$

where the left column refers to the first action, the middle column refers to the second action,
and the right column refers to the third action. Suppose the vector $[a_1, b_1, c_1]$ defines the
first target action and the language being spoken is insensitive to variations in dimension C
when a_1 and b_1 take on the values desired in this case, that is, it doesn't matter whether the
value of C is $c_1, c_2,$ or c_3. The target vector for the first action can then be rewritten $[a_1, b_1, *]$,
where $*$ denotes an "indifferent" or "don't-care" value. An example of a don't-care value
might be the degree of lip rounding when one says "t" in English. The acceptability of "t" is
unaffected by lip rounding. Similarly, if the value of b_2 does not have to be specified in the
context of a_2 and c_2, the second target vector can be rewritten $[a_2, *, c_2]$. Finally, the third target vector can be rewritten $[a_3, b_3, *]$ if c need not be specified exactly in the context of a_3 and
b_3, just as it need not be specified exactly in the context of a_1 and b_1. Owing to the presence
of don't-care values in the target vectors, the values they ultimately take on can be chosen to
optimize the ease with which the other, constrained values are successively produced.

Jordan's method for achieving optimization is to rely on a network whose units work
in parallel and where the information coded in the network is represented through the
strengths of the connections among the units. A network of this kind is a *connectionist* system (Rumelhart & McClelland, 1986).

Jordan's connectionist system is shown in Figure 10.12. It has three types of units: output
units (mentioned above), hidden units, and input units. Hidden units are like interneurons
(see Chapter 3) in that they mediate input and output signals. They are used in Jordan's
model and in other comparable models to ensure nonlinear relations between input-unit

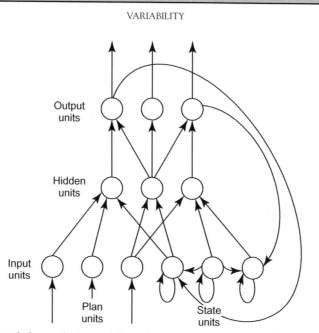

FIGURE 10.12 Network for producing serially ordered speech output. From Jordan, M. I. (1986a). Attractor dynamics and parallelism in a connectionist sequential machine. In C. Clifton, Jr. (Ed.), Proceedings of the 8th Annual Meeting of the Cognitive Science Society, (pp. 531-545). Hillsdale, NJ: Lawrence Erlbaum Associates. With permission.

and output-unit signal strengths. Input units represent the plan to be carried out as well as the current state of the output units. In Jordan's model, disparities between desired outcomes, specified by the plan units, and actual outcomes, produced by output units, are reduced through a method called *back propagation*. When the first target action is $[a_1, b_1, *]$, no alterations are made for the third dimension because the produced value of that dimension, dimension C, does not matter (its value is $*$). However, on the next time step, when $[a_2, *, c_2]$ is the target action, back propagation makes alterations on dimension C so the desired value, c_2, can be produced. The error reduction at this time generalizes to the previous time step, so the value c_2, needed at time 2, tends to be anticipated at time 1, when the target value for dimension C is $*$. Similarly, the value b_3, which is needed at time 3, comes to be anticipated at time 2, when the target value for dimension B is $*$.

What sets this model apart from previous models of coarticulation is that the selection of values is done automatically, without an intelligent overseer. The selection occurs entirely through partial activation of the units corresponding to the don't-care values. Partial activation allows for generalization across time, so the values that were initially unconstrained end up being influenced by values that are required later. The result of the interactions is coarticulation, and the coarticulation generated with the network is similar to what is actually observed. The model predicts forward as well as backward coarticulation effects—that is, effects of preceding as well as forthcoming utterances, as observed in natural speech. Similar effects have been observed as well as in reaching and grasping (Rosenbaum, Cohen, Jax, van der Wel, & Weiss, 2007).

Jordan's work represents an important advance in our understanding of speech production and motor control generally. It shows how a relatively simple network can achieve complex, planned behavior. The model also recasts phonetic features as constraints to be satisfied by the production system, rather than *a posteriori* descriptions of behavior, as in classical phonological theory (Chomsky & Halle, 1968).

HIGH-LEVEL CONTROL OF SPEECH

The discussion so far has been restricted to the production of individual phonemes. Now let us turn to the question of how the various phonemes of succeeding words are selected and ordered. What mechanisms regulate the serial ordering of words, phrases, and the sentences of which they are a part? Research on this question has relied extensively on speech errors, occurring either in spontaneous conversation or in specially designed word games.

Word Games

Pig Latin is a familiar example of a word game. Speakers of Pig Latin transfer the initial consonant or consonant cluster of a word to the end of the word and add an "ay" sound after that. Thus, "scram" becomes "amscray," "truck" becomes "ucktray," and so on. Being able to carry out these transformations indicates the cognitive availability of individual phonemes and phoneme clusters (Halle, 1962). Because it is ungrammatical in Pig Latin to say "cramsay" instead of "amscray" when the root word is "scram," the phoneme cluster is implicated as a distinct functional unit in the representation of speech.

Another example of a word game that reveals the psychological reality of phonemes and phoneme clusters is backward talking (Cowan, Braine, & Leavitt, 1985). People who can talk backward do not simply reverse the order of normal articulatory commands, as if they were running a tape recorder in reverse. Rather, they reverse the sounds within individual syllables, proceeding from one syllable to the next either in the forward direction or in the backward direction, depending on the individual speaker. A backward-talking speaker who produces syllables in the forward direction might transform the sentence "I can talk backward" into "I nac kawt cabdraw." One who produces syllables in the backward direction might say "Cabdraw kawt nac I." An important feature of the speech of backward talkers is that reversed phonemes rarely cross syllable boundaries. Thus "backward" becomes "drawcab" rather than "drawk-ab." This outcome provides evidence for the psychological reality of syllables (Treiman, 1983).

Backward speech also reveals that stress is represented independently of phonemes. Backward talkers usually maintain the temporal ordering of stress relations within a word, even if this alters the original mappings of stresses to syllables within the word. Thus, the un "*con*trast" is usually reversed as "*tsart*noc" rather than "tsart*noc* (Cowan et al., 1985); the stressed syllables are italicized. Maintaining the temporal ordering of stress sug- t stress patterns have the status of autonomous segments in the mind of the speaker. nappings of stresses to phonemes is altered in successive productions of the pho- dramatic slowing of speech production rates, as discussed in Chapter 4 in connection with the parameter remapping effect (Rosenbaum, Weber, Hazelett, & Hindorff, 1986). A related phenomenon was described for handwriting in Chapter 8.

Laboratory Studies of Speaking Speed

Whereas Pig Latin and backward talking are word games that people play on their own, other word games or game-like tasks involving words have been devised specifically for laboratory purposes. These tasks have yielded results complementary to those just considered. For example, subjects in one study (Gordon & Meyer, 1987) learned to associate different four-syllable utterances with different stimuli (Figure 10.13). On each experimental trial, one stimulus was presented, and then, with high probability, either that same stimulus was presented or, with lower probability, one of the other stimuli was presented. Subjects were supposed to produce the utterance designated by the second stimulus as quickly as possible. This meant it was adaptive for the subjects to become highly prepared for the utterance designated by the first stimulus.

The reaction time to say, or begin saying, the test utterance was shortest when it matched the initially prepared utterance, suggesting that subjects did indeed prepare to say the utterance associated with the first signal. In addition and more importantly, when the test utterance did not match the initially prepared utterance, reaction times were shorter when the two utterances had the same hierarchical syllable organization than when they did not. For example, if the initially prepared sequence was "bee-bay-bah-boo," subjects were quicker to say "bah-boo-bee-bay" than to say "bah-bay-boo-bee." The first of these test sequences

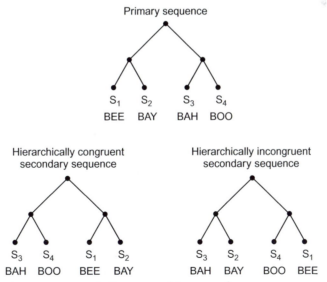

FIGURE 10.13 A primary sequence of utterances and two secondary sequences, one of which is hierarchically congruent with the primary sequence, the other of which is incongruent with the primary sequence. From Gordon, P. C. & Meyer, D. E. (1987). Hierarchical representation of spoken syllable order. In A. Allport, D. MacKay, W. Prinz, & E. Scheerer (Eds.), Language Perception and Production (pp. 445–462). London: Academic Press. With permission.

("bah-boo-bee-bay") is hierarchically congruent with the initially prepared sequence; it simply reverses the order of the first and second syllable pairs. The second test sequence ("bah-bay-boo-bee") is not hierarchically congruent with the initially prepared sequence; it reverses the order of the middle and outer pairs of syllables. The fact that hierarchically congruent sequences are faster than hierarchically incongruent sequences suggests that syllables and syllable pairs are functional units for speech. This conclusion corroborates what we saw earlier in connection with backward speech, and it fits with linguistic analyses of word morphology (word form) (Selkirk, 1982).

Why should syllables be hierarchically organized? One reason is that this form of organization makes it easy to modify words depending on linguistic context. For example, adding or deleting prefixes and suffixes takes advantage of hierarchical organization, as does word contraction (Selkirk, 1982). Another advantage of hierarchical organization is that it allows properties of an entire speech sequence to be specified in a single step. This point was demonstrated in an experiment (Rosenbaum, Gordon, Stillings, & Feinstein, 1987) in which subjects were asked to say one of two equally likely sequences depending on the identity of an auditory signal (see Figure 10.14). In one condition, the two possible sequences consisted of one syllable starting with a hard "g" sound: "gee" versus "goo." In another condition, the two possible sequences consisted of *two* syllables starting with a hard "g" sound: "geebee" versus "gooboo." In a third condition, the two possible sequences consisted of *three* syllables starting with the same hard "g" sound: "geebeedee" versus "gooboodoo." As seen in Figure 10.14, the time to start saying the designated sequence increased with the number of

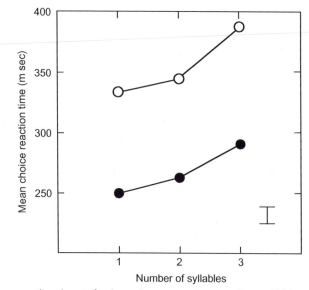

FIGURE 10.14 Mean reaction time to begin saying a one-, two-, or three-syllable sequence when the signal designating each sequence is either compatible (filled dots) or incompatible (empty dots) with its distinguishing vowel. From D. A. Rosenbaum, A. M. Gordon, N. A. Stillings, & M. H. Feinstein (1987). Stimulus-response compatibility in the programming of speech. *Memory & Cognition*, **15**, 217–224. Reprinted by permission of the Psychonomic Society, Inc.

syllables within it. Moreover, the mean choice reaction time for a sequence was affected by its overall compatibility with the signal. The choice reaction time for a sequence was shorter when the signal was compatible with its distinguishing vowel (a high-pitched tone for the "ee" sequence and a low-pitched tone for the "oo" sequence) than when the signal was incompatible with the sequence's distinguishing vowel (a high-pitched tone for the "oo" sequence and a low-pitched tone for the "ee" sequence). The additive relation between sequence length and signal compatibility suggests that the vowel characterizing the entire sequence could be specified in a single processing stage (Sternberg, 1969), as would be expected if the sequence were represented hierarchically and if a vowel assignment could be made for all the syllables at once, at the root of the tree.

The other major result from this study—that reaction time increased with sequence length—also accords with the hierarchical model because initiating a long sequence requires the traversal of many nodes from the root of the tree to the node corresponding to the first overt response (the left-most terminal node) (Johnson, 1970; Rosenbaum, 1985). Even when people are almost entirely sure they will have to produce a previously identified vocal sequence, the time to begin producing the sequence increases with its length (Sternberg, Monsell, Knoll, & Wright, 1978), as discussed in the chapter on keyboarding.

Speech Errors

The physical production of speech is only one stage in the act of conversing. Before the articulators are set into motion, the speaker must formulate a message to be transmitted, the message must be put into words (if they were not already specified lexically), the words must be ordered, and a stress or intonation pattern must be selected. How these functions are achieved before speech is produced has been addressed through the analysis of speech errors. A speech error is an "unintended, nonhabitual deviation from a speech plan" (Dell, 1986, p. 284). Speaking backward is not a speech error, because it is an intended departure from normal speech. Backward speakers do not make the mistake of unintentionally speaking in reverse (Cowan et al., 1985). No case of unintended reverse speaking has been reported in the literature, at least to the best of the author's knowledge.

One of the first analyses of speech errors was provided by Sigmund Freud (1901), who argued that mistakes in speaking express pent-up, unconscious thoughts, many of which are sexual in nature—hence the famous Freudian slip. An example of a Freudian slip would be the following. A person serving as a subject in a psychology experiment is supposed to read aloud nonsense syllables such as "bine foddy." The subject happens to be tested by an attractive, provocatively attired, experimenter. Under this condition, there is a good chance the subject might mistakenly say "fine body" instead of "bine foddy" (Motley, 1980). Such an error would suggest that Freud's theory is correct in some instances. However, because errors of this kind are not inevitable, people are capable of editing what they would otherwise say, albeit imperfectly.

Not all editing of speech is as sexy as Freud argued. Editing also applies, or has been thought to apply, to the work-a-day process of determining the features of ordinary speech. A source of evidence for such basic editing is the observation that verbal slips contain fewer nonwords than words. Baars, Motley, and MacKay (1975) offered evidence for this process by presenting subjects with lists of words, one at a time, to be read silently. The word

RESPOND was presented at some unpredictable point in the sequence, at which time the subject was supposed to say aloud the last word pair presented before the RESPOND prompt. A representative list follows. You should read it as subjects in the Baars et al. (1975) experiment did, covering all the words with a card and sliding the card down the column, word pair by word pair, reading each word pair silently until you come to the word RESPOND, whereupon you should say aloud the last word pair you read. Go ahead.

ball doze
bash door
bean deck
bell dark
darn bore
RESPOND.

Did you say "barn door" rather than "darn bore"? This error occurred on 30% of the trials in the Baars et al. (1975) experiment. If you made this error, or were strongly tempted to do so, you fell prey to a phonological bias to begin the first word with a "b" and the second word with a "d."

Now repeat the procedure with the following list:

big dutch
bang doll
bill deal
bark dog
dart board
RESPOND.

By the time you reached the final pair in this list, you may have again had a phonological bias to start the first word with a "b" and the second word with a "d." Had this bias been realized, you would have said "bart doard." But you probably did not make this error. In the experiment of Baars et al. (1975) it occurred only 10% of the time. Presumably "bart" and "doard" were not produced because they are nonwords, whereas "darn" and "bore," the two error terms in the previous list, are words. The fact that people are more likely to err with words than with nonwords was taken by Baars et al. (1975) to suggest that people edit their speech before producing it. Nonwords are less likely to arise than words in the speaker's mind, so less editing is needed to suppress them.

The latter statement implies that some of the factors contributing to speech errors and their prevention are not Freudian, in the sense of representing suppressed libidonal (sexual) urges. Since many, and perhaps most, speech errors do not pertain to sexual themes, influences of the sort that Freud wrote about are not the only ones that cause slips of the tongue. The generally accepted position among psycholinguists is that speech errors derive from mistakes in the otherwise normal workings of the speech planning and production process. If one accepts this view, the study of speech errors can be embraced as a tool for investigating the normal organization of speech planning and production.

Table 10.4 presents the major types of speech errors that have been recorded in spontaneous conversations. The list is not exhaustive, but it illustrates the variety and regularity of errors that have been documented. There are several noteworthy features of this list. First, a number of linguistic units are involved: entire words, morphemes (the meaning-bearing parts of words, such

TABLE 10.4   Types of Speech Errors[a]

Type	Examples	Unit involved
Sound errors		
Misordering		
Substitution		
Exchange	York library → lork yibrary	Phoneme
	Spill beer → speer bill	Rime constituent
	Snow flurries → flow snurries	Constant cluster
	Clear blue → glear plue	Feature
Anticipation	Reading list → leading list	Phoneme
	Couch is comfortable → comf is …	Syllable or rime
Preservation	Beef noodle → beef needle	Phoneme
Addition		
Anticipatory addition	Eerie stamp → steerie stamp	Consonant cluster
Perseveratory addition	Blue bug → blue blug	Phoneme
Shift	Black boxes → back bloxes	Phoneme
Deletion	Sample state → same sate	Phoneme
Noncontextual errors	Department → jepartment	Phoneme
(substitution, addition,	Winning → winnding	keywords
deletion)	Tremendously → tremely	Syllable
Morpheme errors		
Misordering		
Substitution		
Exchange	Self-destruct instruction → self-instruct de …	Prefix
	Thinly sliced → slicely thinned	Stem
Anticipation	My car towed → my tow towed	Stem
Preservation	Explain…rule insertion → …rule exsertion	Prefix
Shift	G ets it → get its	Inflectional suffix
Addition	Dollars deductible → dedollars deductible	Prefix
	Some weeks → somes weeks	Inflectional suffix
Noncontextual errors	Conclusion → concludment	Derivational suffix
(substitution, addition,	To strain it → to strained it	Inflectional suffix
deletion)	He relaxes → he relax	Inflectional suffix
Word errors		
Misordering		
Substitution		
Exchange	Written a letter to my mother → writing a mother to my letter	Noun
Anticipation	Sun is in the sky → sky is in sky	Noun
Preservation	Class will be about discussing the test → …discussing the class	Noun
Addition	These flowers are purple → these purple flowers are purple	Adjective
Shift	Something to tell you all → something all to tell you	Quantifier
Noncontextual errors		
Substitution	Pass the pepper → pass the salt	Noun
	Liszt's second Hungarian rhapsody → second Hungarian restaurant	Noun
Blend	Athlete/player → athler	Noun
	Taxi/cab → tab	Noun
Addition	The only thing I can do → the only thing	Quantifier
Deletion	I just wanted to ask that → I just wanted to that	Verb

[a]From Dell, 1986.

as the final s that indicates a plural ending), phonemes, consonant clusters, and vowel-consonant combinations. Second, the errors reflect different sorts of disruptions, including misorderings (for example, anticipations, perseverations, shifts, and deletions) and "noncontextual errors" in which the exact source of error is hard to identify (for example, blends). A third feature of the errors is that for those involving interacting units, such as word exchanges (Writing a letter to my mother→Writing a mother to my letter) or phoneme exchanges (York library→Lork yibrary), the units participating in the interaction generally belong to the same linguistic category. For example, they are both words (mother and letter) or both phonemes (L and y).

Researchers who model speech production by studying speech errors have attempted to account for such regularities. An assumption common to virtually all the models (Dell, 1986; Fromkin, 1971; Garrett, 1975; Levelt, 1989; Shattuck-Hufnagle, 1979) is that there are distinct levels of representation for forthcoming sentences. These levels have been referred to as the *semantic* level, the *syntactic* level, the *morphological* level, the *phonological* level, the *phonetic* level, and the *motor* level. The semantic level codes the linguistic meaning of the message the speaker intends to transmit, which may originate prelinguistically, in the mysterious "language of thought." The syntactic level codes word order and other factors affected by the grammatical relation between words. The morphological level codes the details of word formation, such as the presence of prefixes and suffixes. The phonological and phonetic levels break words and their affixes into phonemes and phones, respectively. Finally, the motor level permits the physical realization of the phonetic features that have been selected.

The models that have been proposed differ with respect to the way units are assumed to interact within and between these levels. At one end of the theoretical continuum are models that assume information passes only from high to low levels (Fromkin, 1971; Garrett, 1975; Levelt, 1989; Shattuck-Hoffnagel, 1979). At the other end are models that assume information passes from high to low levels and from low to high levels (Dell, 1986). Models of speech production also vary with respect to the way choices are made about the units to be produced. Dell's (1986) model assumes spreading activation among units, with the choice of units, and so the likelihood of choosing the wrong unit, depending on its level of activation.

An important feature of Dell's model is that it does not require an editing operation to account for the prevalence of word errors over nonword errors. Words are more likely than nonwords because of the pattern of excitation and inhibition among units within and across levels of the network. More traditional models, such as those of Fromkin (1971), Garrett (1975), Levelt (1989), and Shattuck-Hoffnagel (1979), assume that choices among units are entirely rule-governed though they are subject to error. In Garrett's model, for example, if someone says "She's already trunked two packs" instead of "She's already packed two trunks," the error is assumed to result from an incorrect assignment of words to previously defined, but as yet unfilled, word slots. Rules establish that the slots should be filled with words and that both words should be nouns, but the insertion of words into the slots goes awry.

Note that in the above error, the affixes—the -s from trunks and the -ed from packed—attach properly to the switched words. This argues that a distinct morphological level is accessed after syntactic processing has begun.

Phonological processing also appears to occur after morphological processing has been completed. The reason is that phonemes accommodate to new morphological environments. For example, suppose one makes the mistake of substituting the word "outs" for the word "runs" while describing a baseball game. This substitution requires a change in the "hardness" of the final s. The s in "runs" is pronounced like a z, whereas the s in "outs" is pronounced like a hard s. Because the pronunciation that occurs is correct when "runs" switches to "outs," the hardness of the final s is accommodated to the new phonological environment. An error like this suggests that phonological processing follows morphological processing.

BRAIN MECHANISMS UNDERLYING SPEECH

As the preceding discussion has been meant to show, even when the speech production system functions normally, it can occasionally give rise to speech errors. Speech errors that occur when the nervous system is damaged provide another window into the control of speech. If particular characteristics of speech are affected by damage to particular brain sites, one can infer that those sites play some role in controlling the speech characteristics that have been impaired. Additionally, if the impaired aspects of speech correspond to particular, hypothesized stages in the speech production process, one can go a step further and hypothesize that each of the stages is controlled by each of the damaged brain centers.

Over a century ago, a young French neurologist named Paul Broca made an important contribution to the understanding of the brain mechanisms underlying speech. He performed autopsies on patients who had suffered from profound speaking difficulties during their lifetimes. Broca found that the patients' brains had damage to the anterior left temporal lobe. Broca relied on autopsies because when he did this work, in the nineteenth century, methods for localization of brain function, such as fMRI, were not yet available.

The area Broca discovered came to be called Broca's area, and the speech disorder he identified came to be called Broca's aphasia. The hallmark of Broca's aphasia is *telegraphic speech*. The patient speaks in short bursts, usually without function words (prepositions, conjunctions, and determiners). Broca's aphasia is not a disorder of motor control, for Broca's aphasics are able to produce the words that elude them in spontaneous conversation. For example, they can read aloud sentences such as "Two bee oar knot two bee" (Gardner & Zurif, 1975). Another indication that the expressive difficulties of Broca's aphasics are not due to problems with motor control per se is that they also have difficulty generating function words in writing or in sign language, so it is not simply physical output that is damaged in Broca's apahsia. Instead, it is the use of linguistic information.

Recent work on aphasia has focused on the detailed properties of the grammatical capabilities that Broca's aphasics and other aphasics lack. A major issue is whether Broca's aphasics have lost syntactic knowledge or instead have merely lost the ability to call up the necessary syntactic rules when generating speech. An important clue that they possess syntactic knowledge is that they can recognize ungrammatical sentences as such, even when the grammatical errors to which they are exposed deviate only subtly from correct usage (Linbebarger, Schwartz, & Saffran, 1983). Because aphasic patients can pass this test, it follows that they have not simply forgotten their grammar. Instead, they have difficulty implementing the grammar they have stored away for the overt production of language.

Scientists concerned with the neurophysiological control of speech production have adopted a model of speech production that consists of three main stages: planning, programming, and execution (Logemann, 1985). Disorders of planning are referred to as aphasias. Disorders of programming are called speech *apraxias*. Patients with speech apraxias are unable to produce orderly sequences of phonemes though they can physically produce individual phonemes or limited sequences of phonemes. Disorders of speech execution are called *dysarthrias*. Dysarthric speakers are unable to produce the articulatory gestures that allow for individual phonemes (Logemann, 1985). Speech can become temporarily dysarthric, as when one gets drunk and slurs one's speech.

The existence of these distinct kinds of disorders supports the view that there are distinct stages in the production of speech. Distinct areas of the brain have been linked to each type of disorder. Patients with speech apraxia usually have lesions in the secondary motor area, whereas dysarthric patients usually have lesions in the primary motor cortex or the part of the brain stem from which the oro-facial cranial nerves emerge (i.e., the nerves that innervate the mouth and face) (Keller, 1987). Stimulation of the primary motor cortex produces uncontrollable vocalization and slurring of speech (Penfield & Roberts, 1959). Stimulation of the secondary motor cortex produces syllable repetitions and hesitations (Keller, 1987).

As neat as this picture is, it is important to keep in mind that the primary and secondary areas of the motor cortex are not the only brain sites responsible for the programming and execution of speech. Brain stem nuclei are involved as well, and there is evidence that the basal ganglia, cerebellum, and other cortical areas also play a role (Gracco & Abbs, 1987). The complete picture of the brain's role in controlling speech production is therefore predictably complex.

One generalization about the brain's control of speech that has been known for at least a century is that the left cortical hemisphere is specialized for language in most people. Broca recognized this when he saw that most aphasics had damage to the left but not to the right hemisphere. His observation has been replicated many times, though it has also been recognized that left hemispheric control of language is more distinct for right-handed people, whose manual control is usually also centered in the left hemisphere, than for left-handed people.

One of the tantalizing questions raised by the discovery of brain lateralization for speech and manual control is whether it is unique to humans. Some of the most dramatic evidence that it is not comes from studies of the control of bird song.

BIRD SONG

Because people rely on speaking more than singing for everyday communication, more research has been done on speech than on song (but see Harvey, 1985; Sundberg, 1977). Much of the work that has been done on singing has concentrated on bird song. Bird song is an appealing topic for research, not just because of its aesthetic qualities, but also because one can determine how exposure to song at various points in the bird's life affects its ability to sing. For ethical reasons, comparable manipulations cannot be tried with people.

A number of intriguing findings have been obtained through this approach (Hinde, 1970). Work with the chaffinch, a common bird in Europe, has shown that it has a species-characteristic song consisting of several short phrases (see Figure 10.15A). Under normal conditions, very young chaffinches produce a kind of rambling song of indefinite length—a kind of melodic "babble"—which gradually approximates the species-specific song of the adult. Chaffinches reared in isolation develop only a rudimentary form of the species song (see Figure 10.15B), but chaffinches reared in groups develop somewhat more elaborate versions that turn out to be peculiar to the group in which they are raised (see Figure 10.15C). Chaffinches kept in isolation after being exposed to the song of their species but before they themselves can sing are able later to sing a fairly good approximation to the normal species song, but not a perfect rendition of it. On the other hand, groups of chaffinches kept together after being exposed to the species song but before they are able to sing, later sing the song perfectly. Chaffinches reared in isolation who are not exposed to the species song until after the first breeding season usually cannot learn the species song, but chaffinches reared in isolation who are exposed to the species song before the first breeding season usually can learn it. Finally, when chaffinches isolated from birth are exposed to taped songs that differ in various ways from the normal species song, their ability to learn the artificial song depends on

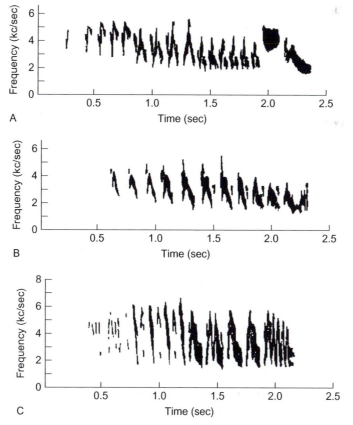

FIGURE 10.15 Song cycle of wild chaffinches (A), of chaffinches reared in isolation (B), and of chaffinches reared in small groups (C). From Hinde, R. A. (1970). The development of bird song. In K. Connolly (Ed.), Mechanisms of motor skill development (pp. 287–304). London: Academic Press. With permission.

its similarity to the species song. This is true even though all the notes in the artificial song are contained in the species song.

These results suggest that the acquisition of bird song depends on an interplay of innate tendencies, environmental conditions, and maturational factors. The role of innate tendencies is suggested by the fact that not all songs that chaffinches are physically able to sing are equally learnable. The role of environmental conditions is suggested by the importance of being exposed to the species song rather than some other song, and of being around other birds after the first breeding season. The importance of maturational factors is suggested by the fact that after the first breeding season, a bird that has never been exposed to a song can never learn to sing it—a true critical period.

The foregoing conclusions are qualitatively similar to conclusions of research on human language acquisition (Carroll, 1986). Children deprived of linguistic input are usually unable to recover from this deprivation if their first exposure to language comes only after puberty, though they have a chance of recovering from the deprivation if their first exposure comes before puberty. Additionally, children deprived of linguistic input who are in the company of other such children sometimes develop a language of their own that obeys many of the basic features of all human languages. Finally, the fact that all human languages may share a number of grammatical features suggests that there are genetic predispositions for the abstract form that human language takes (Chomsky, 1975). Given these similarities between the acquisition of human language and the acquisition of bird song, the brain mechanisms underlying bird song become especially interesting for those interested in human language acquisition. If the study of the bird brain can reveal how heredity, experience, and maturation affect the way birds learn to sing, it may also suggest how those factors affect the way people learn to speak.

In the late 1980's, pathbreaking work was done on the brain mechanisms underlying bird song by Fernando Nottebohm and his colleagues at Rockefeller University in New York City (Nottebohm, 1989). One of this group's notable discoveries was that bird song is primarily controlled in the left hemisphere of the bird's brain. This discovery was made in studies of the canary. The studies involved cutting a nerve—the tracheosyringeal (TS) nerve—that innervates the muscles of the syrinx (the organ for song). Cutting the *right* TS nerve had little effect on the birds' singing ability, but cutting the *left* TS nerve had a deleterious effect. Further work showed that the left TS nerve is controlled by a center in the left hemisphere of the brain. Thus, for canaries, as for humans, the left hemisphere is specialized for the control of vocalization.

Later work yielded an even more startling result. After identifying the left-brain center for bird song, Nottebohm and his co-workers studied the properties of that center during song acquisition. Surprisingly, the volume of the brain center varied according to the intensity of song use. In the spring, when male canaries sang frequently, the center was found to be large, but in the fall, when the same birds sang much less, the center was found to be much smaller.

That the center was involved in song learning became clear through several converging observations. Canaries with large song centers were better singers than canaries with small song centers. Female canaries given testosterone, a male hormone, learned to sing, which they otherwise do not do, and their song centers also grew larger than normal. Finally, male canaries that were castrated, and so were unable to produce testosterone, did not learn to sing, and their song centers failed to grow.

These observations led Nottebohm and his co-investigators to speculate that neurons in the song center might grow and die depending on the waxing and waning of testosterone. Proposing that new neurons grow in the brains of adult canaries represented a challenge to the prevailing view within neuroscience at the time, that new neurons cannot grow in adulthood. To challenge this view, Nottebohm had to prove that changes in the volume of the song center did not simply reflect changes in the size of already existing neurons. Through painstaking work, he and his group showed that neurons do indeed grow in the brains of adult birds.

This work was controversial, but over time the neuroscience community came to accept the idea that new neurons do grow in the adult brain, including the adult brains of humans (Miller, 2007b). The debate subsequently shifted from whether new neuron growth occurs to what its role is in the species under investigation, how and whether that role changes depending on the point in development when the new neurons appear, and how the tasks served by the new neurons are affected. Such work has raised the tantalizing possibility that people with aphasia, speech apraxia, dysarthria, and other impairments might be helped in new ways by the promotion or redirection of neural growth.

Meanwhile, research on the neural control of birdsong has taken flight. It has been discovered that a part of the brain of the zebra finch is devoted to innate babbling, whereas learned songs are represented elsewhere (Aronov, Andalman, & Fee, 2008). A mirror neuron system has also been found to play a role in birdsong learning in swamp sparrows (Miller, 2008), and a specific gene has been found to play a role in the capacity for avian song acquisition in the chaffinch (Chin & Veston, 2007). An especially interesting feature of the latter finding is that the gene thought to play a role in birdsong learning is the same one that may play a role in human language learning (Haesler et al., 2007). People lacking this gene have difficulty learning to speak, though their intellectual and other abilities are normal (Trivedi, 2001).

MOTOR RESONANCE

Earlier in this chapter we considered the motor theory of speech perception in connection with the variability problem of speech perception. The problem was that people hear speech sounds as invariant (belonging to the same category) even though the acoustic properties of the sounds give little hint of their invariance. We briefly considered the hypothesis that subtle motor activity aroused by acoustic input might explain the invariance of speech perception, but we saw that this proposal did not stand up to close scrutiny and that other accounts were necessary.

The motor theory has enjoyed a resurgence of interest, however, though the main focus of interest in the topic has shifted. Instead of focusing on whether motor activity aroused by speech input can explain invariance in speech perception, the focus has shifted to the more general question of whether motor activity is aroused by speech input and if so whether it plays a role in the processing of speech (Galantucci, Fowler, & Turvey, 2006; Massaro, & Chen, 2008).

Several lines of evidence have suggested positive answers to both questions. These sources of evidence have encouraged the belief that perception is affected by *motor resonance*, the tendency of perceptual input to arouse related motor activities. According to the idea that motor resonance is crucial for perception, the motor system resonates to perceptual input and this resonant activity in turn affects what one perceives.

An illustrative study, summarized by Saunders (2008), came from researchers who wondered whether people would hear a word differently depending on the stretch of their facial muscles. The scientists used a sensitive robotic device to stretch participants' facial muscles either in ways that conformed to what the muscles would do if they were involved in producing one word such as "head" or another word such as "had." While the participants' facial muscles were gently and painlessly tugged by the robot, the participants were exposed to single-syllable words such as "head" or "had" and were asked to indicate which word they heard. The participants were more likely to identify the signal as "head" when their facial muscles were pulled in the "head"-producing direction, and they were more likely to identify the signal as "had" when their facial muscles were pulled in the "had"-producing direction. The effects were small but statistically significant. Thus, the state of the facial muscles has some effect on what one hears, consistent with the principle of motor resonance for speech.

Another finding that supports the idea of speech motor resonance takes the form of the *action compatibility effect* (Glenberg & Kaschak, 2002). Glenberg and Kaschak asked what would happen if participants listened to sentences and made inward (toward-the-body) hand movements to indicate that the sentence was sensible, or outward (away-from-the-body) hand movements to indicate that the sentence was not sensible. A priori, there is no reason to expect the direction of hand displacement to have an effect, yet Glenberg and Kaschak found that it does. Participants were quicker to indicate that a sentence like "Open the drawer" was sensible when they made toward-the-body hand movements than when they made away-from-the-body hand movements. Conversely, participants were quicker to indicate that a sentence like "Close the drawer" was sensible when they made away-from-the-body hand movements than when they made toward-the-body hand movements.

These results are hard to explain with a theory of language comprehension in which the understanding of language amounts to nothing more than activation of "symbol nodes" in memory. Such activations may be necessary, but they cannot be the whole story given the action compatibility effect, which suggests that understanding language, or at least understanding language related to action, tends to elicit action tendencies. The action compatibility effect is consistent with the broad and increasingly popular view that cognition is *embodied*, that is, that cognition is largely about, and relies directly on, internal activation of what our bodies do in the physical world (Wilson, 2002).

Now a skeptic might say that action tendencies should only be aroused by a sentence if one has already understood the sentence, so it makes little sense to argue that motor resonance is essential for language understanding. Said another way, motor resonance cannot explain language understanding if it is triggered by such understanding in the first place.

An answer to this challenge is that language understanding is not a perfectly stage-wise process in which all the words of a sentence are identified one by one and then the words are put together to yield a suddenly understood sentence-as-a-whole. Such a theory is tidy but turns out to be ill-supported by data. Research on language understanding has shown that identification of individual words and the assembly of words into understood phrases and sentences is more of a free-for-all, with top-down as well as bottom-up processes at work, and with statistical predictions and other forms of relevant knowledge being used, including physical action tendencies (Spivey, 2007). The action compatibility effect, which has been replicated and extended by others (Zwaan & Taylor, 2006), suggests that physical action tendencies are easily aroused and do indeed play a role in language understanding.

SUMMARY

1. Speaking and singing are usually carried out for communication. Their most important output is acoustic. Speaking and singing have been studied in a wide variety of fields, including psychology, physiology, linguistics, engineering, and speech pathology.
2. Language is made up of words, which in turn are made up of phonemes (sound categories that convey meaning) and phones (sound categories that may but do not necessarily convey meaning). Allophones are distinct phones in a language that are not distinct phonemes, so they do not convey meaning. The elements making up and distinguishing phones are phonetic features.
3. Intonation, stress, and rate also distinguish speech signals.
4. When the same words are spoken at different rates, they are not uniformly slowed down or sped up. As speech speeds up, intonation flattens, extraneous syllables are eliminated, and vowels but not consonants shorten. Speech occurs more quickly than would be possible if each phoneme were prepared only after the preceding phoneme was completed. The articulators move in parallel and anticipate forthcoming phoneme requirements, a phenomenon called *coarticulation*.
5. Besides accounting for the production of phonemes and phones through coarticulation, a theory of speech production must explain why some speech sounds are universally absent. It must also explain how speakers and singers compensate for physical changes in the articulators, for example, while holding a pipe between the teeth.
6. Another challenge is to understand how speakers and singers coordinate vocal production and hearing, both when they learn to speak and when they engage in speaking. Delaying auditory feedback is a method that has been used to address this issue. Stuttering can be induced with delayed auditory feedback. Being deprived of auditory input as a result of deafness can lead to distortions in the way speech is produced.
7. The main topics covered in the chapter on speaking and singing are the vocal tract and articulatory dynamics, the relation between speech and hearing, network models of coarticulation and speech errors, brain mechanisms, bird song, and motor resonance. The last term refers to the tendency of perceptual input to arouse physical action tendencies that in turn affect the way the perceptual input is interpreted.
8. The vocal tract has three subsystems—the respiratory subsystem, the laryngeal subsystem, and the articulatory subsystem. Within the respiratory system, the

diaphragm and external intercostals promote inhalation, and the internal intercostals promote exhalation. The timing of activity in these opposing muscle groups is based on muscle feedback about the volume and change of volume of the lungs, exploitation of the physical mechanics of the lungs and associated machinery, and planning for the speech or singing to come.

9. The larynx, which lies at the base of the throat, serves four main functions: It regulates the characteristic pitch of the voice, it modulates aspiration (accompanying syllable-initial p sounds, for example), it is responsible for whispering, and it controls voicing. Voicing is vocal cord vibration achieved by creating a small distance between the vocal cords atop the larynx, causing them to "buzz" as air is driven through them while producing voiced consonants such as "v." The shape and flexibility of the larynx contributes to the quality of one's singing voice, and the size of the vocal cords, which can increase with the release of testosterone in puberty, can affect how low one's voice can go. Vocal frequency is also modulated by changing the stiffness of the vocal cords.

10. The rich variation of speech sounds depends on the structures above the larynx, including the pharynx (the cavity lying between the larynx and the mouth or oral cavity), the mouth, jaws, and lips, the nasal tract, and the velum (a movable flap connecting the nasal tract and oral cavity).

11. The pharynx allows for the production of some vowels but not others. Fossil evidence has led some investigators to suggest that the vowels produced by human adults have only been produced within the last 35,000 years. Other investigators have argued that speech as we know it has been produced for at least 2 million years.

12. Different vowels are produced by varying the position of the tongue body in the mouth. The main dimensions along which the position of the tongue body vary are up-down and front-back.

13. Different consonants are produced by varying manners of articulation (ways of constricting the air stream in the oral cavity) and places of articulation (locations where the air stream is constricted). It is possible to characterize consonants and vowels by assuming that each one has a distinct manner and place of articulation. The "standard theory" of phonology assumes that each consonant and vowel can be characterized by the presence or absence of features defined by particular place-manner combinations.

14. There is enormous variability in the way speech sounds are produced. The variability is so great that visual inspection of speech spectrograms makes it unclear how people can recognize particular consonants or vowels when produced in different linguistic contexts.

15. A proposed solution to the variability problem mentioned in 14 is embodied in the motor theory of speech perception. The idea here is that listeners recognize speech sounds because heard speech tends to arouse speech production tendencies. According to the motor theory, perceived invariance of speech sounds is due to invariance of articulatory commands. Such articulatory invariance has not been found, however.

16. A hypothesis about how speech sounds can be reliably produced assumes that the articulators aim for specific target positions, with the movement of the articulators toward the target positions being mediated by gamma motor neurons (see Chapter 3). Initial results were promising for this hypothesis, but later results were less so.

17. A hypothesis that was designed to solve the problems that the target hypothesis was designed to solve says that the speech production system attempts to bring the articulators to *relative* positions to permit desired acoustic targets. As predicted by this hypothesis, following external perturbations, there is rapid compensation that preserves relative positions needed for acoustic goals. When other sorts of relative positioning goals are required, as in finger pinching, similar results are obtained.
18. A possible mechanism for achieving invariant relative positioning relies on mutual inhibition between command centers for articulators whose relative positions must be coordinated.
19. A connectionist model with don't-care elements, proposed by Jordan, provides one model of coarticulation. The model anticipates features of forthcoming actions because of generalization to states whose exact values at earlier or later times are irrelevant in the language beyond spoken.
20. Pig Latin and backward speech provide evidence for the psychological reality of syllables and the autonomous representation of stress.
21. Laboratory studies of reaction times to begin speaking when a switch must be made from an initially prepared utterance to another utterance suggest that word syllables are represented hierarchically. Hierarchical organization provides a way of specifying characteristics of an entire word in a single processing step, as shown in reaction time studies where participants chose between verbal alternatives that were equally likely.
22. Speech errors have been used to infer the major stages in the planning and production of words, phrases, and sentences. People are unlikely to produce nonwords when making speech errors—a result that has been interpreted to mean that speakers edit forthcoming utterances, as Freud once proposed. An alternative is that with a parallel distributed processing system that has distinct tiers corresponding to semantic, syntactic, morphological, phonological, phonetic, and motor levels, the prevalence of word errors over nonword errors can arise without the need for editing.
23. Deficits in language production accompanying damage to the brain can be understood by assuming that distinct brain sites are related to distinct stages of language production. Three major types of language dysfunction accompany brain damage—aphasia (a language planning deficit), apraxia (a phoneme sequencing deficit), and dysarthria (a motor execution deficit). Speech is mainly controlled in the left hemisphere, at least for most right-handed individuals.
24. Because it is impossible, for ethical reasons, to vary children's exposure to language, birds have been exposed to the songs of their species in a wide range of conditions. The acquisition of bird song depends on an interplay of hereditary, experiential, and maturational factors. Human language learning also appears to depend on these three factors.
25. Investigations of the neural substrates of the acquisition and control of bird song have revealed several remarkable principles. First, the left hemisphere of the bird's brain is generally specialized for singing, as is true of the human brain's control of language. Second, new neurons appear to grow in the bird's brain when songs are learned. This finding upsets the belief, long held in neuroscience, that during adulthood new neurons do not form in the central nervous system. Mirror neurons seem to play a role in birdsong

learning, and a gene that seems critical for birdsong learning has also been implicated in the learning of human language.

26. Heard speech tends to arouse physical action tendencies, which in turn affects what one hears, a phenomenon called *motor resonance*. One speech-related demonstration of motor resonance is that the state of one's facial muscles has some effect on what one hears. Another is that people can indicate their understanding of sentences more rapidly if their physical responses are compatible with actions described by the sentences than if their physical responses are not compatible with actions described by the sentences (the action compatibility effect). These phenomena are consistent with the notion of embodied cognition, the idea that cognition is largely about, and relies directly on, mental activation of what our bodies can do in the physical environment.

Further Reading

Houde and Jordan (1998) described adaptation to perturbed speech feedback akin to adaptation to perturbed visual feedback via prisms.

Two topics that were not treated here in much detail though they are relevant to speech and singing are language learning and the diagnosis and treatment of speech disorders. Coverage of the first topic can be found in journals such as *Journal of Child Language* and texts such as Hoff (2009) and Hoff and Shatz (2007). Coverage of the second topic can be found in journals such as *Journal of Speech and Hearing Disorders* and *Journal of Speech and Hearing Research* and in texts such as Duffy (2005).

For an erudite review of the recent literature on speech motor control, see Fowler (2007). An important point in this review is that recent analyses of speech errors have gone beyond making diary entries about heard vocal mistakes. Detailed analyses of speech acoustics and articulation have done much to enrich and, to some extent challenge, characterizations of speech errors and their underlying causes.

For recent discussions of the motor theory of speech perception, see Galantucci, Fowler, and Turvey (2006) and Massaro and Chen (2008).

For more information about brain mechanisms underlying language production, see Guenther, Ghosh, and Tourville (2006).

For a review article that focuses on brain mechanisms underlying speech motor resonance, see Pulvermüller (2005).

A phenomenon described in this chapter—the tendency to hear a syllable one way or the other depending on how one's facial muscles are manipulated (Saunders, 2008)—is reminiscent of the McGurk effect, a tendency to hear a syllable different from the one presented acoustically when one is simultaneously shown the speaker's mouth producing a different syllable (McGurk & MacDonald, 1976; Wright & Wareham, 2005).

Journals where research on speaking and singing can be found include *Brain and Language, Brain, Neuropsychologia, Neuropsychology*, and *Journal of Memory and Language*.

Artificial speech recognition is a difficult technical problem, which is why you must interact with your computer via keyboard rather than via speech when you would probably prefer to speak. A classic text on this topic is Rabiner and Juang (1993). Current advances are described at *IEEE Transactions on Audio, Speech & Language Processing* (http://www.ewh.ieee.org/soc/sps/tap/).

C H A P T E R

11

Smiling

O U T L I N E

Physical Control of the Face	364	*Associations Between Expressions and Emotions*	371
Neural Control of the Face	366		
Control of the Upper and Lower Face	366	**Social Interaction**	374
Volitional and Emotional Control	366	*Imitation in Newborns*	375
Left-Right Differences	368	*Imitation in Married Couples*	375
Origins of Emotional Expression	369	**Summary**	377
Innateness and Universality	369		
Causal Connections Between Expressions and Emotions	370	**Further Reading**	378

No other stimulus is more significant to us as social creatures than the human face. Faces have been the subject of countless works of art, both literary and graphic. In everyday life, we look at faces to gather information about others' reactions. The capacity to pick up information from faces is present at a very early age. Newborns are more likely to look at faces than at other sorts of visual stimuli (Fantz, 1961; Kleiner & Banks, 1987), and newborns can discriminate facial expressions within the first 36 hours of life (Field, Woodson, Greenberg, & Cohen, 1982). Faces are also remembered well. People can recognize faces from high-school yearbooks virtually perfectly even if they haven't seen the pictures or the people depicted in them for 70 years or more (Anderson, 1985). No less remarkable is the fact that people can recognize others whom they haven't seen in years despite dramatic facial changes accompanying the aging process. This capacity may be possible because critical facial features remain invariant during aging (Todd, Mark, Shaw, & Pittenger, 1980).

Facial *movement* attracts attention as much, if not more so, than facial *structure*. If faces were static, they would convey much less information than they normally do, as any poker player knows. The mobility of the face allows people to express a wide range of emotions. Efforts to count the emotions expressed by the face have yielded differing estimates (Averill, 1975; Storm & Storm, 1987). On the other hand, there is little disagreement that there is a close link between facial expression and emotions. For this reason, analyzing facial expressions as a means of reflecting emotions is a natural way to approach the topic of facial control.

Although this chapter is called Smiling, that word is only one of many that will be discussed here. Several questions about the control of facial expression will occupy our attention. First, how are facial expressions physically achieved? Second, how are facial expressions neurally controlled? Third, why are particular facial expressions associated with particular emotions? Fourth, what can be learned about the control of the face by studying imitation?

Ironically, although perception of the face has been one of the most widely studied topics in visual perception (Humphreys & Bruce, 1989), the *production* of facial expression has been one of the least studied topics in motor control. The reason may be that research on facial expression has less obvious practical importance than does research on activities with direct physical impact on the environment, such as walking or reaching. Robot *smiling*, to name one possible expression that a robot might display, has received less attention. Curiously, even in fiction dealing with robots, the physiognomy of the robot has tended to be rigid, as if the idea of an expressive machine were too close for comfort. That sentiment is changing, however, as robots are being developed that can smile, look quizzical, and so on (Henig, 2007).

PHYSICAL CONTROL OF THE FACE

In approaching the analysis of facial expression, one of the first issues to be dealt with is how to describe expressions. One possibility is to use everyday terms like "happy," "sad," or "pensive" and to qualify these terms with intensity descriptors like "extremely," "mildly," or "deeply." This approach has been used in some studies (Sackeim & Gur, 1978), but it has proven unreliable because of imperfect agreement about the meanings of the terms. Not everyone knows what is meant by a "pensive" expression or an "extremely sad" or "moderately sad" look, for example. This coding scheme also lacks a description of the face itself, so it is not as useful as one might like for characterizing how the face physically conveys the emotions it does.

Another approach is to seek a detailed physical description of the face and its poses. This method requires elaborate scoring techniques (Blurton-Jones, 1971; Ekman & Friesen, 1975). As many as 44 expressions have been identified (Ekman & Friesen, 1975). It has also been found that some expressions last for minutes at a time whereas others are fleeting, lasting no more than 40 ms (Ekman & Friesen, 1975).

Because facial expressions depend on facial musculature, another method that has been used to characterize facial activity is to describe the activity of the musculature itself, relying on electromyography (EMG) (see Figure 11.1). It has been assumed since Darwin (1872/1965) that there is a close correspondence between facial expressions and the muscles that produce them. Electromyographic recordings have helped confirm this assumption. The recordings have shown that some expressions are produced by many muscles, whereas other expressions are produced by just one muscle. Raising the eyebrows is achieved with two branches

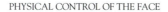

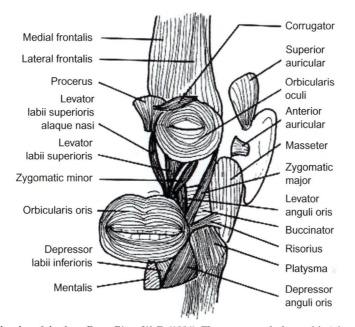

Medial frontalis

Lateral frontalis

Procerus

Levator
labii superioris
alaque nasi

Levator
labii superioris

Zygomatic minor

Orbicularis oris

Depressor
labii inferioris

Mentalis

Corrugator

Superior
auricular

Orbicularis
oculi

Anterior
auricular

Masseter

Zygomatic
major

Levator
anguli oris

Buccinator

Risorius

Platysma

Depressor
anguli oris

FIGURE 11.1 Muscles of the face. From Rinn, W. E. (1984). The neuropsychology of facial expression: A review of the neurological and psychological mechanisms for producing facial expressions. Psychological Bulletin, 95, 52–77. With permission.

of a single muscle, the *frontalis* (Rinn, 1984), but lowering the eyebrows is produced by the collective action of three muscles—the *corrugator*, the *procerus*, and the *depressor supercilii* (part of the orbicularis oculi). In general, a given expression can be produced by one or more muscles, and a given muscle can be involved in conveying one or more expressions.

The analysis of facial muscle activity also provides a way of determining what occurs when a facial expression appears to be a mixture of different expressions—for example, when one tries to conceal sadness with a "brave smile." The *zygomatic major* is responsible for smiling, whereas the *depresser anuli oris* is responsible for down-turning the mouth during sadness. When clear smiling or pouting occurs, there is clear activity of only the *zygomatic major* or *depresser anuli oris*, respectively, but when a "brave smile" is made, both muscles are active (Ekman, Friesen, & O'Sullivan, 1988; Oster & Ekman, 1978).

Electromyography is also useful for clinical purposes. It has been shown that the facial muscles are selectively active when different emotions are induced, even when the face as a whole reveals little or nothing about the patient's emotional state. In one study, patients who were instructed to imagine a happy scene showed increased EMG activity in the muscles normally associated with happy expressions—the *depressor angular oris*, the *zygomatic*, and the *mentalis* muscles. Instructions to imagine sad scenes resulted in increased activity of muscles normally associated with sad expressions (the *corrugators*), and imagination of anger produced increased activity of the *angular oris*, a muscle that horizontally widens the lips (Schwartz, 1982).

NEURAL CONTROL OF THE FACE

The nerve fibers that innervate the facial muscles comprise the seventh cranial, or *facial*, nerve. This nerve divides into three branches that supply the upper, middle, and lower face, respectively. When nerves to the face are unable to function properly as a result of disease, accident, or a genetic disorder known as Möbius syndrome (Miller, 2007a), the affected individual is incapable of changing his or her facial expression.

The facial nerve innervating the left side of the face and the facial nerve innervating the right side of the face originate in opposite sides of the brain stem. Within each facial nerve nucleus, the cell bodies of the facial nerve fibers are organized topographically in a manner similar to the motor homunculus of the cerebral cortex (see Figure 3.12). Distinct regions of the nucleus map onto the upper face, middle face, and lower face. The facial nerve nuclei are driven by higher brain centers, including the motor areas of the cerebral cortex as well as the extra-pyramidal motor system.

Control of the Upper and Lower Face

The upper and lower face differ in their capacity for fine movement. The upper face, encompassing the eyes and forehead, can move up or down but not from side to side. Many but not all people can elevate one eyebrow or the other, but few people can elevate one eyebrow and then the other (Rinn, 1984). Effectors in the lower face, by contrast, can move much more precisely. Thus, the mouth can move up, down, or sidewise, and virtually all people can move just one side of the lower face, as in pulling down the corner of the mouth while leaving the other side still (Rinn, 1984).

These behavioral differences between the upper and lower face can be traced to the way the face muscles are centrally controlled. The parts of the brain stem nucleus of the facial nerve that project to the eyebrows and forehead receive their direct cortical input from the contralateral motor cortex and from the ipsilateral motor cortex (Demyer, 1980). By contrast, the parts of the facial nerve nucleus that innervate the lower half of the face receive all their direct cortical input only from the contralateral motor cortex. Because each side of the lower face is controlled contralaterally, damage to one side of the brain disrupts the motor capacities of the contralateral mouth and chin. By contrast, because each side of the upper face is controlled by both sides of the brain, unilateral brain damage seldom disrupts the motor capacities of the eyebrows or forehead; the intact side of the brain continues to activate those parts of the face (DeMyer, 1980).

Volitional and Emotional Control

Figure 11.2 (left panel) shows an individual attempting to retract both corners of his mouth in response to a verbal command to smile. He could not follow this command. The right panel shows the same man smiling spontaneously in response to an emotionally satisfying event. The man had a tumor in the face region of his right motor cortex. The fact that he could smile spontaneously but not in response to a verbal instruction suggests a

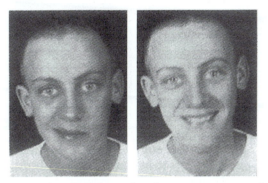

FIGURE 11.2 A verbally instructed smile (left panel) and a spontaneous, emotional smile (right panel) in a patient with a tumor in the face region of the right motor cortex. Reprinted from R.N. DeJong, 1979, The neurologic examination (4th ed.). Copyright © 1979. Harper & Row, Publishers. With permission.

fundamental neurological distinction between volitionally triggered and emotionally triggered facial expressions. The distinction cannot be attributed to different muscles, for the same muscles are involved in smiles that are feigned or genuine.

If the brain has two means of producing facial expressions—a deliberate and a nondeliberate or "emotional" means—one might expect to find a disorder in which patients can make facial expressions in response to verbal instructions but not in response to the patients' own emotional states. Such a syndrome would be complementary to the one just described. The complementary syndrome does exist. One symptom of Parkinson's disease is the so-called *masked face*. Patients with this disorder can move their faces in response to verbal instruction, but their faces do not move spontaneously in response to their own emotional states. Recall that Parkinson's disease is associated with damage to the basal ganglia (see Chapter 3). Masked-face syndrome suggests that the basal ganglia are involved in emotional expression.

Does it follow that emotional expression *originates* in the basal ganglia? No, at best one can say that the communication of emotions is *served by* the basal ganglia. It is known, in fact, that other areas are involved in emotional displays. Patients with *pseudobulbar palsy*, a disorder resulting from lesions of the pathways between the cerebral cortex and the brain stem, often exhibit dramatic emotional displays that are completely involuntary and at variance with the patients' emotional states. Pseudobulbar palsy may result from multiple sclerosis, stroke, or amyotrophic lateral sclerosis (also known as motor neuron disease). Figure 11.3 shows one such patient, a 61-year-old woman with amyotrophic lateral sclerosis, who laughed uncontrollably, though the emotions she reported while laughing were far from mirthful. Ironically, she reported being in pain during these episodes.

A final source of support for the distinction between deliberate and emotional facial expressions comes from the behavior of anencephalic babies. These babies have little or no cerebral cortex, but they often cry and show other emotional displays. In view of their age and lack of higher brain centers, their facial expressions may originate without conscious control, emanating instead from more primitive "emotional" sources (Rinn, 1984).

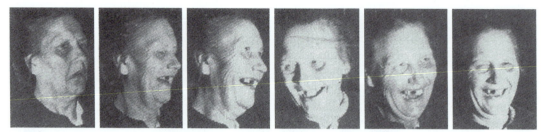

FIGURE 11.3   Uncontrollable laughter in a 61-year-old woman suffering from amyotrophic lateral sclerosis. The pictures show successive stages of laughing, which was completely involuntary and at odds with how the woman reported feeling. From Poeck, K. (1969). Pathophysiology of emotional disorders associated with brain damage. In P. J. Vinken & G. W. Bruyn (Eds.), Handbook of clinical neurology (Vol. 3). New York: American Elsevier. With permission.

Left-Right Differences

Having considered differences between the upper and lower face and differences between emotional and deliberate facial expressions, let us now consider one other distinction that has been drawn in the study of facial motor control—the distinction between the animacy of the left and right sides of the face. According to several authors, the left side of the face is more animated than the right (Bower, 1989; Moscovitch & Olds, 1982; Sackeim, Gur, & Saucy, 1978). What accounts for this left-right difference?

If one is willing to accept the premise, made famous in the popular press, that the left cerebral cortex is analytic while the right cerebral cortex is holistic and emotional, one can say that the left side of the face is more animated than the right side of the face because the left side of the face is primarily controlled by the emotional hemisphere, whereas the right side of the face is primarily controlled by the unemotional hemisphere. There are difficulties with this hypothesis, however. As pointed out by Rinn (1984), emotional expressiveness appears to be controlled by subcortical brain areas, yet only the cortex is thought to be functionally lateralized (Luria, 1973). Rinn also noted that the difference between right face and left face expressiveness is only observed in face-to-face interactions and in situations where people are asked to pose. Left-right differences are not observed when people are unaware of being watched (Ekman, Hager, & Friesen, 1981; Lynn & Lynn, 1938). The latter result makes it difficult to accept the hypothesis that there is a fundamental neurological difference between the emotional expressiveness of the left and right sides of the brain. If the left and right hemispheres truly differed in their capacity for producing emotional expressions, the differences would likely appear no matter how they were being studied.

How then can one account for the fact that the left side of the face appears more expressive than the right side of the face in face-to-face discussions and in poses? Rinn's (1984) answer was that the left hemisphere may be more effective than the right at inhibiting emotions. Behind this proposal is the assumption that the cerebral cortex inhibits impulses arising from lower brain centers, an assumption that is well grounded in neurology (Luria & Homskaya, 1970). An attraction of Rinn's hypothesis is that it accounts for the fact that left-right differences are more pronounced when people are aware of being observed than when they are not. When there is a cost to displaying emotions, the left cerebral cortex exerts its inhibitory influence, but when there is little or no cost in displaying emotions, the inhibition need not occur and the special inhibitory power of the left cerebral cortex is unseen.

ORIGINS OF EMOTIONAL EXPRESSION

Are facial expressions learned or innate? Because many behavioral functions mediated by subcortical centers are inborn (for example, breathing and sucking), and because facial control is largely subcortical, it would be reasonable to hypothesize that facial expressions are inborn as well. Added to this possibility is one that is even more intriguing. If particular expressions are innate, so too may be their corresponding emotions.

Innateness and Universality

How can one tell whether facial behaviors are innate? One way is to determine whether they are universal. If people all over the world display a facial behavior, this outcome would suggest that they share a genetic program for that behavior. Furthermore, if the interpretations of the behaviors were the same across all cultures—that is, if people everywhere saw a given expression as representing the same emotion—this outcome could be taken to suggest that the emotions are universal as well.

These possibilities were pursued by Paul Ekman and his colleagues (1975). In one study, they showed university students from the United States, Japan, Brazil, Chile, and Argentina photographs of people making facial expressions. The participants were asked to pick photographs from the set that best depicted each of several emotions: anger, happiness, fear, surprise, disgust, and sadness. There was a high degree of agreement among the participants. No matter which country they came from, they recognized expressions as conveying the same emotions.

The participants in this experiment shared a literate Western tradition, so their agreement may have stemmed from common experience rather than common genes. To address this possibility, Ekman and his colleagues studied people from isolated, nonliterate cultures in New Guinea and Borneo. The basic approach taken by the investigators was the same as before, though the method was modified to accommodate the illiteracy of the participants. Rather than have the participants read lists of emotion terms, Ekman and his colleagues read the participants brief stories concerning fear, anger, and happiness. They then asked the participants to point to the photograph that best depicted the emotion being described (Figure 11.4). The tribesmen showed virtually complete agreement about the best picture for each story. Furthermore, the pictures they selected for each emotion matched the pictures chosen by Western university students given the same task. Finally, when the tribesmen were asked to show what they would look like if they were protagonists in the stories, the expressions they adopted were later identified by American students as representing the emotions the tribesmen said they wanted to portray.

These results suggest that there is a universal basis for the expression of particular emotions. Nevertheless, one might raise one's eyebrows about this interpretation, wondering whether the universality of emotional expression results from the universality of human

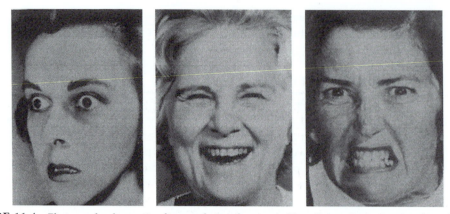

FIGURE 11.4 Photographs shown simultaneously to tribesmen in New Guinea during stories about fear ("She is afraid the pig will bite her"), happiness ("Her friends have come and she is happy"), and anger ("She is angry and is about to fight"). The pictures in the left, middle, and right panels were selected as the best for the surprise story, happiness story, and anger story, respectively. From Ekman, P. (1975). Face muscles talk every language. Psychology Today (September), 35–39. With permission.

experience. Consider a behavior that does not involve the face—breaking a stick with two hands. If people all over the world break sticks bimanually, it would be unnecessary to conclude that there is a genetic program for bimanual stick breaking. What is more likely is that the physical properties of hands and sticks are such that the behavior used to break sticks is independently discovered by people everywhere. Similarly, it is possible that all human cultures adopt the same expressions for the same emotions because of similar environmental or biological demands encountered by people everywhere.

One way to address this alternative hypothesis is to study the facial expressions of babies. If it turns out that babies display the same facial expressions as adults and if the conditions that elicit those expressions are similar to the ones that elicit the comparable expressions in grownups, this outcome would add weight to the genetic argument.

As it turns out, babies throughout the world smile when their needs are met, grimace when in pain, and, in general, make facial expressions like adults in similar circumstances. Even babies who are blind and deaf exhibit these patterns (Freedman, 1964; Goodenough, 1932), making it unlikely that expressions and their meanings are based entirely on experience. This conclusion is further supported by the fact that human expressions are functionally related to animal expressions, as Darwin (1872/1965) argued in *The Expression of the Emotions in Man and Animals*. Menacing looks in humans and animals are similar, as are submissive grins (Andrew, 1965). The human practice of raising the eyebrows may be based on the animal reflex of perking up the ears to unexpected sounds. The same muscles are involved in both behaviors, as you can demonstrate for yourself by looking in the mirror while you raise your eyebrows. When you raise your brows, your ears will rise as well.

Causal Connections Between Expressions and Emotions

Given that facial expressions are likely to have a genetic basis, the finding that there are distinct, primary expressions suggests that there may be genetically distinct, primary emotions. Ekman and Oster (1979) suggested that there are six such emotions: anger, happiness, disgust, sadness, fear, and surprise. To this list might be added two others: interest and shame (Izard, 1977).

Regardless of the exact number or identity of basic emotions (Averill, 1975; Storm & Storm, 1987), curiosity prompts one to wonder about the direction of causation between the expression of emotions and their experience. Do we smile because we are happy or are we happy because we smile?

William James, a founder of American psychology, suggested, along with a contemporary of his named Carl Lange, that emotional experience results from physiological feedback from one's actions. According to the James-Lange theory of emotion (for a review, see Lang, 1994), we do not smile because we are happy, but instead we are happy because we smile. The emotions we experience come from the movements we perform. We may smile when we have learned that something is associated with pleasant events, but the happiness we experience comes from the feedback derived from the movements made at the time, or so says the James-Lange theory.

A report by Ekman, Levenson, and Friesen (1983) provided evidence for this *facial feedback* view. Ekman, Levenson, and Friesen asked people familiar with facial posing (actors and scientists working on facial control) to make specifically defined facial expressions. In one condition, the participants were asked to relive experiences in which particular emotions were strongly experienced. In another condition, the same participants were asked to move particular facial muscles without reference to the emotions that would be signaled by them (Figure 11.5). The question was whether specific patterns of autonomic activity would accompany the expressions. The researchers reasoned that if the production of particular facial expressions gives rise to specific emotions and if those emotions are physiologically indexed by distinct autonomic changes, then specific patterns of autonomic function should be evident when particular poses are made.

The results confirmed the prediction. Measures of heart rate, electrical activity of muscles in the forearm, right- and left-hand temperature, and skin resistance showed distinct changes following different facial expressions. Heart rate was higher in anger and in fear than in happiness, and there was a larger decrease in skin resistance during sadness than during anger or disgust. Furthermore, many of these autonomic changes appeared when subjects made facial poses or relived emotional experiences. The magnitudes of the autonomic changes and the differences among them were more pronounced in the posing condition than in the relived-emotion condition; see also Niedenthal (2007).

These findings support the hypothesis that distinct patterns of autonomic activity are associated with distinct emotions. The findings also support the view that these patterns of autonomic activity can be elicited by distinct patterns of facial activity. Therefore, the results are consistent with the James-Lange theory. They also provide a defense against the argument that autonomic responses are not differentiated enough to allow for the range of emotions we experience (Cannon, 1927).

Associations Between Expressions and Emotions

Why are particular expressions and emotions associated as they are? Why do we smile when we are happy and frown when we are angry? Why don't we smile when we are

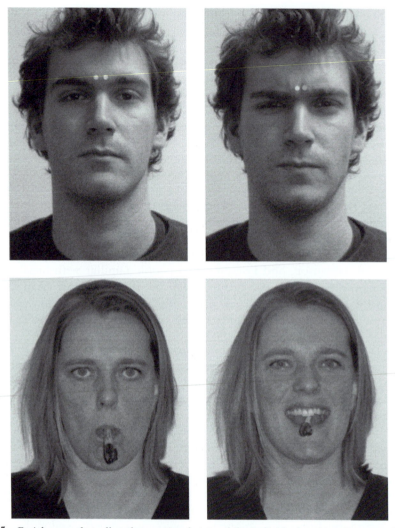

FIGURE 11.5 Facial poses that affect the emotional state of the individual making the poses. With golf tees affixed to his eyebrows, a poser is more likely to experience negative emotion if his brows are furrowed (top right panel) than if his brows are relaxed (top left panel). With a pen held between her teeth (bottom right panel), a person is more likely to experience positive emotion than if she holds the pen between her lips (bottom left panel). From http://www.sciencemag.org/cgi/content/full/316/5827/1002.

enraged or frown when we are ecstatic? The issue is complicated by the fact that some aspects of the expressions we make while experiencing one emotion are also made while experiencing other, incompatible emotions (Andrew, 1965; Konner, 1987). For example, we bare our teeth both when we smile and when we growl.

Darwin (1872/1965) tried to develop an answer to this question by appealing to his theory of natural selection. For Darwin, every emotional display serves, or once served, an adaptive function. Baring the teeth in response to threatened attack, for instance, was an adaptive behavior insofar as potential attackers tended to be scared off by ominous displays. The adaptive value of bared teeth is straightforward. However, the value of other displays is less transparent. What is the adaptive value of pouting, for example?

The need for a theory of emotional expression that had greater predictive power was recognized by an obscure French physician, Israel Waynbaum (1907), who proposed an entirely different view of the relation between emotions and facial activity. As reported by Zajonc (1985), Waynbaum proposed that different facial postures selectively affect the flow of blood to different parts of the brain. Furrowing the brows during intense concentration, for example, may allow more blood to reach the cerebral cortex, which in turn may allow for more effective thinking. The relation between brow furrowing and blood flow is mechanical. During intense concentration, the brows furrow, the frontalis muscle contracts (see Figure 11.1), the eyeballs become a little swollen, and the jawbone protrudes. These changes in the position of the face effectively put a tourniquet on the external carotid artery as well as the facial veins (see Figure 11.6). When these vascular pathways are closed off,

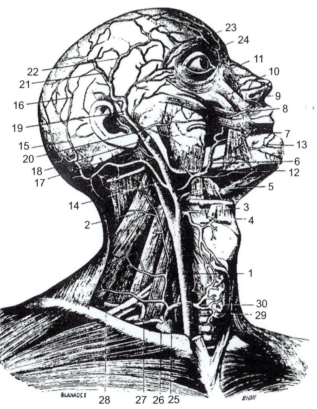

FIGURE 11.6 Circulatory system of the neck and head. The arteries relevant to the Zajonc-Waynbaum theory are (1) the common carotid, (2) the internal carotid, and (3) the external carotid. From Zajonc, R. B. (1985). Emotion and facial efference: A theory reclaimed. Science, 228, 15–21. With permission.

more blood is sent to the cerebral cortex. Perhaps for this reason, when people work hard on intellectual problems they engage in other, seemingly unrelated behaviors like rubbing the chin, chewing the fingernails, or scratching the head. These behaviors may divert more blood to the brain. Elevations of cerebral blood flow have in fact been observed during intense concentration (Ingvar & Risberg, 1967).

Whereas frowning may increase the amount of blood to the brain, smiling may have just the opposite effect. Smiling is partly achieved through contraction of the major zygomatic muscle, which causes the frontal vein to be gorged with blood, indirectly causing blood to be diverted from the carotid artery. Contraction of the corrugator muscles, which also occurs during smiling, blocks the return of blood. During smiling, then, blood flow to the cerebrum may be temporarily blocked, but when this block is released, there can be "a surge of subjectively felt positive effect" (Zajonc, 1985, p. 17). A consequence of the discomfort associated with the rising cerebral blood pressure brought on by laughter, which can viewed as a kind of intense smiling, is that tears may begin to flow, and tears can act as an anesthetic (Frey, DeSota-Johnson, & Hoffman, 1981). Laughing may be healthy, therefore (Cousins, 1984), because it provides a kind of "oxygen bath" for the brain. Sadness, on the other hand, reduces the amount of oxygen in the facial tissues. The cumulative effect may be a prematurely wrinkled, "care-worn" look (Zajonc, 1985).

Waynbaum's theory of facial expression is clever in that it relies on principles of anatomy to explain psychological data, and it provides a way of accounting for seemingly disparate aspects of behavior. Nevertheless, the theory has come under attack. One charge is that it is not disconfirmable (Fridlund & Gilbert, 1985). The mechanical effects of facial muscles on cerebral veins and arteries are intricate, so it is not always clear what effects particular facial expressions have on blood flow to various brain areas. Added to this problem, we do not have a complete understanding of the relation between brain activity and emotional experience. Even if one knows where blood flow in the brain is most intense, it is hard to say with certainty what emotion will follow. Finally, contrary to Waynbaum's theory, the absence of overt facial expression does not preclude emotional experience. Patients with facial paralysis report full-blown sadness, happiness, and other emotions though their overt expressions hardly change (Fridlund & Gilbert, 1985). This outcome is also problematic for the James-Lange theory of emotion.

SOCIAL INTERACTION

Because of the importance of facial expression in interpersonal communication, much of the work on the face has been conducted by social psychologists and students of nonverbal behavior. Some of the issues they have studied include rules for producing expressions in various social circumstances, differences between individuals in their expressiveness and ability to read others' emotional or cognitive states, and the ability to exaggerate or hide one's feelings (Feldman, 1982; Rosenthal, 1979; Siegman & Feldstein, 1987). Another issue that has been studied by social psychologists, which also bears on motor control of the face, is imitation, to which we turn next.

Imitation in Newborns

Field, Woodson, Greenberg, and Cohen (1982) showed that newborns can imitate facial expressions in the first 36 hours of life. Each of 74 babies was held by a model who made distinct facial expressions of happiness, sadness, or surprise (see Figure 11.7). A video camera recorded the model's face, and another camera recorded the baby's face. Later, independent judges viewed the videotapes of the babies, trying to determine which expression the baby was responding to—that is, what face the model was making. The logic of the experiment was that if babies can perceptually discriminate facial expressions and can also imitate those expressions, it should be possible to say which face the model was making based on the baby's expression. The judges could do this quite successfully. They guessed the model's expression with 76% accuracy; 33% was the level expected by chance.

The ability of the judges to tell what expressions the newborns were imitating implies that newborns can discriminate facial expressions and also produce them at will. From this outcome, one can infer that humans are innately equipped with mechanisms for perceiving facial movements, generating complex facial movement patterns, and coordinating the two.

Imitation in Married Couples

With the capacity for imitation present at birth, it is perhaps not surprising that imitation persists through the lifespan. A study by Zajonc, Adelman, Murphy, and Niedenthal (1987) suggests that life-long imitation may affect what faces look like. The impetus for this study was the folk wisdom that the longer couples are married, the more they look alike. Zajonc et al. tested this belief by showing subjects photographs of men and women, side by side. Unknown to the subjects, all the couples were married, and had been married for at least 25 years. The subjects' task was to rate the physical similarity of the two people shown in each stimulus display and guess whether they were married to each other. Only faces were shown in the photographs; the models' bodies were not revealed. Half the photographs came from the couples' first wedding anniversaries; the other half came from the couples' 25th wedding anniversary. The result was that the ratings of the physical similarity of the two members of each couple, and the ratings of the likelihood that the couple was married, were higher for the pictures taken after 25 years of marriage than for the pictures taken after 1 year of marriage.

Why did couples look more similar if they were married longer? Was it perhaps due to common eating habits over 25 years of living together? This seems unlikely, for when the photographed men and women were rank-ordered from heaviest to lightest, the correlation between men and women was higher for pictures taken from the 1-year photographs than for pictures taken from the 25-year photographs. Thus, perceived weight for husbands and wives was more similar when the husbands and wives had been married for a brief time than for a long time. The tendency to see greater physical similarity between older couples was also not due to the couple's experiencing the same climate or living conditions, for all the couples had similar geographic and demographic backgrounds.

The key to understanding the effect was the degree of happiness the couples reported. Zajonc et al. (1987) asked the couples depicted in the photographs to answer questions about

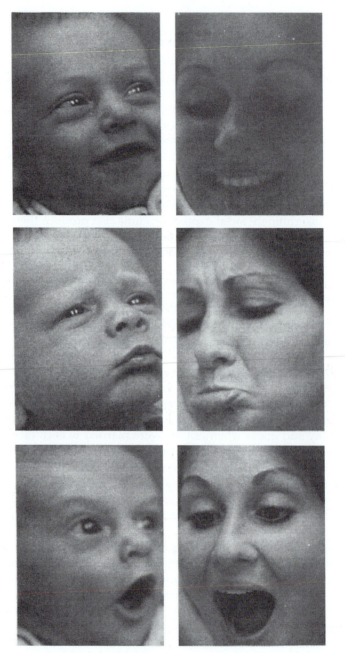

FIGURE 11.7 Imitation of an adult model's expressions of happiness, sadness, and surprise by an infant approximately 36 hours old. From Field, T., Woodson, R., Greenberg, R. & Cohen, D. (1982). Discrimination and imitation of facial expressions by neonates. Science, 218, 179–181. With permission.

their marriages. When Zajonc et al. compared the marital happiness data with the physical similarity data, they found that the higher the couple's reported happiness, the greater the perceived similarity of their faces. In addition, the more similar their attitudes, and the more often they shared worries and concerns, the more similar they appeared. Apparently, couples who are predisposed to share each others' joys and sorrows for long periods of time may tend to imitate each others' facial expressions, promoting empathy and, incidentally, facial similarity.

SUMMARY

1. Faces and facial expressions are recognized from birth and can be remembered for years. Movements of the face are especially important for conveying different emotions. Despite the importance of smiling and other facial activities for social communication, the control of facial expression has been one of the least studied topics in motor control.

2. Facial expressions have been described in terms of the emotions they convey, their detailed physical appearance, and their underlying electromyographic activity. Electromyography has shown that an emotional expression can be achieved with one or more muscles and that expressions can have short or long durations. Mixed expressions such as a "brave smile" are characterized by simultaneous activity of muscles that are usually involved in different, often conflicting, expressions. Imagining emotional states can produce subtle activity in the associated facial muscles.

3. The left and right sides of the face are innervated, respectively, by the left and right facial nerves. The cell bodies of the facial nerves are located in the brain stem and are topographically organized, primarily with respect to the vertical dimension of the face. Damage to the facial nerves due to disease, accident, or genetic disorders such as Möbius syndrome impairs the ability to change facial expressions.

4. The lower part of the face can be moved with greater precision than the upper part of the face. The likely reason is that the lower part of the face is controlled by one side of the brain whereas the upper part of face is controlled by both sides of the brain.

5. Facial expressions can be instigated in a deliberate or nondeliberate ("emotional") fashion. This distinction is suggested by the inability of some patients with motor cortex lesions to smile deliberately, by the inability of some patients with basal ganglia damage (Parkinson's patients) to smile emotionally, and by the inability of some patients with damage to the pathways between the cerebral cortex and brain stem (pseudobulbar palsy) to suppress facial expressions at odds with their reported emotions.

6. The left side of the face is usually more animated than the right. The asymmetry may be due to the greater inhibitory effect of the left compared to the right cerebral hemisphere.

7. Facial expressions appear to be genetically determined, as shown by the fact that they are displayed universally, almost always in the same emotional contexts, and in adults as well as infants, including newborns and infants who are both deaf and blind.

8. The James-Lange theory of emotion holds that we experience emotions based on sensory feedback from our movements. Thus, we are happy because we smile and

not the other way around. Evidence has been obtained in support of this *facial feedback* hypothesis.

9. Why do we smile rather than frown when we are happy? In general, what explains the associations between particular expressions and particular emotions? Two answers have been offered. One is that the links can be traced to behavior patterns from earlier evolutionary times. The other is that different facial expressions selectively affect the flow of blood to different brain areas. Each answer has something to recommend it, but neither is wholly satisfactory.

10. Newborns can imitate facial expressions in the first 36 hours of life. This implies that newborns can perceive and produce distinct expressions and can accurately reproduce the expressions they perceive.

11. Couples who have been married for long periods tend to look more alike than the couples who have been married for 1 year. The source of the greater similarity may be sustained imitation of partners' facial expressions.

Further Reading

For more information about the facial feedback hypothesis, see Niedenthal (2007).

For an investigation of facial expressions during lying, see Porter and Ten Brinke (2008).

For a study of interactions between seeing one's face being touched and feeling one's face being touched, see Serino, Pizzoferrato, and Làdavas (2008).

For a study of similarities between facial movement patterns in blind twins, see Peleg et al. (2006).

For a review of the cognitive neuroscience of emotional and social information processing by the human amygdala, see Adolph (2004).

For information about the neural mechanisms underlying visual face recognition and whether a specialized module exists in the brain for this function, see Kanwisher (2006).

To explore animation of robot faces, see http://www.softimage.com/products/facerobot/.

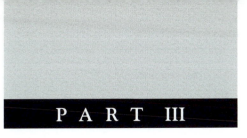

PART III

PRINCIPLES AND PROSPECTS

OUTLINE

Integration	379	**Theories of Human Motor Control**	397
Hitting Oncoming Balls	380	*Dynamical Systems Theory*	400
Golf Putting	383	*Optimization*	405
Walking and Reaching	385	**Innovations**	412
Enactive Cognition	386	*Genetics*	412
More Subtle Manifestations of		*Technology*	415
Cognition in Action	388	**Concluding Remarks**	418
Moving with Others	391		
Motion and Emotion	392	**Summary**	421
Individual Differences	395	**Further Reading**	423

We have covered a lot of ground in this book. After pursuing a general introduction and discussion of the core problems in the field, we reviewed the physiological and psychological foundations of human motor control. Then we discussed several activity systems, including walking, looking, and speaking. More remains to be done, however. In this final chapter, we will look at new lines of work that integrate different activities, we will consider new paths of investigation that integrate motor as well as non-motor activities, and we will glimpse new advances in theorizing about human motor control as well as relevant innovations in genetics and technology. The latter developments signal an exciting future for this already dynamic field.

INTEGRATION

One indication of the maturity of a field is its ability to apply its analytic tools to more complex, and so more ecologically relevant, topics. The field of human motor control has matured in this sense. Although investigators in the field continue to focus on relatively simple skills such as manual aiming (Chapter 7) or tapping at relatively steady rates (Chapter 9), there has also been a push to examine more complex skills. The range of such skills is impressive. Some tasks that have been studied recently include stone knapping (Biryukova & Bril, 2008), bouncing a ball with a tennis racquet (Sternad, Duarte, Katsumata, & Schaal, 2001), juggling (Beek, 1989; Beek & Lewbel, 1995), doing somersaults (Luis & Tremblay, 2008), skiing (Vereijken, Whiting, & Beek, 1992), shooting pistols (Arutyunan, Gurfinkel, & Mirskii , 1968), wielding objects (Carello & Turvey, 2004; Turvey, 1996), swinging hand-held pendulums (Amazeen, Amazeen, & Turvey, 1998; Turvey, 1990), playing golf (Jagacinski, Greenberg, & Liao, 1997), playing the violin (Baader, Kazennikov, & Wiesendanger, 2005), playing the cello (Winold, Thelen, & Ulrich, 1994), playing the guitar (Heijink, & Meulenbroek, 2002), flying airplanes (Gray, 2008), climbing rock faces (Boschker, Bakker, & Michaels, 2002), hula-hooping (Balasubramaniam & Turvey, 2004), and catching baseballs (McLeod & Dienes, 1996).

Of necessity, the work done on any activity, no matter how simple or complex, must focus on selective aspects of that experience. It is impossible to "study everything." A key to success in researching a topic in human motor control, as in any field, is to ask the right questions—that is, to identify the features that are both worthy of investigation and, once investigated, are likely to yield scientific payoffs. In the sections that follow, we will consider some domains where, at least in the author's opinion, the right questions have been asked and useful answers have been found. The list is necessarily selective; many other advances have been made. As in much of this book, the author's aim is to whet your appetite, leaving it to you to pursue your own just desserts.

Hitting Oncoming Balls

One topic that has attracted considerable attention among students of human motor control is the act of hitting an oncoming ball. Some have said this is the hardest perceptual-motor act humans perform. Regardless of whether that statement is true, the claim is certainly provocative.

In batting an oncoming ball, batters are supposed to keep their eyes on the ball. Yet hitting the ball obviously entails more than controlling one's eyes. The hands must be coordinated with the eyes to meet the ball at the right time and at the right place. Further, the bat cannot simply be brought to the location where the eye points, because the oncoming ball often travels faster than the eyes can move (Bahill & LaRitz, 1984). In such cases, the batter must predict, at least implicitly (unconsciously), where the ball will be and when it will get there.

How do batters predict the trajectories of oncoming balls? One way to address this question is to consider the optical information that allows observers to extrapolate a ball's trajectory. As suggested by Lee (1976), the time to contact an object toward which one is moving at constant velocity (or equivalently, the time for an object to contact an observer if it is approaching him or her with constant velocity) happens to equal the inverse of the rate of dilation of the closed optical contour of the object. Said another way, the more quickly the image of the object expands on the retina, the less time there is before the time to contact. Lee assigned the Greek letter τ ("tau") to this time.

Lee's (1976) τ principle, as it is called, implies that it is possible to tell when an object will be contacted by determining the rate at which its image expands. When the image expands at a high rate, time to contact will be short, but when the image expands at a slow rate, time to contact will be long. Birds diving into lakes (Lee & Reddish, 1981), flies landing on tables (Wagner, 1982), and people approaching walls behave as if they are sensitive to this principle (Lee & Thomson, 1982). Batters seem to be sensitive to it as well (Lee, Young, Reddish, Lough, & Clayton, 1983), as are champion table tennis players, at least judging from the fact that they initiate their paddle swings at relatively constant times during the approach of the ball, as would be expected if they began to swing when τ reached a critical value (Bootsma & Van Wieringen, 1988). Still another indication that τ might be used in hitting oncoming balls is that people do better at hitting a ball coming right at them than at indicating when a ball will pass some other point as it travels perpendicular to the line of sight (McLeod, McLaughlin, & Nimmo-Smith, 1986). In the perpendicular case, τ cannot be used; in the direct-line-of-travel case it can be.

Balls do not always travel in straight lines, nor do they always travel directly to the batter, and rarely do they move with constant velocity. All these conditions are required for reliance on τ. Therefore, the τ principle, unadorned, cannot account for determination of time to contact in all the situations where it may potentially be useful. Mindful of this difficulty, some investigators have suggested that other optical cues might be used to establish time to contact as well as place of contact (see Lee et al., 1983; Todd, 1981; Williams, Williams, & Davids, 1999).

To determine when and where a ball will be contacted, batters may need to identify the direction in which the ball will be traveling at the moment of contact. To act on this information, batters must move the bat so it gets to the right place at the right time with adequate force and they must direct the bat so the ball is propelled toward the desired location. Clearly, there are many variables to control, which is perhaps why batting an oncoming ball is viewed as such a demanding task. It is remarkable that batters can hit balls as often as they do. Expert cricket batters can contact 88% of the balls delivered to them within a time window of plus or minus 10 ms, and they can contact 66% of the balls within a time window of plus or minus 5 ms (McLeod et al., 1986). Comparable levels of accuracy are seen in table tennis (Bootsma & Van Wieringen, 1988).

How do batters and table tennis players manage such high levels of performance? One view, traceable to Bernstein's (1967) emphasis on simplifying the degrees of freedom problem, is that they limit the number of variables to be controlled. Evidence consistent with this view has been obtained in studies of champion table tennis players. The forehand drives of these players turn out to have extremely short, and nearly constant, durations (Tyldesley & Whiting, 1975). Thus, a performance variable that could be modulated by changing the duration of the arm swing is kept approximately constant, enabling the players to move their arms as quickly as possible during the forehand strokes. What these players modulate instead of their forehand speed is when they initiate the stroke and in what direction they move the paddle.

Do champion table tennis players fully preprogram their strokes? Such full preprogramming would eliminate the need to correct strokes during their execution based on feedback. On the other hand, fully preprogramming the strokes would take away the opportunity to make corrections while the strokes are under way. Relying on feedback is one of the most important means of solving the degrees of freedom problem, but so is reducing the number of variables to be controlled (Jordan & Rosenbaum, 1989). These two strategies—using feedback and reducing control variables—can be viewed as the "ying and yang" of motor control. In the present context, they might also be called the "ping and pong."

Recent evidence suggests that batting oncoming balls may rely on feedback. Batters almost always do better when they can see the ball throughout its trajectory than when part of the trajectory is obscured (Sharp, 1975; Whiting, Gill, & Stephenson, 1970). If batting strokes were fully preprogrammed, losing sight of the ball in the final part of its flight would not impair performance.

Another source of evidence for the use of feedback during bat swings is the finding that batters can respond rapidly to unexpected perturbations of ball trajectories. When cricket batsmen swing at rapidly approaching balls that unexpectedly strike bumps on the playing surface, the batsmen can alter their ongoing swings in as little as 190 ms (McLeod, 1987). Batters also do better at hitting oncoming balls when they can swing the bat continuously than when they merely have to release a spring-loaded bat of the same size, effectively controlling the release time only (Bootsma, 1989). Times to initiate the bat movement are more variable in the bat-swing condition than in the bat-release condition, suggesting that whatever variability there is in the time to initiate the bat swing is compensated for in the swing phase, perhaps because of feedback correction (Bootsma, 1989).

A final source of evidence for ongoing correction during the act of striking an oncoming ball is that, among champion table tennis players, the variability of the direction of paddle movement is greater at the start of the forehand stroke than at the time the ball is contacted (Bootsma & Van Wieringen, 1988, 1990). Representative curves, which collectively can be said to look like a horse's tail, are shown in Figure 12.1. The convergence at the contact point could reflect preprogramming of the stroke, but detailed analysis of the trajectories suggests that, at least in some players, paddle movement is altered during the swing based on visual monitoring of the ball. This finding is all the more remarkable considering that the paddle sometimes travels as quickly as 800° per second.

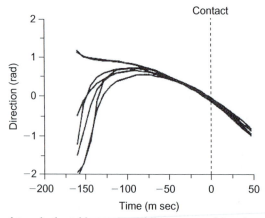

FIGURE 12.1   Direction of travel of a table tennis paddle in seven drives by a top player. From Bootsma, R. J., & Van Wieringen, P. C. (1990). Timing an attacking forehand drive in table tennis. Journal of Experimental Psychology: Human Perception and Performance, 16, 21–29. Copyright ℗ 1990 by the American Psychological Association. Reprinted with permission.

Golf Putting

Whereas the foregoing discussion of hitting oncoming balls concerned the relative contributions of preprogrammed versus corrective control, the following discussion concerns the frame of reference in which movements are controlled. Are movements controlled with respect to *egocentric* frames of reference or with respect to *allocentric* frames of reference (see, e.g., Swinnen, 2002)? Egocentric frames of reference are body-centered, as when you reach for your knee with your hand no matter where your knee is located. Allocentric frames of references are externally centered, as when you reach for a glass occupying a fixed position no matter where you are located relative to the glass. Egocentric frames of reference can be expressed in allocentric terms. Your knee is somewhere in external space, so when you reach for your knee, you may aim for a place in external space that just happens to have your knee at that location. This point shows that it can sometimes be tricky to determine which frame of reference is actually being used, if indeed just *one* frame of reference is being used. More than one frame of reference may be used at a time (Graziano & Gross, 1996).

An everyday activity in which the frame-of-reference issue has been addressed is golf, and in particular, golf putting. The majority of golf strokes are putts. For this reason, a great deal of attention has been paid by golfers and golf aficionados to the way putting is managed or, if one is green on the greens, not managed. Tiger Woods offered this assessment of what should happen in putting:

> Every good putter keeps the head absolutely still from start to finish. Every bad putter I know moves the head to some degree. It's as simple as that. If I move my head even a fraction, it's almost impossible to keep my putting path stable and true. It's hard to hit the ball solidly, too. More than likely I'll open my shoulders on the forward stroke, causing me to pull the putter across the ball from out to in. I practice keeping my head dead still until well after the ball is gone (Woods, 2001, p. 37)

Tiger Woods' words must be taken seriously for he is, arguably, the greatest golfer of all time. What do Tiger Words' comments indicate about the frame of reference for putting? One interpretation is that his comments imply that the head should be stabilized in *allocentric* coordinates, which makes sense from the point of view of keeping the eyes fixed on the ball on the tee, where it occupies a fixed position in the external environment.

A recent study (Lee, Ishikura, Kegel, Gonzalez, & Passmore, 2008) suggests that expert golfers do not behave as Tiger Woods recommends. The data from this study are shown in Figure 12.2. In the case of the relatively unpracticed golfer whose data are shown in Figure 12.2A, the golfer's head moves along with the putter. When the golfer withdraws the putter from the ball and then brings the putter back to the ball, the golfer's head moves in like manner, turning away from the ball at first and then turning back toward the ball as the putter returns. For the skilled golfer whose data are shown in Figure 12.2B, the motion of the head *opposes* the putter. When the putter is withdrawn from the ball, the golfer's head moves toward the ball, and when the putter is brought back to the ball, the golfer's head moves away from the ball.

How should one interpret these results apropos the frame of reference in which head and hand positions are controlled during putting? Lee et al. (2008) argued that skilled golfers control their head and putter movements in an egocentric frame of reference, whereas novices control their head and putter movements in an allocentric frame of reference. The basis for the authors' claim about skilled golfers is that the inverse relation between head position and putter position suggests that the motor system relies on negative coupling between the

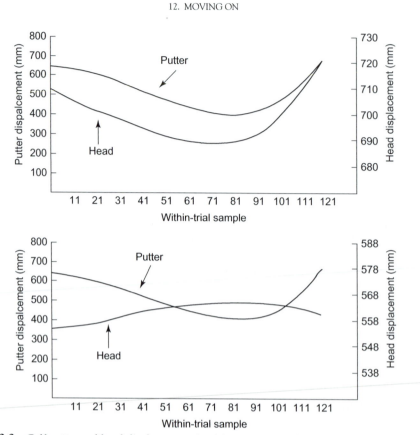

FIGURE 12.2   Golf putter and head displacements (positions over time) for a novice golfer (top) and a skilled golfer (bottom). From Lee, T. D., Ishikura, T., Kegel, S., Gonzalez, D., & Passmore, S. (2008). Head–putter coordination patterns in expert and less skilled golfers. Journal of Motor Behavior, 40, 267–272. With permission.

head and putter. Such negative coupling is defined with respect to an egocentric, or body-centered, frame of reference. Lee et al. argued that the novice golfer, in contrast to the expert golfer, relies on an *allocentric* frame of reference because the positions of the hand and putter are *positively* correlated, as if the positions of the head and hand are jointly governed by their common distance from an external point.

It is interesting to note the similarity between the negative coupling of the head and putter in expert golfers and the negative coupling of the upper and lower lips in the production of sounds requiring bilabial closure. As was seen in Chapter 10, when the lower lip moves up more than usual, the upper lip moves down more than usual, and vice versa. This relation only holds, however, when the speaker tries to achieve bilabial closure, as in saying/ba/or/pa/; it does not hold when the speaker tries to produce a sound that does not require lip closure, as in saying/fa/or/ga/. Drawing on this result, one may speculate that in golf, the transition from novice to expert golf putting involves, at least in part, a change in the appreciation of what variables must be controlled. Specifically, there may be a shift in emphasis from one frame of reference to another.

The idea that there is a change in reference frame accompanying learning is an exciting concept. It is certainly worth pursuing in the future, although in so doing one should remember that this idea has a venerable history in psychology. We encountered the idea earlier in connection with the classic work of Tolman (1948); see Chapter 5. Recall that Tolman showed that, with practice, rats in mazes switch from representations defined in terms of routes to be followed (route maps) to representation of spatial layouts (cognitive maps).

Walking and Reaching

Another domain in which researchers have seen the value of studying the integration of activities is walking and reaching. Historically, these two activities have been studied largely independently, though in everyday life they typically go hand in hand. For example, in supermarkets, shoppers often walk down aisles and pick up items they plan to buy with hardly any pause in their strides.

Apart from casual observations like this, one would expect the control of locomotion and prehension to be well integrated. One reason is that in the case of arboreal creatures such as monkeys and squirrels, scrambling up and down tree trunks and clamoring over branches requires full integration of locomotion and prehension (Thorpe, Holder, & Crompton, 2007). It is difficult to tell where locomotion ends and prehension begins in such activities. Because humans descended from tree-dwelling primates, it is likely that we have similarly integrated control.

A second reason to expect walking and reaching to be well integrated is that the neural structures involved in the control of locomotion and the control of reaching and grasping are near each other in the brain and are closely intertwined (Georgopoulos & Grillner, 1989).

Given these preliminaries, it is surprising that there has been relatively little work on the combined control of locomotion and prehension. Nonetheless, the work that has been done has shown that these two activities are well integrated. An especially interesting study was reported by Marteniuk and Bertram (2001). These investigators compared the transport of an object from one position to another when the person moving the object either stood still or stepped forward (Figure 12.3). When the participant's handpath was plotted in extrinsic or allocentric coordinates the two plots were remarkably similar, as shown in the upper two panels of Figure 12.4), but when the handpaths were plotted in intrinsic or egocentric coordinates the two plots were remarkably *dissimilar*, as shown in the lower two panels Figure 12.4. The simplicity of the handpaths in extrinsic coordinates compared to the complexity of the handpaths in intrinsic coordinates suggests that the motor system strives for simple, direct handpaths in external spatial coordinates, though it does so through complex coordination of the body itself.

A similar conclusion was reached in earlier studies of handpaths performed by seated individuals (Figure 12.5). There (Morasso, 1981) it was found that moving the hand from one location to another was generally achieved with straight handpaths in external coordinates (in-out position versus left-right position). The associated handpaths in intrinsic coordinates (elbow angle versus shoulder angle) were curved. Marteniuk and Bertram's data indicate that the same principle—simpler handpaths in extrinsic coordinates than in intrinsic coordinates—holds even when the entire body moves through the environment. This finding is

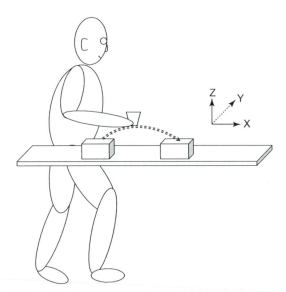

FIGURE 12.3   Walking while reaching for a cup, grasping it, and releasing it. From Marteniuk, R. G. & Bertram, C. P. (2001) Contributions of gait and trunk movement to prehension: Perspectives from world and body-centered coordinates. Motor Control, 5, 151–164. With permission.

truly remarkable. How does the nervous system do this? Answering this question will be an important challenge for future research.

Enactive Cognition

A growing body of research has indicated that motor states are more sensitive to cognitive states than was previously believed. This work has shown that the body is used to aid thinking and that the body reveals states of mind more subtly than one might expect. Cognition, it turns out, is *enactive* (Carlson, 1997; Rosenbaum, Carlson, & Gilmore, 2001; Weimer, 1977).

You will appreciate that the body is used in thinking when you consider the simple act of counting. When you count, you probably say the numbers to yourself. When you count objects before you, you probably point at the objects as you count them. Carlson, Avraamides, Cary, and Strasberg (2007) asked what would happen if participants (university students) tried to count asterisks on a computer screen while the participants either could point to the asterisks or were discouraged from doing so. Carlson et al. found that most participants spontaneously pointed at the asterisks. Carlson et al. also found that this behavior helped improve the speed and accuracy of counting. Participants who were instructed not to point tended to do worse on the counting task than did participants who were not so instructed, and participants who were told not to point engaged in pointing-like behaviors anyway, such as nodding at the asterisks.

Additional findings from the study by Carlson et al. (2007) indicate that being deprived of the ability to move the hands may result in speaking as well as nodding. In another

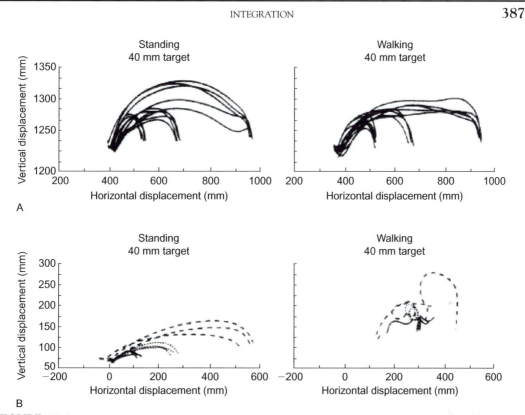

FIGURE 12.4 Handpaths associated with object transport plotted in intrinsic coordinates (top panels) or in extrinsic coordinates (bottom panels) when the person moving the object stood still (left panels) or walked (right panels). From Marteniuk, R. G. & Bertram, C. P. (2001) Contributions of gait and trunk movement to prehension: Perspectives from world and body-centered coordinates. Motor Control, 5, 151–164. With permission.

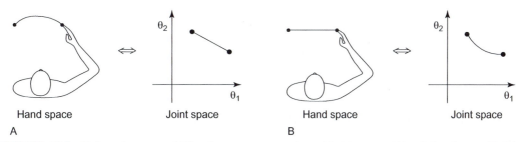

FIGURE 12.5 Trajectories expected if hand movements are planned in joint space (A) or in hand space (B). Joint space is body-centered, intrinsic, or egocentric (words meaning the same thing here), and hand space is allocentric, externally based, or extrinsic (words also meaning the same thing here). From Hollerbach, J. M. & Atkeson, C. G. (1986). Characterization of joint-interpolated arm movements. In H. Heuer & C. Fromm (Ed.), Generation and modulation of action patterns (pp. 41–54). Berlin: Springer-Verlag. With permission.

experiment, Carlson et al. had participants add digits presented on dice-like tokens. All the participants were invited to speak aloud while doing the task, but one group of participants was explicitly forbidden from moving the tokens. Intuitively, one would expect that it helps to be able to move the tokens; having just dealt with a token, it would be helpful to slide it out of the way, for example. The data bore out this expectation. Participants who were not allowed to move the tokens spoke more than those who were allowed to do so. Those in the do-not-move condition said more than those in the you-can-move condition, and what they said was related to counting. They repeated the displayed digits and used terms specifically related to the mathematical operations to be performed such as "plus," "equals," and so on. These results suggest that movements play a role in cognition. When one movement channel is stopped up, we tend to use another. Why we do so is a fascinating question. A promising hypothesis, advocated by Carlson et al., is that we rely on and manipulate the external environment to offload working memory demands.

More Subtle Manifestations of Cognition in Action

Apart from overt, explicit manifestations of cognitive activity, more subtle changes in motor states also accompany cognition. The discovery of these subtle changes has been an exciting advance in the study of human motor control.

Consider walking. This activity seems far removed from high-level mental activity. Indeed, one might expect walking to be completely unaffected by what one is thinking or by "how hard" one is thinking. Yet walking depends on mental activity, as exemplified by the slow, deliberate strides of people lost in thought.

Laboratory studies have confirmed that walking is affected by mental activity. Mulder and colleagues (1993) showed that healthy elderly individuals as well as healthy younger individuals slowed their walking speed while performing a concurrent cognitive task; the elderly individuals slowed more than the younger individuals did. Hausdorff, Balash, and Giladi (2003) showed that gait variability increased when subjects walked while subtracting by 7's from a three-digit number, as in "93, 86, 79, 72, 65, ..." The variability of step lengths grew when participants performed this task as compared to when they could walk with "nothing on their minds." Haggard, Cockburn, Cock, Fordham, and Wade (2000) showed, in like manner, that walking is affected by word generation. Such studies indicate that thinking and walking are functionally related.

Are the rhythmic motions of the legs affected by thought? Could only the visual control of walking be affected by cognitive activity? To the best of the author's knowledge, studies of the integration of walking and cognition have all been done in open walkways where visual guidance is required along with cyclic motions of the legs. Consequently, it is impossible to tell whether visual control of walking or walking per se is affected by the addition of cognitive loads. Other lines of investigation suggest, however, that motor activity per se can be affected by cognitive loads (which is not to say that visual guidance of walking is unaffected).

One of these other lines of investigation concerns balance. If you merely stand still, your sway depend on your mental activity. Representative findings appear in Figure 12.6. Here participants stood on a force platform, a device that made it possible to record the center of pressure of each standing subject at each moment in time. Beneath the participant's feet but

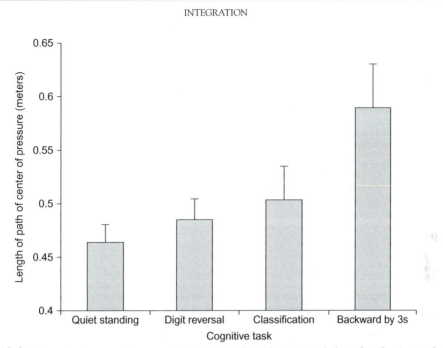

FIGURE 12.6 Amount of sway while engaged in quiet standing, digit reversal, digit classification, and subtracting by 3's. From Pellecchia, G. L. (2003). Postural sway increases with attentional demands of concurrent cognitive task. Gait and Posture, 18, 29–34. With permission.

above the force platform on which the participants stood was a spongy surface that allowed for more body sway than would have been possible had the participant stood on the force platform itself. Pellecchia (2003) measured the length of the path of the center of pressure of the standing subject as an index of sway. She asked how this index changed when participants listened to two-digit numbers and either stood quietly or performed different mental tasks with those numbers. The mental tasks were classifying the two-digit number as odd or even, reversing the two-digit number (e.g., saying "75" in response to "57"), or subtracting by 3's (e.g., having heard "57," saying "54," "51," "48," ...). As seen in Figure 12.6, the length of the center of pressure path differed for these tasks. The length of the path, and so the amount of sway, was smallest during quiet standing, second smallest during odd-even classification, third smallest during digit reversal, and largest during subtracting by 3's. Other studies have also explored the effects of cognitive and perceptual tasks on sway (e.g., Stoffregen et al., 2006, 2007).

The foregoing results help address the question of whether visual guidance alone is affected by cognition. To the extent that the control of sway is not solely reliant on visual guidance, the results suggest that cognition affects movement.

Another line of research supports this conclusion. This other line of study used cyclic behavior of the hands rather than cyclic behavior of the legs. It turns out that swinging pendulums with the two hands (Figure 12.7) is affected by the kinds of manipulations described above (Pellecchia & Turvey, 2001; Pellecchia, Shockley, & Turvey, 2005). Swinging two hand-held pendulums is not a task that heavily relies on visual guidance, so the demonstration

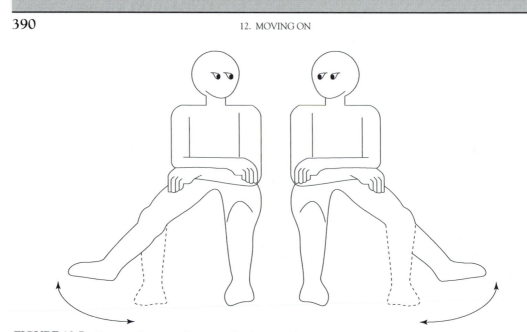

FIGURE 12.7   Two people engaged in mutually observed leg swinging. From Schmidt, R. C., Carello, C. & Turvey, M. T. (1990). Phase transitions and critical fluctuations in the visual coordination of rhythmic movements between people. Journal of Experimental Psychology: Human Perception and Performance, 16, 227–247. With permission.

of cognitive effects on two-hand pendulum swinging gives further support to the idea that there is tight coupling between mental and motor functions.

Yet another line of work that reveals close connections between mental functions and motor functions concerns the use of movement measures to investigate the time course of information processing. We considered this topic briefly in Chapter 9 in connection with reaction times. As reviewed there, reaction times increase as more complex transformations need to be made between stimulus and response.

Understanding the translation of stimuli to responses has been a long sought-after goal of cognitive science. A long tradition of research has been devoted to this topic, yet almost all of it has relied on simple button pressing to record reaction times. Only a handful of researchers have considered the possibility that the dynamics of ongoing movement might provide more information about the translation process. The paucity of such researchers is not due to the logic of this alternative approach being terribly difficult. All one has to do to pursue this approach is to appreciate that instead of relying on a single, punctate measure of the time needed for stimulus-response translation (when a button is pressed), one can use a series of unfolding behaviors to reflect the dynamics of the translation as it takes shape.

One of the few studies that took this approach was by Abrams and Balota (1991). These investigators studied a classically explored topic in cognitive psychology—how people distinguish words from nonwords (the so-called lexical decision task). Traditionally, the lexical decision task has been studied using simple button presses. Participants press one button if the letter string they are shown is a word, or they press another button if the letter string they are shown is a nonword. Reaction times for "yes" button presses are usually shorter for frequent words than for infrequent words.

Abrams and Balota (1991) showed that this word frequency effect extended to ongoing movements. Their participants moved a lever to the left or to the right depending on whether they thought the letters they were shown comprised a word (e.g., left move) or a nonword (e.g., right move). The lever moves began more quickly for high-frequency words than for low-frequency words, corroborating the button-press results. In addition, and of greater interest here, the lever moves also had higher accelerations for high-frequency words than for low-frequency words and were completed more quickly for high-frequency words than for low-frequency words. These effects indicate that the word frequency effect is not limited to response initiation, but extends as well to response completion. Other studies that have taken a similar approach have likewise shown that cognitive processes affect movement completion (Balota & Abrams, 1995; Coles, Gratton, Bashore, Enksen, & Donchin, 1985). Finding that mental states affect ongoing movements opens the door for many new lines of inquiry. Being open to the use of apparatus a bit more complicated than electrical buttons can allow more researchers to pass through this entrance.

Moving with Others

Movements do not only occur when one is alone. They also occur when one is acting with others. Wrestling, shaking hands, and making love all require inter-personal coordination. The control of such joint action is a sexy new line of research in human motor control.

Socially cooperative activity was studied by Schmidt, Carello, and Turvey (1990), who monitored couples sitting beside each other while swinging their legs and watching each other do so (Figure 12.7). The two people's leg swings often entrained. If one person's leg swung back and forth at a relatively high frequency, so did the other person's; if one person's leg swung back and forth at a relatively low frequency, so did the other person's leg; and so on. The phase lags of the two people's legs—where in the swing cycle the two people's legs were at any given time—also tended to be consistent. Finally, and of special note, if the phase lag of the two legs tended to be unstable for the two limbs of one person, it also tended to be unstable for the two limbs of the two people acting together. Thus, the two legs of the people observing each other tended to swing in phase or, if the frequency was sufficiently low, in anti-phase provided the legs began that way. It was as difficult for the two individuals to swing their legs in other phase lags as it is for singly tested individuals to maintain those other phase lags with their own limbs (cf. Schöner & Kelso, 1988).

The study summarized above concerned rhythmic entrainment between people. Is there also *cognitive* entrainment between people? Can one person tell what another person is thinking based on his or her actions? In a trivial sense, the answer, of course, must be yes, for otherwise, we would be unable to communicate at all. We would be unable to understand what other people are thinking based on their words, gestures, facial expressions, or body language. A more subtle form of cognitive entrainment has also been discovered, however, thanks to the insight that useful things can be learned by having people perform reaction time tasks not just as they have done in thousands of traditional studies—alone, in "solitary confinement"—but also in pairs.

Sebanz, Knoblich, and Prinz (2003) tested the hypothesis that sharing a task might be similar to performing the task on one's own. There were two versions of the task—a one-person version and a two-person version. In the one-person version, a solo performer pressed a left button in response to a picture of a *green* ring worn on a pictured, pointing finger. Alternatively, the same solo performer pressed a right button in response to a picture of a *red* ring worn on a pictured, pointing finger. In some trials, the pictured finger pointed to the button to be pressed. In other trials, the pictured finger pointed to the button *not* to be pressed. As expected from traditional reaction time research, reaction times were shorter when the ringed finger pointed to the needed button than when the ringed finger pointed to the unneeded button.

The innovation came in the two-person task. Here each participant was responsible for responding to just one color. The person on the left was responsible for pressing the left button when the green ring appeared but did not have to respond when the red ring was shown. Similarly, the person on the right was responsible for pressing the right button when the red ring was shown but did not have to respond at all when the green ring was shown. (Other subject pairs were tested with the opposite mapping; the mapping of colors to participants was not an important variable.) Reaction times were longer when responses were made to depicted fingers pointing in the wrong direction—in this case, to the other actor who did *not* have to act—than when responses were made to depicted fingers pointing in the correct direction—in this case, to the other actor who *did* have to act. This outcome suggests that the person who had to respond had to suppress the action he or she imagined the other actor might be tempted to make when the finger pointed to him or her. Consistent with this interpretation, when participants were tested *alone* in the same go/no-go task, they were no slower to respond when the finger pointed toward them or when the finger pointed away from them. Therefore, it was not the stimulus itself that accounted for the slowing of reaction times when participants responded to the color of the wrong-pointing finger. Instead and by implication, the slowing was due to the relation between the stimulus and what the stimulus signified for the other person. Knoblich and Sebanz (2006) concluded, in a review of this and related work, that "Action representations are shared even if that leads to a decline in one's own performance . . . people cannot help representing what other people do" [p.101].

Motion and Emotion

The final integrative domain to which we turn is motor control and emotion. We touched on this topic in the last chapter when we focused on smiling and other facial expressions. Smiling, frowning, grimacing, and other facial activities convey emotions, but the face is not the only part of the body that allows emotions to be conveyed. If you sit in your car behind another car waiting for a red light to change green, you can see when the people in the car in front of you are having an argument. Even if you can't hear them and or see their faces, you can infer from their movements that they are in the midst of an altercation. Their movements are rapid, accelerating and decelerating quickly. If minimizing jerk were a constant criterion for motor control, people would move as gracefully when they are upset as when they are calm. The fact that people resort to jabbing their fingers in the air when they are angry shows that minimizing jerk is an optional or "soft" constraint rather than an obligatory or "hard" constraint.

The history of thought about the relation between motion and emotion is long. No less a scholar than Charles Darwin wrote an entire treatise on the relation between movement and the expression of emotion (Darwin, 1872/1965). Nevertheless, surprisingly little research has been done on this topic in modern times. This is ironic considering the strides that have been made in human motor control, both on the methodological and theoretical fronts. This dearth of research is also surprising considering that it has been reported that monkeys with lesions of the motor cortex that are unable to use their upper extremities when apparently calm can sometimes use their upper extremities when apparently upset. The latter result suggests that there are multiple pathways to the motor neurons activating the muscles of the upper extremities.

Just a handful of motor-control studies have been published recently on the non-facial expression of emotion. These studies are worth reviewing to convey the promise of this important line of study.

Pollick, Paterson, Bruderlin, and Sanford (2001) asked participants to carry out drinking movements and knocking movements when the participants were in different affective states induced by exposures to brief stories. Depending on the nature of the stories, the participants were presumed to feel afraid, angry, excited, happy, neutral, relaxed, sad, strong, tired, or weak. Having read the stories, the participants carried out drinking and knocking movements that were recorded with an OPTOTRAK motion tracking system (Northern Digital, Waterloo, Ontario). To enable the OPTOTRAK to record the movements, each participant wore infrared emitting diodes (IREDs) on his or her head, right shoulder, right elbow, right wrist, and right first and fourth metacarpal joints. The positions of the IREDs were recorded. Later, observers were shown movies of the IRED positions in the form of point-light displays. The observers were asked to categorize each point-light display in terms of the emotion it conveyed. The result was that they could do so at a level that differed significantly from chance. Even more remarkably, they could perform better than chance even when the point-light displays were inverted and scrambled in ways that left only the "bare-bone" kinematics.

Figure 12.8 shows a related result from this same paper (Pollick, Paterson, Bruderlin, & Sanford, 2001). Both in Experiment 1, where observers saw unscrambled point-light displays, and in Experiment 2, where observers saw scrambled point-light displays, there was a positive relation between judged emotional activation and average velocity of the moving points of light: The higher the average velocity, the greater the judged emotional activation. Thus, as shown in Figure 12.8, movements connoting anger or excitement had higher average velocities than did movements connoting sadness or fatigue. (Strictly speaking, one might express this relation in terms of average speed rather than average velocity, because velocity, being a vector, can be negative as well as positive, whereas speed, being a scalar, can only be positive or zero.)

The results shown in Figure 12.8 suggest that there are links between emotion and movement, or at least between emotion *activation* and movement. On the other hand, another important feature of movement, how pleasant or unpleasant an emotion is, did not correlate so clearly with any of the kinematic features that Pollick et al. (2001) recorded. Hence, a remaining question is what features of movements correspond to the affective valence (pleasantness) of emotion.

One way of pursuing this question is to ask how emotion affects movement. This question is the opposite of the one posed by Pollick et al. (2001). The idea behind the question just raised is not to determine how well emotions can be inferred from movements, but how movements are affected by actors' emotional states.

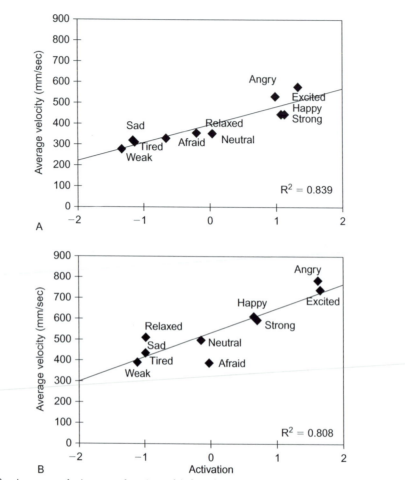

FIGURE 12.8 Average velocity as a function of inferred emotional activation. Adapted from Pollick F.E., Paterson, H.M., Bruderlin A., & Sanford, A.J. (2001). Perceiving affect from arm movement. Cognition, 82, 51–61. With permission.

A moment's reflection will reveal that emotions affect movements. Were this not the case, Pollick could not have obtained the results they did. Still, it is worth contemplating the fact that feeling blue leads to slow "dragging" movements, whereas feeling happy leads to quick "spritely" movements. More work is needed on why these relations exist, especially considering that "as contemporary emotion-performance literature develops, movement scientists remain blissfully unaware of the rapid progression of affective science," to quote from an article that provides an excellent entry to the effects of emotion on motor performance (Coombes, Janelle, & Duley, 2005, p. 425).

As reviewed by Coombes, Janelle, and Duley (2005), motor performance suffers when performers become anxious. The steadiness of performance deteriorates, the precision of performance suffers, and the capacity to pick up peripheral visual cues decreases when people are in states of high anxiety. Given such results, it is clear that movement scientists interested in understanding the factors that affect movement should attend to emotional influences on motor control. Equally important, movement scientists interested in turning their research to the improvement of everyday life—to the reduction of accidents, for example, or to the enhancement of precision in tasks such as sharp shooting or surgery—should pay closer attention to the means by which emotion and motion interact.

One domain where movement scientists can also make useful inroads is in the prevention and treatment of psychogenic motor disorders, such as tics (Rogers, 1992) and debilitating back pain not ascribable to obvious physical causes (Sarno, 2004). The number of work hours lost to low back pain is huge, and the loss to the economy is correspondingly gigantic (Guo, Tanaka, Halperin, & Cameron, 1999). Postural mechanisms are fundamental to motor performance, as has been mentioned a number of times in the present volume, and anticipatory postural adjustments are a constant forerunner of voluntary motor acts. Thus, if one is in a state of virtually endless preparedness for attack, postural muscles may enter a state of virtually endless contraction, leading, quite possibly, to the muscle spasm that is all too familiar to people with chronic back pain. Helping these individuals arrive at a different appreciation of the actual likelihood of threat may be a useful psychological approach to chronic back pain. Similarly, recalling the James-Lange theory of emotion (which says that emotions are interpretations of bodily states rather than the way around—see Chapter 11), it may be helpful to people with chronic back pain to remind them that they are interpreting their back muscle tension as a sign that threat is out there when no threat may actually be present. It may be that, in a real physiological sense, they have nothing to fear but fear itself, as President Franklin Delano Roosevelt once said in another context.

INDIVIDUAL DIFFERENCES

Just as people differ in their perception of how threatening or accommodating the environment is, they differ in their motor and other abilities. Research by Ericsson, Krampe, and Tesch-Romer (1993) has shown that one individual difference—the amount of time people spend in deliberate practice—predicts how likely they are to perform at champion levels. This point was mentioned in Chapter 2. According to the analysis of Ericcson et al., talent by itself does not replace hours of concentrated practice. Still, individuals do differ in how quickly they improve as a function of practice, no matter how deliberate or concentrated their practice may be. Individuals also differ with respect to which activities they choose to practice, deliberately or not. Usually, they pursue activities for which they seem to have a natural inclination. Understanding such individual differences is worthwhile for practical purposes not just to find those who will excel but also to find those who may be especially prone to accidents or other problems.

Inquiring into individual differences also has theoretical value. Differences between individuals provide a way of identifying dimensions of motor control. If the motor system is organized such that it "cares about" independent dimensions A, B, and C, then people good at controlling an aspect of movement corresponding to dimension A may be good, but they don't necessarily have to be good at controlling aspects of movement corresponding to dimensions B or C. Turning this around, motor-control dimensions can be identified by determining those aspects of performance that are consistently or inconsistently achieved within individuals.

This approach has borne fruit in the analysis of timing control (see Chapter 9). Using repetitive tapping, Keele and Ivry (1987) found that maximum rates of tapping by different limbs are correlated within individuals. People who can tap quickly with the hand can also tap quickly with the foot. Likewise, timing accuracy is correlated within people. Individuals who can tap accurately with the foot can tap accurately with the hand. That this ability is based on timing is suggested by the finding that people adept at *producing* time intervals are also adept at *perceiving* time intervals. Furthermore, people skilled at timing are not necessarily good at varying force, and vice versa.

Clumsy children, whose timing abilities would be expected to be deficient, show significantly higher timing variability in rhythmic tapping tasks than do typically developing children (Williams, Woollacott, & Ivry, 1989). When asked to stand on a horizontal platform that can be suddenly displaced (see Chapter 5), clumsy children exhibit patterns of muscle timing that are less functionally suited to restoring balance than do typically developing children (Williams & Woollacott, 1988). In like manner, clumsy children take longer to respond to release of the arm when it is initially held by a mechanical device than do children not classified as clumsy. However, clumsy children and typically developing children take about the same time to make the same response to visual stimuli (Smyth & Glencross, 1986). These results suggest that clumsiness may be a reflection of disturbed proprioception, timing, or both, which is not to say that clumsiness has no other underlying cause. Bumping into obstacles, as clumsy children do, presumably results from lapses of attention as much as from lack of balance or lapses of timing.

Perhaps people who are good at timing or responding to proprioceptive inputs are just more able generally than people who are poor at these tasks. Perhaps they would do better no matter what task they performed. We have already encountered a finding that violates this prediction: Timing accuracy does not predict accuracy of force production. A more general prediction from the general-ability view is that there should be high positive correlations across tasks requiring any arbitrarily selected motor skill. In fact, correlations between motor tasks are usually quite low. In a massive study that made this point, Parker and Fleishman (1960) tested over 200 people on a battery of 50 tasks. The researchers correlated the scores on all pairs of tasks, obtaining each subject's score on one task and each subject's score on another task, after which they calculated the correlation over subjects between the two sets of numbers. This process was repeated for every pair of tasks. Most correlations were below 0.4, which means that less than $0.4^2 = 16\%$ of the variability in one task could be predicted by variability in the other. The few tasks that had higher correlations were so similar that it would have been troubling if their correlations were any lower than they turned out to be. For instance, walking a balance beam 2 meters long versus walking a balance beam 4 meters long had a correlation of 0.85.

Low correlations have been observed in other studies as well. When people were supposed to climb a gymnastics ladder in the middle of a floor and keep the ladder erect for as long as possible, their scores were almost completely uncorrelated with their scores in a task in which they were supposed to balance on a seesaw (Bachman, 1961).

How can one reconcile the fact that, in general, correlations between motor tasks are low, but in some studies, such as the one by Keele and Ivry (1987), fairly high correlations have been obtained? One possibility is that every task draws on a set of abilities and only those tasks that happen to have many abilities in common as well as few differing abilities are likely to yield substantial correlations. Simple tasks, like tapping the finger or toe, presumably use fewer abilities than complex tasks like climbing an unsupported ladder. Thus, high correlations, if they are to appear, are more likely to appear for simple tasks than complex tasks.

Not all simple tasks are well correlated, however, even when their underlying requirements seem similar (Lotter, 1960). Thus, the source of low correlations is still a bit of a mystery. Perhaps abilities within individuals are as variable over time as are abilities among individuals. We all have our good days and bad days, and that source of variability may tend to blur differences among us.

These observations notwithstanding, investigators have found ways to extract from their data hints about the factors that are likely to enable individuals to perform better on some tasks than others. One method, called *factor analysis*, is a statistical technique that lets one isolate factors that account for differences among correlations; the technique can be used even if the highest correlations are low. Based on factor analysis, a number of factors have been suggested, some of which, taken from a review by Schmidt (1988) of the work of Fleishman and his colleagues (Fleishman & Bartlett, 1969), are as follows:

1. *Control precision.* Rapid precise movements must be made with relatively large body segments, as in driving a golf ball.
2. *Multi-limb coordination.* Several limbs must move concurrently and in a coordinated fashion, as in juggling.
3. *Reaction time.* Response must be made as quickly as possible to an expected stimulus, as in starting to sprint in the 50-yard dash.
4. *Finger dexterity.* Precise movements of the hands and fingers are required, as in performing micro-surgery.
5. *Arm-hand steadiness.* Unwanted movements of the upper extremity must be eliminated, as in riflery.

Motor-control factors are not the only ones that predict task success, of course. Other factors that are likely to be important are an individual's physical characteristics, intelligence, and motivation. Being tall helps one play basketball, knowing what to do during surgery helps one be an effective surgeon, and having the desire to succeed is arguably as important for most tasks as is any computational or physical factor. This range of factors—and motivation in particular—has historically been divorced from motor-control research, but a complete account must incorporate all of them.

THEORIES OF HUMAN MOTOR CONTROL

As one collects more data in a domain such as human motor control, one aspires to a theoretical understanding of the data. What overarching principles account for them? Is a general theory of human motor control within reach? If not, have the seeds for such a theory been planted?

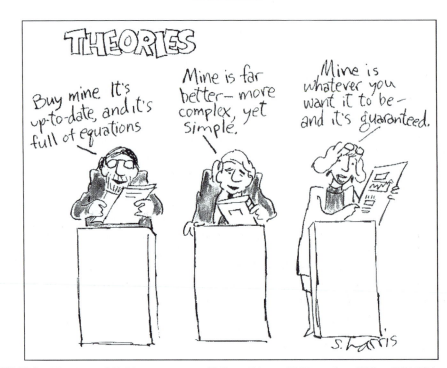

FIGURE 12.9   Theories peddled in a cartoon world. From Science, 23 November, 1990, p. 1117. With permission.

Before turning to examples of theories that have been advanced in this field, it is useful to clarify a few points about the role of theory in science. In the popular mind, scientists engaged in theorizing are often depicted as wooly-headed intellectuals, lost in a haze of chalk as they scribble their arcane equations on blackboards, unaware of, and unconcerned about, the real world. Another stereotype is that scientists propounding theories are egomaniacs, more concerned with self-aggrandizement than with discovery of truth. According to this stereotype, they try to sell their theoretical views to any willing buyer, being little more principled than unscrupulous sales people (Figure 12.9).

Some scientists who develop theories may fit these stereotypes, but most do not. Most theorists in science appreciate that the role of scientific theorizing is intellectually positive. A scientific theory helps in a positive intellectual way by providing a succinctly worded principle or set of principles that serves to predict and also "post-dict" all and only the reliably obtainable data in a field. Predicting data means forecasting replicable data. Post-dicting data means accounting for results that have been obtained in the past, with special weight being given to those results that have been obtained by a number of independent laboratories (i.e., replicated). A theory is *interesting* if it post-dicts reliable data that were not accounted for by other theories and/or if it makes surprising new predictions. A theory is *powerful* if it withstands many attempts to disprove it. Aristotle's theory of physical mechanics was powerful because it took centuries to disprove it, that disproof having come from Isaac Newton. Darwin's theory of evolution is powerful because it has withstood concerted attempts to disprove it for well over a century. The theory of evolution is a *theory* because it is a statement of principle that can never be absolutely proven or disproven, unlike a principle of mathematics or logic. When scientists call some principle a theory, they do not mean to cast doubt on it. This differs from the pejorative statement by Creationists that the principle of evolution is "just a theory" (Angier, 2007).

Two other terms that are often mixed up with "theory" are "hypothesis" and "model." A hypothesis (or as the British would say, *an* hypothesis) is a conjecture about the world, a speculation that a certain mechanism is at play. Hypotheses give rise to predictions. Thus, one might have a hypothesis about why someone does better on one task than another. The hypothesis might be that balance control is responsible for the difference. From the hypothesis, a prediction might be generated: If balance control accounts for the difference, then increasing the difficulty of the balancing act should exaggerate the difference. After data come in, one can say that the results are either consistent or inconsistent with the hypothesis. This procedure is the *hypothetico-deductive* method. A key feature of the hypothetico-deductive method is that one never denies that some other hypothesis might explain one's results. Indeed, some other hypothesis always might be able to do so, at least in principle. Having obtained data consistent with a hypothesis, one tries to generate a new hypothesis that makes a new prediction. The new prediction hopefully differs from the prediction of the hypothesis for which consistent data have already been found.

A *model*, in contrast, to a hypothesis, is a mini-theory. It is a statement of principle applied to a limited domain. The Wing-Kristofferson model of timing (see Chapter 9) is a *model* because it is a statement of principle about the limited task of generating series of time intervals with a sequence of movements. If one said that Wing and Kristofferson had a theory of timing, that statement would be a bit overblown. (On occasion in this book, the author has used the term "theory" in connection with particular models just because the theory term has been associated with those models in the literature.)

Pursuing a theory of human motor control is a laudable aim, for the aim of human motor-control research is to understand, in a broad sense, how people control movement and physical stability. As discussed in Chapter 1, such an understanding will be realized when it becomes possible to predict and control human movement and stability. By this measure, a truly valuable theory of human motor control will be one that leads to the discovery of new useful facts about human motor control. For example, if we can someday significantly curtail the amount of time it takes to learn motor skills, that will be a tremendous advance. Propounding a theory that predicts such a new method is one way that the method might be found. Another way is less theory-bound. It is to more or less "stumble" onto a useful finding by accident or wide-eyed empiricism, keeping one's eyes and ears open for a phenomenon that may prove theoretically and practically important once it has been thought through thoroughly. Cohen and Rosenbaum's (2004) discovery of the grasp-height effect, shown in Figure 7.1, was made this way. The author of this book came home from work one day and saw a toilet plunger standing where it had been left earlier in the day. When he picked it up to return it to its normal storage location, he stopped and asked himself why he grasped it where he did. Keeping pragmatic goals in mind for science, it is important not to be a "theory snob." One should not insist that results are only interesting if they are couched in deep theoretical terms.

We will consider two theories of human motor control in the remainder of this section. One is called dynamical systems theory. The other is called optimization theory. Both are theories in the sense discussed above in that both offer a broad statement of principle.

Dynamical Systems Theory

Dynamical systems theory is an approach to the study of time-varying systems. The main idea is that the state of the system at a given time is a function of the state of the system at earlier times. Furthermore, some *regime* characterizes the time series of the system under study. If the system cycles back and forth endlessly between one state and another, the system can be said to operate under a regime with a *limit-cycle attractor*. If the system cycles back and forth between one state and another but, left to its own devices, settles on a single fixed point, it operates under a regime with a *point attractor*. Other regimes and corresponding attractors can be identified within the dynamical systems perspective. Each regime has an underlying equation.

What makes the dynamical systems approach intriguing for many people is that the equation for a regime may often be deceptively simple relative to the complexity of the events it allows. Depending on the state of the system at a given time, wildly different events may follow, as pointed out by the late Edward Lorenz of MIT, in his famous quip that a butterfly flapping its wings in a forest could trigger a hurricane. Dramatically unpredictable outcomes can arise when the underlying equation is nonlinear, even if the system is deterministic (has no statistical randomness). This concept inspires people to try to predict complex systems like the weather or the stock market. Not surprisingly, dynamical systems theorists can be found on payrolls of meteorology departments and financial consultancies. They also can be found in departments where research is done on human motor control.

Seeing an unexpected transition in a system is often taken as the landmark feature of a dynamical system. This makes any behavioral task that yields an unexpected transition interesting from the perspective of dynamical systems theory. The behavioral task that helped put dynamical systems theory on the map for human motor control was one first studied by Cohen (1971) and then modeled fruitfully by Haken, Kelso, and Bunz (1985). Participants in this task extended their index fingers back and forth, over and over again. In a typical version of the study, subjects held their hands as shown in Figure 12.10A, starting with both index fingers pointing to the right. They then shifted the index fingers so both fingers pointed to the left, then moved both index fingers so they pointed to the right, then returned the fingers to the left, and so on. The movements were carried out in time with a metronome. Subjects could perform the task well, provided the frequency did not get too high. If the frequency got too high, an extraordinary event occurred. The two fingers suddenly pointed *inward* at the same time or pointed *outward* at the same time. From then on, they always pointed in the same direction as they continued to move back and forth.

What was going on here? Haken, Kelso, and Bunz (1985) offered an equation that described the observed series of events. Before we look at the equation, it is important to appreciate the nature of the explanation to come. The explanation offered by Haken, Kelso, and Bunz was descriptive rather than mechanistic. It was descriptive in the sense that these authors merely wished to recount, in quantitative terms, how one could get a series of finger positions like those observed in the experiment. They sought an abstract characterization of the dynamical system being studied, not a physiological pinpointing of the parts of the brain that caused the switch to occur, nor a psychological account of functional mechanisms that

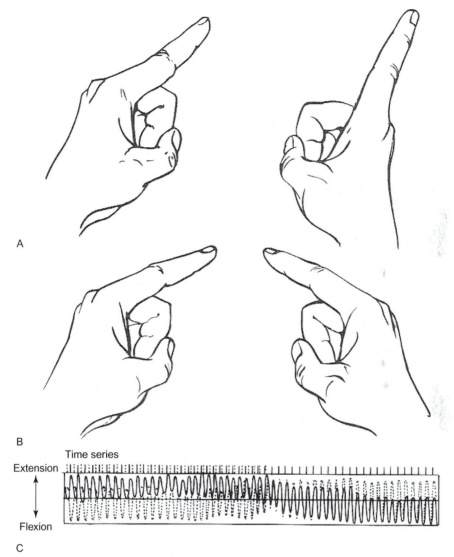

FIGURE 12.10 Coupling of the two index fingers. (A) At low frequency, the two fingers can stay in anti-phase (one finger extending while the other flexes). (B) At high frequency, only an in phase relation can be maintained (both fingers flex or extend). (C) Time series showing the transition from anti-phase to in phase relation as oscillation frequency increases. Position of right finger denoted by a solid curve. Position of left finger denoted by a dashed curve. From Haken, H., Kelso, J. A. S., & Bunz, H. (1985). A theoretical model of phase transitions in human hand movements. Biological Cybernetics, 51, 347–356. With permission.

led to the switch—for example, a possible change from one frame of reference to another as the frequency exceeded some value. The latter explanations would be mechanistic rather than descriptive.

Haken, Kelso, and Bunz (1985) focused on the relative phase of the left and right fingers in this two-finger oscillation task. The relative phase of two oscillators is the difference in their angular positions. If two oscillators vary sinusoidally (see below), if they have the same frequency, and if they start at the same angle, they have 0° relative phase. By contrast, if the first two of the above preconditions are met—the two oscillators vary sinusoidally and they have the same frequency—but if the oscillators start at *different* angles, they have a relative phase equal to that angular difference.

The text to follow in the present paragraph provides a mini-tutorial on what it means to say that an oscillator varies sinusoidally. You can skip this paragraph if you're familiar with sine waves. The sine of an angle inscribed in a circle on the *x-y* plane is the ratio of *y* to the radius of the circle. As the angle increases (i.e., as a dot on the circle goes around and around, typically counterclockwise), the sine of the angle increases, then decreases, then increases, then decreases, and so on. This cyclic variation goes on indefinitely as larger and larger angles are accumulated. For example, 3,600 degrees is ten trips around the circle, assuming 360 degrees per cycle. The rate at which the oscillation continues is captured by the frequency of oscillation (how many degrees are accumulated per unit time). The amplitude of sinusoidal oscillation can be scaled (multiplied by a real number) so the maximum and minimum amplitude can extend over a range other than −1 to 1, which is the default range when the amplitude has a value of 1. The equation for the sine of an angle as a function of time, *t*, is $A\sin(\omega t + \theta)$, where *A* denotes the scaling amplitude, the Greek letter ω ("omega") denotes frequency (the change in angle per unit time, with 1 s being the time unit typically used), and the Greek letter θ ("theta") denotes the phase or starting angle. Because the units of ω are degrees or radians per time (*t*), time cancels out when ω is multiplied by *t*. As noted above, there are 360 degrees per cycle (by convention only) or 2π radians (i.e., 2π "radiuses"). When two sinusoidal oscillators are running at once, the difference in their θ values is their relative phase.

Relative phase provides a convenient measure of coordination in the two-finger oscillation task studied by Haken, Kelso, and Bunz (1985). As shown in Figure 12.10C, relative phase switches from 180° to 0° as the driving frequency (the frequency of the metronome) increases and reaches a critical frequency. Near the critical frequency, coordination becomes highly unstable, as shown in Figure 12.11. The standard deviation of the relative phase of the two fingers "explodes" at or near the critical frequency, provided the fingers start in the anti-phase mode (180° relative phase) and provided the driving frequency approaches the critical frequency from a low value. (The standard deviation of a set of numbers is the square root of the average of the squared deviations of the numbers from their arithmetic mean.) The increased standard deviation preceding the phase transition is called *critical fluctuation*. Phase transitions do not occur, and critical fluctuations do not occur, if the fingers first oscillate with 0° relative phase. Critical fluctuations occur if the frequency starts high and then decreases, but critical fluctuations do *not* occur if the frequency starts low and then increases. This exemplifies *hysteresis*, or directional dependence in an observed transition. Hysteresis is exemplified when the output of a system depends on the direction of change of some input to the system. A thermostat allows for hysteresis if it is designed to turn on the heat at one temperature and turn off the heat at another temperature. In the two-finger oscillation context, hysteresis implies that 0° relative phase is an attractor, constituting a stable state for this system, whereas 180° relative phase is a less stable state for this system. No other relative phase is as stable as 0° or 180°.

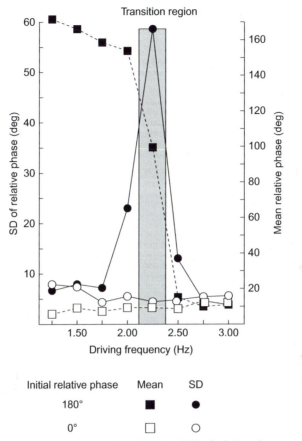

FIGURE 12.11 Mean relative phase and standard deviation (SD) of relative phase as a function of driving frequency for two-finger oscillations begun with 180 degree relative phase. Driving frequency increased in the experiment. Each point of the graph corresponds to an average of ten samples. Adapted from Haken, H. & Wunderlin, A. (1990). Synergetics and its paradigm of self-organization in biological systems. In H. T. A. Whiting, O. G. Meijer, & P. C. van Wieringen (Eds.), The natural-physical approach to movement control (pp. 1–36). Amsterdam: VU University Press. With permission.

The regime that gives rise to the pattern of two-finger behavior is captured by a simple equation,

$$V(\Phi) = -a\cos(\Phi) - b\cos(2\Phi), \tag{12.1}$$

where the Greek letter Φ ("phi") denotes relative phase, a and b are real numbers, $V(\Phi)$ denotes potential energy as a function of Φ, and cos refers to cosine. The cosine of an angle inscribed in a circle on the x-y plane is the ratio of x to the radius of the circle. The series of cosines for a series of successive angles has a phase lag of 180 degrees relative to the series of sines for the series of those same successive angle. Potential energy is illustrated by a rock perched on the edge of a high cliff. The rock has greater potential for conversion to high kinetic energy the higher the cliff on which it is perched. The variation in the rock's

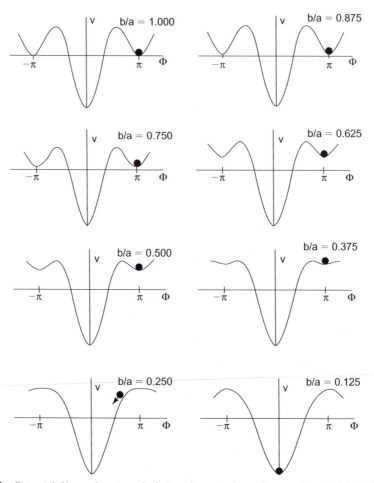

FIGURE 12.12   Potential, V, as a function of relative phase, Φ, depending on the ratio b/a in the equation $V(\Phi)$ $= -a\cos(\Phi) - b\cos(2\Phi)$. From Schmidt, R. C., Carello, C. & Turvey, M. T. (1990). Phase transitions and critical fluctuations in the visual coordination of rhythmic movements between people. Journal of Experimental Psychology: Human Perception and Performance, 16, 227–247. With permission.

potential energy as a function of cliff height is called the *potential landscape*. One can look at the potential landscape, $V(\Phi)$, as a function of the ratio b/a; see Figure 12.12. Doing so shows that when b/a equals 1, the potential landscape has two local minima, or two places where the landscape dips to a place lower than its immediate neighbors. As b/a approaches 0.125, the potential landscape has just one local minimum. Between these two values, the potential landscape undergoes a kind of seismic shift. A marble occupying the higher local minimum when b/a equals 1 "rolls" to the single local minimum that exists when b/a equals 0.125. However, a marble occupying the *lower* local minimum when b/a equals 1 remains in that one local minimum when b/a goes to 0.125. If one allows b/a to decrease as frequency goes up, one can use Equation 12.1—the so-called Haken-Kelso-Bunz equation—to model the data from the two-finger oscillation task. Viewing the marble as the state of the system, one sees that the system can be in either of two stable states, one corresponding to $\Phi = 180°$ ($b/a = 1$) and one corresponding to $\Phi = 0°$ ($b/a = 0.125$). If the system begins in the stable state $\Phi = 0°$ ($b/a = 0.125$), it remains there as frequency increases (as b/a shifts from 1 to 0.125). This simple mathematical excursion provides a descriptive account of the behavior depicted in Figure 12.10. It illustrates the dynamical systems approach in the context where that approach was introduced to most researchers in the field of human motor control.

Since its introduction, the dynamical systems approach has been pursued by many investigators interested in a wide range of tasks. The aim in their studies has been to uncover the underlying equation that provides the most succinct account of their data. Not all investigators pursuing the dynamical systems approach have been content to strive for as abstract a description as the one embodied in the Haken-Kelso-Bunz equation, however. Other investigators have sought equations whose terms are clearly connected to causal mechanisms. For example, some investigators who have studied the stability of rhythmic tapping with the two hands when different phase lags are required have hypothesized, on the basis of their best-fitting equations, that there are patterns of excitatory and inhibitory connections between coupled neural oscillators (Yaminishi, Kawato, & Suzuki, 1980). Similar modeling attempts have been based on two-handed swinging of two pendulums (see Figure 12.13), whose dynamical systems equations have been based on classical physics, where it has long been known that when two pendulums are suspended from a common beam, their swinging motions tend to be coupled. Such coupling is also manifested in people when they swing two pendulums with their two hands. Interestingly, cognitive factors also affect the observed swinging motions (Pellecchia & Turvey, 2001; Pellecchia, Schockley, & Turvey, 2003, 2005). The cognitive effects can be expressed within the dynamical systems equations characterizing the observed time series.

A final point about the dynamical systems approach is that it has practical applications, as has been demonstrated most dramatically in studies of the fluctuations of time intervals between behavioral events of interest. For example, in applications of dynamical systems theory to the study of the heart, it has been found that a perfectly regular heartbeat is a harbinger of cardiac *illness*, not cardiac *health*. In research on walking, analyses of statistical fluctuations of inter-step times have shown that it is possible to distinguish elderly people who are likely to fall from elderly people who are unlikely to fall, it is possible to distinguish Parkinson's patients who are likely to freeze in their gait from Parkinson's patients who are unlikely to freeze in their gait, and it is possible to distinguish people engaged in intense cognitive activities (e.g., subtracting by 7's) while walking from people not so engaged. For a review of this work, including coverage of the mathematical techniques used to carry it out, see Hausdorff (2007).

Optimization

The second major theory that has emerged in human motor control is rooted in optimization. Optimization is the practice of maximizing or minimizing variables. If one is running a business, one wants to maximize profits and minimize costs. Similarly, if one is "running a body"—moving arms, legs, eyes, and a mouth, and trying, for the most part, to keep steady—one wants to maximize desirable variables and minimize undesirable variables.

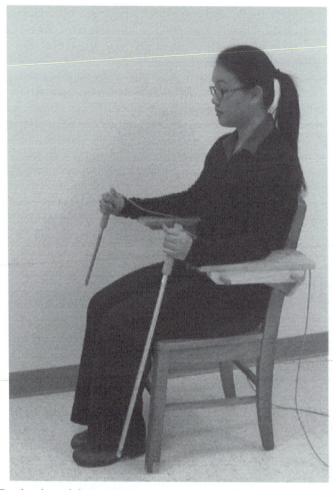

FIGURE 12.13 Two-hand pendulum swinging setup used by Pellechia, Schockley, and Turvey (2005). The pendulums were swung back and forth in the left arm's and right arm's parasaggital planes (parallel to the "nose plane") through rotation of the wrists. Note that in the depicted condition, the lengths of the two rods differ. From Pellechia, G.L., Shockley, K., & Turvey, M.T. (2005). Concurrent cognitive task modulates coordination dynamics. Cognitive Science, 29, 531–557. With permission.

Many researchers in the field of motor control have suggested that optimization is the cornerstone of motor control (e.g., Todorov & Jordan, 2002; Todorov, 2004). As befits this argument, the optimization approach has become one of the dominant approaches to theorizing about motor control.

   We have already encountered some examples of the optimization approach in this book, having referred to criteria that may be optimized in human motor control. One criterion we have referred to is smoothness of movement, as captured, most famously, in the minimum jerk principle (Hogan, 1984; Hogan & Flash, 1987). Another criterion we have referred to is minimizing movement time in Fitts' aiming task (Chapter 7). In connection with that aiming task, we considered the optimized submovement model of Meyer et al., 1988), which claimed that performers find the best series of movements for reaching a target in the least amount of time given that the standard deviation of the movement endpoints they produce is assumed to increase as velocity increases. Meyer et al. showed that Fitts' law can be derived from these assumptions. In similar fashion, Harris and Wolpert (1998) argued that the bell-shaped speed profile for positioning movements, rationalized by the minimum-jerk model, can be derived from an optimization approach in which the variable to be optimized is movement endpoint variance.

As the last paragraph illustrates, several issues arise when one takes an optimization approach. One is what variable or variables are optimized. Plainly, those variables change as a function of the task to be performed. If one is trying to reach a target as quickly as possible, then time is, perforce, the value to be minimized. However, if one is trying to draw the most beautiful line possible from one point to another while painting, minimization of time is not the most important criterion.

There has been a lot of debate about which variable is the one that is "really being optimized" by the motor system. For intelligent discussions of this matter, see Stein (1982) and Engelbrecht (2001). This debate is a bit unfortunate because it potentially misses the point that the essence of motor control is the capacity for flexibility in defining task goals. The same individual can pound a nail or stroke a baby's cheek. No single optimization criterion applies to all the tasks performed by this person or anyone. As tasks change, so do the criteria being optimized. From this perspective, representations of tasks can be viewed as internal mappings of optimization criteria that may be rank-ordered or weighted differently depending on the task to be accomplished. Switching between tasks, which takes measurable amounts of time (Koch, 2005; Monsell, 2003), may entail re-ranking or re-weighting optimization criteria for the next task to be performed (Jax, Rosenbaum, Vaughan, & Meulenbroek, 2003; Rosenbaum, Meulenbroek, Vaughan, & Jansen, 2001).

Another issue raised by the preceding discussion is whether optimization of one variable can make it appear that some other variable is being optimized. This is a more useful topic than the issue of what is "truly optimized." If two variables seem to be optimized, it is possible that one of them actually is being optimized and the other comes for free.

Being open to the possibility that fewer variables are being controlled than first meets the eye is attractive because one prefers to have a scientific theory with few components rather than many. The latter principle was articulated by the fourteenth century English logician and Franciscan friar William of Okham, who wrote in Latin: "Pluralitas non est ponenda sine necessitate," or "Plurality should not be posited without necessity." Putting this into colloquial English, "Keep it simple, stupid!"

An elegant theory of optimization should be as simple as possible. Yet there is a trade-off between how simple a theory should be and how complex should be the phenomena the theory explains. Theories occupy an imaginary space whose axes are theory complexity on the one hand and number of explained phenomena on the other (Figure 12.14). Most scientists who subscribe to the parsimony dictum of William of Okham—that dictum often being referred to as "Ockham's razor"—strive for the upper left region of the theory space shown in Figure 12.14. The upper left region is where the most phenomena are explained with the fewest assumptions or parameters. In practice, theory builders generally veer away from the upper left corner as they make do with their less-than-optimal theories. The more

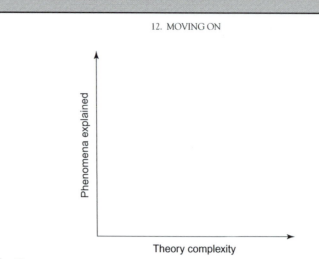

FIGURE 12.14 Theory space.

conservative they are about theorizing, the more they head down to the lower left corner of the space, where theories explain relatively few phenomena and have correspondingly few assumptions or parameters. Where a theorist (or theory) ends up in the space is largely a matter of taste. How the theory is received by the scientific community is also largely a matter of taste. There is no consensus on where a theory should optimally be within the imaginary space of theories shown in Figure 12.14, except for the widespread agreement that the upper left region is the "holy grail." Darwin's theory is an example of a theory in the "holy grail" region of theory space.

Some controversy about the best place to be in theory space has played out in theorizing about the control of reaching and grasping. Smeets and Brenner (1999) proposed that decisions about where to grasp an object reflect optimization of two main criteria: minimizing jerk and grasping the object so the forces applied to the object are perpendicular to the object's surface. With these simple ideas, Smeets and Brenner could account for an impressive range of results concerning the kinematics of reaching and grasping. On the other hand, it was also possible to account for the same set of results with a more complete theory of motor control that also explained more phenomena (Rosenbaum et al., 1995, 2001). Preferring the simpler model, as Smeets and Brenner (2002) did, is a matter of taste.

The theory of motor control referred to above (Rosenbaum et al., 1995, 2001) relies on optimization, and in this regard is similar to other theories of motor control. Because the theory relies on many of the facts reviewed in this book and relies as well on the general style of argumentation that has been used in this volume, the theory is reviewed here in a bit more detail. Other theories are pointed to in the Further Reading section at the end of this chapter. The author's review of the theory adduced by his colleagues and him is not meant to imply that he thinks his theory is the best one out there, nor the most influential.

Figure 12.15 presents an image that helps explain the theory. The image illustrates the difference between two ways of saving images for purposes of computer animation. One saves every image. The other saves a mix of complete images, which serve as keyframes, and incomplete images, which serve as "way stations" between the keyframes. These way-stations or interframes provide the basis for showing motion in real-time movies. The method that uses keyframes and interframes (known as lossless compression) uses less

Interframes only (.avi format)

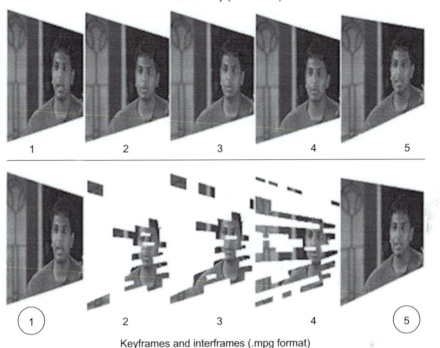

Keyframes and interframes (.mpg format)

FIGURE 12.15 Two methods of computer animation. Top: Storing every frame completely. Bottom: Using keyframes along with interframes that only contain successive differences. From public domain website http://nicky-guides.digital-digest.com/keyframes.htm.

computer memory than storing every image, making it preferable from a memory-storage perspective. Using compression is also preferable from a planning perspective, because it uses levels of control.

This difference between keyframes and interframes is illustrated by the way cartoon animators create animated cartoons. It is common for master cartoonists to draw keyframes and then for lower-level cartoonists to draw the interframes between those higher-level frames. Computer animation relies on a similar approach, with interframes containing limited image data permitting realistic-looking transition (apparent motions) between the keyframes.

The theory to be reviewed claims that a similar process is used by the human motor system for generating movements, or at least for generating positioning movements. The main idea is that when a movement must be made from one location to another, a target position of the body, or a *goal posture*, is identified, and then a movement to that goal posture is determined (see also Kim, Gillespie, & Martin, 2007; Park, Singh, & Martin, 2006; Scheidt & Ghez, 2007). The goal posture is akin to a keyframe. The series of postures to be adopted on the way to the keyframe is akin to the series of interframes. Which goal posture is adopted depends on the task to be performed. Typically, the most important criterion for defining a goal posture for manual positioning is bringing the hand acceptably close to a target location. Another important criterion that often arises is avoiding obstacles. If an obstacle on the way to the target is a rotating electric saw, avoiding that obstacle is clearly the most important criterion. On the other hand, if an obstacle on the way to the target is a set of hanging beads, avoiding that obstacle may be unnecessary. Both the goal posture and the movement to the goal posture are determined, in the theory, according to such criteria.

Still other criteria can be taken into account in motor planning, and the theory allows for those other criteria. For example, an important criterion may be minimizing rotation of joints that have costly motion costs (Rosenbaum et al., 1995). Figure 12.16 shows how this criterion plays out in the theory. The artificial creature shown here brings the hand from an outstretched position to a point in front of the knee when the simulated creature either has normal mobility of the hip, shoulder, and elbow (top panel) or has reduced mobility of

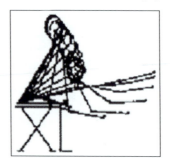

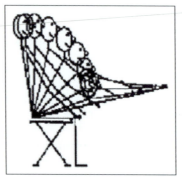

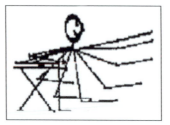

FIGURE 12.16 Reaches that bring the hand from an outstretched position to a point before the knee or vice versa in an artificial creature with normal mobility of the hip, shoulder, and elbow (top panel), reduced mobility of the elbow (middle panel), and reduced mobility of the hip (bottom panel). From Rosenbaum, D. A., Loukopoulos, L. D., Meulenbroek, R. G. M., Vaughan, J., & Engelbrecht, S. E. (1995). Planning reaches by evaluating stored postures. Psychological Review, 102, 28–67. With permission.

the elbow (middle panel) or hip (bottom panel). In the computer program used to generate these simulations, the costs of rotating the joints over a unit angular distance (1 degree of rotation) were comparable when the hip, shoulder, and elbow had normal mobility, but the cost of rotating the elbow was greatly elevated when the mobility of the elbow was reduced. Likewise, the cost of rotating the hip was greatly elevated when the mobility of the hip was reduced. Given these differences in theoretical parameters, goal postures were found that minimized rotation of the elbow when the cost of elbow rotation was high. Similarly, goal postures were found that minimized rotation of the hip when the cost of hip rotation was high. Just a single number was changed in the computer program used to generate these simulations, namely, the cost of rotation of the elbow or hip joint, and the simulated actor moved in the dramatically different ways shown in Figure 12.16. The simplicity of the change in the program that brought about these large behavioral differences is encouraging from the point of view of Ockham's razor. It is encouraging to see an adaptive change in performance achieved through simple, straightforward means.

Figure 12.17 shows another simulation result from the theory. Here is shown a complex reach-and-grasp movement with an obstacle-avoidance component included (Rosenbaum et al., 2001). The simulation was designed to achieve what any normally performing adult or older child can do: reach for a glass of orange juice, say, after bringing the hand around an unwanted object. To achieve the simulation, a goal posture was found that ensured closure of the hand around the desired object, along with a move to that goal posture that ensured avoidance of contact by any part of the body with the unwanted object. Additional

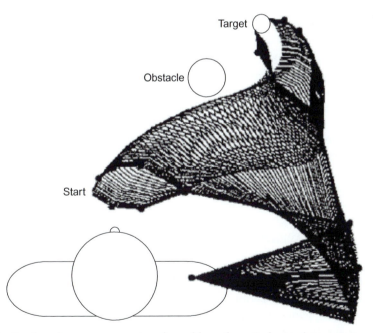

FIGURE 12.17 Reach-and-grasp movement performed by a theoretical actor from a start position around an obstacle and to a target. From Rosenbaum, D. A., Meulenbroek, R. G., Vaughan, J., & Jansen, C. (2001). Posture-based motion planning: Applications to grasping. Psychological Review, 108, 709–734. With permission.

optimization criteria were use to move smoothly in the sense discussed above and to rely on joints that had low costs of rotation. A complex trajectory could be formed by satisfying these multiple optimization criteria. The fact that more optimization criteria were required to achieve obstacle-avoiding movements than to achieve straight-ahead movements fits with the fact that toddlers and young children continue to spill their milk for years after they have managed to reach and grasp objects with no obstacle present. The theory says that obstacle avoidance is more complicated than direct reaches. More generally, the success of the theory both in generating realistic, adaptive simulations and in predicting as well as post-dicting data (Rosenbaum & Dawson, 2004; Rosenbaum, Vaughan, Meulenbroek, Jax, & Cohen, 2009) suggests that it holds promise for future theorizing about human motor control. Insofar as the theory instantiates the optimization approach, that approach seems to the author to be an approach with much potential.

INNOVATIONS

As the field of human motor control has moved into the twenty-first century, it has witnessed major innovations. Thinking back to the methods that were available as recently as the late 1980s, when the first edition of this book was prepared, one's head spins at the pace and drama of the advances that have made. In the remaining sections, we will look at two domains where such innovations have come to the fore: genetics and technology.

Genetics

Hardly any field in science has witnessed such dramatic progress in the past few years as genetics. Among the challenges that work in genetics has addressed are possible improvements in population-wide motor abilities. The term "population-wide" refers, here, to the distribution of motor abilities across all people. Because some motor disabilities have genetic origins (e.g., Huntington's disease), identifying genes responsible for those disorders may enable future generations to encounter those disabilities with lower frequency, either via genetic screening or via genetic modification. Similarly, because some motor *talents* have genetic origins (e.g., the prevalence of fast-twitch fibers, which may promote fast sprinting), identifying genes responsible for "creating champions" may make it possible for more people to excel in sports and other activities.

The field of genetics is large, intricate, and fast-moving, and what follows is just a sketch of a few studies that have caught the author's eye. All the studies point to the importance of genetics in human motor control. Genetics is one of the many fields for which the author has but a passing familiarity.

Two methods allow genetic influences to be uncovered in the study of movement and stability. One is focusing on behaviors that clearly bear the stamp of biological inheritance. The other is identifying genes themselves.

If one pursues the first method, focusing on behaviors that reflect biological hand-me-downs from preceding generations, one need not deny the importance of experience. Both Nature (genes) and Nurture (experience) are important, with the contribution of each being mediated by the other. Still, the contribution of Nature has turned out to be surprisingly strong in some cases.

Consider the "hand walkers" of Turkey. At first, one may be skeptical that any group of human adults could really have problems walking. Yet it turns out these people really are hobbled, as shown in a NOVA program on the Public Broadcasting System (PBS) devoted to this topic (http://www.pbs.org/wgbh/nova/allfours/). These siblings inherited genes that compromised their ability to stand or locomote. The fact that these genetically related individuals can hardly walk or stand, though they can move about nimbly on all fours, suggests that some gene or set of genes turned off the normal walking ability in these people. By implication, some gene or set of genes enables the rest of us to walk and stand as we do.

Another, more subtle, example of genetic influences on locomotion comes from Icelandic horses (Figure 12.18). Thanks to the relative isolation of Iceland from other countries, after horses were brought to Iceland from Scandinavia and continental Europe, Icelandic horses in-bred. As often happens with in-breeding, a trait was then accentuated. In this case, that trait was behavioral. Icelandic horses perform the same four gaits as other horses—walking, trotting, cantering, and galloping—but they also perform a gait that is unique to them—*tölting*. Virtually no amount of training with other horses enables them to adopt this gait, yet Icelandic horses tölt with nary a neigh.

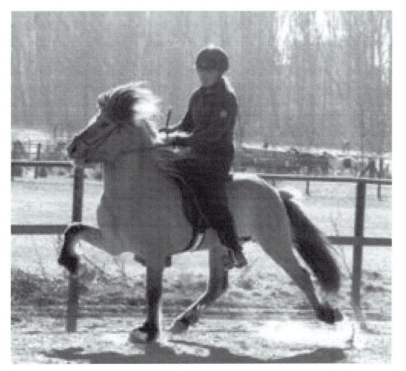

FIGURE 12.18 Icelandic horse performing the tölt, a gait unique to this breed. From http://en.wikipedia.org/wiki/Icelandic_horse.

Just as tölting seems to reflect the presence of special genes, tongue trilling also appears to mirror genetic heritage. Prompting this statement are observations of the author's non-identical twin daughters, Nora and Sarah Kroll-Rosenbaum. These two women are decidedly different. One is much taller than the other, one has much lighter hair than the other, and so on. Beyond these physical differences, these sororal twins differ cognitively and with respect to a specific behavioral ability. Sarah can roll her r's with flare, but Nora cannot roll her r's to save her soul. In this respect, Nora is like her dad, whereas Sarah is like her mom, who can trill *rrrremarkably*. Nora and Sarah were raised together. Nothing in their upbringing explains the difference in their trilling. Sarah didn't hear more Spanish than Nora, wasn't given more training in speech, and, in general, had no more of a trilling early life than her sister. Apparently, different genes were passed down to these two individuals, making it possible for one to trill and one to not. Why there should be such genes is unanswerable. Nonetheless, this example highlights the surprising ways that genes seem to allow and disallow for particular behaviors. *How* they do so, apart from *why* they do so, is an important question for future research.

Let us turn to the second method for implicating genetic sources of behavioral control, acknowledging that the last example is merely anecdotal. Some already-completed research has shown that distinct, identified genes affect the expression of specific behaviors as well as propensities to exhibit whole complexes of behaviors.

One example was the discovery of a gene linked to *trichotillomania*, a psychiatric condition in which afflicted individuals compulsively pull out their own hair (http://news.bbc. co.uk/1/hi/health/5381232.stm). Trichotillomania is often accompanied by other symptoms, such as anxiety, depression, obsessive compulsive disorder, and Tourette's syndrome, a pattern of behavior marked by seemingly uncontrollable tics and occasional verbal outbursts, including shouts of profanity in some cases (Leckman & Cohen, 1999). The researchers who found the affected gene (Zuchner et al., 2006) identified a mutation in a gene called SLITKR1, which had previously been linked to Tourette's. The researchers discovered the SLITKR1 mutation in a family for whom trichotillomania runs rampant.

Discovering such a gene has a useful basic-science and clinical effect. The useful basic-science effect is to buttress the claim that specific behaviors can have specific genetic sources. The useful clinical effect is shifting the burden of explanation for a compulsive behavior from the traditional realm of personality-based psychology to genetics. Not all psychiatric disorders have direct genetic causes, of course, but some do. Finding a gene for a psychiatric disorder opens the possibility that other genes may lead to other psychiatric disorders either directly or indirectly. In the indirect case, genes may predispose individuals to experience events in ways that cause them to pull out their hair, figuratively or literally.

The final example of a genetic basis for a behavior or class of behaviors comes from speech and kindred activities. Regarding speech control, there is perhaps no more contentious claim in cognitive science than the one advanced by the linguist Noam Chomsky (1968) that humans have a distinct gene for language. There has been much debate about this claim (e.g., Pinker, 1995). It is not the place of a book like this to adjudicate this thorny issue. Instead, we can consider the more modest hypothesis that particular genes have something to do with particular aspects of speech and speech-like behaviors. Recent evidence accords with this hypothesis, an outcome that says nothing, strictly speaking, about Chomsky's more sweeping claim that a single mutation allowed language to spring forth in

Homo sapiens. (The author happens to believe that a *series* of mutations rather than a single mutation led to the development of language as we know it.)

One link between genes and speech was obtained by studying the genetic makeup of a family that, like the hand walkers of Turkey, has a specific impairment. That impairment is language-related. Members of this family have difficulty speaking and engaging in other language-related tasks, though, as far as the author knows, they are otherwise normal. Through painstaking work, a team of geneticists found that people in this family have a mutation in a specific gene, FOXP2 (Trivedi, 2001).

The same gene has shown up in other contexts. Mice with movement sequencing difficulties also have a mutation of the FOXP2 gene (Teramitsu & White, 2008). In birds, or more specifically in zebra finches, injection of a chemical that interferes with FOXP2 leads to impairments in song learning. Some of the syllables in the birds' song become garbled, and other difficulties arise in mimicking the serial structure of songs to which these birds are exposed. This outcome, like the one reported above concerning movement sequencing in mice, suggests that the FOXP2 gene may have to do with the sequencing of behavior or the acquisition of behavior sequencing rather than with language per se.

Technology

As we review innovations in human motor control, we turn next to recent advances in technology. Before touting these new advances, it is worth noting that the innovations to be discussed are similar to previous technological innovations in motor control, such as the development of the movie camera. The similarity lies in the fact that the advances were inspired by challenges in the field. It turns out, for example, that the movie camera was not inspired by the desire to make home movies or by the expectation that fortunes could be made by producing blockbuster cinemas in Hollywood, for Hollywood as such did not yet exist in the late nineteenth century. It is interesting to note that the governor of California at that time—one Leland Stanford—offered a prize to anyone who could offer proof, one way or the other, about a hotly debated topic of that era: When a horse gallops, are all its feet ever off the ground? The motion picture camera was invented to help resolve this issue and to reap the prize money that Stanford was offering (Newhall, 1999).

In pursuit of the prize, Muybridge (1887/1957) developed a camera that could take pictures at a very rapid rate. With this new camera, Muybridge filmed people and animals engaged in everyday activities, such as descending stairs (Figure 12.19). Through his work, Muybridge not only helped resolve the "gallop poll" issue of the time, showing that all of a horse's hooves are aloft at once, he also opened the world's eyes to the enchanting world of events that are too fleeting to be seen with the naked eye. People in the late nineteenth century feasted their eyes on motion patterns like the one in Figure 12.19, where nudity was used to permit naturalistic observation rather than voyeurism. (The author's intent here is equally noble!) People interested in movement set out to "analyze" the movement patterns that Muybridge exposed, but truth be told, little in the way of detailed kinematic measures came from this activity, at least to the best of the author's knowledge. Later technological advances enabled such detailed analyses. It is to the growth of this more up-to-date technology that we turn next.

On the day the author began work on this section (October 15, 2008), a news report was broadcast on National Public Radio (NPR) about a technological advance in the treatment

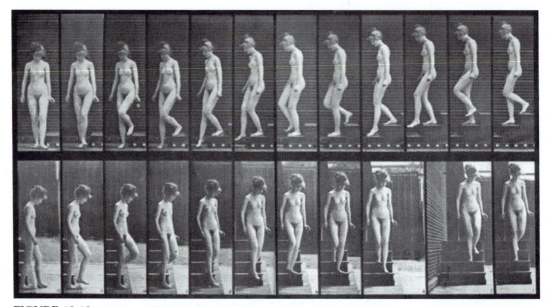

FIGURE 12.19 Woman walking down stairs, from a motion picture taken by Eadweard J. Muybridge (April 9, 1830–May 8, 1904). From http://en.wikipedia.org/wiki/Image:Muybridge-1.jpg.

of paralysis (http://www.npr.org/templates/story/story.php?storyId = 95774683). The fact that NPR carried a story on this topic reflects the wide interest in this problem. Although the story could have been carried on the day this section was being written by chance alone, the odds of its happening were higher than one might think, for the media have carried many such stories in recent years, reflecting not only the interest in the topic but also the relatively high rate at which strides have been made on this front.

The method described in the NPR story was developed by Moritz, Perlmutter, and Fetz (2008) at the University of Washington. Their method entailed recording from neurons in the brain and sending those signals to a computer that then sent electrical signals to the wrist muscles of the monkeys from whom the brain signals were obtained. Anesthetic administered beforehand to the monkeys prevented the brain's efferent signals from reaching the wrist muscles directly, via the spinal cord. Under this circumstance, when the monkeys tried to play a simple video game, they initially had little control over the visual feedback they received; they could not move the cursor at all, let alone move it in desired ways. Over time, however, they could move their hands via a computer-mediated detour provided for them. Thus, they were able to activate their brains so the signals that happened to be picked up in their brains had desired effects on their hand muscles; the spinal cord was not involved. Bypassing the spinal cord in this way might prove useful for patients whose spinal cords have been severed or damaged in other ways.

Another feature of this method makes it especially promising. Other investigators have recorded from the brain and transmitted the picked-up signals, or transformations of those signals, to the muscles. However, in those other studies, efforts were made to use signals that the brain normally uses to activate the muscles (see Blakeslee, 2008). This approach has face validity: If the brain normally generates a movement with a particular pattern of efferent signals, it is sensible to try to replicate that pattern when one is using technology to trigger the movement. There has been some success with this approach, owing partly to the orderliness of population codes (see Chapter 3). For example, much publicity surrounded the demonstration that paralyzed individuals could move a robot arm by thinking about the movements they wanted the robot arm to make (see Blakeslee, 2003). The trick that made such thought to action possible was reliance on the motor cortex's population code. However, relying on the ordinary signal patterns of the brain to activate muscles is daunting. The patterns are often far more complicated than one would like (Olson, Hu, & He, 2005). Thus, no matter how great one's appreciation may be of the elegance and simplicity of population coding, it may be difficult in practice to harness such coding to bypass severed or damaged spinal cords.

The method developed by Moritz, Perlmutter, and Fetz (2008) sidestepped the challenge of finding normal signal patterns used by the brain to effect movement. Rather than hunting for those patterns, Moritz et al. let the brain learn anew. "If you're so smart," Moritz et al. essentially said to the brain, "then you figure it out!" True to form, the brain did indeed learn to generate novel commands to move the body as desired, at least judging from the initial findings of Moritz and colleagues. Hopefully, this promising start will come to fruition for the aid of people (and animals) with paralysis or other movement difficulties.

Getting the brain to speak to muscles without relying on the spinal cord is just one example of recent technological advances in human motor control. Some other examples follow.

One is using computers to assist in rehabilitation. People who have reduced movement abilities caused by stroke can be assisted with robots (Volpe et al., 2008). A typical setup is shown in Figure 12.20. Here a stroke patient is assisted in making manual positioning

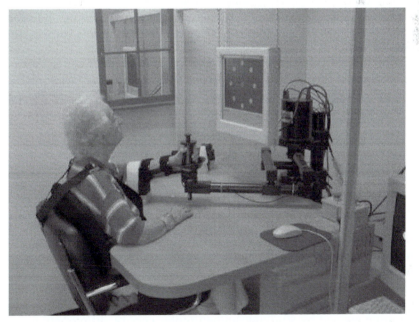

FIGURE 12.20   Robot-assistive rehabilitation therapy. From http://www.jneuroengrehab.com/content/figures/1743-0003-1-5-1.jpg

movements. The idea behind the therapy is to have the robot contribute to the patient's movement attempts, doing so substantially in the early stages of rehabilitation and then, hopefully, doing so less and less as the therapy continues.

Robots used for assisting movement are governed by computers, and computers have also been used for rehabilitation with virtual reality (VR). Here patients are immersed in an artificial visual world through which they are transported in ways that depend on the movements they make. The idea behind the approach is to vary the gain of the system (i.e., the degree to which the patient's movements result in apparent movement through the virtual world). Changing the gain may provide a motivational "carrot" to patients, encouraging them to move more than they might do otherwise, or it may provide a motivational "stick," discouraging patients from moving as much as they do.

Yet another extension of computer technology is decentralization of clinical diagnosis. Thanks in part to Michael J. Fox, the youthful-looking Hollywood actor who, ironically, was stricken with Parkinson's disease at a relatively early age, efforts have been made to allow patients who are physically distant from medical diagnosticians to have their symptoms checked remotely. Camcorders and other electronic devices can be used to send behavioral and other data from the client's site to the physician, where the doctor can diagnose the patient's condition and later, in the course of therapy, monitor the patient's recovery. One can imagine that this method could also be used for coaching. Children in rural regions could take violin lessons with music faculty at urban conservatories. For an example of this approach, see http://www.columbia.edu/cu/news/01/01/zukerman.html.

Avoiding long trips to one's doctor or to one's coach conserves energy, and conserving energy is another technological advance in human motor control. Whenever movements are made, energy is lost. For example, when cars are driven, a great deal of energy is lost through heat dissipation. Heat is also generated during running and other activities. Generally, bodies dissipate large amounts of energy that are often wasted and would be good to recover.

Figure 12.21 shows two examples of engineering advances that have addressed this need. In one case, energy lost from a bouncing backpack is harvested for other purposes, such as powering a radio or light. In another case, energy from walkers' legs is gathered for similar purposes.

CONCLUDING REMARKS

One wonders how much energy could be recovered from the keystrokes made in writing a book like this, the end of which is approaching. Much energy was expended in preparing this second edition of *Human Motor Control*. The author hopes you feel energized by your exposure to this field. A great deal remains to be learned about how we control the movement and stability of our bodies, however. It will be up to you and others in the next generation to push the field forward.

Toward that goal, it may be helpful to end with a particularly powerful example of things that can be learned by studying human motor control. To prepare for the example, consider the fact that Daniel Kahneman of Princeton University received the Nobel Prize

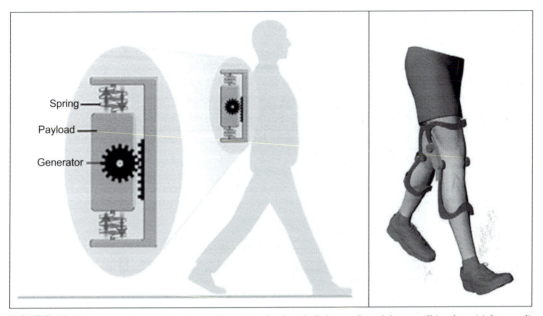

FIGURE 12.21   Energy harvesting from a bouncing backpack (left panel) and from walking legs (right panel). Left panel from Kuo, A. D. (2005). Harvesting energy by improving the economy of human walking. Science, 309, 1686–1687. With permission. Right panel from Donelan, J. M., Li, Q., Naing, V., Hoffer, J. A., Weber, D. J., & Kuo, A. D. (2008). Biomechanical energy harvesting: Generating electricity during walking with minimal user effort. Science, 319, 807–810. With permission.

in Economics for showing that people make economic decisions in ways that depart from what would be expected from classical optimization theory (Figure 12.22). Kahneman, along with Amos Tversky, who could not receive the Nobel Prize with Kahneman because of his untimely death—the Prize is only given to living people—showed that people make economic decisions in ways that depend heavily on the ways the problems are posed. Kahneman and Tversky also showed that people are strongly biased to avoid loss, even if, objectively, doing so fails to optimize total gains (Kahneman & Tversky, 2000; Tversky & Kahneman, 1974).

Research in human motor control has turned the tables on this claim in a surprising way. Julia Trommershäuser and her colleagues at New York University and Giessen University (Germany) have shown, contrary to what one would expect from the Nobel-prize-winning research of Kahneman and Tversky, that people can actually make optimal, or nearly optimal, choices in perceptual-motor tasks (Trommershäuser, Landy, & Maloney, 2006; Trommershäuser, Maloney, & Landy, 2008). In the experiments of Trommershäuser and her colleagues, participants were asked to move the hand as quickly as possible to a target region, denoted with a green circle, but *not* to move the hand to a nearby penalty region, denoted with a red circle. The locations of the target and penalty regions were varied, as were the gains and losses that accrued from bringing the hand to either region (or to another neutral region). Trommershäuser et al. showed that participants' choices of places to aim for were optimal or nearly optimal from the standpoint of maximizing gains. The decisions that

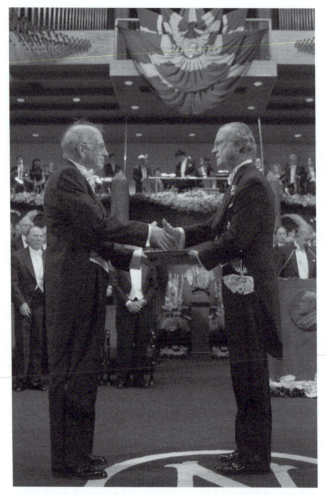

FIGURE 12.22   Daniel Kahneman (left) receiving the Nobel Prize for Economics in 2002. From http://
nobelprize.org/nobel_prizes/economics/laureates/2002/kahneman-photo.html

had to be made in the "aiming game" of Trommershäuser and colleagues were mathematically identical to the ones that Kahneman and Tversky focused on. In both domains, the task
was a lottery, defined in a formal, mathematical sense.

The fact that people can make choices optimally in the context of perceptual-motor
tasks but not in the context of intellectual, verbal, tasks is stunning. The implication is
that the perceptual-motor system is brilliant. If the verbal system could take cues from the
perceptual-motor system, we might all be a little smarter. Apart from that possibility, the
research of Trommershäuser and her co-workers, like so much of the research summarized
here, shows that the more closely we study human motor control, the more deeply we
should revere it.

SUMMARY

1. Research in human motor control includes complex tasks such as hitting oncoming balls and putting golf balls.

2. Striking an oncoming ball requires prediction of the ball's flight. Determining when the ball will arrive can, under certain conditions, be based on how quickly the image of the ball expands. Controlling the striking movement appears, in the case of forehand attacks by top table tennis players, to be simplified by modulating the time when the stroke begins as well as the direction of the stroke. Some correction of the stroke based on visual feedback may also occur while the stroke is in progress.

3. Studies of golf putting indicate that the positions of the hand and putter are positively correlated in novice golfers but are negatively correlated in expert golfers. This result has been taken to mean that novice golfers rely on an allocentric (external) frame of reference to coordinate their head and putter movements, whereas expert golfers rely on an egocentric (personal) frame of reference to coordinate their head and putter movements.

4. Walking and reaching are well coordinated in humans, perhaps owing to the fact that humans are likely to have evolved from tree-dwelling ancestors. Handpaths for object transports during walking are remarkably similar to handpaths for object transports during standing, at least when the handpaths are plotted in extrinsic spatial coordinates.

5. Cognition is enactive. In an experiment that supported this claim, it was found that people had greater difficulty counting objects if they could not point at the objects than if they could.

6. More subtle or indirect indications of coupling between thought and action have come from studies that explored the role of cognitive states on motor performance. Walking variability increases and body sway increases when people are engaged in more complex cognitive tasks. The swinging of handheld pendulums also depends on cognitive states, as does the unfolding of movements made to indicate cognitively mediated decisions.

7. We move with others, as required for social communication, carrying pianos down staircases, sexual reproduction, and other things. Research on joint action indicates that we are remarkably attuned to others, as manifested in our movements. We swing our legs in time with others and take others' perspectives even when engaged in quite low-level cognitive tasks such as performing reaction time tasks with others.

8. Motion and emotion are tightly linked. Abstract kinematic features of movement can be used to judge levels of emotion activation, even if the valence of the emotion (how pleasant or unpleasant it is) cannot be judged on the basis of kinematics alone. Being emotionally stressed can have negative impact on movement and may lead to chronic back pain.

9. Individual differences have been demonstrated in response speed, timing accuracy, precision of force production, finger dexterity, arm-hand steadiness, and other factors. Clumsy children appear to be deficient in timing ability and proprioception. Within the normal population, it has proven difficult to find good predictors of grace versus awkwardness.

10. Theories, hypotheses, models, and predictions all play important roles in the science of human motor control, as in all branches of science. Theories are succinctly worded

general principles. Hypotheses are conjectures about ways that things happen in specific tasks or situations. Models are detailed, typically mathematical, "mini-theories" developed for restricted domains. Predictions are forecasts from theories, hypotheses, or models. The hypothetico-deductive method is the procedure of determining whether data are consistent with predictions. Theories can make post-dictions as well as predictions. A new post-diction is a new account of previously obtained results.

11. One theoretical approach to human motor control has taken the form of dynamical systems theory. Here the aim is to describe change in terms of underlying equations that typically are nonlinear and, as a result, can give rise to sudden changes and other "chaotic" phenomena. The dynamical system approach has been pursued in the analysis of bimanual coordination, the analysis of heart rate, the analysis of walking, and other arenas. The mathematical techniques in dynamical systems analyses sometimes enable investigators to identify subtle effects that might go unnoticed otherwise.

12. Another influential theoretical approach is optimization. Here one maximizes wanted values and minimizes unwanted values. Many models of human motor control have taken an optimization approach. A theory that relies on this approach uses principles akin to those used in computer animation, where movements are treated as transitions between goal postures.

13. Genetics has advanced in leaps and bounds in recent years, and a growing body of work indicates that the control of leaps and bounds, among other motor activities, might have a strong genetic basis. Behavioral differences among individuals within families can be traced to genetic sources, as in non-identical twins raised in the same household with clear differences in specific motor abilities (e.g., the ability to roll r's). Similarly, behavioral differences among breeding stocks can be traced to genes, as in horses capable of unusual gaits. Specific genes have also been linked to specific behaviors such as hair pulling as well as the capacity to learn or express behavioral sequences, including those involving language.

14. Technology has also advanced significantly in the service of the understanding of human motor control and the treatment of motor disorders. By recording electrical signals from the brain and transmitting those signals to computers and amplifiers for further transmission to muscles or robots, it has become possible to bypass severed spinal cords and overcome other movement limitations. Additional technological advances include robot-assisted movements, the use of virtual reality in rehabilitation, and the harvesting of energy from biological motion.

15. Much as our ability to perform adaptively in the physical world demonstrates that we know physics implicitly, our ability to aim for targets and avoid nearby obstacles turns out to reflect an ability to optimize gains over losses. The specific context in which that optimization ability was manifested is analogous to one where deliberate, verbally mediated decision making has proven to be suboptimal. This outcome highlights the remarkable intelligence that is brought to bear in human motor control.

Further Reading

For more information about frames of reference in human motor control, a topic that was brought up in this chapter in connection with golf putting, see Elliott and Conolly (1984), Gallistel (1999), and Gilmore and Johnson (1997).

Research on golf has been pursued by other investigators besides Lee et al. (2008). Richard Jagacinski of Ohio State University is a leading investigator in this field. See, for example, Jagacinski, Greenberg, and Liao (1997).

In connection with links between emotion and movement, Chen and Bargh (1999) reported that inward and outward movements were made at different speeds when people verified sentences with different emotional valences. Outward movements were made more quickly for verifying sentences describing events one wished to "push away," whereas inward movements were made more quickly for verifying sentences describing events one wished to "embrace." This outcome is similar to the action compatibility effect of Glenberg and Kaschak (2002), described in Chapter 10.

In connection with links between movement and cognition, some studies have focused on the deliberate slowing of movements that occur when people try to coordinate their physical actions with the receipt of information for forthcoming decisions (Shin & Rosenbaum, 2002; Sohn & Carlson, 2003). These studies highlight the importance of scheduling of tasks in performance.

For a popular treatment of dynamical systems theory, see Gleick (1988). A wealth of information is available about dynamical systems theory via the world-wide web. Some important recent references concerning dynamical systems theory and the psychology of motor control were presented by Erlhagen and Schöner (2002), Gilden (2001), Van Orden, Holden, and Turvey (2003), and Warren (2006). Turvey (2007) offered a review of the dynamical systems perspective for human movement science.

An important idea in dynamical systems theory is *self-organization*, the notion that things come together in an organized fashion without an executive or architect doing the organizing. This idea is appealing because invoking an executive or architect begs the question of how s/he knows what should be done. On the other hand, finding contexts in which to study and demonstrate self-organization can be difficult. Merely proclaiming that one's theory illustrates self-organization can be misleading. In any case, one especially nice illustration of self-organization is the spontaneous entrainment of hundreds of people applauding with a well-defined rhythm in a European concert hall (Néda, Ravasz, Brechet, Vicsek, & Barabási, 2000).

Theories of motor control have sometimes been implemented in neural network models. See papers by Bullock and colleagues (Bullock & Grossberg, 1988, 1989; Bullock, Grossberg, & Mannes, 1993) and Cruse and colleagues (Cruse, Kindermann, Schumm, Dean, & Schmitz, 1998; Cruse, Steinkühler, & Burkamp, 1998), as well as the many cutting-edge reports from the laboratory of Mitsuo Kawato, where the robotic air hockey player shown in Figure 1.1 was developed (http://www.cns.atr.jp/~kawato/). For example, Franklin, Burdet, Tee, Osu, Chew, Milner, and Kawato (2008) proposed a simple method for learning stable, accurate, and efficient movements. Other theories have also taken a computational approach (e.g., Guigon, Baraduc, & Desmurget, 2007; Morasso & Sanguineti, 1995).

This chapter reviewed findings implicating genetic bases for particular behaviors. In this connection it was recently reported that blind twins show similar facial movement patterns in emotionally comparable situations (Peleg et al., 2006). Tracy and Matsumoto (2008) similarly reported that blind athletes competing in Special Olympics display "proud" and "ashamed" movement patterns (holding the arms high or hunching the shoulders downward) following competitive performance that would typically be associated with pride or shame. Presuming that these movement patterns were not explicitly taught to the blind athletes, the authors suggested, as did Peleg et al. in their study of facial expressions in blind twins, that there are strong genetic bases for many of the behaviors we display.

An area of technological advance not mentioned in the main text is the automatic recognition of biological motion patterns. A colleague of the author's at Penn State, Yanxi Liu, has made important contributions to this domain. For information about her physics-based approach, see Liu, Collins, and Tsin (2004) or go to her website: http://www.cse.psu.edu/people/yanxi. The journal *IEEE Transactions on Pattern Analysis and Machine Intelligence* presents cutting-edge research on automatic motion recognition.

A very readable treatment of genetics and language can be found in a book by Kenneally (2007).

References

Abbs, J. H. (1986). Invariance and variability in speech production: A distinction between linguistic intent and its neuromotor implementation. In J. S. Perkell & D. H. Klatt (Eds.), *Invariance and variability in speech processes* (pp. 202–219). Hillsdale, NJ: Erlbaum.

Abbs, J. H., Gracco, V. L., & Cole, K. J. (1984). Control of multimovement coordination: Sensorimotor mechanisms in speech motor programming. *Journal of Motor Behavior, 16*, 195–231.

Abend, W., Bizzi, E., & Morasso, P. (1982). Human arm trajectory formation. *Brain, 105*, 331–348.

Abrams, R. A., Meyer, D. E., & Kornblum, S. (1989). Speed and accuracy of saccadic eye movements: Characteristics of impulse variability in the oculomotor system. *Journal of Experimental Psychology: Human Perception and Performance, 15*, 529–543.

Abrams, R. A., Meyer, D. E., & Kornblum, S. (1990). Eye-hand coordination: Oculomotor control in rapid aimed limb movements. *Journal of Experimental Psychology: Human Perception and Performance, 16*, 248–267.

Abrams, R. A., & Balota, D. A. (1991). Mental chronometry: Beyond reaction time. *Psychological Science, 2*, 153–157.

Accot, J., Zhai, S. (2001). Scale effects in steering law tasks. Proceedings of ACM CHI 2001 Conference on Human Factors in Computing Systems, 1–8.

Acredolo, L. (1988). Infant mobility and spatial development. In J. Stiles-Davis, M. Kritchevsky, & U. Bellugi (Eds.), *Spatial Cognition: Brain Bases and Development* (pp. 157–166). Hillsdale, NJ: Erlbaum.

Acredolo, L. P., Addams, A., & Goodwyn, S. W. (1984). The role of self-produced movement and visual tracking in infant spatial orientation. *Journal of Experimental Child Psychology, 38*, 312–327.

Adam, J. J., Mol, R., Pratt, J., & Fischer, M. H. (2006). Moving farther but faster: An exception to Fitts's Law. *Psychological Science, 17*, 794–798.

Adams, J. A. (1971). A closed-loop theory of motor learning. *Journal of Motor Behavior, 3*, 111–149.

Adams, J. A. (1976). Issues for a closed-loop theory of motor learning. In G. E. Stelmach (Ed.), *Motor control: Issues and trends* (pp. 87–107). New York: Academic Press.

Adams, J. A. (1984). Learning of movement sequences. *Psychological Bulletin, 96*, 3–28.

Adams, N. (1996). *Piano lessons.* New York: Delta.

Adolph, K. E. (2008). Learning to move. *Current Directions in Psychological Science, 17*, 213–218.

Adolph, K. E. (2000). Specificity of learning: Why infants fall over a veritable cliff. *Psychological Science, 11*, 290–295.

Adolph, K. E., Vereijken, B., & Denny, M. A. (1998). Learning to crawl. *Child Development, 69*, 1299–1312.

Adolph, R. (2004). Processing of emotional and social information by the human amygdala. In M. S. Gazzaniga (Ed.), *The cognitive neurosciences III* (pp. 1017–1030). Cambridge, MA: Bradford/MIT Press.

Aebischer, P., & Kato, A. C. (007). Playing defense against Lou Gehrig's disease. *Scientific American, 297*(5), 86–93.

Aflalo, T. N., & Graziano, M. (2007). Relationship between unconstrained arm movements and single-neuron firing in the macaque motor cortex. *Journal of Neuroscience, 27*, 2760–2780.

Aglioti, S., DeSouza, J. F., & Goodale, M. A. (1995). Size-contrast illusions deceive the eye but not the hand. *Current Biology, 5*, 679–685.

Akmajian, A., Demers, R. A., & Harnish, R. W. (1979). *Linguistics: An introduction.* Cambridge, MA: MIT Press.

Albus, J. S. (1981). *Brains, behavior, and robotics.* Peterborough, NH: BYTE Books.

Alexander, R. M. (1984). Walking and running. *American Scientist, 72*, 348–354.

Alexander, R. M. (1992). *Exploring biomechanics.* New York: W. H. Freeman.

Allopenna, P. D., Magnuson, J. S., & Tanenhaus, M. K. (1998). Tracking the time course of spoken word recognition using eye movements: Evidence for continuous mapping models. *Journal of Memory and Language, 38*, 419–439.

Allport, A., MacKay, D., Prinz, W., & Scheerer, E. (Eds.), (1987). *Language perception and production.* London: Academic Press.

Allum, J. H., & Pfaltz, C. R. (1985). Visual and vestibular contribution to pitch sway stabilization in the ankle muscles of normals and patients with bilateral peripheral vestibular deficits. *Experimental Brain Research, 58*, 82–94.

Alpern, M. (1957). The position of the eye during prism vergence. *American Journal of Opthalmology, 57*, 345–353.

Alpern, M. (1972). Eye movements. In D. Jameson, & L. Hurvich, (Eds.) *Handbook of Sensory Physiology: Vol. VII/4* (pp. 303–330). Berlin: Springer.

Amato, I. (1989). The finishing touch: Robots may lend a hand in the making of Steinway pianos. *Science News, 135,* 108–109.

Amazeen, E. L., Amazeen, P. G., & Turvey, M. T. (1998). Dynamics of human intersegmental coordination: Theory and research. In D. A. Rosenbaum & C. E. Collyer (Eds.), *Timing of behavior* (pp. 237–259). Cambridge, MA: MIT Press.

Anderson, D. I., Campos, J. J., & Barbu-Roth, M. A. (2004). A developmental perspective on visual proprioception. In G. Bremner & A. Slater (Eds.), *Theories of Infant Development* (pp. 30–69). Malden, MA: Blackwell.

Anderson, J. R. (1985). *Cognitive psychology and its implications* (2nd ed). New York: W. H. Freeman.

Andres, M., Olivier, E., & Badets, A. (2008). Actions, words, and numbers: A motor contribution to semantic processing? *Current Directions in Psychological Science, 17,* 313–317.

André-Thomas, A., & Autgarden, T. (1966). *Locomotion from pre- to postnatal life.* Lavenham, Suffolk: Spastics Society.

Andrew, R. J. (1965). The origins of facial expressions. *Scientific American, 213*(4), 88–94.

Angel, R. W., Alston, W., & Garland, H. (1970). Functional relations between the manual and oculomotor control systems. *Experimental Neurology, 27,* 248–257.

Angier, N. (2007). *The canon—A whirligig tour of the beautiful basics of science.* New York: Houghton Mifflin Company.

Angier, N. (2008). Reflections on the simple mirror. The Global Edition of The New York Times, Thursday, July 24, 2008, p. 10.

Annett, J., Annett, M., Hudson, P. T., & Turner, A. (1979). The control of movement in the preferred and nonpreferred hands. *Quarterly Journal of Experimental Psychology, 31,* 641–652.

Annett, J., Golby, C. W., & Kay, H. (1958). The measurement of elements in an assembly task: the information output of the human motor system. *Quarterly Journal of Experimental Psychology, 10,* 1–11.

Anson, J. G. (1982). Memory drum theory: Alternative tests and explanations for the complexity effects on simple reaction time. *Journal of Motor Behavior, 14,* 228–246.

Arbib, M. A., Iberall, T., & Lyons, D. (1985). Coordinated control programs for movements of the hand. In A. W. Goodwin & I. Darian-Smith (Eds.), *Hand function and the neocortex* (pp. 111–129). Berlin: Springer-Verlag.

Aronov, D., Andalman, A. S., & Fee, M. S. (2008). A specialized forebrain circuit for vocal babbling in the juvenile songbird. *Science, 320,* 631–634.

Arshavsky, Y. I., Kots, Y. M., Orlovskii, G. N., Rodionov, I. M., & Shik, M. L. (1965). Investigation of the biomechanics of running by the dog. *Biofizika, 10,* 665–672.

Arterberry, M., Yonas, A., & Bensen, A. S. (1989). Self-produced locomotion and the development of responsiveness to linear perspective and texture gradients. *Developmental Psychology, 25,* 976–982.

Arutyunyan, G. H., Gurfinkel, V. S., & Mirskii, M. L. (1968). Investigation of aiming at a target. *Biophysics, 13,* 536–538.

Asanuma, H. (1981). The pyramidal tract. In V. B. Brooks (Ed.)*Handbook of physiology, Section 1: The nervous system. Motor conrol: Vol. II* (pp. 703–733). Bethesda, MD: American Physiological Society.

Asatryan, D. G., & Feldman, A. G. (1965). Functional tuning of the nervous system with control of movement or maintenance of a steady posture, I. *Biophysics, 10,* 925–935.

Aschersleben, G., & Prinz, W. (1995). Synchronizing actions with events: The role of sensory information. *Perception & Psychophysics, 57,* 305–317.

Aslin, R. N., Ciuffreda, K. J., Dannemiller, J. L., Banks, M. S., Stephens, B. R., Hartmann, E. E., et al. (1983). Eye movements of preschool children. *Science, 222,* 74–77.

Attneave, F., & Benson, B. (1969). Spatial coding of tactual stimulation. *Journal of Experimental Psychology, 81,* 216–222.

Augustyn, J. S., & Rosenbaum, D. A. (2006). Metacognitive control of action: Preparation for aiming reflects knowledge of Fitts' Law. *Psychonomic Bulletin & Review, 12,* 911–916.

Averill, J. (1975). A semantic atlas of emotional concepts. *Catalog of Selected Documents in Psychology, 5,* 330.

Baader, A. P., Kazennikov, O., & Wiesendanger, M. (2005). Coordination of bowing and fingering in violin playing. *Cognitive Brain Research, 23,* 436–443.

Baars, B. J., Motley, M. T., & MacKay, D. G. (1975). Output editing for lexical status in artifically elicited slips of the tongue. *Journal of Verbal Learning and Verbal Behavior, 14,* 382–391.

Baber, C. (2003). *Cognition and tool use: Forms of engagement in human and animal use of tools.* London: Taylor & Francis.

Bacher, L. F. (1998). A kinematic analysis of spontaneous arm movements in infants under different conditions of visual attention during the transition to reaching. *Dissertation Abstracts International: Section B: The Sciences and Engineering, 59,* 3088.

Bachman, J. C. (1961). Specificity vs. generality in learning and performing two large muscle motor tasks. *Research Quarterly, 32,* 3–11.

Baddeley, A. D., & Hitch, G. (1974). Working memory. In G. H. Bower (Ed.)*Psychology of Learning and Motivation: Vol. 8* (pp. 47–89). New York: Academic Press.

Baddeley, A. D., & Lieberman, K. (1980). Spatial working memory. In R. Nickerson (Ed.), *Attention and Performance VIII*. Hillsdale, NJ: Lawrence Erlbaum Associates, pp. 521–539.

Bahill, A. T., & LaRitz, T. (1984). Why can't batters keep their eyes on the ball? *American Scientist, 72,* 249–253.

Bahill, A. T., & Stark, L. (1979). The trajectories of saccadic eye movements. *Scientific American, 1,* 108–117.

Bai, D. L., & Bertenthal, B. I. (1992). Locomotor status and the development of spatial search skills. *Child Development, 63,* 215–226.

Balasubramaniam, R., & Turvey, M. T. (2004). Coordination modes in the multi-segmented dynamics of hula-hooping. *Biological Cybernetics, 90,* 176–190.

Baldissera, F., Hultborn, H., & Illert, M. (1981). Integration in spinal neuronal systems. In V. B. Brooks (Ed.)*Handbook of physiology, Section 1: Vol. II, Part 1* (pp. 509–597). Baltimore: Williams & Wilkins.

Balota, D. A., & Abrams, R. A. (1995). Mental chronometry: beyond onset latencies in the lexical decision task. *Journal of Experimental Psychology: Learning, Memory & Cognition, 21,* 1289–1302.

Bandura, A. (1986). *Social functions of thought and action: A social cognitive theory*. Englewood Cliffs, NJ: Prentice Hall.

Barlow, H. (1952). Eye movements during fixation. *Journal of Physiology (London), 116,* 290–306.

Bartlett, F. C. (1932). *Remembering*. London: Cambridge University Press.

Basmajian, J. V. (1974). *Muscles alive: Their functions revealed by electromyography* (3rd ed). Baltimore: Williams & Wilkins.

Bassili, J. N. (1979). Emotion recognition: The role of facial movement and the relative importance of upper and lower areas of the face. *Journal of Personality and Social Psychology, 37,* 2049–2058.

Bayley, N. (1969). *Bayley scales of infant development*. New York: Psychological Corporation.

Beamish, D., Bhatti, S. A., Mackenzie, I. S., & Wu, J. (2006). Fifty years later: A neurodynamic explanation of Fitts' law. *Journal of the Royal Society Interface, 22,* 649–654.

Beatty, J. (1982). Task-evoked pupillary responses, processing load, and the structure of processing resources. *Psychological Bulletin, 91,* 276–292.

Becker, W., & Fuchs, A. F. (1969). Further properties of the human saccadic system: Eye movements and correction saccades with and without visual fixation points. *Vision Research, 9,* 1247–1258.

Becker, W., & Jurgens, R. (1979). An analysis of the saccadic system by means of double step stimuli. *Vision Research, 19,* 967–983.

Beek, P. J. (1989). *Juggling dynamics*. Amsterdam: Free University Press.

Beek, P. J., Lewbel, A. (1995). The science of juggling. Scientific American, November, 93–97.

Beggs, W. D., & Howarth, C. I. (1972). The movement of the hand towards a target. *Quarterly Journal of Experimental Psychology, 24,* 448–453.

Beilock, S. L., & Holt, L. (2007). Embodied preference judgments: Can likeability be driven by the motor system? *Psychological Science, 18,* 51–57.

Beilock, S. L., Bertenthal, B. I., McCoy, A. M., & Carr, T. H. (2004). Haste does not always make waste: Expertise, direction of attention, and speed versus accuracy in performing sensorimotor skills. *Psychonomic Bulletin & Review, 11,* 373–379.

Belen'kii, V., Gurfinkel, V. S., & Pal'tsev, Y. I. (1967). Elements of control of voluntary movements. *Biofizika, 10,* 135–141.

Bengtsson, S. L., Csikszentmihalyi, M., & Ullen, F. (2007). Cortical regions involved in the generation of musical structures during improvisation in pianists. *Journal of Cognitive Neuroscience, 19*(5), 830–842.

Benson, J. B., & Užgiris, I. C. (1985). Effect of self-initiated locomotion on infant search activity. *Developmental Psychology, 21,* 923–931.

Berkenblit, M. B., Feldman, A. G., & Fucson, O. I. (1986). Adaptability of innate motor patterns and motor control. *Behavioral and Brain Sciences, 9,* 585–638.

Berko, J. (1958). The child's learning of English morphology. *Word, 14,* 150–177.

Berkowitz, A. L., & Ansari, D. (2008). Generation of novel motor sequences: The neural correlates of musical improvisation. *Neuroimage, 41*(2), 535–543.

Bernal, G., & Berger, S. M. (1976). Vicarious eyelid conditioning. *Journal of Personality and Social Psychology, 34,* 62–68.

Bernstein, N. (1967). *The coordination and regulation of movements*. London: Pergamon.

Bertelson, P. (1965). Serial choice reaction-time as a function of response versus signal-and-response repetition. *Nature, 205,* 217–218.

Bertenthal, B. I., Rose, J. L., & Bai, D. L. (1997). Perception-action coupling in the development of visual control of posture. *Journal of Experimental Psychology: Human Perception and Performance, 23,* 1631–1643.

Berthier, N. E. (1996). Learning to reach: A mathematical model. *Developmental Psychology, 32,* 811–823.

Berthoz, A., & Melvill Jones, G. (Eds.), (1985). *Adaptive mechanisms in gaze control*. New York: Elsevier.

Bhat, A. N., & Galloway, J. C. (2006). Toy-oriented changes during early arm movements: Hand kinematics. *Infant Behavior and Development, 29,* 358–372.

Biguer, B., Jeannerod, M., & Prablanc, C. (1982). The coordination of eye, head, and arm movements during reaching at a single visual target. *Experimental Brain Research, 46,* 301–304.

Biguer, B., Jeannerod, M., & Prablanc, C. (1985). The role of position of gaze in movement accuracy. In M. I. Posner & O. S. Marin (Eds.), *Attention and Performance XI: Mechanisims of attention* (pp. 407–424). Hillsdale, NJ: Lawrence Erblbaum Associates.

Binder, M. D., Kroin, J. S., Moore, G. P., & Stuart, D. G. (1977). The response of Golgi tendon organs to single motor unit contractions. *Journal of Physiology, 271,* 337–349.

Bird, G., & Heyes, C. M. (2005). Effector-dependent learning by observation of a finger movement sequence. *Journal of Experimental Psychology: Human Perception and Performance, 31,* 262–275.

Bird, G., Osman, M., Saggerson, A., & Heyes, C. M. (2005). Sequence learning by action, observation, and action observation. *British Journal of Psychology, 96,* 371–388.

Birnholz, J. (1981). The development of human fetal eye movement patterns. *Science, 213,* 679–681.

Biryukova, E. V., & Bril, B. (2008). Organization of goal-directed action at a high level of motor skill: The case of stone knapping in India. *Motor Control, 12,* 181–209.

Bizzi, E., & Mussa-Ivaldi, F. A. (1989). Geometrical and mechanical issues in movement planning and control. In M. I. Posner (Ed.), *Handbook of Cognitive Science* (pp. 769–792). Cambridge, MA: MIT Press.

Bizzi, E. (1974). The coordination of eye-head movements. *Scientific American, 10,* 100–106.

Bizzi, E., Mussa-Ivaldi, F. A., & Giszter, S. (1991). Computations underlying the execution of movement: A biological perspective. *Science, 253,* 287–291.

Blake, R., & Shiffrar, M. (2007). Perception of human motion. *Annual Review of Psychology, 58,* 47–73.

Blakemore, S. J., Wolpert, D. M., & Frith, C. D. (1998). Central cancellation of self-produced tickle sensation. *Nature Neuroscience, 1,* 635–640.

Blakemore, S. J., Wolpert, D. M., & Frith, C. D. (2002). Abnormalities in the awareness of action. *Trends In Cognitive Sciences, 6*(6), 237–242.

Blakeslee, S. (October 19, 2003). In pioneering Duke study, monkey think, robot do. NY Times (Science section).

Blakeslee, S. (January 15, 2008). Monkey's thoughts propel robot, a step that may help humans. New York Times. http://www.nytimes.com/2008/01/15/science/15robo.html.

Bliss, J. C., Hewitt, D. V., Crane, P. K., Mansfield, P. K., & Townsend, J. T. (1966). Information available in brief tactle presentations. *Perception & Psychophysics, 1,* 273–283.

Bonnet, M., Decety, J., Jeannerod, M., & Requin, J. (1997). Mental simulation of an action modulates the excitability of spinal reflex pathways in man. *Cognitive Brain Research, 5,* 221–228.

Bonnet, M., & Requin, J. (1982). Long loop and spinal reflexes in man during preparation for directional hand movements. *Journal of Neuroscience, 2,* 90–96.

Bootsma, R. J. (1989). Accuracy of perceptual processes subserving different perception-action systems. *Quarterly Journal of Experimental Psychology, 41A,* 489–500.

Bootsma, R. J., & Van Wieringen, P. C. (1988). Visual control of an attacking forehand drive in table tennis. In O. G. Meijer & K. Roth (Eds.), *Complex motor behavior: The motor-action controversy* (pp. 189–199). Amsterdam: North-Holland.

Bootsma, R. J., & Van Wieringen, P. C. (1990). Timing an attacking forehand drive in table tennis. Human Perception and Performance. *Journal of Experimental Psychology, 16,* 21–29.

Bosbach, S., Cole, J., Prinz, W., & Knoblich, G. (2005). Inferring another's expectations from action: The role of peripheral sensation. *Nature Neuroscience, 8,* 1295–1297.

Boschker, M. S., Bakker, F. C., & Michaels, C. F. (2002). Memory for the functional characteristics of climbing walls: Perceiving affordances. *Journal of Motor Behavior, 34,* 25–36.

Botvinik, M. (2004). Probing the neural basis of body ownership. *Science, 305,* 782–783.

Botvinick, M., & Cohen, J. (1998). Rubber hands 'feel' touch that eyes see. *Nature, 391,* 756.

Bouma, H., & Bouwhuis, D. G. (Eds.), (1984). *Attention and Performance X: Control of language processes.* London: Lawrence Erlbaum Associates.

Bousset, S., & Zattara, M. (1981). A sequence of postural movements precedes voluntary movement. *Neuroscience Letters, 22,* 263–270.

Bousset, S., & Zattara, M. (1981). A sequence of postural movements precedes voluntary movement. *Neuroscience Letters, 22,* 263–270.

Bower, B. (1989). Baby faces show the right side of emotion. *Science News, 135,* 149.

Bower, G. H., Clark, M., Lesgold, A., & Winzenz, D. (1969). Hierarchical retrieval schemes in recall of categorized word lists. *Journal of Verbal Learning and Verbal Behavior, 8,* 323–443.

Bower, T. G. R. (1972). Object perception in infants. *Perception, 1,* 15–30.

Bower, T. G. R. (1974). *Development in infancy.* San Francisico, CA: W. H. Freeman.

Bower, T. G. R. (1982). *Development in infancy* (2nd ed). San Francisco: W. H. Freeman.

Bower, T. G. R., Broughton, J. M., & Moore, M. K. (1970). Demonstration of intention in the reaching behavior of neonate humans. *Nature, 228,* 679–681.

Brady, M., Hollerbach, J. M., Johnson, T. L., Lozano-Perez, T., & Mason, M. T. (Eds.), (1982). *Robot motion: Planning and control.* Cambridge, MA: The MIT Press.

Bramble, D. M., & Carrier, D. R. (1983). Running and breathing in mammals. *Science, 219,* 251–256.

Brass, M., Bekkering, H., & Prinz, W. (2001). Movement observation affects movement execution in a simple response task. *Acta Psychologica, 106,* 3–22.

Brass, M., & Haggard, P. (2007). To do or not to do: The neural signature of self-control. *Journal of Neuroscience, 27,* 9141–9145.

Brebner, J., Shephard, M., & Cairney, P. (1972). Spatial relations and S-R compatibility. *Acta Psychologica, 36,* 1–15.

Bridgeman, B. (1983). Mechanisms of space constancy. In A. Hein & M. Jeannerod (Eds.), *Spatially oriented behavior* (pp. 263–279). New York: Springer-Verlag.

Bridgeman, B. (2007). Efference copy and its limitations. *Computers in Biology and Medicine, 37,* 924–929.

Bridgeman, B., Kirch, M., & Sperling, A. (1981). Segregation of cognitive and motor aspects of visual information using induced motion. *Perception & Psychophysics, 29,* 336–342.

Brindley, G. S., & Merton, P. A. (1960). The absence of position sense in the human eye. *Journal of Physiology, 153,* 127–130.

Brinkman, C. (1981). Lesions in supplementary motor area interfere with a monkey's performance of a bimanual co-ordination task. *Neuroscience Letters, 27,* 267–270.

Brinkman, C. (1984). Supplementary motor area of the monkey's cerebral cortex: Short- and long-term deficits after unilateral ablation and the effects of subsequent callosal section. *Journal of Neuroscience, 4,* 918–929.

Brinkman, J., Porter, R., & Norman, J. (1983). Plasticity of motor behavior in monkeys with crossed forelimb nerves. *Science, 220,* 438–440.

Brody, J. E. (1988). Personal health: For those at risk of developing Huntington's, an anguished decision on testing for the disorder. The New York Times, August 25, B17.

Brooks, V. B. (Ed.). (1981). *Handbook of physiology, Section 1: Vol. II, Part 1.* Baltimore: Williams & Wilkins.

Brooks, V. B. (1986). *The neural basis of motor control.* New York: Oxford University Press.

Brown, E. L., & Deffenbacher, K. (1979). *Perception and the senses.* New York: Oxford University Press.

Brown, L. E., Kroliczak, G., Demonet, J.-F., & Goodale, M. A. (2008). A hand in blindsight: Hand placement near target improves size perception in the blind visual field. *Neuropsychologia, 46,* 786–802.

Brunia, C. H. M. (1999). Neural aspects of anticipatory behavior. *Acta Psychologica, 101,* 213–242.

Bryan, W. L., & Harter, N. (1897). Studies in the physiology and psychology of the telegraphic language. *Psychological Review, 4,* 27–53.

Buchanan, J. J., & Kelso, J. A. S. (1999). To switch or not to switch: Recruitment of degrees of freedom stabilizes biological coordination. *Journal of Motor Behavior, 31,* 126–144.

Buchanan, J. J., Kelso, J. A. S., DeGuzman, G. C., & Ding, M. (1996). The spontaneous recruitment and suppression of degrees of freedom in rhythmic hand movements. *Human Movement Science, 16,* 1–32.

Buchanan, J. J., Park, J.-H., & Shea, C. H. (2006). Target width scaling in a repetitive aiming task: switchingbetween cyclical and discrete units of action. *Experimental Brain Research, 175,* 710–725.

Buchthal, F., & Schmalbruch, M. (1980). Motor unit of mammalian muscle. *Physiological Reviews, 60,* 90–142.

Bullock, D., & Grossberg, S. (1988). Neural dynamics of planned arm movements: Emergent invariants and speed-accuracy properties during trajectory formation. *Psychological Review, 95,* 49–90.

Bullock, D., & Grossberg, S. (1989). VITE and FLETE: Neural modules for trajectory formation and postural control. In W. A. Hershberger (Ed.)*Volitional action* (pp. 253–297). Amsterdam: North-Holland/Elsevier.

Bullock, D., Grossberg, S. Adaptive neural networks for control of movement trajectories invariant under speed and force rescaling. Human Movement Science. 1991; 10:3–53.

Bullock, D., Grossberg, S., & Mannes, C. (1993). A neural network model for cursive script production. *Biological Cybernetics, 70,* 15–28.

Buonomano, D. V., & Merzenich, M. M. (1998). Cortical plasticity: From synapses to maps. *Annual Review of Neuroscience, 21,* 149–186.

Burdet, E., Osu, R., Franklin, D. W., Milner, T. E., & Kawato, M. (2001). The central nervous system stabilizes unstable dynamics by learning optimal impedance. *Nature, 414,* 446–449.

Butsch, R. L. C. (1932). Eye movements and the eye-hand span in typewriting. *Journal of Educational Psychology, 23,* 104–121.

Butterworth, B. (Ed.). (1980). *Language Production, Vol. 1: Speech and talk.* London: Academic Press.

Butterworth, B. (Ed.). (1983). *Language Production, Vol. 2: Development, writing and other language processes.* London: Academic Press.

Butterworth, B., & Grover, L. (1990). Joint visual attention, manual pointing, and preverbal communication in human infancy. In M. Jeannerod (Ed.), *Attention and Performance XIII* (pp. 605–624). Hillsdale, NJ: Lawrence Erlbaum Associates.

Buxbaum, L. J. (2001). Ideomotor Apraxia: A call to action. *Neurocase, 7,* 445–458.

Buxbaum, L. J., Sirigu, A., Schwartz, M. F., & Klatzky, R. (2003). Cognitive representations of hand posture in ideomotor apraxia. *Neuropsychologia, 41,* 1091–1113.

Calvo-Merino, B., Glaser, D. E., Grezes, J., Passingham, R. E., & Haggard, P. (2005). Action observation and acquired motor skills: An fMRI study with expert dancers. *Cerebral Cortex, 15,* 1243–1249.

Campbell, F. W., & Wurtz, R. H. (1978). Saccadic omission: Why we do not see a grey-out during a saccadic eye movement. *Vision Research, 18,* 1297–1303.

Campos, J. J., Anderson, D. I., Barbu-Roth, M. A., Hubbard, E. M., Hertenstein, M. J., & Witherington, D. (2000). Travel broadens the mind. *Infancy, 1,* 149–219.

Cannon, W. B. (1927). The James-Lange theory of emotions: A critical examination and an alternative theory. *American Journal of Psychology, 39,* 106–124.

Carello, C., & Turvey, M. T. (2004). Physics and psychology of the muscle sense. *Current Directions in Psychological Science, 13,* 25–28.

Carew, T. J. (1985). Posture and locomotion. In E. R. Kandel & J. H. Schwartz (Eds.), *Principles of neural science* (2nd ed) (pp. 478–486). New York: Elsevier/North-Holland.

Carlson, R. A. (1997). *Experienced cognition.* Mahwah, NJ: Lawrence Erlbaum Associates.

Carlson, R. A., Avraamides, M. N., Cary, M., & Strasberg, S. (2007). What do the hands externalize in simple arithmetic? *Journal of Experimental Psychology: Learning, Memory, and Cognition, 33,* 747–756.

Carlton, L. G. (1981). Processing visual feedback information for movement control. *Journal of Experimental Psychology: Human Perception and Performance, 7,* 1019–1030.

Carnahan, H., McFadyen, B. J., Cockell, D. L., & Halverson, A. H. (1996). The combined control of locomotion and prehension. *Neuroscience Research Communications, 19,* 91–100.

Carpenter, R. H. S. (1977). *Movements of the eyes.* London: Pion.

Carpenter, W. B. (1852). On the relation of mind and matter. British and Foreign Medico-chirurgical Review.

Carpenter, W. G. (1884). *Principles of mental physiology, with their applications to the training and discipline of the mind and study of its morbid conditions.* New York: Appleton.

Carroll, D. W. (1986). *Psychology of language.* Monterey, CA: Brooks/Cole.

Carson, L. M., & Wiegand, R. L. (1979). Motor schema formation and retention in young children: A test of Schmidt's schema theory. *Journal of Motor Behavior, 11,* 247–251.

Carterette, E. C., & Friedman, M. P. (Eds.), (1976). *Handbook of perception. Vl. VII: Language and speech.* New York: Academic Press.

Chaffin, R. (2002). *Practicing perfection: Memory and piano performance.* Mahwah, NJ: Lawrence Erlbaum Associates.

Chaffin, R., & Imreh, G. (2002). Practicing perfection: Piano performance as expert memory. *Psychological Science, 13,* 342–349.

Chao, E. Y. S., An, K. N., Cooney, W. P., & Linscheid, R. L. (1989). *Biomechanics of the hand: A basic research study.* New Jersey: World Scientific.

Chase, W. G., & Simon, H. A. (1973). The mind's eye in chess[need page numbers]. In W. G. Chase (Ed.), *Visual information processing.* New York: Academic Press.

Chen, M., & Bargh, J. A. (1999). Nonconscious approach and avoidance behavioral consequences of the autonomic evaluation effect. *Personality and Social Psychology Bulletin, 25,* 215–224.

Cheney, P. D., & Fetz, E. E. (1984). Corticomotoneuronal cells contribute to long-latency stretch reflexes in the rhesus monkey. *Journal of Physiology, 349,* 249–272.

Chevreul, M. E. (1833). Lettre a M Ampere sur une classe particulaires. *Rev. des deux mondes. 2nd series, 2,* 258–266.

Chin, G., & Veston, J. (2007). Learning to sing. *Science, 318,* 1835.

Choi, J. T., & Bastian, A. J. (2007). Adaptation reveals independent control networks for human walking. *Nature Neuroscience, 10,* 1055–1062.

Chomsky, N. (1968). *Language and mind.* New York: Harcourt Brace Jovanovich.

Chomsky, N. (1975). *Reflections on language.* New York: Pantheon.

Chomsky, N., & Halle, M. (1968). *The sound pattern of English.* New York: Harper and Row.

Church, R. M. (2003). A concise guide to scalar timing theory. In W. H. Meck (Ed.), *Functional and neural mechanisms of interval timing* (pp. 3–22). Boca Raton, FL: CRC Press.

Church, R. M. (2006). Behavioristic, cognitive, biological, and quantitative explanations of timing. In E. A. Wasserman & T. R. Zentall (Eds.), *Comparative cognition: Experimental explorations of animal intelligence* (pp. 3–19). Oxford: Oxford University Press.

Churchland, P. S. (1986). *Neurophilosophy.* Cambridge, MA: MIT Press.

Ciuffreda, K. J., & Tannen, B. (1995). *Eye movement basics for the clinician.* St. Louis: Mosby.

Clark, F. J., & Burgess, P. R. (1975). Slowly adapting receptors in the cat knee joint: Can they signal joint angle? *Journal of Neurophysiology, 38,* 1448–1463.

Claxton, L. J., Keen, R., & McCarty, M. E. (2003). Evidence of motor planning in infant reaching behavior. *Psychological Science, 14,* 354–356.

Clearfield, M. W. (2004). The role of crawling and walking experience in infant spatial memory. *Journal of Experimental child Psychology, 89,* 214–241.

Cohen, A. H., Rossignol, S., & Grillner, S. (Eds.), (1988). *Neural control of rhythmic movements in vertebrates.* New York: Wiley.

Cohen, D. J., & Bennett, S. (1997). Why can't most people draw what they see? *Journal of Experimental Psychology: Human Perception and Performance, 23,* 609–621.

Cohen, L. (1971). Synchronous bimanual movements performed by homologous and non-homologous muscles. *Perceptual and Motor Skills, 32,* 639–643.

Cohen, R. G. (2008). Ready for action: Fixational limb movements reveal forthcoming voluntary movements. Unpublished doctoral dissertation, Pennsylvania State University, University Park, PA.

Cohen, R. G., & Rosenbaum, D. A. (2004). Where objects are grasped reveals how grasps are planned: Generation and recall of motor plans. *Experimental Brain Research, 157,* 486–495.

Cohen, R. G., & Rosenbaum, D. A. (2007). Directional bias of limb tremor prior to voluntary movement. *Psychological Science, 18,* 8–12.

Cole, K. J., Gracco, V. L., & Abbs, J. H. (1984). Autogenic and nonautogenic sensorimotor actions in the control of multiarticulate hand movements. *Experimental Brain Research, 56,* 582–585.

Coles, M. G. H., Gratton, G., Bashore, T. R., Enksen, C. W., & Donchin, E. (1985). A psychophysiological investigation of the continuous flow model of human information processing. *Journal of Experimental Psychology: Human Perception and Performance, 11,* 529–553.

Collard, R., & Povel, D.-J. (1982). Theory of serial pattern production: Tree traversals. *Psychological Review, 85,* 693–707.

Collewijn, H. (1981). The optokinetic system. In B. L. Zuber (Ed.), *Models of oculomotor behavior and control* (pp. 111–137). Boca Raton, FL: CRC Press, Inc.

Collewijn, H., & Kowler, E. (2008). The significance of microsaccades for vision and oculomotor control. *Journal of Vision, 8,* 1–21.

Collewijn, H., Martins, A. J., & Steinman, R. M.CohenB. (Ed.). (1981). *Vestibular and oculomotor physiology: Vol. 3.* New York: New York Academy of Sciences, p. 312.

Collewijn, H., Martins, A. J., & Steinman, R. M. (1983). Compensatory eye movements during active and passive head movements: Fast adaptation to changes in visual magnification. *Journal of Physiology, 340,* 259–286.

Collewijn, H., van der Steen, J., & Steinman, R. (1985). Human eye movements associated with blinks and prolonged eye closure. *Journal of Neurophysiology, 54,* 11–27.

Collier, G. L., & Ogden, R. T. (2004). Adding drift to the decomposition of simple isochronous tapping: An extension of the Wing-Kristofferson model. *Journal of Experimental Psychology: Human Perception and Performance, 30,* 853–872.

Collins, S., Ruina, A., Tedrake, R., & Wisse, M. (2005). Efficient bipedal robots based on passive-dynamic walkers. *Science, 307,* 1082–1085.

Conrad, R. (1965). Acoustic confusions in immediate memory. *British Journal of Psychology, 55,* 75–84.

Delcomyn, F. (1975). Neural basis of rhythmic behavior in animals. *Science, 210,* 492–498.

Cooke, J. D. (1980). The organization of simple, skilled movements. In G. E. Stelmach & J. Requin (Eds.), *Tutorials in motor behavior* (pp. 199–212). Amsterdam: North-Holland.

Coombes, S. A., Janelle, C. M., & Duley, A. R. (2005). Emotion and motor control: Movement attributes following affective picture processing. *Journal of Motor Behavior, 37,* 425–436.

Cooper, W. E. (1983). Introduction. In W. E. Cooper (Ed.), *Cognitive aspects of skilled typewriting* (pp. 1–38). New York: Springer-Verlag.

Coover, J. E. (1923). A method of teaching typewriting based upon a psychological analysis of expert typing. *National Educational Association, 61,* 561–567.

Coquery, J.-M. (1978). Role of active movement in control of afferent input from skin in cat and man. In G. Gordon (Ed.), *Active touch.* Oxford: Pergamon.

Coren, S. (1986). An efferent component in the visual perception of direction and extent. *Psychological Review, 93,* 391–410.

Costello, J. M. (Ed.). (1985). *Speech disorders in adults.* San Diego: College Hill Press.

Côté, L., & Crutcher, M. D. (1985). Motor functions of the basal ganglia and diseases of transmitter metabolism. In E. R. Kandel & J. H. Schwartz (Eds.), *Principles of neural science* (2nd ed) (pp. 523–535). New York: Elsevier.

Cousins, N. (1984). *The healing heart.* New York: Avon.

Cowan, N. (1988). Evolving conceptions of memory storage, selective attention, and their mutual constraints within the human information-processing system. *Psychological Bulletin, 104,* 163–191.

Cowan, N., Braine, M. D. S., & Leavitt, L. A. (1985). The phonological and metaphonological representation of speech: Evidence from fluent backward talkers. *Journal of Memory and Language, 24,* 679–698.

Craft, J. L., & Simon, J. R. (1970). Processing symbolic information from a visual display: Interference from an irrelevant directional cue. *Journal of Experimental Psychology, 83,* 415–420.

Craig, J. J. (1986). *Introduction to robotics*. Reading, MA: Addison-Wesley.

Craik, K. J. W. (1943). *The nature of explanation*. London: Cambridge University Press.

Craske, B., & Craske, J. D. (1986). Oscillator mechanisms in the human motor system: Investigating their properties using the after-contraction effect. *Journal of Motor Behavior, 18*, 117–145.

Cromer, R. F. (1983). Hierarchical planning disability in the drawings and constructions of a special group of severely aphasic children. *Brain and Cognition, 2*, 144–164.

Crossman, E. R. F. W. (1959). A theory of the acquisition of speed skill. *Ergonomics, 2*, 153–166.

Crossman, E. R. F. W., & Goodeve, P. J. (1963/1983). Feedback control of hand-movement and Fitts' Law. *Quarterly Journal of Experimental Psychology, 35A*, 251–278.

Cruse, H. (1986). Constraints for joint angle control of the human arm. *Biological Cybernetics, 54*, 125–132.

Cruse, H., Kindermann, T., Schumm, M., Dean, J., & Schmitz, J. (1998). Walknet-a biologically inspired network to control six-legged walking. *Neural Networks, 11*, 1435–1447.

Cruse, H., Steinkühler, U., & Burkamp, C. (1998). MMC-a recurrent neural network which can be used as manipulable body model. In R. Pfeifer, B. Blumberg, J.-A. Meyer, & S. Wilson (Eds.), *From animal to animats 5* (pp. 381–389). Cambridge, MA: MIT Press.

Crutcher, M. D., & DeLong, M. R. (1984). Single cell studies of the primate putamen. II. Relations to direction of movement and pattern of muscular activity. *Experimental Brain Research, 53*, 244–258.

Cutting, J. E. (1986). *Perception with an eye for motion*. Cambridge, MA: Bradford/MIT.

Cutting, J. E., & Proffitt, D. R. (1981). Gait perception as an example of how we may perceive events. In R. D. Walk & H. L. Pick (Eds.), Jr., *Intersensory perception and sensory integration* (pp. 249–273) Plenum.

Daniloff, R., & Moll, K. (1968). Coarticulation of lip rounding. *Journal of Speech and Hearing Research, 11*, 707–721.

Daprati, E., Franck, N., Georgieff, N., Proust, J., Pacherie, E., Dalery, J., et al. (1997). Looking for the agent: An investigation into consciousness of action and self-consciousness in schizophrenic patients. *Cognition, 65*, 71–86.

Darainy, M., Towhidkhah, F., & Ostry, D. J. (2007). Control of hand impedance under static conditions and during reaching movement. *Journal of Neurophysiology, 97*, 2676–2685.

Darwin, C. J., Turvey, M. T., & Crowder, R. G. (1972). An auditory analogue of the Sperling partial report procedure: Evidence for brief auditory storage. *Cognitive Psychology, 6*, 41–60.

Darwin, C. R. (1872/1965). *The expression of the emotions in man and animals*. Chicago: University of Chicago Press (Original work published in 1872).

David, P. (1985). Clio and the economics of QWERTY. American Economic Review. (May). [Cited in The Stanford Observer, April 1985, p.4]

Davidson, A. G., Chan, V., O'Dell, R., & Schieber, M. H. (2007). Rapid changes in throughput from single motor cortex neurons to muscle activity. *Science, 318*, 1934–1937.

Deakin, J. M., & Cobley, S. (2003). An examination of the practice environments in figure skating and volleyball: A search for deliberate practice. In J. Starkes & K. A. Ericsson (Eds.), *Expert performance in sports: Advances in research on sport expertise* (pp. 9–113). Champaign, IL: Human Kinetics.

Decety, J., & Jeannerod, M. (1995). Mentally simulated movements in virtual reality: Does Fitts's law hold in motor imagery? *Behavioral Brain Research, 72*, 127–134.

Deecke, L., Scheid, P., & Kornhuber, H. H. (1969). Distribution of readiness potential, pre-motion positivity, and motor potential of the human cerebral cortex preceding voluntary finger movements. *Experimental Brain Research, 7*, 158–168.

deGroot, A. D. (1965). *Thought and choice in chess*. The Hague: Mouton.

Dehaene, S. (1997). *The number sense: How the mind creates mathematics*. New York: Oxford University Press.

DeJong, R. N. (1967). *The neurologic examination*. New York: Harper & Row.

Dell, G. S. (1986). A spreading activation theory of retrieval in sentence production. *Psychological Review, 93*, 283–321.

Dell'Osso, L. F., & Daroff, R. B. (1981). Clinical disorders of ocular movement. In B. L. Zuber (Ed.), *Models of oculomotor behavior and control* (pp. 233–256). Boca Raton, FL: CRC Press, Inc.

de Lussanet, M. H. E., Smeets, J. B. J., & Brenner, E. (2001). The effect of expectations on hitting moving targets: Influence of the preceding target's speed. *Experimental Brain Research, 137*, 246–248.

de Lussanet, M. H. E., Smeets, J. B. J., & Brenner, E. (2002). The relation between task history and movement strategy. *Behavioral Brain Research, 129*, 51–59.

Demaire, C., Honoré, J., & Coquery, J. M. (1984). Effects of ballistic and tracking movements on spinal proprioceptive and cutaneous pathways in man. In S. Kornblum & J. Requin (Eds.), *Preparatory states and processes* (pp. 201–216). Hillsdale, NJ: Erlbaum.

Demyer, W. (1980). *Technique of the neurologic examination*. New York: McGraw-Hill.

Denier van der Gon, J. J., & Thuring, J. Ph. (1965). The guiding of human writing movements. *Kybernetik, 2*, 145–148.

DeRenzi, E., Motti, F., & Nichelli, P. (1980). Imitating gestures: A quantitative approach to ideomotor apraxia. *Archives of Neurology, 37*, 6–10.

Desmedt, J. E. (1981). *Motor unit types, recruitment and plasticity in health and disease. (Progress in clinical neurophysiology)* (Vol. 9). Basel: Karger.

Deutsch, J. A., & Clarkson, J. K. (1959). Nature of the vibrato and the control loop in singing. *Nature, 183*, 167–168.

Dickinson, M. H., Farley, C. T., Full, R. J., Keohl, M. A., Kram, R., & Lehman, S. (2000). How animals move: An integrative view. *Science, 288*, 100–106.

Diedrichsen, J., Hazeltine, E., Kennerley, S., & Ivry, R. B. (2000). Moving to directly cued locations abolishes spatial interference during bimanual actions. *Psychological Science, 12*, 493–498.

Ditchburn, R. W. (1973). *Eye movements and visual perception.* Oxford: Clarendon Press.

Dodge, R. (1900). Visual perception during eye movement. *Psychological Review, 7*, 454–465.

Doidge, N. (2007). *The brain that changes itself.* New York: Viking.

Donelan, J. M., Li, Q., Naing, V., Hoffer, J. A., Weber, D. J., & Kuo, A. D. (2008). Biomechanical energy harvesting: Generating electricity during walking with minimal user effort. *Science, 319*, 807–810.

Drachman, D. B. (1983). Myasthenia gravis: Immunobiology of a receptor disorder. *Trends in the Neurosciences, 6*, 446–451.

Duff, S., & Sainburg, R. (2007). Lateralization of motor adaptation reveals independence in control of trajectory and steady-state position. *Experimental Brain Research, 179*, 551–561.

Duffy, J. R. (2005). *Motor speech disorders: Substrates, differential Diagnosis, and management.* Mosby.

Duhamel, J.-R., Colby, C. L., & Goldberg, M. E. (1992). The updating of the representation of visual space in parietal cortex by intended eye movements. *Science, 255*, 90–92.

Easton, D. E., & Shor, R. E. (1976). An experimental analysis of the Chevreul pendulum illusion. *Journal of General Psychology, 95*, 111–125.

Easton, T. A. (1972). On the normal use of reflexes. *American Scientist, 60*, 591–599.

Eccles, J. (1977). Cerebellar function in the control of movement. In F. Rose (Ed.), *Physiological aspects of clinical neurology* (pp. 157–178). Oxford: Blackwell.

Edelman, S., & Flash, T. (1987). A model of handwriting. *Biological Cybernetics, 57*, 25–36.

Ehrsson, H. H., Geyer, S., & Naito, E. (2003). Imagery of voluntary movement of fingers, toes, and tongue activates corresponding body-part-specific motor representations. *Journal of Neurophysiology, 90*, 3304–3316.

Ehrsson, H. H., Holmes, N. P., & Passingham, R. E. (2005). Touching a rubber hand: Feeling of body ownership is associated with activity in multisensory brain areas. *Journal of Neuroscience, 25*, 10564–10573.

Ehrsson, H. H., Spence, C., & Passingham, R. E. (2004). That's my hand! Activity in the premotor cortex reflects feeling of ownership of a limb. *Science, 305*, 875–877.

Einhauser, W., Stout, J., Koch, C., & Carter, O. (2008). Pupil dilation reflects perceptual selection and predicts subsequent stability in perceptual rivalry. *Proceedings of the National Academy of Sciences, 105*, 1704–1709.

Ekman, P. (1975). Face muscles talk every language. Psychology Today (September), 35–39.

Ekman, P., & Friesen, W. V. (1975). *Unmasking the face.* Englewood Cliffs, NJ: Prentice-Hall.

Ekman, P., Friesen, W. V., & O'Sullivan, M. (1988). Smiles when lying. *Journal of Personality and Social Psychology, 54*, 414–420.

Ekman, P., Hager, J. C., & Friesen, W. V. (1981). The symmetry of emotional and deliberate facial actions. *Psychophysiology, 18*, 101–106.

Ekman, P., Levenson, R. W., & Friesen, W. V. (1983). Autonomic nervous system activity distinguishes among emotions. *Science, 221*, 1208–1210.

Ekman, P., & Oster, H. (1979). Facial expressions of emotion. *Annual Review of Psychology, 30*, 527–554.

Ekman, P., & O'Sullivan, M. (1991). Who can catch a liar? *American Psychologist, 46*, 913–920.

El'ner, A. N. (1973). Possibilities of correcting the urgent voluntary movements and the associated postural activity of human muscles. *Biophysics, 18*, 966–971.

Elbert, T., Pantev, C., Weinbruch, C., Rockstroh, B., & Taub, E. (1995). Increased cortical representation of the fingers of the left hand. *Science, 270*, 305–307.

Elble, R. J., & Koller, W. C. (1990). *Tremor.* Baltimore, MD: Johns Hopkins University Press.

Elliott, D., Helsen, W. F., & Chua, R. (2001). A century later: Woodworth's (1899) two-component model of goal-directed aiming. *Psychological Bulletin, 127*, 342–357.

Elliott, J. M., & Conolly, K. J. (1984). A classification of manipulative hand movements. *Developmental Medicine and Child Neurology, 26*, 238–296.

Ellis, A. (1979). Slips of the pen. *Visible Language, 13*, 265–282.

Emmorey, K. (2002). *Language, cognition, and the brain: Insights from sign language research.* Hillsdale, NJ: Erlbaum.

Engbert, R., & Kliegl, R. (2003). Microsaccades uncover the orientation of covert attention. *Vision Research, 43*, 1035–1045.

Engelbrecht, S. E. (2001). Minimum principles in motor control. *Journal of Mathematical Psychology, 45,* 497–542.

Enocka, R. M. (1988). *Neuromechanical basis of kinesiology.* Champaign, IL: Human Kinetics Books.

Enocka, R. M., & Stuart, D. G. (1984). Henneman's size principle: Current issues. *Trends in the Neurosciences, 7,* 226–227.

Epelboim, J., Steinman, R. M., Kowler, E., Pizlo, Z., Erkelens, C. J., & Collewijn, H. (1997). Gaze-shift dynamics in two kinds of sequential looking tasks. *Vision Research, 37,* 2597–2607.

Erickson, R. P. (1984). On the neural bases of behavior. *American Scientist, 72,* 233–241.

Ericsson, K. A., Krampe, R. T., & Tesch-Romer, C. (1993). The role of deliberate practice in the acquisition of expert performance. *Psychological Review, 100,* 363–406.

Erlhagen, W., & Schöner, G. (2002). Dynamic field theory of movement preparation. *Psychological Review, 109,* 545–572.

Essock, E. A., & Siqueland, E. R. (1981). Discrimination of orientation by human infants. *Perception, 10,* 245–253.

Essock, E. A., & Siqueland, E. R. (1981). Discrimination of orientation by human infants. *Perception, 10,* 245–253.

Estes, W. K. (1972). An associative basis for coding and organization in memory. In A. W. Melton & E. Martin (Eds.), *Coding processes in human memory* (pp. 161–190). Washington, DC: V. H. Winston.

Evarts, E. V. (1967). Representation of movement and muscles by pyramidal tract neurons of the precentral motor cortex. In M. D. Yahr & D. P. Purpura (Eds.), *Neurophysiological basis of normal and abnormal motor activities.* New York: Raven Press.

Evarts, E. V. (1981). Role of motor cortex in voluntary movements in primates. In: V. B. Brooks (Ed.), Handbook of physiology, Section 1: The nervous system, Vol II. Motor control (1083–1120). Bethesda, MD: American Physiological Society.

Evarts, E., & Tanji, J. (1976). Reflex and intended responses in motor cortex pyramidal tract neurons of monkey. *Journal of Neurophysiology, 39,* 1069–1108.

Fackelmann, K. A. (1989). Drug slows Parkinson's progression [one page article]. *Science News, 136*(6), 84.

Fagard, J. (2000). Linked proximal and distal changes in the reaching behavior of 5– to 12–month old human infants grasping objects of different sizes. *Infant Behavior & Development, 23,* 317–329.

Fajen, B. R., & Warren, W. H. (2003). Behavioral dynamics of steering, obstacle avoidance, and route selection. *Journal of Experimental Psychology: Human Perception and Performance, 29,* 343–362.

Fallang, B., Daugstad, O. D., & Hadders-Algra, M. (2000). Goal directed reaching and postural control in supine position in healthy infants. *Behavioural Brain Research, 115,* 9–18.

Fantz, R. (1961). The origin of form perception. *Scientific American, 204*(5), 66–72.

Feldman, A. G. (1986). Once more on the equilibrium-point hypothesis (Lambda Model) for motor control. *Journal of Motor Behavior, 18,* 17–54.

Feldman, A., & Latash, M. L. (2005). Testing hypotheses and the advancement of science: Recent attempts to falsify the equilibrium point hypothesis. *Experimental Brain Research, 161,* 91–103.

Feldman, R. S. (Ed.). (1982). *Development of nonverbal behavior in children.* New York: Springer-Verlag.

Feltz, D., & Landers, D. M. (1983). The effects of mental practice on motor skill learning and performance: A meta-analysis. *Journal of Sports Psychology, 5,* 25–57.

Fendrick, P. (1937). Hierarchical skills in typewriting. *Journal of Educational Psychology, 28,* 609–620.

Fenn, W. O. (1938). The mechanics of muscle contraction in man. *Journal of Applied Physics, 9,* 165–177.

Fetter, M., Misslisch, H., & Tweed, D. (Eds.), (1997). *Three-dimensional kinematics of eye-, head-, and limb-movements.* Chur, Switzerland: Harwood Academic Publishers.

Field, J. (1977). Coordination of vision and prehension in young infants. *Child Development, 48,* 97–103.

Field, T., Woodson, R., Greenberg, R., & Cohen, D. (1982). Discrimination and imitation of facial expressions by neonates. *Science, 218,* 179–181.

Finkbeiner, M., Song, J. H., & Nakayama, K. (2008). Engaging the motor system with masked orthographic primes: A kinematic analysis. *Visual Cognition, 16,* 11–22.

Fischer, B., & Breitmeyer, B. (1987). Mechanisms of visual attention revealed by saccadic eye movements. *Neuropsychologia, 25,* 73–83.

Fischman, J. (1987). Graphology: The write stuff? *Psychology Today, 7,* 11.

Fischman, M. G., Stodden, D. F., & Lehman, D. M. (2003). The end-state comfort effect in bimanual grip selection. *Research Quarterly for Exercise and Sport, 74,* 17–24.

Fischman, M. G., Christina, R. W., & Anson, J. G. (2008). Memory drum theory's C movement: Revelations from Franklin Henry. *Research Quarterly for Exercise and Sport, 79,* 312–318.

Fitts, P. M. (1964). Perceptual-motor skill learning. In A. W. Melton (Ed.), *Categories of human learning* (pp. 243–285). New York: Academic Press.

Fitts, P. M. (1954). The information capacity of the human motor system in controlling the amplitude of movement (Reprinted in Journal of Experimental Psychology: General, 121, 262–269, 1992). *Journal of Experimental Psychology, 47,* 381–391.

Fitts, P. M., & Deininger, R. L. (1954). S-R compatibility: Correspondence among paired elements with stimulus and response codes. *Journal of Experimental Psychology, 48*, 483–491.

Fitts, P. M., & Peterson, J. R. (1964). Information capacity of discrete motor responses. *Journal of Experimental Psychology, 67*, 103–112.

Flanagan, J. R., & Johansson, R. S. (2003). Action plans used in action observation. *Nature, 424*, 769–771.

Flanagan, J. R., Tresilian, J. R., & Wing, A. M. (1993). Coupling of grip force and load force during arm movements with grasped objects. *Neuroscience Letters, 152*, 53–56.

Flash, T., & Hogan, N. (1985). The coordination of arm movements: An experimentally confirmed mathematical model. *The Journal of Neuroscience, 5*, 1688–1703.

Fleishman, E. A., & Bartlett, C. J. (1969). Human abilities. *Annual Review of Psychology, 20*, 349–380.

Fleishman, E. A., & Parker, R. F., Jr. (1962). Factors in the retention and relearning of perceptual motor skill. *Journal of Experimental Psychology, 64*, 215–226.

Fodor, J. A. (1983). *The modularity of mind.* Cambridge, MA: MIT Press.

Foley, J. D. (1987). Interfaces for advanced computing. *Scientific American, 257*(4), 127–135.

Forssberg, H., Grillner, S., & Rossignol, S. (1975). Phase dependent reflex reversal during walking in chronic spinal cats. *Brain Research, 55*, 247–304.

Forssberg, H., Johnels, B., & Steg, G. (1984). Is parkinsonian gait caused by a regression to an immature walking pattern? *Advances in Neurology, 40*, 375–379.

Fowler, C. A. (2007). Speech production. In M. G. Gaskell (Ed.), *The Oxford Handbook of Psycholinguistics* (pp. 489–502). New York: Oxford University Press.

Fowler, C. A., & Turvey, M. T. (1978). Skill acquisition: A event approach for the optimum of a function of several variables. In G. E. Stelmach (Ed.), *Information processing in motor control and learning.* New York: Academic Press.

Fox, R., & McDaniel, C. (1982). The perception of biological motion by human infants. *Science, 218*(29), 486–487.

Franklin, D. W., Burdet, E., Tee, K. P., Osu, R., Chew, C.-M., Milner, T. E., et al. (2008). CNS learns stable, accurate, and efficient movements using a simple algorithm. *Journal of Neuroscience, 28*, 11165–11173.

Franklin, D. W., Liaw, G., Milner, T. E., Osu, R., Burdet, E., & Kawato, M. (2007). Endpoint stiffness of the arm is directionally tuned to instability in the environment. *Journal of Neuroscience, 27*, 7705–7716.

Franz, E. A., Zelaznik, H. N., Swinnen, S., & Walter, C. (2001). Spatial conceptual influences on the coordination of bimanual actions: When a dual task becomes a single task. *Journal of Motor Behavior, 33*, 103–112.

Franz, E., Eliassen, J., Ivry, R., & Gazzaniga, M. (1996). Dissociation of spatial and temporal coupling in the bimanual movements of callosotomy patients. *Psychological Science, 7*, 306–310.

Franz, V. (2001). Action does not resist visual illusions. *Trends in Cognitive Sciences, 5*, 457–459.

Fraser, C., & Wing, A. M. (1981). A case study of reaching by a user of a manually-operated artificial hand. *Prosthetics and Orthotics International, 5*, 151–156.

Freed, C. R., & Yamamoto, B. K. (1985). Regional brain dopamine metabolism: A marker fo the speed, direction, and posture of moving animals. *Science, 229*, 62–65.

Freedman, D. G. (1964). Smiling in blind infants and the issue of innate vs. acquired. *Journal of Child Psychology and Psychiatry, l5*, 171–184.

Freeman, R. N. (1987). The apraxias, purposeful motor behavior, and left-hemisphere function. In W. Prinz & A. F. Sanders (Eds.), *Cognition and motor processes* (pp. 29–50). Berlin: Springer-Verlag.

Freud, S. (1901/1966). *Psychopathology of everyday life (A. Tyson, Trans.).* London: Benn (Original work published in 1901).

Frey, W. H., II, DeSota-Johnson, D., & Hoffman, C. (1981). *Journal of Ophthalmology, 92*, 559–578.

Fridlund, A. J., & Gilbert, A. N. (1985). Emotions and facial expression. *Science, 230*, 607–608.

Frith, C. D., Blakemore, S. J., & Wolpert, D. M. (2000). Explaining the symptoms of schizophrenia: Abnormalities in the awareness of action. *Brain Research Reviews, 31*, 336–357.

Fromkin, V. A. (Ed.). (1973). *Speech errors as linguistic evidence.* The Hague: Mouton.

Fromkin, V. A. (Ed.). (1980). *Errors in linguistic performance.* New York: Academic Press.

Fry, D. B. (1970). Prosodic phenomena. In: B. Malberg (Ed.), Manual of phonetics. (Chapter 12). Amsterdam: North-Holland Press.

Fuchs, A. (1967). Saccadic and smooth pursuit eye movements in the monkey. *Journal of Physiology (London), 191*, 609–631.

Fuchs, A. F., & Melton, A. W. (1974). Effects of frequency of presentation and stimulus length on retention in the Brown-Peterson paradigm. *Journal of Experimental Psychology, 103*, 629–637.

Fuchs, A., & Ron, S. (1968). An analysis of rapid eye movements of sleep in the monkey. *Electroencephalography and Clinical Neurophysiology, 25*, 244–251.

Fucson, O. I., Berkenblit, M. B., & Feldman, A. G. (1980). The spinal frog takes into account the scheme of its body during the wiping reflex. *Science, 209*, 11261–11263.

Fujii, N., & Graybiel, A. M. (2003). Representation of action sequence boundaries by macaque prefrontal cortical neurons. *Science*, *301*, 1246–1249.

Fujisaki, H. (1983). Dynamic characteristics of voice fundamental frequency in speech and singing. In P. F. MacNeilage (Ed.), *The production of speech* (pp. 39–55). New York: Springer-Verlag.

Fuller, D. C. (1943). Reading factors in typewriting. Unpublished doctoral dissertation. Graduate School of Education, Harvard University.

Galantucci, B., Fowler, C. A., & Turvey, M. T. (2006). The motor theory of speech perception reviewed. *Psychonomic Bulletin & Review*, *13*, 361–377.

Gallistel, C. R. (1980). *The organization of action*. Hillsdale, NJ: Erlbaum.

Gallistel, C. R. (1999). Coordinate transformations in the genesis of directed action. In B. M. Bly & D. E. Rumelhart (Eds.), *Cognitive Science* (pp. 1–42). San Diego: Academic Press.

Galloway, J. C., & Thelen, E. (2003). Feet first: Object exploration in human infants. *Infant Behavior and Development*, *27*, 107–112.

Galton, F. (1979). *Hereditary genius: An inquiry into its laws and consequences*. London: Julian Friedman Publishers (Originally published in 1869).

Gardner, H., & Zurif, E. (1975). Bee but not be: Oral reading of single words in aphasia and alexia. *Neuropsychologia*, *13*, 181–190. Garland, H. T., & Angel, R. W. (1972). Modulation of tactile sensitivity during movement. *Neurology*, *24*, 361.

Garrett, M. F. (1975). The analysis of sentence production. In G. H. Bower (Ed.)*Psychology of learning and motivation: Vol. 9*. New York: Academic Press.

Garrett, M. F. (1982). Production of speech: Observations from normal and pathological language use. In A. Ellis (Ed.), *Normality and pathology in cognitive functions*. London: Academic Press.

Gaskell, M. G. (Ed.). (2007). *The Oxford Handbook of Psycholinguistics*. New York: Oxford University Press.

Gauthier, G. M., Vercher, J.-L., Mussa Ivaldi, F., & Marchetti, E. (1988). Oculo-manual tracking of visual targets: Control learning, coordination control and coordination model. *Experimental Brain Research*, *73*, 127–137.

Gawande, A. (June 30 2008). The itch. *The New Yorker*, 58–65.

Gazzaniga, M. S. (Ed.). (2004). *The cognitive neurosciences III*. Cambridge, MA: Bradford/MIT Press.

Gelfan, S., & Carter, S. (1967). Muscle sense in man. *Experimental Neurology*, *18*, 469–473.

Gelfand, I. M., Gurfinkel, V. S., Tsetlin, M. L., Shik, M. L. (1966). Problems in analysis of movements. In: I. M. Gelfand, V. S. Gurfinkel, S. V. Fomin, M. L. Tsetlin (Eds.), Models of the structural functional organization of certain biological systems. (pp. 330–345). (American translation, 1971). Cambridge, MA: MIT Press.

Gentner, D. R. (1987). Timing of skilled motor performance: Tests of the proportional duration model. *Psychological Review*, *94*, 255–276.

Gentner, D. R., Grudin, J., Conway, E. (1980). Finger movements in transcription typing. La Jolla, CA: University of California, San Diego, Center for Human Information Processing, (Technical Report 8001).

Gentner, D. R., Larochelle, S., & Grudin, J. (1988). Lexical, sublexical, and peripheral effects in skilled typewriting. *Cognitive Psychology*, *20*, 524–548.

Gentner, D. R., & Norman, D. A. (1984). The typist's touch. *Psychology Today*, *8*, 66–72.

Georgopoulos, A. P., & Grillner, S. (1989). Visuomotor coordination in reaching and locomotion. *Science*, *245*, 1209–1210.

Georgopoulos, A. P., Kalaska, J. F., & Massey, J. T. (1981). Spatial trajectories and reaction times of aimed movements: Effects of practice, uncertainty, and change in target location. *Journal of Neurophysiology*, *46*, 725–743.

Georgopoulos, A. P., Lurito, J. T., Petrides, M., Schwartz, A. B., & Massey, J. T. (1989). Mental rotation of the neuronal population vector. *Science*, *243*, 234–236.

Georgopoulos, A. P., Schwartz, A. B., & Kettner, R. E. (1986). Neuronal population coding of movement direction. *Science*, *233*, 1416–1419.

Gergely, G., Bekkering, H., & Kiraly, I. (2002). Rational imitation in preverbal infants. *Nature*, *415*, 755.

Geschwin, N. (1965). The disconnexion syndrome in animals and man. *Brain*, *88*, 237–294.

Ghez, C. (1985). Voluntary movement. In E. R. Kandel & J. H. Schwartz (Eds.), *Principles of neural science* (2nd ed) (pp. 487–501). New York: Elsevier.

Gibbon, J., Allan, L. (Eds.), Timing and time perception. (pp. 183–192). New York: New York Academy of Sciences.

Gibson, E. J. (1987). What does infant perception tell us about theories of perception? *Journal of Experimental Psychology: Human Perception and Performance*, *13*, 515–523.

Gibson, J. J. (1933). Adaptation after-effect and contrast in perception of curved lines. *Journal of Experimental Psychology*, *16*, 1–31.

Gibson, J. J. (1933). Adaptation after-effect and contrast in perception of curved lines. *Journal of Experimental Psychology*, *16*, 1–31.

Gibson, J. J. (1962). Observations on active touch. *Psychological Review*, *69*, 477–491.

Gibson, J. J. (1950). *Perception of the visual world*. Boston: Houghton-Mifflin.

Gibson, J. J. (1966). *The senses considered as perceptual systems*. Boston: Houghton-Mifflin.

Gibson, J. J. (1979). *The ecological approach to visual perception*. Boston: Houghton-Mifflin.

Gielen, C. C. A. M., Vrijenhoek, E. J., & Flash, T. (1997). Principles for the control of kinematically redundant limbs. In M. Fetter, H. Misslisch, & D. Tweed (Eds.), *Three-dimensional kinematics of eye-, head-, and limb-movements* (pp. 285–297). Chur, Switzerland: Harwood Academic Publishers.

Gilbert, D. (July 24, 2006). He Who Cast the First Stone Probably Didn't. New York Times Op-Ed. http://www.nytimes.com/2006/07/24/opinion/24gilbert.html?_r=1&sq=he%20who%20cast%20the%20first%20stone&st=cse&oref=slogin&scp=1&pagewanted=print

Gilbert, P. F. C., & Thach, W. T. (1977). Purkinje cell activity during motor learning. *Brain Research, 128*, 309–328.

Gilden, D. L. (2001). Cognitive emissions of 1/f noise. *Psychological Review, 108*, 33–56.

Gilman, S., Bloedel, J. R., & Lechtenberg, R. (1981). *Disorders of the cerebellum*. Philadelphia: Davis.

Gilmore, R. O., Baker, T. J., & Grobman, K. H. (2004). Stability in young infants' discrimination of optic flow. *Developmental Psychology, 40*, 259–270.

Gilmore, R. O., & Johnson, M. H. (1997). Body-centered representations for visually-guided action emerge during early infancy. *Cognition, 65*, B1–B9.

Glass, A. L. (2004). *Cognition*. Mason, OH: Thompson Custom Publishing.

Gleick, J. (1988). *Chaos: Making a new science*. New York: Penguin.

Gleitman, H. (1981). *Psychology*. New York: W. W. Norton.

Glenberg, A. M., & Kaschak, M. P. (2002). Grounding language in action. *Psychonomic Bulletin & Review, 9*, 558–565.

Glencross, D. J. (1980). Levels and strategies of response organization. In G. E. Stelmach & J. Requin (Eds.), *Tutorials in motor behavior*. Amsterdam: North-Holland.

Glover, S. R. (2002). Visual illusions affect planning but not control. *Trends In Cognitive Sciences, 6*, 288–292.

Glover, S., Rosenbaum, D. A., Graham, J., & Dixon, P. (2004). Grasping the meaning of words. *Experimental Brain Research, 154*, 103–108.

Goldfield, E. C., Kay, B. A., & Warren, W. H. (1993). Infant bouncing: The assembly and tuning of action systems. *Child Development, 64*, 1128–1142.

Goldin-Meadow, S. (1999). The role of gesture in communication and thinking. *Trends in Cognitive Sciences, 3*, 419–429.

Goldin-Meadow, S., & Wagner, S. M. (2005). How our hands help us learn. *Trends in Cognitive Sciences, 9*, 234–241.

Goldman-Eisler, F. (1968). *Psycholinguistics: Experiments in spontaneous speech*. New York: Academic Press.

Goleman, D. (1989). New breed of robots have the human touch. The New York Times, August 1, page C1.

Gomi, H., & Kawato, M. (1996). Equilibrium-point control hypothesis examined by measured arm stiffness during multijoint movement. *Science, 272*, 117–120.

Goodenough, F. L. (1932). Expression of the emotions in a blind-deaf child. *Journal of Abnormal and Social Psychology, 27*, 328–333.

Goodman, D. G., & Kelso, J. A. S. (1980). Are movements prepared in parts? Not under compatible (naturalized) conditions. *Journal of Experimental Psychology: General, 109*, 475–495.

Goodnow, J. (1977). *Children drawing*. Cambridge, Massachusetts: Harvard University Press.

Goodnow, J. J., & Levine, R. (1973). The grammar of action: Sequence and syntax in children's copying. *Cognitive Psychology, 4*, 82–98.

Goodwin, G. M., McCloskey, D. J., & Matthews, P. B. C. (1972). The contribution of muscle afferents to kinaesthesia shown by vibration-induced illusions of movement and by the effect of paralysing joint afferents. *Brain, 95*, 705–748.

Gopher, D., Karis, D., & Koenig, W. (1985). The representation of movement schemas in long-term memory: Lessons from the acquisition of a transcription skill. *Acta Psychologica, 60*, 105–1134.

Gordon, A. M., Forssberg, H., Johansson, R. S., & Westling, G. (1991a). Integration of haptically acquired size information in the programming of the precision grip. *Experimental Brain Research, 83*, 483–488.

Gordon, A. M., Forssberg, H., Johansson, R. S., & Westling, G. (1991b). Integration of sensory information during the programming of precision grip: Comments on the contributions of visual size cues. *Experimental Brain Research, 85*, 226–229.

Gordon, A. M., Forssberg, H., Johansson, R. S., & Westling, G. (1991c). Visual size cues in the programming and control of manipulative forces during precision grip. *Experimental Brain Research, 83*, 477–482.

Gordon, F. R., & Yonas, A. (1976). Sensitivity to binocular depth information in infants. *Journal of Experimental Child Psychology, 22*, 413–422.

Gordon, J., & Ghez, C. (1994). Accuracy of planar reaching movements: I. Independence of direction and extent variability. *Experimental Brain Research, 99*, 97–111.

Gordon, P. C., & Meyer, D. E. (1987a). Control of serial order in rapidly spoken syllable sequences. *Journal of Memory and Language, 26*, 300–321.

Gordon, P. C., & Meyer, D. E. (1987b). Hierarchical representation of spoken syllable order. In A. Allport, D. MacKay, W. Prinz, & E. Scheerer (Eds.), *Language*

Perception and Production (pp. 445–462). London: Academic Press.

Goslow, G. E., Reinking, R. M., & Stuart, D. G. (1973). The cat step cycle: Hind limb joint angles and muscle lengths during unrestrained locomotion. *Journal of Morphology, 141*, 1–42.

Gouras, P. (1985a). Oculomotor system. In E. R. Kandel & J. H. Schwartz (Eds.), *Principles of neural science* (Second Ed) (pp. 571–583). New York: Elsevier.

Gouras, P. (1985b). Physiological optics, accommodation, and stereopsis. In E. R. Kandel & J. H. Schwartz (Eds.), *Principles of neural science* (Second Ed) (pp. 865–875). New York: Elsevier.

Gracco, V. L., & Abbs, J. H. (1987). Programming and execution processes of speech movement control: Potential neural correlates. In E. Keller (Ed.), *Motor and sensory processes of language* (pp. 163–201). Hillsdale, NJ: Lawrence Erlbaum Associates.

Grafton, S. T., Hazeltine, E., & Ivry, R. B. (1995). Functional mapping of sequence learning in noraml humans. *Journal of Cognitive Neuroscience, 7*, 497–510.

Gray, R. (2008). Multisensory information in the control of complex motor actions. *Current Directions in Psychological Science, 17*, 244–248.

Gray, R., Beilock, S. L., & Carr, T. H. (2007). "As soon as the bat met the ball, I knew it was gone": Outcome prediction, hindsight bias, and the representation and control of action in expert and novice baseball player. *Psychonomic Bulletin & Review, 14*, 669–675.

Graziano, M. S. A., & Cooke, D. F. (2006). Parietofrontal interactions, personal space, and defensive behaviour. *Neuropsychologia, 44*, 2621–2635.

Graziano, M. S., & Gross, C. G. (1994). Mapping space with neurons. *Current Directions in Psychological Science, 3*, 164–167.

Graziano, M. S., & Gross, C. G. (1996). Multiple pathways for processing visual space. In T. Inui & J. L. McClelland (Eds.), *Attention and Performance XVI: Information integration* (pp. 181–207). Cambridge, MA: MIT Press.

Graziano, M. S., Taylor, C. S. R., & Moore, T. (2002). Complex movements evoked by microstimulation of precentral cortex. *Neuron, 34*, 841–851.

Grealy, M. A., & Shearer, G. F. (2008). Timing processes in motor imagery. *European Journal of Cognitive Science, 20*, 867–892.

Greenwald, A. G. (1970). Sensory feedback mechanisms in performance control: With special reference to the ideo-motor mechanism. *Psychological Review, 77*, 73–99.

Greer, K. L., & Green, D. W. (1983). Context and motor control in handwriting. *Acta Psychologica, 54*, 205–215.

Gregory, R. L. (1973). *Eye and brain* (Second Edition). New York: McGraw-Hill.

Gribble, P. L., Everling, S., Ford, K., & Mattar, A. (2002). Hand-eye coordination for rapid pointing movements. Arm movement direction and distance are specified prior to saccade onset. *Experimental Brain Research, 145*, 372–382.

Grigg, P. (1976). Responses of joint afferent neurons in cat medial articular nerve to active and passive movements of the knee. *Brain Research, 118*, 482–485.

Grillner, S. (1981). Control of locomotion in bipeds, tetrapods, and fish. In V. B. Brooks (Ed.)*Handbook of Physiology, Section 1: The Nervous System, Vol. II, Motor Control* (pp. 1179–1236). Bethesda, MD: American Physiological Society.

Grondin, S. (Ed.). (2008). *Psychology of Time*. Bingley, U.K: Emerald.

Grosjean, M., Knoblich, G., & Shiffrar, M. (2007). Fitts's Law holds for action perception. *Psychological Science, 18*, 95–99.

Grossberg, S. (Ed.). (1987a). *The adaptive brain, I. Cognition, learning, reinforcement, and rhythm.* Amsterdam: Elsevier/North-Holland.

Grossberg, S., & Kuperstein, M. (1989). *Neural dynamics of sensory-motor control: Expanded Edition.* New York: Pergamon Press.

Grudin, J. G. (1983). Error patterns in novice and skilled typists. In W. E. Cooper (Ed.), *Cognitive aspects of skilled typewriting* (pp. 121–143). New York: Springer-Verlag.

Guenther, F. H., Ghosh, S. S., & Tourville, J. A. (2006). Neural modeling and imaging of the cortical interactions underlying syllable production. *Brain and Language, 96*, 280–301.

Guenther, F. H., Hampson, M., & Johnson, D. (1998). A theoretical investigation of reference frames for the planning of speech movements. *Psychological Review, 105*, 611–633.

Guiard, Y. (1993). On Fitts's and Hooke's laws: Simple harmonic movement in upper-limb cyclical aiming. *Acta Psychologica, 82*, 139–159.

Guigon, E., Baraduc, P., & Desmurget, M. (2007). Computational motor control: Redundancy and invariance. *Journal of Neurophysiology, 97*, 331–347.

Gunilla, R., Oberg, E., & Divac, I. (1981). Cognition and the control of movement. *Trends in NeuroScience, 4*, 122–124.

Guo, H. R., Tanaka, S., Halperin, W. E., & Cameron, L. L. (1999). Back pain prevalence in US industry and estimates of lost workdays. *American Journal of Public Health, 89*, 1029–1035.

Guthrie, B. L., Porter, J. D., & Sparks, D. L. (1983). Corollary discharge provides accurate eye position to the oculomotor position. *Science, 221*, 1193–1195.

Hackley, S. A., & Valle-Inclán, F. (2003). Which stages of processing are speeded by a warning signal? *Biological Psychology, 64*, 27–45.

Haesler, S., Rochefort, C., Georgi, B., Licznerski, P., Osten, P., & Scharff, C. (2007). Incomplete and Inaccurate Vocal Imitation after Knockdown of FoxP2 in Songbird Basal Ganglia Nucleus Area X 10.1371/journal.pbio.0050321. *PLoS Biology, 5*(12), e321.

Haggard, P. (1998). Planning of action sequences. *Acta Psychologica, 99*, 201–215.

Haggard, P., Cockburn, J., Cock, J., Fordham, C., & Wade, D. (2000). Interference between gait and cognitive tasks in a rehabilitating neurological population. *Journal of Neurology, Neurosurgery, and Psychiatry, 69*, 479–486.

Haggard, P., & Cole, J. (2007). Intention, attention and the temporal experience of action. *Consciousness and Cognition, 16*, 211–220.

Haggard, P., & Libet, B. (2001). Conscious intention and brain activity. *Journal of Consciousness Studies, 8*(11), 47–63.

Haggard, P., & Richardson, J. (1996). Spatial patterns in the control of human arm movements. *Journal of Experimental Psychology: Human Perception and Performance, 22*, 42–62.

Haken, H. (1977). *Synergetics: An introduction.* Berlin: Springer-Verlag.

Haken, H. (1983). *Advanced synergetics.* Berlin: Springer-Verlag.

Haken, H., Kelso, J. A. S., & Bunz, H. (1985). A theoretical model of phase transitions in human hand movements. *Biological Cybernetics, 51*, 347–356.

Haken, H., & Wunderlin, A. (1990). Synergetics and its paradigm of self-organization in biological systems. In H. T. A. Whiting, O. G. Meijer, & P. C. van Wieringen (Eds.), *The natural-physical approach to movement control* (pp. 1–36). Amsterdam: VU University Press.

Hale, B. D. (1982). The effects of internal and external imagery on muscular and ocular concomitants. *Journl of Sports Psychology, 4*, 379–387.

Halle, M. G. (1962). Phonology in generative grammar. *Word, 18*, 54–72.

Halle, M. G., & Clements, G. N. (1983). *Problem book in phonetics.* Cambridge, MA: MIT Press.

Hallet, P. E., & Lightstone, A. D. (1975). Saccadic eye movements to stimuli triggered by prior saccades. *Vision Research, 16*, 99–106.

Hallett, M., Shahani, B. T., & Young, R. R. (1975a). EMG analysis of stereotyped voluntary movements in man. *Journal of Neurology, Neurosurgery, and Psychiatry, 38*, 1154–1162.

Hallett, M., Shahani, B. T., & Young, R. R. (1975b). EMG analysis of patients with cerebellar deficits. *Journal of Neurology, Neurosurgery, and Psychiatry, 38*, 1163–1169.

Hammond, P. H. (1956). The influences of prior instruction to the subject on an apparently involuntary neuromuscular response. *Journal of Physiology, 132*, 17–18P.

Hansen, R. M., & Skavenski, A. A. (1985). Accuracy of spatial localization near the time of saccadic eye movements. *Vision Research, 25*, 1077–1082.

Hansen, S., Elliott, D., & Khan, M. A. (2008). Quantifying the variability of three-dimensional aiming movements using ellipsoids. *Motor Control, 12*, 241–251.

Hardyck, C., & Petrinovich, L. F. (1977). Left-handedness. *Psychological Bulletin, 84*, 385–404.

Harris, C. M., & Wolpert, D. M. (1998). Signal-dependent noise determines motor planning. *Nature, 394*, 780–784.

Harvey, N. (1985). Vocal control in singing: A cognitive approach. In P. Howell, I. Cross, & R. West (Eds.), *Musical structure and cognition*, p. 289. London: Academic Press.

Hasan, Z. (1986). Optimized movement trajectories and joint stiffness in unperturbed, inertially loaded movements. *Biological Cybernetics, 53*, 373–382.

Hasegawa, A., McCutcheon, M., Wolf, M., & Fletcher, S. (1976). Lip and jaw coordination during the production of of/f, v/in English. *Journal of the Acoustical Society of America, S84*, 59.

Hausdorff, J. M., Balash, J., & Giladi, N. (2003). Effects of cognitive challenge on gait variability in patients with Parkinson's disease. *Journal of Geriatric Psychiatry and Neurology, 16*, 53–58.

Hausdorff, J. M. (2007). Gait dynamics, fractals and falls: Finding meaning in the stride-to-stride fluctuations of human walking. *Human Movement Science, 26*, 555–589.

Hay, L. (1984). The development of movement control. In M. M. Smyth & A. M. Wing (Eds.), *The psychology of human movement* (pp. 241–267). London: Academic Press.

Hayhoe, M., & Ballard, C. (2005). Reaching in natural behavior. *Trends in Cognitive Sciences, 9*, 188–194.

Heathcote, A., Brown, S., & Mewhort, D. J. K. (2000). The power law repealed: The case for an exponential law of practice. *Psychonomic Bulletin and Review, 7*, 185–207.

Heijink, H., & Meulenbroek, R. G. (2002). On the complexity of classical guitar playing: Functional adaptations to task constraints. *Journal of Motor Behavior, 43*, 339–351.

Heilman, K. M., & Roth, L. J. (1985). Apraxia. In K. M. Heilman & E. Valenstein (Eds.), *Clinical neuropsychology* (Second Edition) (pp. 131–150). New York: Oxford.

Hein, A. (1974). Prerequisite for development of visually guided reaching in the kitten. *Brain Research, 71*, 259–263.

Held, R. (1965). Plasticity in sensory-motor systems. *Scientific American, 213*(5), 84–94. Helmholtz, H. (1866/1962). *Handbook of physiological optics*. New York: Dover (Translation of Handbuch der physiologischen Optik. Hamburg: Voss.).

Henderson, S. E., & Sugden, D. A. (1992). *Movement assessment battery for children*. London: Psychological Corporation.

Henig, R. M. (2007). The real transformers. The New York Times Magazine, July 29, pp 28–55.

Henis, E. A., & Flash, T. (1995). Mechanisms underlying the generation of averaged modified trajectories. *Biological Cybernetics, 72*, 407–419.

Henneman, E., Somjen, G., & Carpenter, D. (1965). Excitability and inhibitability of motoneurons of different size. *Journal of Neurobiology, 28*, 599–620.

Henry, F. M., & Rogers, D. E. (1960). Increased response latency for complicated movements and a "memory drum" theory of neuromotor reaction. *Research Quarterly, 31*, 448–458.

Herman, R., Herman, R., & Maulucci, R. (1981). Visually triggered eye-arm movements in man. *Experimental Brain Research, 42*, 392–398.

Herman, R., Wirta, R., Bampton, S., & Finley, F. R. (1976). Human solutions for locomotion: I. Single limb analysis. In R. Herman, S. Grillner, P. Stein, & D. Stuart (Eds.), *Neural control of locomotion* (pp. 13–49). New York: Plenum.

Herron, J., Galin, D., Johnstone, J., & Ornstein, R. E. (1979). Cerebral specialization, writing posture, and motor control of writing in left-handers. *Science, 205*, 1285–1289.

Hess, E. (1975). *The tell-tale eye: How your eyes reveal hidden thoughts*. New York: Van Nostrand Reinhold.

Heuer, H. (1982a). Binary choice reaction time as a criterion of motor equivalence. *Acta Psychologica, 50*, 35–47.

Heuer, H. (1982b). Binary choice reaction time as a criterion of motor equivalence: Further evidence. *Acta Psychologica, 50*, 49–60.

Heuer, H. (1988). Testing the invariance of relative timing: Comment on Gentner (1987). *Psychological Review, 95*, 552–557.

Heyman, K. (2007). Hippocampal cells help rats think ahead (one page article). *Science, 318*, 900.

Hick, W. E. (1952). On the rate of gain of information. *Quarterly Journal of Experimental Psychology, 4*, 11–26.

Higgins, C. I., Campos, J. J., & Kermoian, R. (1996). Effect of self-produced locomotion on infant postural compensation to optic flow. *Developmental Psychology, 32*, 836–841.

Hinde, R. A. (1970). The development of bird song. In K. Connolly (Ed.), *Mechanisms of motor skill development* (pp. 287–304). London: Academic Press.

Ho, L., & Shea, J. G. (1978). Effects of relative frequency of knowledge of results on retention of a motor skill. *Perceptual and Motor Skills, 46*, 859–866.

Hockett, C. F. (1955). A manual of phonology. In, International Journal of American Linguistics (Memoir II). Baltimore: Waverly Press.

Hoff, E. (2009). *Language Development* (4th ed). Belmont, California: Wadsworth/Cengage Learning.

Hoff, E., & Shatz, M. (Eds.), (2007). *Handbook of language development*. Oxford, England: Blackwell Publishers.

Hoffman, J. H., & Roffwarg, H. P. (1983). Modifying oculomotor activity in awake subjects increases the amplitude of eye movements during REM sleep. *Science, 220*, 1074–1076.

Hofsten, C. (1979). Development of visually guided reaching: The approach phase. *Journal of Human Movement Studies, 5*, 150–178.

Hofsten, C.von. (1979). Development of visually guided reaching: The approach phase. *Journal of Human Movement Studies, 5*, 150–178.

Hofsten, C.von (1980). Predictive reaching for moving objects by human infants. *Journal of Experimental Child Psychology, 30*, 369–392.

Hofsten, C.von., & Rönnqvist, L. (1988). Preparation for grasping an object: A developmental study. *Journal of Experimental Psychology: Human Perception and Performance, 14*, 610–621.

Hofsten, C.von., & Rönnqvist, L. (1993). The structuring of neonatal arm movements. *Child Development, 64*, 1046–1057.

Hogan, N. (1984). An organizing principle for a class of voluntary movements. *The Journal of Neuroscience, 4*, 2745–2754.

Hogan, N., & Flash, T. (1987). Moving gracefully: Quantitative theories of motor coordination. *Trends in the Neurosciences, 10*(4), 170–174.

Hogan, N., & Sternad, D. (2007). On rhythmic and discrete movements: Reflections, definitions and implications for motor control. *Experimental Brain Research, 181*, 13–30.

Holding, D. H. (Ed.). (1989). *Human skills* (2nd ed). Chichester: John Wiley & Sons.

Hollerbach, J. M. (1981). An oscillation theory of handwriting. *Biological Cybernetics, 39*, 139–156.

Hollerbach, J. M., & Atkeson, C. G. (1986). Characterization of joint-interpolated arm movements. In H. Heuer & C. Fromm (Eds.), *Generation and modulation of action patterns* (pp. 41–54). Berlin: Springer-Verlag.

Hollerbach, J. M., Moore, S. P., & Atkeson, C. G. (1987). Workspace effect in arm movement kinematics derived by joint interpolation. In G. N. Gantchev, B. Dimitrov, & P. Gatev (Eds.), *Motor Control* (pp. 197–208). Plenum.

Holmes, G. (1939). The cerebellum of man. *Brain, 62,* 1–30.

Holst, E.von. (1973). *The behavioural physiology of animal and man: The collected papers of Erich von Holst* (Vol. 1). London: Methuen Ltd.

Holst, E.von. (1939). Die relative Koordiatnion als PhŠnomenon und als Methode zentral-nervŠse Funktionsanalyze [English translation in Holst, E. von. (1973). Relative coordination as a phenomenon and as a method of analysis of central nervous functions. In The behavioural physiology of animal and man: The collected papers of Erich von Holst (Vol. 1) [R. Martin, Translator]. London: Methuen. *Erg. Physiol., 42,* 228–306.

Holst, E.von., & Mittelstaedt, H. (1950). Das Reafferenzprinzip (English translation in Holst, E. von (1973). The reafference principle. The behav_ioral physiology of animals and man: The collected papers of Erich von Holst (Vol. 1) [R. Martin, Translator]. London: Methuen. *Wechselwirkungen zwis_chen Zentralnervensystem und Peripherie. Naturwissenschaften, 37,* 464–476.

Hommel, B., Musseler, J., Aschersleben, G., & Prinz, W. (2001). The Theory of Event Coding (TEC): A framework for perception and action planning. *Behavioral And Brain Sciences, 24,* 849–937.

Hooker, D. (1938). The origin of the grasping movement in man. *Proceedings of the American Philosophical Society, 79,* 587–606.

Hopkins, B., & Rönnqvist, L. (2002). Facilitating postural control: Effects on the reaching behavior of 6–month-old infants. *Developmental Psychobiology, 40,* 168–182.

Houde, J. F., & Jordan, M. I. (1998). Sensorimotor adaptation in speech production. *Science, 20,* 1213–1216.

Houk, J., & Henneman, E. (1967). Responses of Golgi tendon organs to active contractions of the soleus muscle of the cat. *Journal of Neurophysiology, 30,* 466–481.

Hughes, A. E. (1966). *Self-analysis from your handwriting.* New York: Grosset & Dunlap.

Hughes, C. (1996). Planning problems in autism at the level of motor control. *Journal of Autism and Developmental Disorders, 26,* 99–107.

Hughes, C. M., & Franz, E. A. (2007). Goal-related planning constraints in bimanual grasping and placing of objects. *Experimental Brain Research, 188,* 541–550.

Hughes, O., & Abbs, J. H. (1976). Labial-mandibular coordination in the production of speech: Implications for the operation of motor equivalence. *Phonetica, 44,* 199–221.

Hulse., Fowler, H., & Honig, K. (Eds.), (1978). *Cognitive processes in animal behavior.* Hillsdale, NJ: Erlbaum.

Hulse, S. H. (1978). Cognitive structure and serial pattern learning by animals. In S. Hulse, H. Fowler, & K. Honig (Eds.), *Cognitive processes in animal behavior* (pp. 311–340). Hillsdale, NJ: Erlbaum.

Humphrey, D. R. (1986). Representation of movements and muscles within the primate precentral motor cortex: Historical and current perspectives. *Federation Proceedings, 45,* 2687–2699.

Humphreys, G. W., & Bruce, V. (1989). *Visual cognition.* Hillsdale, NJ: Lawrence Erlbaum Associates.

Huxley, A. F. (1974). Review lecture: Muscular contraction. *Journal of Physiology, 243,* 1–43.

Hyde, J. E. (1959). Some characteristics of voluntary human ocular movements in the horizontal plane. *American Journal of Ophthalmology, 48,* 85–94.

Hyman, R. (1953). Stimulus information as a determinant of reaction time. *Journal of Experimental Psychology, 45,* 188–196.

Iansek, R., & Porter, R. (1980). The monkey globus pallidus: Neuronal discharge properties in relation to movement. *Journal of Physiology (London), 301,* 439–455.

Imamizu, H., Miyauchi, S., Tamada, T., Sasaki, Y., Takino, R., Putz, B., et al. (2000). Human cerebellar activity reflecting an acquired internal model of a new tool. *Nature, 403,* 192–195.

Ingvar, D. H., & Risberg, J. (1967). Increase of regional cerebral blood flow during mental effort in normals and in patients with focal brain disorders. *Experimental Brain Research, 3,* 195–211.

Inhoff, A. W. (1986). Preparing sequences of saccades under choice reaction conditions: Effects of sequence length and context. *Acta Psychologica, 61,* 211–228.

Inhoff, A. W., Rosenbaum, D. A., Gordon, A. M., & Campbell, J. A. (1984). Stimulus-response compatibility and motor programming of manual response sequences. *Journal of Experimental Psychology: Human Perception and Performance, 10,* 724–733.

Ito, M. (1984). *The cerebellum and neural control.* New York: Raven Press.

Ivry, R. B., & Hazeltine, R. E. (1995). Perception and production of temporal intervals across a range of durations: Evidence for a common timing mechanism. *Journal of Experimental Psychology: Human Perception and Performance, 21,* 3–18.

Ivry, R. B. (1996). The representation of temporal information in perception and motor control. *Current Opinion in Neurobiology, 6,* 851–857.

Ivry, R. B., Keele, S. W., & Diener, H. C. (1988). Dissociation of the lateral and medial cerebellum in movement timing and movement execution. *Experimental Brain Research, 73,* 167–180.

Izard, C. E., & Dougherty, L. M. (1982). Two comple-mentary systems for measuring facial expressions in infants and children. In C. E. Izard (Ed.), *Measuring emotions in infants and children*. Cambridge, England: Cambridge University Press.

Izard, C. E. (1977). *Human emotions*. New York: Plenum.

Jacobson, E. (1931). Electrical measurement of neu-romuscular states during mental activities: VI. A note on mental activities concerning an amputated limb. *American Journal of Physiology, 43*, 122–125.

Jagacinski, R. J., & Flach, J. M. (2003). *Control theory for humans: Quantitative approaches to modeling perform-ance*. Mahwah, NJ: L. Erlbaum Associates.

Jagacinski, R. J., Greenberg, N., & Liao, M. J. (1997). Tempo, rhythm, and aging in golf. *Journal of Motor Behavior, 29*, 159–173.

Jagacinski, R. J., Marshburn, E., Klapp, S. T., & Jones, M. R. (1988). Tests of parallel versus integrated structures in polyrhythmic tapping. *Journal of Motor Behavior, 20*, 416–442.

Jagacinski, R., & Glass, B. (1980). Fitts' Law and the microstructure of rapid discrete movements. *Journal of Experimental Psychology: Human Perception and Performance, 6*, 309–320.

James, W. (1890). *Principles of psychology*. New York: Holt.

Jankowska, E., & Lindstrom, S. (1971). Morphology of interneurones mediating Ia reciprocal inhibition of motoneurones in the spinal cord of the cat. *Journal of Physiology, 226*, 805–823.

Jax, S. A., & Rosenbaum, D. A. (2007). Hand path prim-ing in manual obstacle avoidance: Evidence that the dorsal stream does not only control visually guided actions in real time. *Journal of Experimental Psychology: Human Perception and Performance, 33*, 425–441.

Jax, S. A., Rosenbaum, D. A., & Vaughan, J. (2007). Extending Fitts' Law to manual obstacle avoidance. *Experimental Brain Research, 180*, 775–779.

Jax, S. A., Rosenbaum, D. A., Vaughan, J., & Meulenbroek, R. G. J. (2003). Computational motor control and human factors: Modeling movements in real and possible environments. *Human Factors, 45*, 5–27.

Jeannerod, M. (1981). Intersegmental coordination during reaching at natural objects. In J. Long & A. Baddeley (Eds.), *Attention and Performance IX* (pp. 153–169). Hillsdale, NJ: Erlbaum.

Jeannerod, M. (1984). The timing of natural prehen-sion movement. *Journal of Motor Behavior, 26*(3), 235–254.

Jeannerod, M. (1988). *The neural and behavioral organi-zation of goal-directed movements*. Oxford: Oxford University Press.

Jeannerod, M. (1995). Mental imagery in the motor con-text. *Neuropsychologia, 33*, 1419–1432.

Jeka, J. J., & Lackner, J. R. (1994). Fingertip contact influ-ences human postural control. *Experimental Brain Research, 100*, 495–502.

Jenkins, W. M., Merzenich, M. M., Ochs, M. T., Allard, T., & Guic-Robles, E. (1990). Functional reorganiza-tion of primary somatosensory cortex in adult owl monkeys after behaviorally controlled tactile stimu-lation. *Journal of Neurophysioogy, 63*, 82–104.

Johansson, G. (1973). Visual perception of biological motion and a model for its analysis. *Perception & Psychophysics, 14*, 201–211.

Johansson, R. S., & Westling, G. (1988). Programmed and triggered actions to rapid load changes dur-ing precision grip. *Experimental Brain Research, 271*, 1–15.

Johnson, A., & Redish, A. D. (2007). Neural ensembles in CA3 transiently encode paths forward of the ani-mal at a decision point. *Journal of Neuroscience, 27*, 12176–12189.

Johnson, N. F. (1970). The role of chunking and organi-zation in the process of recall. In G. H. Bower (Ed.)*Psychology of learning and motivation: Vol. 4*. New York: Academic Press.

Johnson, P. (1984). The acquisition of skill. In M. M. Smyth & A. M. Wing (Eds.), *The psychology of human movement* (pp. 215–240). London: Academic Press.

Johnson, R., Wicks, G. G., & Ben-Sira, D. (1981). Practice in the absence of knowledge of results: Motor skill retention. Unpublished manuscript, University of Minnesota.

Johnson-Frey, S. H. (2003). What's so special about human tool use? *Neuron, 39*, 201–204.

Jones, L. A., & Lederman, S. J. (2006). *Human hand func-tion*. New York: Oxford University Press.

Jones, M. R. (1981). A tutorial on some issues and methods in serial pattern research. *Perception & Psychophysics, 30*, 492–504.

Jones, M. R. (1981). A tutorial on some issues and methods in serial pattern research. *Perception & Psychophysics, 30*, 492–504.

Jordan, M. I. (1986a). Attractor dynamics and paral-lelism in a connectionist sequential machine. In C. Clifton (Ed.), Jr, *Proceedings of the 8th Annual Meeting of the Cognitive Science Society* (pp. 531–545). Hillsdale, NJ: Lawrence Erlbaum Associates.

Jordan, M. I. (1986b). Serial order: A parallel, distributed processing approach. Technical Report 8604. La Jolla, CA: University of California, San Diego, Institute for Cognitive Science.

Jordan, M. I., & Rosenbaum, D. A. (1989). Action[Also appeared as COINS Technical Report #88–26, Computer and Information Science Department,

University of Massachusetts, Amherst, March 1988.]. In M. I. Posner (Ed.), *Foundations of cognitive science* (pp. 727–767). Cambridge, MA: MIT Press.

Jordan, S. (1970). Ocular pursuit as a function of visual and proprioceptive stimulation. *Vision Research, 10*, 775–780.

Joseph, R. (1999). Frontal lobe psychopathology: Mania, depression, confabulation, catatonia, perseveration, obsessive compulsions and schizophrenia. *Psychiatry, 62*, 138–172.

Kaas, J. H. (1991). Plasticity of sensory and motor maps in adult mammals. *Annual Review of Neuroscience, 14*, 137–167.

Kagan, J. (1971). *Change and continuity in infancy.* New York: Wiley.

Kahneman, D., & Beetty, J. (1966). Pupil diameter and load on memory. *Science, 154*, 1583–1585.

Kahneman, D., & Tversky, A. (Eds.), (2000). *Choices, values & frames.* New York: Cambridge University Press.

Kakei, S., Hoffman, D. S., & Strick, P. L. (1999). Muscle and movement representations in the primary motor cortex. *Science, 285*, 2316–2319.

Kalat, J. W. (1984). *Biological psychology* (2nd ed). Belmont, CA: Wadsworth.

Kaminski, T., & Gentile, A. M. (1986). Joint control strategies and hand trajectories in multijoint pointing movements. *Journal of Motor Behavior, 189*, 261–278.

Kamon, E., & Gormley, J. (1968). Muscular activity pattern for skilled performance and during learning of a horizontal bar exercise. *Ergonomics, 11*, 345–357.

Kandel, E. R. (2006). *In search of memory.* New York: W. W. Norton & Co.

Kandel, E. R., Schwartz, J. H., & Jessell, T. M. (Eds.), (2000). *Principles of neural science* (4th ed). New York: McGraw Hill.

Kantowitz, B. H., & Sorkin, R. D. (1983). *Human factors: Understanding people-system relationships.* New York: John Wiley & Sons.

Kanwisher, N. (2006). What's in a face? *Science, 311*, 617–618.

Kaufman, L. (1984). *Sight and mind.* New York: Oxford University Pres.

Kavšek, M. (2003). Development of depth and object perception in infancy. In S. Gudrun & L. Helmut (Eds.), *The development of face processing* (pp. 35–52). Ashland, OH: Hogrefe & Huber Publishers.

Keele, S. W. (1968). Movement control in skilled motor performance. *Psychological Bulletin, 70*, 387–403.

Keele, S. W. (1981). Behavioral analysis of movement. In: V. B. Brooks (Ed.), Handbook of physiology: Section 1. The Nervous System. Vol. II. Motor Control, Part 2 (pp. 1391–1414). Baltimore: American Physiological Society.

Keele, S. W. (1986). Motor control. In J. K. Boff, L. Kaufman, & J. P. Thomas, (Eds.) *Handbook of human perception and performance: Vol. II.* New York: Wiley.

Keele, S. W. (1987). Sequencing and timing in skilled perception and action: An overview. In A. Allport, D. MacKay, W. Prinz, & E. Scheerer (Eds.), *Language Perception and Production* (pp. 463–487). London: Academic Press.

Keele, S. W., & Ivry, R. I. (1987). Modular analysis of timing in motor skill. In G. H. Bower (Ed.)*The psychology of learning and motivation: Vol. 21* (pp. 183–228). San Diego: Academic Press, Inc.

Keele, S. W., Pokorny, R. A., Corcos, D. M., & Ivry, R. (1985). Do perception and motor production share common timing mechanisms: A correlation analysis. *Acta Psychologica, 60*, 173–191.

Keele, S. W., & Posner, M. I. (1968). Processing visual feedback in rapid movement. *Journal of Experimental Psychology, 77*, 155–158.

Keele, S. W., & Summers, R. J. (1976). The structure of motor programs. In G. E. Stelmach (Ed.), *Motor control: Issues and trends* (pp. 109–142). New York: Academic Press.

Keetch, K. M., Schmidt, R. A., Lee, T. D., & Young, D. E. (2005). Especial skills: Their emergence with massive amounts of practice. *Journal of Experimental Psychology: Human Perception and Performance, 31*, 970–978.

Keller, E. (1987). The cortical representation of motor processes of speech. In E. Keller & M. Gopnik (Eds.), *Motor and sensory processes of language* (pp. 125–162). Hillsdale, NJ: Lawrence Erlbaum Associates.

Keller, E. & Gopnik, M. (Eds.), Motor and sensory processes of language. Hillsdale, NJ: Lawrence Erlbaum Associates.

Keller, P. E. (2008). Joint action in music performance. In F. Morganti, A. Carassa, & G. Riva (Eds.), *Enacting intersubjectivity: A cognitive and social perspective on the study of interactions* (pp. 205–221). Amsterdam: IOS Press.

Keller, P. E., Wascher, E., Prinz, W., Waszak, F., Koch, I., & Rosenbaum, D. A. (2006). Differences between intention-based and stimulus-based actions. *Journal of Psychophysiology, 20*, 9–20.

Kelso, J. A. S. (1981). Contrasting perspectives on order and regulation in movement. In J. Long & A. Baddeley (Eds.), *Attention and performace IX* (pp. 437–457). Hillsdale, New Jersey: Lawrence Erlbaum Associates.

Kelso, J. A. S. (1984). Phase transitions and critical behavior in human bimanual coordination. *American Journal of Physiology: Regulatory, Integrative and Comparative, 246*, R1000–R1004.

Kelso, J. A. S., & Holt, D. G. (1980). Exploring a vibratory system analysis of human movement production. *Journal of Neurophysiology, 43*, 1183–1196.

Kelso, J. A. S., & Holt, K. G. (1980). Exploring a vibratory systems analysis of human movement production. *Journal of Neurophysiology, 435,* 1183–1196.

Kelso, J. A. S., Putnam, C. A., & Goodman, D. (1983). On the space-time structure of human interlimb co-ordination. *Quarterly Journal of Experimental Psychology, 35A,* 347–375.

Kelso, J. A. S., & Schöner, G. (1988). Self-organization of coordinative movement patterns. *Human Movement Science, 7,* 27–46.

Kelso, J. A. S., & Stelmach, G. E. (1976). Central and peripheral mechanisms in motor control. In G. E. Stelmach (Ed.), *Motor control: Issues and trends* (pp. 1–40). New York: Academic Press.

Kelso, J. A. S., Southard, D. L., & Goodman, D. (1979). On the nature of human interlimb coordination. *Science, 203,* 1029–1031.

Kelso, J. A. S., Southard, D. L., & Goodman, D. (1979). On the co-ordination of two-handed movements. *Journal of Experimental Psychology: Human Perception and Performance, 5,* 229–238.

Kelso, J. A. S., Tuller, B., & Harris, K. S. (1983). A "dynamic pattern" perspective on the control and coordination of movement. In P. F. MacNeilage (Ed.), *The production of speech* (pp. 137–173). New York: Springer-Verlag.

Kelso, J. A. S., Tuller, B., Vatikiotis-Bateson, E., & Fowler, C. A. (1984). Functionally specific articulatory cooperation following jaw perturbations during speech: Evidence for coordinative structures. *Journal of Experimental Psychology: Human Perception and Performance, 10,* 812–832.

Kenneally, C. (2007). *The first word – The search for the origins of language.* New York: Penguin.

Kennedy, J. M. (1983). What can we learn about pictures from the blind? *American Scientist, 71,* 19–26.

Kennedy, J. M., & Juricevic, I. (2006). Blind man draws using diminution in three dimensions. *Psychonomic Bulletin & Review, 13,* 506–509.

Kermoian, R., & Campos, J. J. (1988). Locomotor experience: A facilitator of spatial cognitive development. *Child Development, 59,* 908–917.

Kerr, B. A., & Langolf, G. D. (1977). Speed of aiming movements. *Quarterly Journal of Experimental Psychology, 29,* 475–481.

Kerr, R. (1973). Movement time in an underwater environment. *Journal of Motor Behavior, 5,* 175–178.

Kim, H. H., Gillespie, R. B., & Martin, B. J. (2007). Head movement control in visually guided tasks: Postural goal and optimality. *Computers in Biology and Medicine, 37,* 1009–1019.

Klapp, S. T. (1977a). Reaction time analysis of programmed control. *Exercise and sport sciences reviews, 5,* 231–253.

Klapp, S. T. (1977b). Response programming, as assessed by reaction time, does not establish commands for particular muscles. *Journal of Motor Behavior, 9,* 301–312.

Klapp, S. T. (1979). Doing two things at once: The role of temporal compatibility. *Memory and Cognition, 7,* 375–381.

Klapp, S. T., Hill, M. D., Tyler, J. G., Martin, Z. E., Jagacinski, R. J., & Jones, M. R. (1985). On marching to two different drummers: Perceptual aspects of the difficulties. *Journal of Experimental Psychology: Human Perception and Performance, 11,* 814–827.

Klatzky, R. L., & Lederman, S. J. (1985). Hand movements: A window to haptic object recognition. Paper presented at the Twenty-sixth Annual Meeting of the Psychonomoic Society. Boston.

Kleiner, K. A., & Banks, M. (1987). Stimulus energy does not account for 2–month-olds' face preferences. *Journal of Experimental Psychology: Human Perception and Performance, 13,* 594–600.

Kleinholdermann, U., Brenner, E., Franz, V. H., & Smeets, J. B. (2007). Grasping trapezoidal objects. *Experimental Brain Research, 180,* 415–420.

Klemmer, E. T. (1957). Simple reaction time as a function of time uncertainty. *Journal of Experimental Psychology, 54,* 195–200.

Kluger, J. (2007). Rewiring the brain. *Time, 170*(11), 46–47.

Knoblich, G., & Sebanz, N. (2006). The social nature of perception and action. *Current Directions in Psychological Science, 15,* 99–104.

Knoblich, G., Thornton, I. M., Grosjean, M., & Shiffrar, M. (2006). *Human body perception from the inside out.* New York: Oxford University Press.

Koch, I. (2005). Sequential task predictability in task switching. *Psychonomic Bulletin & Review, 12,* 107–113.

Kolers, P. A. (1976). Reading a year later. *Journal of Experimental Psychology: Human Learning and Memory, 2,* 554–565.

Konner, M. (1987). The enigmatic smile. *Psychology Today, 21*(3), 42–44.

Koretz, J. F., & Handelman, G. H. (1989). How the human eye focuses. *Scientific American, 259*(1), 92–99.

Kornblum, S. (1965). Response competition and/or inhibition in two choice reaction time. *Psychonomic Science, 2,* 55–56.

Kornmuller, A. E. (1930). Eine experimentelle Anesthesie der auberen Augenmuskein am Menschen und ihre Auswirkungen. *Journal für Psycyhologie und Neurologie, 41,* 354–366.

Koshland, G. F., & Hasan, Z. (2000). Electromyographic responses to a mechanical perturbation applied during impending arm movements in different directions: one-joint and two-joint conditions. *Experimental Brain Research, 132,* 485–499.

Kots, Y. M., & Syrovegnin, A. V. (1966). Fixed set of variants of interactions of the muscles of two joints in the execution of simple voluntantry movements. *Biophysics, 11,* 1212–1219.

Kowler, E., & Martins, A. J. (1983). Eye movements of preschool children. *Science, 215,* 997–999.

Kowler, E., & Steinman, R. M. (1979). The effect of expectations on slow oculomotor control – I. Periodic target steps. *Vision Research, 19,* 619–632.

Kowler, E., & Steinman, R. M. (1981). The effect of expectations on slow oculomotor control – III. Guessing unpredictable target displacements. *Vision Research, 21,* 191–203.

Kozhevnikov, V. A., & Chistovich, L. (1965). *Speech: Articulation and perception.* Moscow-Leningrad: Nauka (Translation available from the Joint Publication Research Sercice, United States Department of Commerce, Washington, D. C.).

Krakauer, J. W., Ghilardi, M.-F., & Ghez, C. (1999). Independent learning of internal models for kinematic and dynamic control of reaching. *Nature Neuroscience, 2,* 1026–1031.

Kroll, J. F., & Potter, M. C. (1984). Recognizing words, pictures, and concepts: A comparison of lexical, object, and reality decisions. *Journal of Verbal Learning and Verbal Behavior, 23,* 39–66.

Kubler, A., Kotchoubey, B., Kaiser, J., Wolpaw, J. R., & Bierbaumer, N. (2001). Brain-computer communication: Unlocking the locked in. *Psychological Bulletin, 127,* 358–375.

Kugler, P. G. (1986). A morphological perspective on the origin and evolution of movement patterns. In M. G. Wade & H. T. A. Whiting (Eds.), *Motor skills acquisition in children: Aspects of coordination and control* (pp. 459–525). The Hague: Martinus Nijhoff.

Kugler, P. N., & Turvey, M. T. (1987). *Information, natural law and self-assembly of rhythmic movements: A study in the similitude of natural law.* Hillsdale, NJ: Lawrence Erlbaum Associates.

Kunde, W., & Weigelt, M. (2005). Goal congruency in bimanual object manipulation. *Journal of Experimental Psychology: Human Perception and Performance, 31,* 145–156.

Kuo, A. D. (2005). Harvesting energy by improving the economy of human walking. *Science, 309,* 1686–1687.

Kuypers, H. G. (1973). The anatomical organization of the descending pathways and their contributions to motor control especially in primates. In J. E. Desmedt (Ed.)*New developments in electromyography and clinical neurophysiology: Vol. 3.* Basel: Karger.

Kvalseth, T. O. (1980). An alternative to Fitts' law. *Bulletin of the Psychonomic Society, 16,* 371–373.

Kvalseth, T. O. (1980). An alternative to Fitts' law. *Bulletin of the Psychonomic Society, 16,* 371–373.

Laabs, G. J. (1973). Retention characteristics of different reproduction cues in motor short-term memory. *Journal of Experimental Psychology, 100,* 168–177.

Lackner, J. R., & Dizio, P. (1994). Rapid adaptation to Coriolis force perturbations of arm trajectory. *Journal of Neurophysiology, 72,* 299–313.

Lackner, J. R., & Evanoff, J. N. (1977). Smooth pursuit eye movements elicited by somatosensory stimulation. *Neuroscience Letters, 4,* 43–48.

Lackner, J. R., & Zabkar, J. J. (1977). Proprioceptive information about target location suppresses autokinesis. *Vision Research, 17,* 1225–1229.

Lacquaniti, F., & Maioli, C. (1989). The role of preparation in tuning anticipatory and reflex responses during catching. *Journal of Neuroscience, 9,* 134–148.

Lacquaniti, F., & Soechting, J. F. (1984). Behavior of the stretch reflex in a multi-jointed limb. *Brain Research, 311,* 161–166.

Lacquaniti, F., Terzuolo, C., & Viviani, P. (1983). The law relating the kinematic and figural aspects of drawing movements. *Acta Psychologica, 54,* 115–130.

Lacquaniti, F., Terzuolo, C., & Viviani, P. (1984). Global metric properties and preparatory processes in drawing movements. In S. Kornblum & J. Requin (Eds.), *Preparatory states and processes* (pp. 357–370). Hillsdale, NJ: Lawrence Erlbaum Associates.

Ladefoged, P. (1967). *Three areas of experimental phonetics.* New York: Oxford University Press.

Ladefoged, P., DeClerk, J., Lindau, M., & Papçun, G. (1972). An auditory-motor theory of speech production. *UCLA Working Papers in Linguistics, 22,* 48–75.

Ladefoged, P., Silverstein, R., & Papcun, G. (1973). Interruptibility of speech. *Journal of the Acoustical Society of America, 54,* 1105–1108.

Lafont, D. (2007). Towards a new hitting model in tennis. *Journal of Performance Analysis in Sport, 7,* 106–116.

Lagerspetz, K., Nygård, M., & Strandvik, C. (1971). The effects of training in crawling on the motor and mental development of infants. *Scandinavian Journal of Psychology, 12,* 192–197.

Lakoff, G. (2004). Don't think of an elephant: Know your values and frame the debate.

Lang, P. J. (1994). The varieties of emotional experience: A meditation on James-Lange theory. *Psychological Review, 101,* 211–221.

Langolf, G. D., Chaffin, D. B., & Foulke, J. A. (1976). An investigation of Fitts' Law using a wide range of movement amplitudes. *Journal of Motor Behavior, 8,* 113–128.

Larochelle, S. (1983). Some aspects of movements in skilled typewriting. In H. Bouma & D. G. Bouhuis

(Eds.), *Attention and Performance X* (pp. 43–54). Hillsdale, NJ: Erlbaum.

Lashley, K. S. (1917). The accuracy of movement in the absence of excitation from the moving organ. *American Journal of Physiology, 43,* 169–194.

Lashley, K. S. (1951). The problem of serial order in behavior. In L. A. Jeffress (Ed.), *Cerebral mechanisms in behavior* (pp. 112–131). New York: Wiley.

Latash, M. (2008b). *Synergies.* Champaign, IL: Human Kinetic.

Latash, M. L. (2008a). *Neurophysiological basis of movement* (2nd ed). Champaign, IL: Human Kinetics.

Latash, M. L., Scholz, J. P., & Schöner, G. (2007). Toward a new theory of motor synergies. *Motor Control, 11,* 276–308.

Latour, P. L. (1962). Visual thresholds during eye movements. *Vision Research, 2,* 261–262.

Laubrock, J., Engbert, R., & Kliegl, R. (2005). Microsaccade dynamics during covert attention. *Vision Research, 45,* 721–730.

Laubrock, J., Engbert, R., & Kliegl, R. (2007). Microsaccades are an index of covert attention. *Psychological Science, 18,* 364–366.

Lawrence, D. G., & Hopkins, D. A. (1972). Developmental aspects of pyramidal motor control in the rhesus monkey. *Brain Research, 40,* 117–118.

Leckman, J. F., & Cohen, D. J. (1999). *Tourette's Syndrome—Tics, Obsessions, Compulsions: Developmental Psychopathology and Clinical Care.* New York: John Wiley & Sons.

Lee, B. S. (1950). Effects of delayed speech feedback. *Journal of the Acoustical Society of America, 22,* 824–826.

Lee, D. N., & Reddish, P. E. (1981). Plummeting gannets: A paradigm of ecological optics. *Nature, 293,* 293–294.g.

Lee, D. N. (1976). A theory of visual control of braking based on information about time-to-collision. *Perception, 5,* 437–459.

Lee, D. N., & Aronson, E. (1974). Visual proprioceptive control of standing in human infants. *Perception & Psychophysics, 15,* 529–532.

Lee, D. N., & Lishman, J. R. (1975). Visual proprioceptive control of stance. *Journal of Human Movement Studies, 1,* 87–95.

Lee, D. N., Lishman, J. R., & Thomson, J. (1982). Regulation of gait in long jumping. *Journal of Experimental Psychology, 8,* 448–459.

Lee, D. N., & Thomson, J. A. (1982). Vision in action: The control of locomotion. In D. J. Ingle, M. A. Goodale, & R. J. W. Mansfield (Eds.), *Analysis of visual behavior* (pp. 411–433). Cambridge, MA: MIT.

Lee, D. N., Young, D. S., Reddish, P. E., Lough, S., & Clayton, T. M. (1983). Visual timing in hitting an accelerating ball. *Quarterly Journal of Experimental Psychology, 35A,* 333–346.

Lee, T. D., Blandin, Y., & Proteau, L. (1996). Effects of task instructions and oscillation frequency on bimanual coordination. *Psychological Research, 59,* 10–106.

Lee, T. D., Ishikura, T., Kegel, S., Gonzalez, D., & Passmore, S. (2008). Head–putter coordination patterns in expert and less skilled golfers. *Journal of Motor Behavior, 40,* 267–272.

Legge, D., & Barber, P. J. (1976). *Information and skill.* London: Methuen.

Legge, D., Steinberg, H., & Summerfield, A. (1964). Simple measures of handwriting as indices of drug effects. *Perceptual and Motor Skills, 18,* 549–558.

Lehman, R. S. (1965). Eye-movements and the autokinetic illusion. *American Journal of Psychology, 78,* 490–492.

Lehmkuhl, G., & Poeck, K. (1981). A disturbance in the conceptual organization of actions in patients with ideational apraxia. *Cortex, 17,* 153–158.

Leonard, J. A. (1959). Tactual choice reactions. *Quarterly Journal of Experimental Psychology, 11,* 76–83.

Leonard, J. A., & Newman, R. C. (1964). Formation of higher habits. *Nature, 203,* 550–551.

Lessenberry, D. D. (1928). *Analysis of errors.* Syracuse, New York: L. C. Smith and Corona Typewriters, School Department [Reprinted in A. Dvorak, N. Merrick, W. Dealey, & G. Ford (1936). Typewriting behavior. New York: American Book Company.].

Levelt, W. (1989). *Speaking.* Cambridge, MA: MIT Press.

Levy, J. (1972). Autokinetic illusion: A systematic review of theories, measures, and independent variables. *Psychological Bulletin, 78,* 457–474.

Levy, J. (1982). Handwriting posture and cerebral organization: How are they related? *Psychological Bulletin, 91,* 589–608.

Levy, J., & Reid, M. L. (1976). Variations in writing posture and cerebral organization. *Science, 194,* 337–339.

Liao, M. J., Jagacinski, R. J., & Greenberg, N. (1997). Quantifying the performance limitations of older and younger adults in a target acquisition task. *Journal of Experimental Psychology: Human Perception and Performance, 23,* 1644–1664.

Liberman, A. M., Cooper, F. S., Shankweiler, D. P., & Studdert-Kennedy, M. G. (1967). Perception of the speech code. *Psychological Review, 74,* 431–461.

Libet, B., Gleason, C. A., Wright, E. W., & Pearl, D. K. (1983). Time of conscious intention to act in relation to onset of cerebral activity (Readiness-Potential). *Brain, 106,* 623–642.

Lieberman, P. (1984). *The biology and evolution of language.* Cambridge, MA: Harvard.

Limb, C. J., & Braun, A. R. (2008). Neural substrates of spontaneous musical performance: an FMRI study of jazz improvisation. *PLoS ONE, 3,* e1679.

Lindblom, B. (1983). Economy of speech gestures. In P. F. MacNeilage (Ed.), *The production of speech* (pp. 217–245). New York: Springer-Verlag.

Lindblom, B., Lubker, J., & Gay, T. (1979). Formant frequencies of some fixed-mandible vowels and a model of speech motor programming by predictive simulation. *Journal of Phonetics, 7,* 147–161.

Lindblom, B. & Sundberg, J. (1971, August). Neurophysiological representation of speech sounds. Paper presented at the XVth World Congress of Logopedics and Phoniatrics. Buenos Aires, Argentina.

Lindblom, B., & Sundberg, J. (1971). Acoustical consequences of lip, tongue, jaw and larynx movements. *Journal of the Acoustical Society of America, 50,* 1166–1179.

Linebarger, M. C., Schwartz, M. F., & Saffran, E. M. (1983). Sensitivity to grammatical structure in so-called agrammatic aphasics. *Cognition, 13,* 361–392.

Lisberger, S. G. (1988). The neural basis for learning of simple motor skills. *Science, 242,* 728–735.

Liu, Y., Collins, R., & Tsin, Y. (2004). A Computational Model for Periodic Pattern Perception Based on Frieze and Wallpaper Groups. *IEEE Transactions on Pattern Analysis and Machine Intelligence, 26,* 354–371.

Llinas, R. (1981). Electrophysiology of the cerebellar networks. In: V. B. Brooks (Ed.), Handbook of physiology, Section 1: The nervous system, Vol II. Motor conrol (831–875). Bethesda, MD: American Physiological Society.

Lockman, J. J., & Ashmead, D. H. (1983). Asynchronies in the development of manual behavior. In P. Lipsitt, & C. K. Rovee-Collier, (Eds.) *Advances in infancy research: Vol. 2* (pp. 114–136). Norwood, NJ: Ablex.

Lockman, J. J., Ashmead, D. H., & Bushnell, E. W. (1984). The development of anticipatory hand orientation during infancy. *Journal of Experimental Child Psychology, 37,* 176–186.

Loeb, G. E. (1985). Motorneurone task groups: Coping with kinematic heterogeneity. *Journal of Experimental Biology, 115,* 137–146.

Loftus, E. R., & Loftus, G. R. (1980). On the permanence of stored information in the human brain. *American Psychologist, 35,* 409–420.

Logan, G. D. (1982). On the ability to inhibit complex movements: A stop-signal study of typewriting. *Journal of Experimental Psychology: Human Perception and Performance, 8,* 778–792.

Logan, G. D. (1983). Time, information, and the various spans in typewriting. In W. E. Cooper (Ed.), *Cognitive aspects of skilled typewriting.* New York: Springer-Verlag.

Logan, G. D., & Cowan, W. B. (1984). On the ability to inhibit thought and action: A theory of an act of control. *Psychological Review, 91,* 295–327.

Logan, G. D., & Zbrodoff, J. (1998). Stroop-type interference: Congruity effects in color naming with typewritten responses. *Journal of Experimental Psychology: Human Perception and Performance, 24,* 978–992.

Logemann, J. A. (1985). Assessment and treatment of articulatory disorders in adults: State of the art. In J. M. Costello (Ed.), *Speech disorders in adults* (pp. 3–19). San Diego, CA: College-Hill Press.

Long, J. (1976). Visual feedback and skilled keying: Differential effects of masking the printed copy and the keyboard. *Ergonomics, 19,* 93–110.

Lotter, W. S. (1960). Interrelationships among reaction times and speeds of movement in different limbs. *Research Quarterly, 31,* 147–155.

Luce, R. D. (1986). *Response times: Their role in inferring elementary mental organization.* New York: Oxford University Press.

Luis, M., & Tremblay, L. (2008). Visual feedback use during a back tuck somersault: Evidence for optimal visual feedback utilization. *Motor Control, 12,* 210–218.

Luria, A. R., & Homskaya, E. D. (1970). Frontal lobes and the rgulation of arousal processes. In D. I. Mostofsky (Ed.), *Attention: Contemporary theory and analysis.* New York: Appleton-Century-Crofts. Luria, A. R. (1973). *The working brain.* New York: Basic Books.

Lynn, J. G., & Lynn, D. R. (1938). Face-hand laterality in relation to personality. *Journal of Abnormal and Social Psychology, 33,* 291–322.

MacKay, D. G. (1981). The problem of rehearsal or mental practice. *Journal of Motor Behavior, 13,* 274–285.

MacKay, D. G. (1982). The problem of flexibility, fluency, and speed-accuracy trade-off in skilled behavior. *Psychological Review, 89,* 483–506.

MacKay, D. G. (1987). *The organization of perception and action: A theory for language and other cognitive skills.* New York: Springer-Verlag.

MacKay, D. G., & Bowman, R. W. (1969). On producing the meaning in sentences. *American Journal of Psychology, 82,* 23–39.

MacKay, D. M. (1970). Elevation of visual theshold by displacement of retinal image. *Nature (London), 225,* 90–92.

MacKenzie, C. L., & Iberall, T. (1994). *The grasping hand.* Amsterdam: North-Holland.

MacKenzie, C. L., Marteniuk, R. G., & Dugas, C. (1987). 3-dimensional movement trajectories in Fitts task: Implications for control. *Quarterly Journal of Experimental Psychology Section A-Human Experimental Psychology, 39,* 629–647.

MacLeod, C. (1991). Half a century of research on the Stroop effect: An integrative review. *Psychological Bulletin, 109,* 163–203.

Macmillan, D. L. (1975). A physiological analysis of walking in the American lobster (Homarus americanus).

Philosophical Transactions of the Royal Society of London, 270, 1–59.

MacNeilage, P. F. (1970). Motor control of serial ordering of speech. *Psychological Review, 77,* 182–196.

MacNeilage, P. F. (1980). Distinctive features of speech control. In: G. E. Stelmach, J. Requin (Eds.), Tutorials in motor behavior. Amsterdam: North-Holland.

MacNeilage, P. F. (Ed.). (1983). *The production of speech.* New York: Springer-Verlag.

MacNeilage, P. F., & DeClerk, J. L. (1969). On the motor control of coarticulation in CVC monosyllables. *Journal of the Acoustical Society of America, 45,* 1217–1233.

MacNeilage, P. F., Krones, R., & Hanson, R. (1969). Closed-loop control of the initiation of jaw movement for speech. Paper presented at the meeting of the Acoustical Society of America, San Diego.

MacNeilage, P. F., & Ladefoged, P. (1976). The production of speech and language. In E. C. Carterette, & M. P. Friedman, (Eds.) *Handbook of perception: Vol. VII* (pp. 75–120). New York: Academic Press.

MacNeilage, P. F., Rootes, T. P., & Chase, R. A. (1967). Speech production and perception in a patient with severe impairment of somesthetic perception and motor control. *Journal of Speech and Hearing Research, 10,* 449–467.

Magill, R. A. (1989). *Motor learning* (3rd ed). Dubuque, Iowa: Wm. C. Brown.

Manetto, C., & Lidsky, T. I. (1989). The effects of movements on caudate sensory responses. *Neuroscience Letters, 96,* 295–299.

Margaria, R. (1976). *Biomechanics and energetics of muscular exercise.* Oxford: Clarendon Press.

Margolin, D. I. (1984). The neuropsychology of writing and spelling: Semantic, phonological, motor, and perceptual processes. *Quarterly Journal of Experimental Psychology, 36A,* 459–489.

Margolin, D. I., & Wing, A. M. (1983). Agraphia and micrographia: Clinical manifestations of motor programming and performance disorders. *Acta Psychologica, 54,* 263–283.

Marlsen-Wilson, W., & Tyler, L. K. (1980). The temporal structure of spoken language understanding. *Cognition, 8,* 1–71.

Marr, D. (1969). A theory of cerebellar cortex. *Journal of Physiology (London), 202,* 437–470.

Marr, D. (1982). *Vision.* San Francisco: W. H. Freeman.

Marsden, C. D. (1982). The mysterious functions of the basal ganglia: The Robert Warternberg Lecture. *Neurology, 32,* 514–539.

Marsden, C. D., Merton, P. A., & Morton, H. B. (1973). Is the human stretch reflex cortical rather than spinal? *Lancet, 1,* 759–761.

Marsden, C. D., Merton, P. A., & Morton, H. B. (1977). Disorders of movement in cerebellar disease in man.

In F. C. Rose (Ed.), *Physiological aspects of clinical neurology.* Oxford: Blackwell.

Marsden, C. D., Obeso, J. A., & Rothwell, J. C. (1983). The function of the antagonist muscle during fast limb movements in man. *Journal of Physiology (London), 335,* 1–13.

Marsden, C. D., Rothwell, J. C., & Day, B. L. (1983). Long-latency automatic responses to muscle stretch in man: Origin and function. In: J. E. Desmedt (Ed.), Advances in Neurology, 39, 509–539.

Marsden, C. D., Rothwell, J. C., & Dell, B. L. (1984). The use of peripheral feedack in the control of movement. *Trends in the Neurosciences, 7,* 253–257.

Marteniuk, R. G., & Bertram, C. P. (2001). Contributions of gait and trunk movement to prehension: Perspectives from world and body-centered coordinates. *Motor Control, 5,* 151–164.

Marteniuk, R. G., MacKenzie, C. L., Jeannerod, M., Athenes, S., & Dugas, C. (1987). Constraints on human arm movement trajectories. *Canadian Journal of Psychology, 4,* 365–378.

Mason, A. H., & MacKenzie, C. L. (2005). Grip forces when passing an object to a partner. *Experimental Brain Research, 163,* 173–187.

Massaro, D. W., & Chen, T. (2008). The motor theory of speech perception revisited. *Psychonomic Bulletin & Review, 15,* 453–454.

Massion, J. (1984). Postural changes accompanying voluntary movements: Normal and pathological aspects. *Human Neurobiology, 2,* 261–267.

Mather, G. (2006). *Foundations of perception.* Sussex: Psychology Press.

Matin, L. (1972). Eye movements and perceived visual direction. In: D. Jameson, L. Hurvich (Eds.), Handbook of sensory physiology. Vol. 7. (pp. 331-380). Berlin: Springer.Matin, E. (1974). Saccadic suppression. Psychological Bulletin, 81, 899–918.

Matin, L., Stevens, J. K., & Picoult, E. (1983). Perceptual consequences of experimental extraocular muscle paralysis. In A. Hein & M. Jeannerod (Eds.), *Spatially oriented behavior* (pp. 243–262). New York: Springer-Verlag.

Matthews, P. B. C. (1972). *Mammalian muscle receptors and their central actions.* London: Arnold.

Matthews, P. B. C., & Rushworth, G. (1958). The discharge from muscle spindles as an indicator of g efferent paralysis by procaine. *Journal of Physiology, 140,* 421–426.

Matthews, P. B. C., & Simmonds, A. (1974). Sensations of finger movement elicited by pulling upon flexor tendons in man. *Journal of Physiology, 239,* 27–28.

Mayer, E. J. (1895/1972). *Movement.* New York: Arno Press & New York Times (Originally published, 1895).

Mays, L. E., & Sparks, D. L. (1980). Saccades are spatially, not retinocentrically, coded. *Science, 208,* 1163–1165.

McAuley, J. D., Jones, M. R., Holub, S., Johnston, H. M., & Miller, N. S. (2006). The time of our lives: Lifespan development of timing and event tracking. *Journal of Experimental Psychology: General, 135,* 348–367.

McBride, E., & Rothstein, A. (1979). Mental and physical practice and the learning and retention of open and closed skills. *Perceptual and Motor Skills, 49,* 359–365.

McCarty, M. E., & Ashmead, D. H. (1999). Visual control of reaching and grasping in infants. *Developmental Psychology, 35,* 620–631.

McCarty, M. E., Clifton, R. K., & Collard, R. R. (1999). Problem solving in infancy: the emergence of an action plan. *Developmental Psychology, 35*(4), 1091–1101.

McCarty, M. E., Clifton, R. K., & Collard, R. R. (2001). The beginnings of tool use by infants and toddlers. *Infancy, 2,* 233–256.

McCarty, M. E., & Keen, R. (2005). Facilitating problem-solving performance among 9-and 12-month-old infants. *Journal of Cognition and Development, 6*(2), 209.

McCormick, D. A., & Thompson, R. F. (1984). Cerebellum: Essential involvement in the classically conditioned eyelid response. *Science, 223,* 296–299.

McDonald, P. V., van Emmerik, R. E., & Newell, K. M. (1989). The effects of practice on limb kinematics in a throwing task. *Journal of Motor Behavior, 21,* 245–264.

McGraw, M. B. (1943). *Neuro-muscular maturation of the infant.* New York: Columbia University Press.

McGurk, H., & MacDonald, J. (1976). Hearing lips and seeing voices. *Nature, 264,* 746–748.

McIntyre, J., Zago, M., Berthoz, A., & Lacquaniti, F. (2001). Does the brain model Newton's laws? *Nature Neuroscience, 4,* 693–694.

McLeod, P. (1987). Visual reaction time and high-speed ball games. *Perception, 16,* 49–59.

McLeod, P., & Dienes, Z. (1996). Do fielders know where to go to catch the ball or only how to get there? *Journal of Experimental Psychology: Human Perception and Performance, 22,* 531–543.

McLeod, P., McLaughlin, C., & Nimmo-Smith, I. (1986). Information encapsulation and automaticity: Evidence from the visual control of finely-timed actions(Pages...) [still to be entered in ref. list]. In M. Posner & O. Marin (Eds.), *Attention and Performance XI.* Hillsdale, NJ: Lawrence Erlbaum Associates.

McMahon, T. A. (1984). *Muscles, reflexes, and locomotion.* Princeton, NJ: Princeton University Press.

Mechsner, F., Kerzel, D., Knoblich, G., & Prinz, W. (2001). Perceptual basis of bimanual coordination. *Nature, 414,* 69–73.

Meck, W. H. (Ed.). (2003). *Functional and neural mechanisms of interval timing.* Boca Raton, FL: CRC Press.

Medendorp, W. P., Goltz, H. C., & Vilis, T. (2006). Directional selectivity of BOLD activity in human posterior parietal cortex for memory-guided double-step saccades. *Journal of Neurophysiology, 95,* 1645–1655.

Meijer, O. G., & Roth, K. (Eds.), (1988). *Complex motor behavior: The motor-action controversy.* Amsterdam: Elsevier Science.

Merton, P. A. (1972). How we control the contraction of our muscles. *Scientific American, 226*(5), 30–37.

Merzenich, M. M., Nelson, R. J., Stryker, M. P., Cynder, M. S., Shoppmann, A., & Zook, J. M. (1984). Somatosensory cortical map changes following digit amputation in adult monkeys. *Journal of Comparative Neurology, 224,* 591–605.

Meulenbroek, R. G. J., Rosenbaum, D. A., Thomassen, A. J. W. M., Loukopoulos, L. D., & Vaughan, J. (1996). Adaptation of a reaching model to handwriting: How different effectors can produce the same written output, and other results. *Psychological Research/Psychologische Forschung, 59,* 64–74.

Meulenbroek, R. G. J., Rosenbaum, D. A., Jansen, C., Vaughan, J., & Vogt, S. (2001). Multijoint grasping movements: Simulated and observed effects of object location, object size, and initial aperture. *Experimental Brain Research, 138,* 219–234.

Meulenbroek, R. G., Rosenbaum, D. A., Thomassen, A. J., & Schomaker, L. R. (1993). Limb-segment selection in drawing behavior. *Quarterly Journal of Experimental Psychology, 46A*(2), 273–299.

Meulenbroek, R. G. J., & Thomassen, A. J. W. M. (1991). Stroke-direction preferences in drawing and handwriting. *Human Movement Science, 10,* 247–270.

Meyer, D. E., Abrams, R. A., Kornblum, S., Wright, C. E., & Smith, J. E. K. (1988). Optimality in human motor performance: Ideal control of rapid aimed movements. *Psychological Review, 95,* 340–370.

Meyer, D. E., Osman, A. M., Irwin, D. E., & Yantis, S. (1988). Modern mental chronometry. *Biological Psychology, 26,* 3–67.

Meyer, D. E., Smith, J. E. K., Kornblum, S., Abrams, R. A., & Wright, C. E. (1990). Speed-accuracy tradeoffs in aimed movements: Toward a theory of rapid voluntary action. In M. Jeannerod (Ed.), *Attention and Performance XIII.* Hillsdale, NJ: Lawrence Erlbaum Associates.

Meyer, D. E., Smith, J. E. K., & Wright, C. E. (1982). Models for the speed and accuracy of aimed movements. *Psychological Review, 89,* 449–482.

Meyers, J. (1967). Retention of balance coordination learning as influenced by extended lay-offs. *Research Quarterly, 38,* 72–78.

Miall, R. C. (2007). Walking the walk. *Nature Neuroscience, 10,* 940–941.

Miceli, G., Silveri, C., & Caramazza, A. (1985). Cognitive analysis of a case of pure dysgraphia. *Brain and Language, 25*, 187–212.

Miller, G. (2007a). The mystery of the missing smile. *Science, 316*, 826–827.

Miller, G. (2007b). Spying on new neurons in the human brain. *Science, 318*, 899–900.

Miller, G. (2008). Mirror neurons may help songbirds stay in tune. *Science, 319*, 269.

Miller, G. A. (1956). The magical number seven plus or minus two: Some limits on our capacity for processing information. *Psychological Review, 63*, 81–97.

Miller, G. A. (1981). *Language and speech*. New York, San Francisco: Freeman.

Miller, G. A., Galanter, E., & Pribram, K. H. (1960). *Plans and the structure of behavior*. New York: Holt, Rinehart, & Winston.

Miller, J., & Low, K. A. (2001). Motor processes in simple, go/no-go, and choice reaction time tasks: A psychophysiological analysis. *Journal of Experimental Psychology: Human Perception and Performance, 27*(2), 266–289.

Miller, J., & Navon, D. (2002). Global precedence and response activation: Evidence from LRPs. *The Quarterly Journal of Experimental Psychology, 55A*(1), 289–310.

Miller, J., Ulrich, R., & Rinkenauer, G. (1999). Effects of stimulus intensity on the lateralized readiness potential. *Journal of Experimental Psychology: Human Perception and Performance, 25*, 1454–1471.

Miller, N. (1986). *Dyspraxia and its management*. London: Croom Helm.

Miller, S., & Van der Meeche, F. G. (1975). Locomotion in cat: Hypothesis for interlimb coordination. *Brain Research, 91*, 255–269.

Milner, A. D., & Goodale, M. A. (1995). *The visual brain in action*. New York: Oxford University Press.

Milner, B. (1965). Memory disturbance after bilateral hippocampal lesions. In P. M. Milner & S. E. Glickman (Eds.), *Cognitive processes and the brain*. Princeton: Van Nostrand.

Minas, S. C. (1978). Mental practice of a complex perceptual motor skill. *Journal of Human Movement Studies, 4*, 102–107.

Mitra, S., & Turvey, M. T. (2004). A rotation invariant in 3-D reaching. *Journal of Experimental Psychology: Human Perception and Performance, 30*, 163–179.

Moar, I., & Bower, G. H. (1983). Inconsistencies in spatial knowledge. *Memory & Cognition, 11*, 107–113.

Moll, K. L., & Daniloff, R. G. (1971). Investigation of the timing of velar movements during speech. *Journal of the Acoustical Society of America, 50*, 678–684.

Monsell, S. (2003). Task switching. *Trends in Cognitive Sciences, 7*, 134–140.

Morasso, P. (1981). Spatial control of arm movements. *Experimental Brain Research, 42*, 223–227.

Morasso, P., & Sanguineti, V. (1995). Self-organizing body schema for motor planning. *Journal of Motor Behavior, 27*, 52–66.

Moritz, C. T., Perlmutter, S. I., & Fetz, E. E. (2008). Direct control of paralyzed muscles by cortical neurons. Nature, Published online 15 October 2008.

Moscovitch, M., & Olds, J. (1982). Asymmetries in spontaneous facial expressions and their possible relation to hemispheric specialization. *Neuropsychologia, 20*, 71–81.

Moscovitch, M., & Smith, L. C. (1979). Differences in neural organization between individuals with inverted and noninverted handwriting postures. *Science, 205*, 710–713.

Motley, M. T. (1980). Verification of "Freudian slips" and semantic prearticulatory editing via laboratory-induced spoonerisms. In V. A. Fromkin (Ed.), *Errors in linguistic performance* (pp. 133–147). New York: Academic Press.

Mottet, D., & Bootsma, R. J. (1999). The dynamics of goal-directed rhythmical aiming. *Biological Cybernetics, 80*, 235–245.

Mottet, D., Guiard, Y., Ferrand, T., & Bootsma, R. J. (2001). Two-handed performance of a rhythmical Fitts task by individuals and dyads. *Journal of Experimental Psychology: Human Perception and Performance, 27*, 1275–1286.

Mountcastle, V. B., Lynch, J. C., Georgopoulos, A., Sakata, H., & Acuna, C. (1975). Posterior parietal association cortex of the monkey: Command functions for operations within extrapersonal space. *Journal of Neurophysiology, 38*, 871–908.

Mulder, T., Berndt, H., Pauwels, J., & Nienhuis, B. (1993). Sensorimotor adaptability in the elderly and disabled. In G. E. Stelmach & V. Homberg (Eds.), *Sensorimotor impairment in the elderly* (pp. 413–426). Netherlands: Kluwer Academic Publishers.

Munhall, K. G., & Ostry, D. J. (1983). Mirror-image movements in typing. In W. E. Cooper (Ed.), *Cognitive aspects of skilled typewriting* (pp. 247–257). New York: Springer-Verlag.

Munte, T. F., Altenbuller, E., & Janke, I. (2002). The musician's brain as a model of neuroplasticity. *Nature Reviews Neuroscience, 3*, 473–478.

Murray, G. K., Veijola, J., Moilanen, K., Miettunen, J., Glahn, D. C., Cannon, T. D., Jones, P. B., et al. (2006). Infant motor development is associated with adult cognitive categorisation in a longitudinal birth cohort study. *Journal of Child Psychology and Psychiatry, 47*, 25–29.

Mussa-Ivaldi, F. A. (1988). Do neurons in the motor cortex encode movement direction? An alternative hypothesis. *Neuroscience Letters, 91*, 106–111.

Muybridge, E. (1887/1957). *Animals in motion*. New York: Dover.

Nashner, L. M. (1976). Adapting reflexes controlling the human posture. *Experimental Brain Research, 26,* 59–72.

Nashner, L. M., & McCollum, G. (1985). The organization of human postural movements: A formal basis and experimental synthesis. *The Behavioral and Brain Sciences, 8,* 135–172.

Nashner, L. M., Woollacott, M., & Tuma, G. (1979). Organization of rapid responses to postural and locomotor-like perturbations of standing man. *Experimental Brain Research, 36,* 463–476.

Néda, Z., Ravasz, E., Brechet, Y., Vicsek, T., & Barabási, A.-L. (2000). The sound of many hands clapping. *Nature, 403,* 849–850.

Needham, D. M. (1971). *Machina Carnia: The biochemistry of muscular contraction in its historical development.* Cambridge: Cambridge University Press.

Neisser, U. (1967). *Cognitive psychology.* New York: Appleton-Century-Crofts.

Nelson, W. L. (1983). Physical principles for economies of skilled movements. *Biological Cybernetics, 46,* 135–147.

Neves, D. M., & Anderson, J. R. (1981). Knowledge compilation: Mechanisms for the automatization of cognitive skills. In J. R. Anderson (Ed.), *Cognitive skills and their acquisition* (pp. 57–84). Hillsdale, NJ: Erlbaum.

Newcombe, N. S., & Huttenlocher, J. (2003). *Making space: The development of spatial representation and reasoning.* Cambridge, MA: The MIT Press.

Newell, A. M., & Rosenbloom, P. S. (1981). Mechanisms of skill acquisition and the law of practice. In J. R. Anderson (Ed.), *Cognitive skills and their acquisition.* Hillsdale NJ: Erlbaum.

Newell, K. M. (1985). Skill learning. In D. H. Holding (Ed.), *Human skills* (pp. 203–226). Chichester: John Wiley & Sons.

Newell, K. M. (1996). Change in movement and skill: Learning, retention, and transfer. In M. Latash & M. Turvey (Eds.), *Dexterity and its development* (pp. 393–432). Hillsdale, NJ: Erlbaum.

Newell, K. M., & Carlton, L. G. (1988). Force variability in isometric responses. *Journal of Experimental Psychology: Human Perception and Performance, 14,* 37–44.

Newell, K. M., & Vaillancourt, D. E. (2001). Dimensional change in motor learning. *Human Movement Science, 20,* 695–715.

Newell, K. M., & van Emerick, R. E. A. (1989). The acquisition of coordination: Preliminary analysis of learning to write. *Human Movement Science, 8,* 17–32.

Newhall, B. (1999). *The history of photography: From 1839 to the present* (5th ed). New York: Museum of Modern Art.

Newman, C., Atkinson, J., & Braddick, O. (2001). The development of reaching and looking preferences in infants to objects of different sizes. *Developmental Psychology, 37,* 561–572.

Niedenthal, P. (2007). Embodying emotion. *Science, 316,* 1002–1005.

Nissen, M. J., & Bullemer, P. (1987). Attentional requirements of learning: Evidence from performance measures. *Cognitive Psychology, 19,* 1–32.

Nooteboom, S. G. (1970). The target theory of speech production. *IPO Annual Progress Report, 5,* 51–55.

Norman, D. A. (1981). Categorization of action slips. *Psychological Review, 88,* 1–15.

Norman, D. A. (1988). *The psychology of everyday things.* New York: Basic Books.

Nottebohm, F. (1989). From bird song to neurogensis. *Scientific American, 260*(2), 74–79.

O'Keefe, J., & Nadel, L. (1978). *The hippocampus as a cognitive map.* New York: Oxford University Press.

Ohala, J. J. (1983). The origin of sound patterns in vocal tract constraints. In P. F. MacNeilage (Ed.), *The production of speech* (pp. 189–216). New York: Springer-Verlag.

Ohlsson, S. (1992). The learning curve for writing books: Evidence from Professor Asimov. *Psychological Science, 3,* 380–383.

Ohman, S. E. G. (1966). Coarticulation in VCV utterances: Spectrographic measurements. *Journal of the Acoustical Society of America, 39,* 151–168.

Oldfield, R. C. (1971). The assessment and analysis of handedness: The Edinburgh inventory. *Neuropsychologia, 9,* 97–113.

Oliveira, F., & Ivry, R. B. (2008). The representation of action: Insights from bimanual coordination. *Current Directions In Psychological Science, 17,* 130–135.

Olsen, R. A. & Murray, R. A. III. (1976). Finger motion in typing texts of varying complexity. Proceedings of the 6th Congress of the International Ergonomic Association (pp. 446–450).

Olson, B. P., Hu, S. J., & He, J. (2005). Closed-loop cortical control of direction using support vector machines. *IEEE Transactions on Neural Systems and Rehabilitation Engineering, 13,* 72–80.

Olton, D. S. (1979). Mazes, maps, and memory. *American Psychologist, 34,* 583–596.

Osman, A., Kornblum, S., & Meyer, D. E. (1990). Does motor programming necessitate response execution? *Journal of Experimental Psychology: Human Perception and Performance, 16,* 183–198.

Oster, H., & Ekman, P. (1978). Facial behavior in child development. In W. A. Collins (Ed.) *Minnesota symposium on child psychology: Vol. 11.* Hillsdale, NJ: Erlbaum.

Ostry, D. J. (1983). Determinants of interkey times in typing. In W. E. Cooper (Ed.), *Cognitive aspects of skilled typewriting* (pp. 225–246). New York: Springer-Verlag.

Osu, R., Uno, Y., Koike, Y., & Kawato, M. (1997). Possible explanations for trajectory curvature in multijoint arm movements. *Journal of Experimental Psychology: Human Perception and Performance, 23,* 890–913.

Owen, A. M., Coleman, M. R., Boly, M., Davis, M. H., Laureys, S., & Pickard, J. D. (2006). Detecting awareness in the vegetative state (one page article). *Science, 313,* 1402.

Paillard, J. (1949). Quelques donnés psychophysiologiques relatives au déclenchment de la commade mortirce [Some psychophysiological data relating to the triggering of motor commands.]. *L'Annee Psychologique, 48,* 28–47.

Paillard, J., & Brouchon, M. (1968). Active and passive movements in the calibration of position sense. In S. J. Freedman (Ed.), *The neuropsychology of spatially oriented behavior* (pp. 37–55). Homewood, IL: Dorsey.

Palazzolo, J. J., Ferraro, M., Krebs, H. I., Lynch, D., Volpe, B. T., & Hogan, N. (2007). Stochastic estimation of arm mechanical impedance during robotic stroke rehabilitation. *IEEE Transactions On Neural Systems And Rehabilitation Engineering, 15,* 94–103.

Palmer, C. (2005). Sequence memory in music performance. *Current Directions in Psychological Science, 14,* 247–250.

Palmer, C., & Pfordresher, P. Q. (2003). Incremental planning in sequence production. *Psychological Review, 110,* 683–712.

Park, W., Singh, D., & Martin, B. (2006). A memory-based model for planning target reach postures in the presence of obstructions. *Ergonomics, 49,* 1565–1580.

Parker, J. F. & Fleishman, E. A. (1960). Ability factors and component performance measures as predictors of complex tracking behavior. Psychological Monographs, 74 (Whole No. 503).

Parkinson, J., & Khurana, B. (2007). Temporal order of strokes primes letter recognition. *Quarterly Journal of Experimental Psychology, 60,* 1265–1274.

Pascual-Leone, A., & Merabet, L. B. (2005). The plastic human brain cortex. *Annual Review of Neuroscience, 28,* 377–401.

Pashler, H., Ramachandran, V. S., & Becker, M. (2006). *Psychonomic Bulletin & Review, 13,* 954–957.

Patla, A. E., & Vickers, J. N. (1997). Where and when do we look as we approach and step over an obstacle in the travel path? *NeuroReport, 8,* 3661–3665.

Pavese, A., & Buxbaum, L. J. (2002). Action matters: The role of action plans and object affordances in selection for action. *Visual Cognition, 9,* 559–560.

Pearson, K. R. (1976). The control of walking. *Scientific American, 235*(6), 72–86.

Peleg, G., Katzir, G., Peleg, O., Kamara, M., Brodsky, L., Hel-Or, H., Keren, D., & Nevo, E. (2006). Hereditary family signature of facial expression. *Proceedings of the National Academy of Sciences, 103,* 15921–15926.

Pellecchia, G. L. (2003). Postural sway increases with attentional demands of concurrent cognitive task. *Gait and Posture, 18,* 29–34.

Pellecchia, G. L., Shockley, K., & Turvey, M. T. (2005). Concurrent cognitive task modulates coordination dynamics. *Cognitive Science, 29,* 531–557.

Pellecchia, G. L., & Turvey, M. T. (2001). Cognitive activity shifts the attractors of bimanual coordination. *Journal of Motor Behavior, 33,* 9–15.

Penfield, W., & Rasmssen, T. (1950). *The cerebral cortex of man: A clinical study of localization of function.* New York: MacMillan.

Penfield, W., & Roberts, L. (1959). *Speech and brain mechanisms.* New York: Atheneum.

Peper, C. E., Beek, P. J., & van Wieringen, P. C. W. (1995). Multifrequency coordination in bimanual tapping: Aymmetrical coupling and signs of supercriticality. *Journal of Experimental Psychology: Human Perception and Performance, 21,* 1117–1138.

Perkell, J. S. & Klatt, D. H. (Eds.), Invariance and variability in speech processes. Hillsdale, NJ: Erlbaum.

Peschel, E. R., & Peschel, R. E. (1987). Medical insights into the castrati in opera. *Amercian Scientist, 75,* 578–583.

Peters, M. (1977). Simultaneous performance of two motor activities: The factor of timing. *Neuropsychologia, 15,* 461–465.

Pew, R. W. (1966). Acquisition of hierarchical control over the temporal organization of a skill. *Journal of Experimental Psychology, 71,* 764–771.

Pew, R. W., & Rosenbaum, D. A. (1988). Human motor performance: Computation, representation, and implementation. In R. C. Atkinson, R. J. Herrnstein, G. Lindzey, & R. D. Luce (Eds.), *Stevens' Handbook of Experimental Psychology* (Second Edition) (pp. 473–509)). New York: Wiley.

Pew, R. W., & Rosenbaum, D. A. (1988). Human motor performance: Computation, representation, and implementation. In R. C. Atkinson, R. J. Herrnstein, G. Lindzey, & R. D. Luce (Eds.), *Stevens' Handbook of Experimental Psychology* (Second Edition) (pp. 473–509). New York: Wiley.

Pfordresher, P. Q., Palmer, C., & Jungers, M. K. (2007). Speed, accuracy, and serial order in sequence production. *Cognitive Science, 26,* 1–37.

Phillips, C. G., & Porter, R. (1977). *Corticospinal neurones: Their role in movement.* London: Academic Press.

Piaget, J. (1970). *Science of education and the psychology of the child (D. Coltman, Trans.).* Oxford, England: Orion.

Pinker, S. (1995). *The language instinct*. New York: HarperPerenniel.

Plamondon, R., & Alimi, A. M. (1997). Speed/accuracy trade-offs in target-directed movements. *Behavioral and Brain Sciences, 20*, 279–303.

Plamondon, R., & Lamarche, F. (1986). Modelization of handwriting: A system approach. In H. S. Kao, G. P. van Galen, & R. Hoosain (Eds.), *Graphonomics: Contemporary research in handwriting* (pp. 169–183). Amsterdam: North-Holland.

Poeck, K. (1969). Pathophysiology of emotional disorders associated with brain damage. In P. J. Vinken, & G. W. Bruyn, (Eds.) *Handbook of clinical neurology: vol. 3*. New York: American Elsevier.

Poizner, H., Klima, E. S., & Bellugi, U. (1987). *What the hands reveal about the brain*. Cambridge, MA: MIT Press/Bradford Books.

Polanyi, M. (1964). *Personal knowledge*. New York: Harper & Row.

Polit, A., & Bizzi, E. (1978). Processes controlling arm movements in monkeys. *Science, 201*, 1235–1237.

Polit, A., & Bizzi, E. (1979). Characteristics of motor programs underlying arm movements in monkeys. *Journal of Neurophysiology, 42*, 183–194.

Poldrak, R. A., Prabakharan, V., Seger, C., & Gabrieli, J. D. (1999). Striatal activation during cognitive skill learning. *Neuropsychology, 13*, 564–574.

Pollack, G. H. (1983). The cross-bridge theory. *Physiological Reviews, 63*, 1049–1130.

Pollick, F. E., Paterson, H. M., Bruderlin, A., & Sanford, A. J. (2001). Perceiving affect from arm movement. *Cognition, 82*, B51–B61.

Popescu, F., Hidler, J. M., & Rymer, W. Z. (2003). Elbow impedance during goal-directed movements. *Experimental Brain Research, 152*, 17–28.

Porter, S., & Ten Brinke, L. (2008). Reading between the lies: Identifying concealed and falsified emotions in universal facial expressions. *Psychological Science, 19*, 508–514.

Posner, M. I. (1967). Characteristics of visual and kinesthetic memory codes. *Journal of Experimental Psychology, 75*, 103–107.

Posner, M. I. (1978). *Chronometric explorations of mind*. Hillsdale, NJ: Lawrence Erlbaum Associates.

Posner, M. I., Nissen, M. J., & Klein, R. (1976). Visual dominance: An information-processing account of its origins and significance. *Psychological Review, 83*, 157–171.

Potter, J. M. (1980). What was the matter with Dr. Spooner? In V. A. Fromkin (Ed.), *Errors in linguistic performance* (pp. 13–34) New York: Academic Press.

Potter, M. C., Kroll, J. F., & Harris, C. (1980). Comprehension and memory in rapid sequential reading. In R. S. Nickerson (Ed.), *Attention and performance VIII* (pp. 395–417). Hillsdale, NJ: Erlbaum.

Povel, D.-J., & Collard, R. (1982). Structural factors in patterned finger tapping. *Acta Psychologica, 52*, 107–124.

Powers, W. T. (1973). *Behavior: The control of perception*. Chicago: Aldine.

Prablanc, C., Echallier, J. F., & Jeannerod, M. (1979). Optimal response of eye and hand motor systems in pointing at a visual target. I. Spatio-temporal characteristics of arm and hand movements and their relationshiops when varying the amount of information. *Biological Cybernetics, 35*, 113–124.

Pratt, J., Chasteen, A. L., & Abrams, R. A. (1994). Rapid aimed limb movements: Age-differences and practice effects in component submovements. *Psychology and Aging, 9*, 325–334.

Pritchard, R. M. (1961). Stabilized images on the retina. *Scientific American, 204*, 72–78.

Prochazka, A. (1989). Sensorimotor gain control: A basic strategy of motor systems? *Progress in Neurobiology, 33*, 281–307.

Proctor, R. W., & Reeve, T. G. (Eds.), (1989). *Stimulus-response compatibility: An integrated perspective*. Amsterdam: North-Holland.

Proctor, R. W., & Van Zandt, T. (1994). *Human factors in simple and complex systems*. Boston: Allyn & Bacon.

Proffitt, D. R. (2006). Distance perception. *Current Directions in Psychological Science, 15*, 131–135.

Proffitt, D. R., Bhalla, M., Gossweiler, R., & Midgett, K. (1995). Perceiving geographical slant. *Psychonomic Bulletin & Review, 2*, 409–428.

Proteau, L., Marteniuk, R. G., & Lévesque, L. (1992). A sensorimotor basis for motor learning: Evidence indicating specificity of practice. *Quarterly Journal of Experimental Psychology, 44A*, 557–575.

Pulvermüller, F. (2005). Brain mechanisms linking language and action. *Nature Reviews Neuroscience, 6*, 576–582.

Purves, D., & Lotto, R. B. (2003). *Why we see what we do: An empirical theory of vision*. Sunderland, MA: Sinauer Associates.

Pylyshyn, Z. W. (1981). The imagery debate: Analog media versus tacit knowledge. *Psychological Review, 88*, 16–45.

Rabbitt, P. M. A. (1978). Detection of errors by skilled typists. *Ergonomics, 21*, 945–958.

Rabbitt, P. M. A., & Vyas, S. M. (1970). An elementary preliminary taxonomy for some errors in laboratory choice RT tasks. *Acta Psychologica, 33*, 56–76.

Rabbitt, P. M. A., Vyas, S. M., & Fearnley, S. (1975). Programming sequences of complex responses. In P. M. A. Rabbitt & S. Dornic (Eds.), *Attention and performance V*. London: Academic Press.

Rabiner, L. R., & Juang, B. H. (1993). *Fundamentals of speech recognition*. Englewood Cliffs, NJ: Prentice-Hall.

Raibert, M. H. (1977). Motor control and learning by the state-space model. Technical Report AI- TR-439, Artificial Intelligence Laboratory, MIT.

Raibert, M. H., & Sutherland, I. E. (1983). Machines that walk. *Scientific American, 248*(1), 44–53.

Ramachandran, V. S., & Blakeslee, S. (1998). *Phantoms in the brain*. New York: William Morrow and Company, Inc.

Ramachandran, V. S., & Rogers-Ramachandran, D. (1996). Synaesthesia in phantom limbs induced with mirrors. *Proceedings Of The Royal Society Of London Series B-Biological Sciences, 263*, 377–386.

Rashbass, C. (1961). The relationship between saccadic and smooth tracking eye movements. *Journal of Physiology (London), 159*, 326–338.

Rashbass, C. (1981). Reflexions on the control of vergence. In B. L. Zuber (Ed.), *Models of oculomotor behavior and control* (pp. 139–148). Boca Raton, FL: CRC Press, Inc.

Rayner, K., & Pollatsek, A. (2006). Eye-movement control in reading. In M. J. Traxler & M. A. Gernsbacher (Eds.), *Handbook of Psycholinguistics, Second Edition* (pp. 613–658). Amsterdam: Elsevier.

Rayner, K., Foorman, B. R., Perfetti, C. A., & Pesetsky, D. (2001). How psychological science informs the teaching of reading. *Psychological Science in the Public Interest, 2*, 31–74.

Redding, G. M., & Wallace, B. (1997). *Adaptive spatial alignment*. Mahwah, N.J.: Lawrence Erlbaum Associates.

Redding, G. M., & Wallace, B. (2008). Intermanual transfer of prism adaptation. *Journal of Motor Behavior, 40*, 246–262.

Reeve, T. G., & Proctor, R. W. (1984). On the advance preparation of discrete finger responses. *Journal of Experimental Psychology: Human Perception and Performance, 10*, 541–553.

Reina, G. A., & Schwartz, A. B. (2003). Eye-hand coupling during closed-loop drawing: Evidence of shared motor planning? *Human Movement Science, 22*, 137–152.

Repp, B. H. (1999). Control of expressive and metronomic timing in pianists. *Journal of Motor Behavior, 31*, 145–164.

Repp, B. (2005). Sensorimotor synchronization: A review of the tapping literature. *Psychonomic Bulletin & Review, 12*, 969–992.

Repp, B. H., & Knoblich, G. (2004). Perceiving action identity: How pianists recognize their own performances. *Psychological Science, 15*, 604–609.

Restle, F. (1970). Theory of serial pattern learning: Structural trees. *Psychological Review, 77*, 481–495.

Rhodes, B. J., Bullock, D., Verwey, W. B., Averbeck, B. B., & Page, M. P. A. (2004). Learning and production of

movement sequences: Behavioral, neurophysiological, and modeling perspectives. *Human Movement Science, 23*, 699–746.

Richards, W. (1968). Visual suppression during passive eye movement. *Journal of the Optical Society of America, 58*, 1559.

Richardson, A. (1967a). Mental practice: A review and discussion I. *Research Quarterly, 38*, 95–107.

Richardson, A. (1967b). Mental practice: A review and discussion II. *Research Quarterly, 38*, 262–273.

Rieger, M. (2004). Automatic keypress activation in skilled typing. *Journal of Experimental Psychology: Human Perception and Performance, 30*, 555–565.

Rieser, J. J., Pick, H. L., Ashmead, D. H., & Garing, A. E. (1995). Calibration of human locomotion and models of perceptual-motor organization. *Journal of Experimental Psychology: Human Perception and Performance, 21*, 480–497.

Rinn, W. E. (1984). The neuropsychology of facial expression: A review of the neurological and psychological mechanisms for producing facial expressions. *Psychological Bulletin, 95*, 52–77.

Rizzolatti, G., & Craighero, L. (1998). From spatial attention to attention to objects: An extension of the premotor theory of attention. *Revue De Neuropsychologie, 8*, 155–174.

Rizzolatti, G., Riggio, L., & Sheliga, B. M. (1994). Space and selective attention. In C. Umilta & M. Moscovitch (Eds.), *Attention and Performance, XV* (pp. 231–265). Cambridge USA: MIT Press.

Robinson, D. A. (1964). The mechanics of human saccadic eye movement. *Journal of Physiology (London), 174*, 245–264.

Robinson, D. A. (1968). The oculomotor control system: A review. *Proceedings of the Institute of Electrical Engineers, 56*, 1032–1047.

Robinson, D. A. (1981). Control of eye movements. In Handbook of physiology, Section I: The nervous system, 2. Bethesda, MD: American Physiological Society.

Rochat, P. (1992). Self-sitting and reaching in 5- to 8-month old infants: The impact of posture and its development on early eye-hand coordination. *Journal of Motor Behavior, 24*, 210–220.

Rochat, P., & Goubet, N. (1995). Development of sitting and reaching in 5- to 6-month-old infants. *Infant Behavior and Development, 18*, 53–68.

Rochat, P., Goubet, N., & Senders, S. J. (1999). To reach or not to reach? Perception of body effectivities by young infants. *Infant and Child Development, 8*, 129–148.

Rock, I. (1983). *The logic of perception*. Cambridge, MA: MIT Press.

Rock, I., & Harris, C. S. (1967). Vision and touch. *Scientific American, 216*(5), 96–104.

Roeltgin, D. (1985). Agraphia. In K. M. Heilman & E. Valenstein (Eds.), *Clinical neuropsychology* (Second edition) (pp. 75–96). New York: Oxford University Press.

Rogers, D. M. (1992). *Motor disorder in psychiatry: Towards a neurological psychiatry*. New York: J. Wiley & Sons.

Roland, P. E., Larsen, B., Lassen, N. A., & Skinhoj, E. (1980). Supplementary motor area and other cortical areas in organizaiton of voluntary movements in man. *Journal of Neurophysiology*, 43, 118–136.

Rosenbaum, D. A. (1975). Perception and extrapolation of velocity and acceleration. *Journal of Experimental Psychology: Human Perception and Performance*, 1, 395–403.

Rosenbaum, D. A. (1980). Human movement initiation: Specification of arm, direction, and extent. *Journal of Experimental Psychology: General*, 109, 444–474.

Rosenbaum, D. A. (1983). Central control of movement timing. *The Bell System Technical Journal (Special Human Factors and Behavioral Sciences issue)*, 62, 1647–1657. Rosenbaum, D. A. (1983). The movement precuing technique: Assumptions, applications, and extensions. In R. A. Magill (Ed.), *Memory and control of action* (pp. 231–274). Amsterdam: North-Holland.

Rosenbaum, D. A. (1985). Motor programming: A review and scheduling theory. In H. Heuer, U. Kleinbeck, & K.-M. Schmidt (Eds.), *Motor behavior: Programming, control, and acquisition* (pp. 1–33). Berlin: Springer-Verlag.

Rosenbaum, D. A. (1987a). Hierarchical organization of motor programs. In S. Wise (Ed.), *Neural and Behavioral Approaches to Higher Brain Functions* (pp. 45–66). New York: Wiley.

Rosenbaum, D. A. (1987b). Successive approximations to a model of human motor programming. In G. H. Bower (Ed.)*Psychology of learning and motivation: Vol. 21* (pp. 153–182). Orlando, FL: Academic Press.

Rosenbaum, D. A. (1991). *Human motor control*. San Diego: Academic Press.

Rosenbaum, D. A. (2002). Time, space, and short term memory. *Brain and Cognition*, 48, 52–65.

Rosenbaum, D. A. (2005). The Cinderella of psychology: The neglect of motor control in the science of mental life and behavior. *American Psychologist*, 60, 308–317.

Rosenbaum, D. A. (2007). *MATLAB For Behavioral Scientists*. Mahwah, NJ: Lawrence Erlbaum Associates.

Rosenbaum, D. A. (2008). Reaching and walking: Reaching distance costs more than walking distance. *Psychonomic Bulletin & Review*, 15, 1100–1104.

Rosenbaum, D. A., Carlson, R. A., & Gilmore, R. O. (2001). Acquisition of intellectual and perceptual-motor skills. *Annual Review of Psychology*, 52, 453–470.

Rosenbaum, D. A., Cohen, R. G., Jax, S. A., van der Wel, R., & Weiss, D. J. (2007). The problem of serial order in behavior: Lashley's legacy. *Human Movement Science*, 26, 525–554.

Rosenbaum, D. A., Cohen, R. G., Meulenbroek, R. G., & Vaughan, J. (2006). Plans for grasping objects. In M. Latash & F. Lestienne (Eds.), *Motor Control and Learning Over the Lifespan* (pp. 9–25). New York: Springer.

Rosenbaum, D. A., & Dawson, A. M. (2004). The motor system computes well but remembers poorly. *Journal of Motor Behavior*, 36, 390–392.

Rosenbaum, D. A., Dawson, A. M., & Challis, J. H. (2006). Haptic tracking permits bimanual independence. *Journal of Experimental Psychology: Human Perception and Performance*, 32, 1266–1275.

Rosenbaum, D. A., Gordon, A. M., Stillings, N. A., & Feinstein, M. H. (1987). Sitmulus-response compatibility in the programming of speech. *Memory & Cognition*, 15, 217–224.

Rosenbaum, D. A., Inhoff, A. W., & Gordon, A. M. (1984). Choosing between movement sequences: A hierarchical editor model. *Journal of Experimental Psychology: General*, 113, 372–393.

Rosenbaum, D. A., & Jorgensen, M. J. (1992). Planning macroscopic aspects of manual control. *Human Movement Science*, 11, 61–69.

Rosenbaum, D. A., Kenny, S., & Derr, M. A. (1983). Hierarchical control of rapid movement sequences. *Journal of Experimental Psychology: Human Perception and Performance*, 9, 86–102.

Rosenbaum, D. A., & Kornblum, S. (1982). A priming method for investigating the selection of motor responses. *Acta Psychologica*, 51, 223–243.

Rosenbaum, D. A., Loukopoulos, L. D., Meulenbroek, R. G. M., Vaughan, J., & Engelbrecht, S. E. (1995). Planning reaches by evaluating stored postures. *Psychological Review*, 102, 28–67.

Rosenbaum, D. A., Marchak, F., Barnes, H. J., Vaughan, J., Slotta, J., & Jorgensen, M. (1990). Constraints for action selection: Overhand versus underhand grips. In M. Jeannerod (Ed.), *Attention and Performance XIII: Motor representation and control* (pp. 321–342). Hillsdale, NJ: Lawrence Erlbaum Associates.

Rosenbaum, D. A., Meulenbroek, R. G., Vaughan, J., & Jansen, C. (2001). Posture-based motion planning: Applications to grasping. *Psychological Review*, 108, 709–734.

Rosenbaum, D. A., & Patashnik, O. (1980). A mental clock-setting process revealed by reaction times. In G. E. Stelmach & J. Requin (Eds.), *Tutorials in motor behavior* (pp. 487–499). Amsterdam: North-Holland Publishing Co.

Rosenbaum, D. A., van Heugten, C., & Caldwell, G. C. (1996). From cognition to biomechanics and back:

The end-state comfort effect and the middle-is-faster effect. *Acta Psychologica, 94*, 59–85.

Rosenbaum, D. A., Vaughan, J., Barnes, H. J., Marchak, F., & Slotta, J. (1990). Constraints on action selection: Overhand versus underhand grips. In M. Jeannerod (Ed.), *Attention and Performance XIII* (pp. 321–342). Hillsdale, NJ: Lawrence Erlbaum Associates.

Rosenbaum, D. A., Vaughan, J., Jorgensen, M. J., Barnes, H. J., & Stewart, E. (1993). Plans for object manipulation. In D. E. Meyer & S. Kornblum (Eds.), *Attention and performance XIV — A silver jubilee: Synergies in experimental psychology, artificial intelligence and cognitive neuroscience* (pp. 803–820). Cambridge: MIT Press, Bradford Books.

Rosenbaum, D. A., Vaughan, J., Meulenbroek, R. G. J., Jax, S., & Cohen, R. (2009). Smart moves: The psychology of everyday perceptual-motor acts. In E. Morsella, J. A. Bargh, & P. M. Gollwitzer (Eds.), *Oxford Handbook of Human Action* (pp. 121–135). New York: Oxford University Press.

Rosenbaum, D. A., Weber, R. J., Hazelett, W. M., & Hindorff, V. (1986). The parameter remapping effect in human performance: Evidence from tongue twisters and finger fumblers. *Journal of Memory and Language, 25*, 710–725.

Rosenthal, R. (Ed.). (1979). *Skill in nonverbal communication: Individual differences.* Cambridge, MA: Oelgeschlager, Gunn, & Hain, Publishers, Inc.

Rosenzweig, M. R., & Leiman, A. L. (1982). *Physiological psychology.* Lexington, Massachusetts: D. C. Heath.

Rossetti, Y., Jacquin-Courtois, S., Rode, G., Ota, H., Michel, C., & Boisson, D. (2004). Does action make the link between number and space representation? Visuo-manual adaptation improves number bisection in unilateral neglect. *Psychological Science, 15*, 426–430.

Rossetti, Y., Rode, G., Pisella, L., Farné, A., Li, L., Boisson, D., et al. (1998). Prism adaptation to a rightward optical deviation rehabilitates left hemispatial neglect. *Nature, 395*, 166–169.

Rossini, P.M., Barker, A.T., Berardelli, A., Caramia, M.D., Caruso, G., Cracco, R.Q., et al., (1994). Noninvasive electrical and magnetic stimulation of the brain, spinal-cord and roots-basic principles and procedures for routine clinical-application-Report of an IFCN committee. Electroencephalography and Clinical Beurophysiology, 91, 79–92

Rothbart, M. K. (1981). Measurement of temperament in infancy. *Child Development, 52*, 569–578.

Rothbart, M.K. (1989). Behavioral approach and inhibition. Perspectives on behavioral inhibition: The John D. and Catherine T. MacArthur Foundation series on mental health and development, 139–157.

Rothwell, J. C. (1987). *Control of human voluntary movement.* London: Croom-Helm.

Rovee, C. K., & Fagan, J. W. (1976). Extended conditioning and 24–hour retention in infants. *Journal of Experimental Child Psychology, 21*, 1–11.

Rumelhart, D. E., & McClelland, J. L. (1986). *Parallel distributed processing: Explorations in the microstructure of cognition.* Cambridge, MA: MIT.

Rumelhart, D. E., & Norman, D. A. (1982). Simulating a skilled typist: A study of skilled cognitive-motor performance. *Cognitive Science, 6*, 1–36.

Ryan, E. D. (1962). Retention of stabilometer and pursuit rotor skills. *Research Quarterly, 33*, 593–598.

Ryan, E. D. (1965). Retention of stabilometer performance over extended periods of time. *Research Quarterly, 36*, 46–51.

Sabes, P. N., & Jordan, M. I. (1997). Obstacle avoidance and a perturbation sensitivity model for motor planning. *The Journal of Neuroscience, 15*, 7119–7128.

Sackeim, H. A., & Gur, R. C. (1978). Lateral asymmetry in intensity of emotional expression. *Neuropsychologia, 16*, 473–481.

Sackeim, H. A., Gur, R. C., & Saucy, M. C. (1978). Emotions are expressed more intensely on the left side of the face. *Science, 202*, 443–446.

Sahrmann, S. A., & Norton, B. J. (1977). The relationship of voluntary movement to spasticity in the upper motor neuron syndrome. *Annals of Neurology, 2*, 460–465.

Sainburg, R. L. (2002). Evidence for a dynamic dominance hypothesis of handedness. *Experimental Brain Research, 142*, 241–258.

Sainburg, R. (2005). Handedness: Differential specializations for control of trajectory and position. *Exercise and Sport Sciences Reviews, 33*, 206–213.

Salinas, E., & Their, P. (2000). Gain modulation: A major computational principle of the central nervous system. *Neuron, 27*, 15–21.

Saltzman, E., & Kelso, J. A. S. (1987). Skilled actions: A task dynamic approach. *Psychological Review, 94*, 84–106.

Saltzman, E. (1979). Levels of sensorimotor representation. *Journal of Mathematical Psychology, 20*, 91–163.

Sappey, P. (1888/89). *Traité d'Anatomie Descriptive.* Paris: Delahaye Lecrosnier.

Sarno, J. E. (2004). *Healing back pain: The mind-body connection.* New York: Warner Books.

Sasaki, K., Gemba, H., & Mizuno, N. (1982). Cortical field potnetials preceding visually initiated hand movements and cerebellar actions in the monkey. *Experimental Brain Research, 46*, 29–36.

Saslow, M. G. (1967). Effects of components of displacement-step stimuli upon latency of saccadic eye movement. *Journal of the Optical Society of America, 57*, 1024–1029.

Saunders, F. (2008). Touching the listener. *American Scientist, 96*(2: March-April), 111.

Savelsbergh, G. J. P., & van der Kamp, J. (1993). The coordination of infant's reaching, grasping, catching and posture: A natural physical approach. In G. J. P. Savelbergh (Ed.), *Advances in Psychology* (pp. 289–317). New York: Elsevier.

Sawashima, M., & Hirose, H. (1983). Laryngeal gestures in speech production. In P. F. MacNeilage (Ed.), *The production of speech* (pp. 11–38). New York: Springer-Verlag.

Schack, T., & Mechsner, F. (2006). Representation of motor skills in human long-term memory. *Neuroscience Letters, 391,* 77–81.

Schall, J.D. & Boucher L. (2007). Executive control of gaze by the frontal lobes. *Cognitive Affective and Behavioral Neuroscience, 7(4):* 396–412.

Scheidt, R. A., & Ghez, C. (2007). Separate adaptive mechanisms for controlling trajectory and final position in reaching. *Journal of Neurophysiology, 98,* 3600–3613.

Schieber, M. H. (2001). Constraints on somatotopic organization in the primary motor cortex. *Journal of Neurophysiology, 86,* 2125–2143.

Schmahmann, J. D. (2000). *MRI Atlas of the Human Cerebellum.* San Diego, CA: Academic Press.

Schmahmann, J. D., Anderson, C. M., Newton, N., & Ellis, R. (2001). The function of the cerebellum in cognition, affect and consciousness: Empirical support for the embodied mind. *Conscious Emotion, 2,* 273–309.

Schmidt, R. A. (1968). Anticipation and timing in human motor performance. *Psychological Bulletin, 70,* 631–646.

Schmidt, R. A. (1975). A schema theory of discrete motor skill learning. *Psychological Review, 82,* 225–260.

Schmidt, R. A. (1976). The schema as a solution to some persistent problems in motor learning theory. In G. E. Stelmach (Ed.), *Motor control: Issues and trends* (pp. 41–65). New York: Academic Press.

Schmidt, R. A. (1982). *Motor control and learning.* Champaign, Illinois: Human Kinetics Publishers.

Schmidt, R. A. (1988). *Motor control and learning* (Second Edition). Champaign, Illinois: Human Kinetics Publishers.

Schmidt, R. A., & Bjork, R. A. (1992). New conceptualizations of practice: Common principles in three paradigms suggest new concepts for training. *Psychological Science, 3,* 207–214.

Schmidt, R. A., & Lee, T. D. (2005). *Motor control and learning – A behavioral emphasis* (4th Ed). Champaign, Illinois: Human Kinetics.

Schmidt, R. A., Zelaznik, H. N., Hawkins, B., Frank, J. S., & Quinn, J. T., Jr. (1979) Motor output variability: A theory for the accuracy of rapid motor acts. *Psychological Review, 86,* 415–451.

Schmidt, R. C., Carello, C., & Turvey, M. T. (1990). Phase transitions and critical fluctuations in the visual coordination of rhythmic movements between people. *Journal of Experimental Psychology: Human Perception and Performance, 16,* 227–247.

Scholz, J. P., Kelso, J. A. S., & Schöner, G. (1987). Nonequilibrium phase transitions in coordinated biological motion: Critical slowing down and switching time. *Physics Letters, 123,* 390–394.

Scholz, J. P., & Schöner, G. (1999). The uncontrolled manifold concept: Identifying control variables for a functional task. *Experimental Brain Research, 126,* 289–306.

Schöner, G. (1990). Dynamic theory of coordination of discrete movement. *Biological Cybernetics, 63,* 257–270.

Schöner, G., & Kelso, J. A. S. (1988). Dynamic pattern generation in behavioral and neural systems. *Science, 239,* 1513–1520.

Schutter, D. J., & van Honk, J. (2005). The cerebellum on the rise in human emotion. *The Cerebellum, 4,* 290–294.

Schwartz, A. B. (1994). Direct cortical representation of drawing. *Science, 265,* 540–542.

Schwartz, A., Ebner, T., & Bloedel, J. (1987). Responses of interposed and dentate nuerons to perturbations of the locomotor cycle. *Experimental Brain Research, 67,* 323–338.

Schwartz, G. E. (1982). Psychophysiological patterning and emotion revisited: A systems perspective. In C. E. Izard (Ed.), *Measuring emotions in infants and children.* Cambridge, England: Cambridge University Press.

Scott, C. M., & Ringel, R. L. (1971). Articulation without oral sensory control. *Journal of Speech and Hearing Research, 14,* 804–814.

Scott, S. H., Gribble, P. L., Graham, K. M., & Cabel, D. W. (2001). Dissociation between hand motion and population vectors from neural activity in motor cortex. *Nature, 413,* 161–165.

Scoville, W. B., & Milner, B. (1957). Loss of recent memory after bilateral hippocampal lesions. *Journal of Neurology, Neurosurgery, and Psychiatry, 20,* 11–21.

Seashore, C. E. (1938). *Psychology of music.* New York: McGraw Hill.

Sebanz, N., Knoblich, G., & Prinz, W. (2003). Representing others' actions: Just like one's own? *Cognition, 88,* 11–21.

Selkirk, E. O. (1982). *The syntax of words.* Cambridge, MA: MIT Press.

Sen, M. G., Yonas, A., & Knill, D. C. (2001). Development of infants' sensitivity to surface contour information for spatial layout. *Perception, 30,* 167–176.

Serino, A., Pizzoferrato, F., & Làdavas, E. (2008). Viewing a face (especially one's own face) being touched enhances tactile perception on the face. *Psychological Science, 19*(5), 434–438.

Shadmehr, R., & Wise, S. P. (2005). *The computational neurobiology of reaching and pointing*. Cambridge, MA: MIT Press.

Shaffer, L. H. (1973). Latency mechanisms in transcription. In S. Kornblum (Ed.), *Attention and performance IV*. New York: Academic Press.

Shaffer, L. H. (1975). Multiple attention in continuous verbal tasks. In P. M. Rabbitt & S. Dornic (Eds.), *Attenion and performance V*. London: Academic Press.

Shaffer, L. H. (1975a). Control processes in typing. *Quarterly Journal of Experimental Psychology, 27,* 419–432.

Shaffer, L. H. (1975b). Multiple attention in continuous verbal tasks. In P. M. Rabbitt & S. Dornic (Eds.), *Attention and performance V*. London: Academic Press.

Shaffer, L. H. (1984a). Timing in musical performance. In J. Gibbon & L. Allan (Eds.), *Timing and time perception* (pp. 420–428). New York: New York Academy of Sciences.

Shaffer, L. H. (1984b). Timing in solo and duet piano performances. *Quarterly Journal of Experimental Psychology, 36A,* 577–595.

Shannon, C. E., & Weaver, W. (1949). *The mathematical theory of communication*. Urbana, IL: University of Illinois Press.

Shapiro, D. C., Zernicke, R. F., Gregor, R. J., & Diestel, J. D. (1981). Evidence for generalized motor programs using gait pattern analysis. *Journal of Motor Behavior, 13,* 33–47.

Sharp, R. H. (1975). Skill in fast ball games: Some input considerations. Unpublished doctoral dissertation. University of Leeds, Leeds, Yorkshire, England.

Shattuck-Hufnagle, S. (1979). Speech errors as evidence for a serial order mechanism in sentence production. In W. E. Cooper & E. C. T. Walker (Eds.), *Sentence processing: Psycholinguistic studies presented to Merrill Garrett* (pp. 295–342). Hillsdale, NJ: Erlbaum.

Shea, J. B., & Morgan, R. L. (1979). Contextual interference effects on acquisition, retention, and transfer of a motor skill. *Journal of Experimental Psychology: Human Learning and Memory, 5,* 179–187.

Shepard, R. N., & Cooper, L. (1982). *Mental images and their transformations*. Cambridge, MA: MIT Press/Bradford Books.

Sheridan, M. R. (1979). A reappraisal of Fitts' law. *Journal of Motor Behavior, 11,* 179–188.

Sherrington, C. S. (1906). *Integrative action of the nervous system*. New York: Scribner.

Shik, M. L., Severin, F. V., & Orlosky, G. N. (1966). Control of walking and running by means of electrical stimulation of the mid-brain. *Biophysics, 11,* 756–765.

Shin, J. C. (2008). The procedural learning of action order is independent of temporal learning. *Psychological Research, 72,* 376–386.

Shin, J., & Rosenbaum, D. A. (2002). Reaching while calculating: Scheduling of cognitive and perceptual-motor processes. *Journal of Experimental Psychology: General, 131,* 206–219.

Shirley, M. M. (1931). *The first two years: A study of twenty-five babies, Vol. I. Postural and locomotor development*. Minneapolis: University of Minnesota Press.

Shumway-Cook, A., & Woollacott, M. (2006). *Motor control: Translating research into clinical practice*. Philadelphia: Lippincott Williams & Wilkins.

Siegman, A. W., & Feldstein, S. (Eds.), (1987). *Nonverbal behavior and communication* (Second Edition). Hillsdale, NJ: Lawrence Erlbaum Associates.

Simon, H. A. (1972). Complexity and the representation of patterned sequences of symbols. *Psychological Review, 79,* 369–382.

Simon, J. R. (1990). The effect of an irrelevant directional cue on human information processing. In R. W. Proctor & T. G. Reeve (Eds.), *Stimulus-response compatibility: An integrated perspective* (pp. 31–86). Amsterdam: North-Holland.

Sirigu, A., Duhamel, J-R., Cohen, L., Pillon, B., Dubois, B., & Agid, Y. (1996). The mental representation of hand movements after parietal cortex damage. *Science, 273,* 1564–1568.

Skavenski, A. A. (1972). Inflow as a source of extraretinal eye position information. *Vision Research, 12,* 221–229.

Skavenski, A. A., & Hansen, R. M. (1978). Role of eye position information in visual space perception. In J. Senders, D. Fisher, & R. Monty (Eds.), *Eye movements and the higher psychological functions* (pp. 15–34). Hillsdale, NJ: Erlbaum.

Skavenski, A. A., Haddad, G., & Steinman, R. M. (1972). The extraretinal signal for the visual perception of direction. *Perception & Psychophysics, 11,* 287–290.

Skoglund, S. (1956). Anatomical and physiological studies of knee joint innervation in the cat. *Acta Physiologica Scandinavica, 36*(Supplement 124), 1–101.

Slater-Hammel, A. T. (1960). Reliability, accuracy, and refractoriness of a transit reaction. *Research Quarterly, 31,* 217–228.

Sloboda, J. A. (1983). The communication of musical metre in piano performance. *Quarterly Journal of Experimental Psychology, 35A,* 377–396.

Smeets, J. B. J., & Brenner, E. (1999). A new view on grasping. *Motor Control, 3,* 237–271.

Smeets, J. B., & Brenner, E. (2002). Does a complex model help to understand grasping? *Experimental Brain Research, 144,* 132–135.

Smeets, J. B., & Brenner, E. (2006). 10 years of illusions. *Journal of Experimental Psychology: Human Perception and Performance, 32,* 1501–1504.

Smith, E. E., & Kosslyn, S. M. (2007). *Cognitive Psychology.* Pearson Prentice Hall.

Smith, L. B., Thelen, E., Titzer, R., & McLin, D. (1999). Knowing in the context of acting: The task dynamics of the A-not-B error. *Psychological Review, 106,* 235–260.

Smith, L. C., & Moscovitch, M. (1979). Writing posture, hemispheric control of movement and cerebral dominance in individuals with inverted and noninverted hand postures during writing. *Neuropsychologia, 17,* 637–644.

Smyth, M. M. (1984). Memory for movements. In M. M. Smyth & A. M. Wing (Eds.), *The psychology of human movement* (pp. 83–117). London: Academic Press.

Smyth, M. M., & Mason, U. C. (1997). Planning and execution of action in children with or without developmental coordination disorder. *Journal of Child Psychology and Psychiatry, 38,* 1023–1037.

Smith, S. M., Brown, H. O., Toman, J. E. P., & Goodman, L. S. (1947). Lack of cerebral effect of d-Tubercurarine. *Anesthesiology, 8,* 1–14.

Smith, T. S. & Lee, C. Y. (1971). Peripheral feedback mechanisms in speech production models. Paper presented at the VII International Congress of Phonetic Sciences, Montreal (August).

Smith, W. M., McCrary, J. M., & Smith, K. U. (1960). Delayed visual feedback and behavior. *Science, 132,* 1013–1014.

Smyth, M. M., & Pendleton, L. R. (1989). Working memory for movements. *Quarterly Journal of Experimental Psychology, 41A,* 235–250.

Smyth, T. R., & Glencross, D. J. (1986). Information processing deficits in clumsy children. *Australian Journal of Psychology, 38,* 13–22.

Soechting, J. F., & Flanders, M. (1989). Sensorimotor representations for pointing to targets in three-dimensional space. *Journal of Neurophysiology, 62,* 582–594.

Soechting, J. F., Buneo, C. A., Herrmann, U., & Flanders, M. (1995). Moving effortlessly in three dimensions: Does Donders' Law apply to arm movement? *Journal of Neuroscience, 15,* 6271–6280.

Soechting, J. F., & Lacquaniti, F. (1981). Invariant characteristics of a pointing movement in man. *Journal of Neuroscience, 1,* 710–720.

Sohn, M. A., & Carlson, R. A. (2003). Implicit temporal tuning of working memory strategy during cognitive skill acquisition. *American Journal of Psychology, 116,* 239–256.

Sokolov, A. N. (1972). *Inner speech and thought.* New York: Plenum Press.

Sommer, M. A. (2007). The feeling of looking. *Nature Neuroscience, 10,* 538–540.

Sparks, D. L. (1996). Testing the predictions of different models of the saccadic system. In R. Caminiti, K.-P. Hoffmann, F. Lacquaniti, & J. Altman (Eds.), *Vision and movement: Mechanisms in the cerebral cortex* (pp. 107–116). Strasbourg, France: Human Frontier Science Program.

Sparks, D. L., & Mays, L. E. (1983). Role of the monkey superior colliculus in the spatial localization of saccade targets. In A. Hein & M. Jeannerod (Eds.), *Spatially oriented behavior* (pp. 63–85). New York: Springer-Verlag.

Spelke, E., Hirst, W., & Neisser, U. (1976). Skills of divided attention. *Cognition, 4,* 215–230.

Spencer, J. P., Smith, L. B., & Thelen, E. (2001). Tests of a dynamic systems account of the A-not-B error: The influence of prior experience on the spatial memory abilities of two-year-olds. *Child Development, 72,* 1327–1346.

Spencer, R. M. C., Zelaznik, H. N., Diedrichsen, J., & Ivry, R. B. (2003). Disrupted timing of discontinuous but not continuous movements by cerebellar lesions. *Science, 300,* 1437–1439.

Sperling, G. A. (1960). The information available in brief visual presentation. Psychological Monographs, 74, Whole No. 498.

Sperry, R. W. (1950). Neural basis of the spontaneous optokinetic response produced by visual inversion. *Journal of Comparative and Physiological Psychology, 43,* 482–489.

Spivey, M. (2007). *The continuity of mind.* New York: Oxford University Press.

Squire, L. R. (1987). *Memory and brain.* New York: Oxford University Press.

Stark, L. (1968). *Neurological control systems: Studies in bioengineering.* New York: Plenum.

Stein, R. B. (1982). What muscle variable(s) does the nervous system control in limb movements? *Brain and Behavioral Sciences, 5,* 535–577.

Steinbach, M. J., & Held, R. (1968). Eye tracking of observer-generated target movements. *Science, 161,* 187–188.

Steinbach, M. J., & Smith, D. R. (1981). Spatial localization after strabismus surgery: Evidence for inflow. *Science, 213,* 1407–1409.

Steinman, R. M. (1986). The need for an eclectic, rather than systems, approach to the study of the primate oculomotor system. *Vision Research, 26,* 101–112.

Steinman, R. M., Haddad, G. M., Skavenski, A. A., & Wyman, D. (1973). Miniature eye movement. *Science, 181,* 810–819.

Stelmach, G. E., & Teulings, H-L. (1983). Response characteristics of prepared and restructured handwriting. *Acta Psychologica, 54,* 51–67.

Sternad, D., Duarte, M., Katsumata, H., & Schaal, S. (2001). Bouncing a ball: Tuning into dynamic stability. *Journal of Experimental Psychology: Human Perception And Performance, 27,* 1163–1184.

Sternberg, S. (1969). The discovery of processing stages: Extensions of Donders' method. In W. G. Koster (Ed.), *Attention and performance II* (pp. 276–315). Amsterdam: North-Holland.

Sternberg, S., Monsell, S., Knoll, R. L., & Wright, C. E. (1978). The latency and duration of rapid movement sequences: Comparisons of speech and typewriting. In G. E. Stelmach (Ed.), *Information processing in motor control and learning* (pp. 117–152). New York: Academic Press.

Stetson, R. H. (1951). *Motor phonetics.* Amsterdam: North-Holland.

Stevens, J. A. (2005). Interference effects demonstrate distinct roles for visual and motor imagery during the mental representation of human action. *Cognition, 95,* 329–350.

Stevens, K. N. (1983). Design features of speech sound systems. In P. F. MacNeilage (Ed.), *The production of speech* (pp. 247–261). New York: Springer-Verlag.

Stillings, N. A., Feinstein, M. H., Garfield, J. L., Rissland, E. L., Rosenbaum, D. A., Weisler, S. E., et al. (1987). *Cognitive science: An introduction.* Cambridge, MA: Bradford/MIT Press.

Stoffregen, T. A., Bardy, B. G., Bonnet, C. T., & Pagulayan, R. J. (2006). Postural stabilization of visually guided eye movements. *Ecological Psychology, 18,* 191–222.

Stoffregen, T. A., Hove, P., Bardy, B. G., Riley, M., & Bonnet, C. T. (2007). Postural stabilization of perceptual but not cognitive performance. *Journal of Motor Behavior, 39,* 126–138.

Storm, C., & Storm, T. (1987). A taxonomic study of the vocabulary of emotions. *Journal of Personality and Social Psychology, 53,* 805–816.

Strayer, D. L., & Drews, F. A. (2007). Cell-phone–induced driver distraction. *Current Directions in Psychological Science, 16,* 128–131.

Strelow, E. R. (1985). What is needed for a theory of mobility: Direct perception and cognitive maps— Lessons from the blind. *Psychological Review, 92,* 226–248.

Stroop, J. R. (1935). Studies of interference in serial verbal reactions. *Journal of Experimental Psychology, 18,* 643–662.

Summers, J. J. (1975). The role of timing in motor program representation. *Journal of Motor Behavior, 7,* 229–241.

Summers, J., Rosenbaum, D. A., Burns, B., & Ford, S. (1993). Production of polyrhythms. *Journal of Experimental Psychology: Human Perception and Performance, 19,* 416–428.

Sundberg, J. (1977). The acoustics of the singing voice. *Scientific American, 3:*82–91.

Swinnen, S. P. (2002). Intermanual coordination: From behavioural principles to neural-network interactions. *Nature Reviews Neuroscience, 3,* 350–361.

Swinnen, S. P., Heuer, H., & Casaer, P. (Eds.), (1994). *Interlimb coordination: Neural, dynamical, and cognitive constraints.* San Diego: Academic Press.

Tanaka, H., Krakauer, J. W., & Qian, N. (2006). An optimization principle for determining movement duration. *Journal of Neurophysiology, 95,* 3875–3886.

Tanenhaus, M. K., Spivey-Knowlton, M., Eberhard, K., & Sedivy, J. (1995). *Science, 268,* 1632–1634.

Tanenhaus, M., Magnuson, J., Dahan, D., & Chambers, C. (2000). Eye movements and lexical access in spoken-language comprehension: Evaluating a linking hypothesis between fixations and linguistic processing. *Journal of Psycholinguistic Research, 29,* 557–580.

Tastevin, J. (1937). En partant de l'expérience d'Aristote. *L'Encephale, 1,* 57–84.

Taub, E., & Berman, A. J. (1968). Movement and learning in the absence of sensory feedback. In S. J. Freeman (Ed.), *The neuropsychology of spatially oriented behavior* (pp. 173–192). Homewood, IL: Dorsey.

Taub, E., & Uswatt, G. (2006). Constraint induced movement therapy: Answers and questions after two decades of research. *NeuroRehabilitation, 21,* 93–95.

Taylor-Clarke, M., Kennett, S., & Haggard, P. (2002). Vision modulates somatosensory cortical processing. *Current Biology, 12,* 233–236.

Teichner, W. H., & Krebs, M. J. (1972). Laws of simple visual reaction time. *Psychological Review, 79,* 344–358.

Teitelman, R. (1984). Stepping out. *Forbes, June 18,* 154–157.

Temprado, J. J., Zanone, P. G., Monno, A., & Laurent, M. (2001). A dynamical framework to understand performance trade-offs and interference in dual tasks. *Journal of Experimental Psychology: Human Perception & Performance, 27,* 1303–1313.

Teramitsu, I., & White, S. (2008). Motor Learning: The FoxP2 Puzzle Piece. *Current Biology, 18*(8), R336.

Terzuolo, C. A., & Viviani, P. (1980). Determinants and characteristics of motor patterns used for typing. *Neuroscience, 5,* 1085–1103.

Teulings, H-L., Thomassen, A. J., & van Galen, G. P. (1983). Preparation of partly precued handwriting movements: The size of movement units in handwriting. *Acta Psychologica, 54,* 165–177.

Thelen, E. (1983). Learning to walk is still an "old" problem: A reply to Zelazo. *Journal of Motor Behavior, 15*(2), 139–161.

Thelen, E. (1995). Motor development: A new synthesis. *American Psychologist, 50,* 79–95.

Thelen, E., Bradshaw, G., & Ward, J. A. (1981). Spontaneous kicking in month-old infants: Manifestations of a human central locomotor program. *Behavioral and Neural Biology, 32,* 45–53.

Thelen, E., Corbetta, D., & Spencer, J. P. (1996). Development of reaching during the first year: Role of movement speed. *Journal of Experimental Psychology: Human Perception and Performance, 22,* 1059–1076.

Thelen, E., Corbetta, D., Kamm, K., & Spencer, J. P. (1993). The transition to reaching: Mapping intention and intrinsic dynamics. *Child Development, 64*(4), 1058–1098.

Thelen, E., & Fisher, D. M. (1982). Newborn stepping: An explanation for a "disappearing" reflex. *Developmental Psychology, 18,* 760–775.

Thelen, E., Kelso, J. A. S., & Fogel, A. (1987). Self-organizing systems and infant motor development. *Developmental Review, 7,* 39–65.

Thiel, E. V., Meulenbroek, R. G. J., & Hulstijn, W. (1998). Path curvature in workspace and in joint space: Evidence for coexisting coordinative rules in aiming. *Motor Control, 2,* 331–351.

Thomassen, A. J., & Teulings, H.-L. (1985). Time, size, and shape in handwriting: Exploring spatio-temporal relationships at different levels. In J. A. Michon & J. B. Jackson (Eds.), *Time, mind, and behavior* (pp. 253–263). Berlin: Springer.

Thorndike, E. L. (1911). *Animal intelligence.* New York: Hafner.

Thorndike, E. L. (1927). The law of effect. *American Journal of Psychology, 39,* 212–222.

Thorpe, S. K., Holder, R. L., & Crompton, R. H. (2007). Origin of human bipedalism as an adaptation for locomotion on flexible branches. *Science, 316,* 1328–1331.

Tipper, S., Howard, L., & Jackson, S. (1997). Selective reaching to grasp: Evidence for distractor interference effects. *Visual Cognition, 4,* 1–38.

Tipper, S. P., Lortie, C., & Baylis, G. C. (1992). Selective reaching: evidence for action-centered attention. *Journal of Experimental Psychology: Human Perception and Performance, 18,* 891–905.

Todd, J. T. (1981). Visual information about moving objects. *Journal of Experimental Psychology: Human Perception and Performance, 7,* 795–810.

Todd, J. T., Mark, L. S., Shaw, R. E., & Pittenger, J. B. (1980). The perception of human growth. *Scientific American, 242*(2), 132–144.

Todorov, E. (2004). Optimality principles in sensorimotor control. *Nature Neuroscience, 7,* 907–915.

Todorov, E., & Jordan, M. I. (2002). Optimal feedback control as a theory of motor coordination. *Nature Neuroscience, 5,* 1226–1235.

Tolman, C. E. (1948). Cognitive maps in rats and man. *Psychological Review, 55,* 189–208.

Touwen, B. C. (1971). A study on the development of some motor phenomena in infancy. *Developmental Medicine and Child Neurology, 13,* 435–446.

Tracy, J. L., & Matsumoto, D. (2008). The spontaneous expression of pride and shame: Evidence for biologically innate nonverbal displays. *Proceeding of the National Academy of Sciences, 105,* 11655–11660.

Treiman, R. (1983). The structure of spoken syllables: Evidence from novel word games. *Cognition, 15,* 49–74.

Trivedi, B. P. (2001). Scientists identify a language gene. National Geographic Today. http://news.nationalgeographic.com/news/pf/17562866.html.

Trommershäuser, J., Landy, M. S., & Maloney, L. T. (2006). Humans rapidly estimate expected gain in movement planning. *Psychological Science, 11,* 981–988.

Trommershäuser, J., Maloney, L. T., & Landy, M. S. (2008). Decision making, movement planning and statistical decision theory. *Trends in Cognitive Science, 12,* 291–297.

Tuller, B., Turvey, M. T., & Fitch, H. L. (1982). The Bernstein perspective: II. The concept of muscle linkage or coordinative structure. In J. A. S. Kelso (Ed.), *Human motor behavior* (pp. 253–281). Hillsdale, NJ: Erlbaum.

Turvey, M. T. (1977). Preliminaries to a theory of action with reference to vision. In R. Shaw & J. Bransford (Eds.), *Perceiving, acting, and knowing.* Hillsdale, NJ: Erlbaum.

Turvey, M. T. (1990). Coordination. *American Psychologist, 45*(8), 938–953.

Turvey, M. T. (1990). The challenge of a physical account of action: A personal view. In H. T. A. Whiting, O. G. Meijer, & P. C. van Wieringen (Eds.), *The natural-physical approach to movement control* (pp. 57–93). Amsterdam: VU University Press.

Turvey, M. T. (1996). Dynamic touch. *American Psychologist, 51,* 1134–1152.

Turvey, M. T. (2007). Action and perception at the level of synergies. *Human Movement Science, 26,* 657–697.

Tversky, A., & Kahneman, D. (1974). Judgment under uncertainty: Heuristics and biases. *Science, 185,* 1124–1131.

Twitchell, T. E. (1970). Reflex mechanisms and the development of prehension. In K. Connolly (Ed.), *Mechanisms of motor skill development* (pp. 25–45). London: Academic Press.

Tyldesley, D. A., & Whiting, H. T. A. (1975). Operational timing. *Journal of Human Movement Studies, 1,* 172–177.

Ungerleider, L. G., & Mishkin, M. (1982). Two cortical visual systems. In D. J. Engle, M. A. Goodale, &

R. J. Mansfield (Eds.), *Analysis of visual behavior* (pp. 549–586). Cambridge, MA: MIT Press.

Vallbo, A. B. (1970). Slowly adapting muscle receptors in man. *Acta Physiologica Scandinavica, 78*, 315–333.

van der Stigchel, S., & Theeuwes, J. (2006). Our eyes deviate away from a location where a distractor is expected to appear. *Experimental Brain Research, 169*, 338–349.

van der Stigchel, S., Meeter, M., & Theeuwes, J. (2006). Eye movement trajectories and what they tell us. *Neuroscience & Biobehavioral Reviews, 30*, 666–679.

van der Wel, R., Eder, J. R., Mitchel, A. D., Walsh, M. W., & Rosenbaum, D. A. (2009). Trajectories emerging from discrete versus continuous processing models in phonological competitor tasks: A commentary on Spivey, Grosjean, and Knoblich (2005). *Journal of Experimental Psychology: Human Perception and Performance, 35*, 588–594.

van der Wel, R. P., Fleckenstein, R., Jax, S., & Rosenbaum, D. A. (2007). Hand path priming in manual obstacle avoidance: Evidence for abstract spatio-temporal forms in human motor control. *Journal of Experimental Psychology: Human Perception and Performance, 33*, 1117–1126.

van der Wel, R. P., & Rosenbaum, D. A. (2007). Coordination of locomotion and prehension. *Experimental Brain Research, 176*, 281–287.

van Mourik, A., & Beek, P. (2004). Discrete and cyclical movements: Unified dynamics or separate control? *Acta Psychologica, 117*, 121–138.

Van Orden, G. C., Holden, J. G., & Turvey, M. T. (2003). Self-organization of cognitive performance. *Journal of Experimental Psychology: General, 132*, 331–350.

van Rossum, J. H. A. (1990). Schmidt's schema theory: The empirical base of the variability of practice hypothesis (a critical analysis). *Human Movement Science, 9*, 387–435.

Van Sommers, P. (1984). *Drawing and cognition: Descriptive and experimental studies of graphic production processes.* Cambridge: Cambridge University Press.

Van Sommers, P. (1986). How the mind draws. *Psychology Today, May*, 62–66.

Vaughan, J. (1983). Saccadic reaction time in visual search. In K. Rayner (Ed.), *Eye movements in reading* (pp. 397–411). New York: Academic Press.

Vereijken, B., Whiting, H. T. A., & Beek, W. J. (1992). A dynamic-systems approach to skill acquisition. *Quarterly Journal Of Experimental Psychology Section A-Human Experimental Psychology, 45*, 323–344.

Vickers, J. N. (2007). *Perception, Cognition, and Decision Training—The Quiet Eye In Action.* Urbana, IL: Human Kinetics.

Vince, M. A., & Welford, A. T. (1967). Time taken to change the speed of a response. *Nature, 213*, 532–533.

Viviani, P., & Terzuolo, C. (1980). Space-time invariance in learned motor skills. In G. E. Stelmach & J. Requin (Eds.), *Tutorials in motor behavior* (pp. 525–533). Amsterdam: North-Holland.

Vogel, S. (1989). In the blink of an eye. *Discover, 2*, 62–64.

Volkmann, F. C. (1976). Saccadic suppression: A brief review. In R. A. Monty & J. W. Senders (Eds.), *Eye movements and psychological processes* (pp. 73–84). Hillsdale, NJ: Erlbaum.

Volkmann, F. C., Riggs, L. A., & Moore, R. K. (1980). Eyeblinks and visual suppression. *Science, 207*, 900–902.

Volkmann, F. C., Schick, A. M., & Riggs, L. A. (1969). Time course of visual inhibition during voluntary saccades. *Journal of the Optical Society of America, 58*, 562–569.

Volpe, B. T., Lynch, D., Eykman-Berland, A., Ferraro, M., Galgano, M., Krebs, H. I., et al. (2008). Intensive sensorimotor arm training mediated by therapist or robot improves hemiparesis in patients with chronic stroke. *Neurorehabilitation and Neural Repair, 22*, 305–310.

von Holst, E., & Mittelstaedt, H. (1950). Das Reafferenzprinzip. Die Naturwissenschaften, 37, 464–474. (English translation in P. C. Dodwell (Ed.), (1980), Perceptual processing: Stimulus equivalence and pattern recognition. New York: Appleton-Century-Crofts.

Von Holst, E., & Mittelstaedt, H. (1950). Das Reafferenzprinzip. Wechselwirkungen zwischen Zentralnervensystem und Peripherie. Naturwissenschaften, 37, 464–476. (English translation in Holst, E. von (1973). The reafference principle. The behavioral physiology of animals and man: The collected papers of Erich von Holst (Vol. 1) [R. Martin, Translator] (pp. 139–173). London: Methuen.

Vorberg, D., & Hambuch, R. (1978). On the temporal control of rhythmic performance. In J. Requin (Ed.), *Attention and Performance VII.* Hillsdale, NJ: Erlbaum.

Vorberg, D., & Hambuch, R. (1984). Timing of two-handed rhythmic performance. In J. Gibbon & L. Allan (Eds.), *Timing and time perception* (pp. 390–406). New York: New York Academy of Sciences.

Vredenbregt, J., & Koster, W. G. (1971). Analysis and synthesis of handwriting. *Philips Technical Review, 32*, 73–78.

Wagner, H. (1982). Flow-field variables trigger landing in flies. *Nature, 297*, 147–148.

Wallace, R. J. (1971). Stimulus-response compatibility and the idea of a response code. *Journal of Experimental Psychology, 88*, 354–360.

Walsh, V., & Cowey, A. (2000). Transcranial magnetic stimulation and cognitive neuroscience. *Nature Reviews Neuroscience, 1,* 73–79.

Wang, J., & Sainburg, R. L. (2007). The dominant and nondominant arms are specialized for stabilizing different features of task performance. *Experimental Brain Research, 178,* 565–570.

Wang, X., Zhang, M., Cohen, I. S., & Goldberg, M. E. (2007). The proprioceptive representation of eye position in monkey primary somatosensory cortex. *Nature Neuroscience, 10,* 640–646.

Wann, J. (1987). Trends in refinement and optimization of fine-motor trajectories: Observations from an analysis of the handwriting of primary school children. *Journal of Motor Behavior, 19,* 13–37.

Wann, J., Nimmo-Smith, I., & Wing, A. (1988). Relation between velocity and curvature in movement: Equivalence and divergence between a power law and minimum-jerk model. *Journal of Experimental Psychology: Human Perception and Performance, 14,* 622–637.

Warren, R. M., & Warren, R. P. (1970). Auditory illusions and confusions. *Scientific American, 23,* 30–36.

Warren, W. H., Jr. (2006) The dynamics of perception and action. *Psychological Review, 113,* 358–389.

Warren, W. H., Jr. (1984) Perceiving affordances: Visual guidance of stair climbing. *Journal of Experimental Psychology: Human Perception and Performance, 10,* 683–703.

Waszak, F., Wascher, E., Keller, P., Koch, I., Aschersleben, G., Rosenbaum, D., & Prinz, W. (2005). Intention-based and stimulus-based mechanisms in action selection. *Experimental Brain Research, 162,* 346–356.

Waynbaum, I. (1907). *La physionomie humaine: Son mÄcanisme et son rÖle social.* Paris: Alcan.

Webb, W. B. (1973). Sleep and dreams. In B. B. Wolman (Ed.), *Handbook of General Psychology.* Englewood Cliffs, NJ: Prentice-Hall.

Wegner, D. M. (2002). *The Illusion of Conscious Will.* Cambridge, MA: MIT Press.

Wegner, D. M., Ansfield, M., & Pilloff, D. (1998). The putt and the pendulum: Ironic effects of the mental control of action. *Psychological Science, 9,* 196–199.

Weigelt, M., Kunde, W., & Prinz, W. (2006). End-state comfort in bimanual object manipulation. *Experimental Psychology, 53,* 143–148.

Weimer, W. B. (1977). A conceptual framework for cognitive psychology: Motor theories of the mind. In R. Shaw & J. Bransford (Eds.), *Perceiving, acting, and knowing: Toward an ecological psychology* (pp. 267–311). Hillsdale, NJ: Erlbaum.

Weinrich, M., & Wise, S. (1982). Premotor cortex of the monkey. *Journal of Neuroscience, 2,* 1329–1345.

Weiskrantz, L., Warrington, E. K., Sanders, M. D., & Marshall, J. (1974). Visual capacity in the hemianopic field following a restricted occipital ablation. *Brain, 97,* 709–728.

Weiss, D. J., Wark, J. D., & Rosenbaum, D. A. (2007). Monkey see, monkey plan, monkey do: The end-state comfort effect in cotton-top tamarins (Saguinus Oedipus). *Psychological Science, 18,* 1063–1068.

Welford, A. T. (Ed.). (1980). *Reaction times.* London: Academic Press.

Welsh, T. N., & Elliott, D. (2004). Movement trajectories in the presence of a distracting stimulus: Evidence for a response activation model of selective reaching. *Quarterly Journal of Experimental Psychology, 57A,* 1031–1057.

Welsh, T. N., & Pratt, J. (2008). Actions modulate attentional capture. *Quarterly Journal of Experimental Psychology, 61,* 968–976.

Wentworth, N., Benson, J. B., & Haith, M. M. (2000). The development of infants' reaches for stationary and moving targets. *Child Development, 71,* 576–601.

West, L. J., & Sabban, Y. (1982). Hierarchy of stroking habits at the typewriter. *Journal of Applied Psychology, 67,* 370–376.

Westheimer, G. H. (1954). Eye movement responses to a horizontally moving visual stimulus. *Archives of Ophthalmology, 52,* 932–943.

Westheimer, G. H., & Conover, D. W. (1954). Smooth eye movements in the absence of a moving visual stimulus. *Journal of Experimental Psychology, 47,* 283–284.

White, B. L., Castle, P., & Held, R. (1964). Observations on the development of visually directed reaching. *Child Development, 35,* 349–364.

Whiting, H. T. A. (1989). Toward a cognitive psychology of human movement. In P. C. W. van Wieringen & R. J. Bootsma (Eds.), *Catching up: Selected essays of H. T. A. Whiting* (pp. 195–230). Amsterdam: Free University Press.

Whiting, H. T. A., Gill, E. B., & Stephenson, J. M. (1970). Critical time intervals for taking in flight information in a ball-catching task. *Ergonomics, 13,* 265–272.

Wickelgren, W. A. (1969). Context-sensitive coding, associative memory, and serial order in (speech) behavior. *Psychological Review, 76,* 1–15.

Wickens, D. (1938). The transference of conditioned excitation and conditioned inhibi_tion from one muscle group to the antagonistic group. *Journal of Experimental Psychology, 22,* 101–123.

Wiesendanger, M. (1981). Organization of secondary motor areas of cerebral cortex. In V. B. Brooks (Ed.)*Handbook of physiology, Section 1: The nervous system, Vol II. Motor control* (pp. 1121–1147). Bethesda, MD: American Physiological Society.

Wiesendanger, M. (1987). Initiation of voluntary movements and the supplementary motor area In

H. Heuer & C. Fromm (Eds.), *Generation and modulation of aciton patterns* (pp. 3–13). Berlin: Springer-Verlag.

Williams, A. M., Williams, J. G., & Davids, K. (1999). Visual perception and action in sport. Van Nostrand Reinhold.

Williams, H. G., & Woollacott, M. H. (1988). Characteristics of neuromuscular responses underlying posture control in clumsy children. Neuroscience Abstracts, 14, 66. {Editor: This is a one-page paper.}

Williams, H. G., Woollacott, M. H., & Ivry, R. (1989). Timing and motor control in clumsy children. Neuroscience Abstracts, 15, 1334.

Willingham, D. B. (1998). A neuropsychological theory of motor skill learning. *Psychological Review, 105,* 558–584.

Willingham, D. B., Wells, L. A., Farrell, J. M., & Stemwedel, M. E. (2000). Implicit motor sequence learning is represented in response locations. *Memory & Cognition, 28,* 366–375.

Willingham, D. T. (2004). *Cognition -- The Thinking Animal* (Second Edition). Upper Saddle River, NJ: Pearson/Prentice Hall.

Wilson, M. (2002). Six views of embodied cognition. *Psychonomic Bulletin & Review, 9*(4), 625–636.

Wing, A. (1978). Response timing in handwriting. In G. E. Stelmach (Ed.), *Information processing in motor control and learning* (pp. 153–172). New York: Academic Press.

Wing, A. M. (1980). The long and short of timing in response sequences. In G. E. Stelmach & J. Requin (Eds.), *Tutorials in motor behavior* (pp. 469–486). Amsterdam: North-Holland.

Wing, A. M., & Beek, P. J. (2002). Movement timing: A tutorial. In W. Prinz & B. Hommel (Eds.), *Common mechanisms in perception and action* (pp. 202–226). Oxford: Oxford University Press.

Wing, A. M., Haggard, P., & Flanagan, R. (Eds.), (1996). *Hand and brain: Neurophysiology and psychology of hand movement.* San Diego: Academic Press.

Wing, A., Keele, S. W., & Margolin, D. I. (1984). Motor disorder and the timing of repetitive movements. In J. Gibbon & L. Allan (Eds.), *Timing and time perception* (pp. 183–192). New York: New York Academy of Sciences.

Wing, A. M., & Kristofferson, A. B. (1973). Response delays and the timing of discrete motor responses. *Perception & Psychophysics, 14,* 5–12.

Wing, A. M., Nimmo-Smith, I., & Eldridge, M. A. (1983). The consitency of cursive letter formation as a function of position in the word. *Acta Psychologica, 54,* 197–204.

Wing, A. M., Turton, A., & Fraser, C. (1986). Grasp size and accuracy of approach in reaching. *Journal of Motor Behavior, 18,* 245–260.

Winold, H., Thelen, E., & Ulrich, B. D. (1994). Coordination and control in the bow arm movements of highly skilled cellists. *Ecological Psychology, 6,* 1–31.

Winstein, C. J., & Schmidt, R. A. (1989). Sensorimotor feedback. In D. H. Holding (Ed.), *Human skills* (Second Edition) (pp. 17–47). Chichester: John Wiley & Sons.

Wise, S. P., & Desimone, R. (1988). Behavioral neurophysiology: Insights into seeing and grasping. *Science, 242,* 736–741.

Wishart, J. G., Bower, T. G. R., & Dunkeld, J. (1978). Reaching in the dark. *Perception, 7,* 507–512.

Witherington, D. C. (2005). The development of prospective grasping control between 5 and 7 months: A longitudinal study. *Infancy, 7,* 143–161.

Witt, J. K., Ashe, J., & Willingham, D. T. (2008). An egocentric frame of reference in implicit motor sequence learning. *Psychological Research, 72,* 542–552.

Witt, J. K., Linkenauger, S. A., Bakdash, J. Z., & Proffitt, D. R. (2008). Putting to a bigger hole: Golf performance relates to perceived size. *Psychonomic Bulletin & Review, 15,* 581–585.

Witt, J. K., Proffitt, D. R., & Epstein, W. (2005). Tool use affects perceived distance but only when you intend to use it. *Journal of Experimental Psychology: Human Perception and Performance, 31,* 880–888.

Wolpert, D. M., & Flanagan, J. R. (2001). Motor prediction. *Current Biology, 11,* 729–732.

Woods, T. (2001). *How I play golf.* New York: Warner Books.

Woodworth, R. S. (1899). The accuracy of voluntary movement. *Psychological Review, 3,* 1–119.

Woodworth, R. S. (1938). *Experimental Psychology.* New York: Holt.

Woodworth, R. S., & Schlosberg, H. (1954). *Experimental Psychology* (Second Edition). New York: Holt.

Woollacott, M. H., Debu, B., & Mowatt, M. (1987). Neuromuscular control of posture in the infant and child: Is vision dominant? *Journal of Motor Behavior, 19,* 167–186.

Wright, D., & Wareham, G. (2005). Mixing sound and vision: The interaction of auditory and visual information for earwitnesses of a crime scene. *Legal and Criminological Psychology, 10,* 103–108.

Wulf, G. (2007). *Attention and motor skill learning.* Champaign, IL: Human Kinetics.

Wulf, G., Hoss, M., & Prinz, W. (1999). Instructions for motor learning: Differential effects of internal versus external focus of attention. *Journal of Motor Behavior, 30,* 169–179.

Wurtz, R. H., Goldberg, M. E., & Robinson, D. L. (1982). Brain mechanisms of visual attention. *Scientific American, 246*(6), 124–135.

Yakolev, P., & Lecours, A. (1967). The myelogenetic cycles of regional maturation of the brain. In A. Minkowski (Ed.), *Regional development of the brain in early life*. Philadelphia: F. A. Davis & Co.

Yamada, H. (1983). Certain problems associated with the design of input keyboards for Japanese writing. In W. E. Cooper (Ed.), *Cognitive aspects of skilled typewriting* (pp. 305–407). New York: Springer-Verlag.

Yaminishi, J., Kawato, M., & Suzuki, R. (1980). Two coupled oscillators as a model for the coordinated finger tapping by both hands. *Biological Cybernetics, 37*, 219.

Yarbus, A. L. (1967). *Eye movements and vision*. New York: Plenum.

Yonas, A., & Granrud, C. E. (1985). Reaching as a measure of infants' spatial perception. In G. Gottlieb & N. A. Krasnegor (Eds.), *Measurement of Audition and Vision in the First Year of Postnatal Life* (pp. 301–322). Norwood, NJ: Ablex.

Yonas, A., Petterson, L., & Lockman, J. J. (1979). Young infants' sensitivity to optical information for collision. *Canadian Journal of Psychology, 33*, 268–276.

Young, S., Chau, T., & Pratt, J. (2008). Choosing the fastest movement: Perceiving speed-accuracy tradeoffs. *Experimental Brain Research, 185*, 681–688.

Yu, H., Russell, D. M., & Sternad, D. (2003). Task–effector asymmetries in a rhythmic continuation task. *Journal of Experimental Psychology, 29*, 616–630.

Zahariev, M., & MacKenzie, C. (2007). Grasping at 'thin air': Multimodal contact cues for reaching and grasping. *Experimental Brain Research, 180*, 69–84.

Zajonc, R. B. (1985). Emotion and facial efference: A theory reclaimed. *Science, 228*, 15–21.

Zajonc, R. B., Adelman, P. K., Murphy, S. T., & Niedenthal, P. M. (1987). Convergence in the physical appearance of spouses. *Motivation and emotion, 11*, 335–346.

Zatsiorsky, V. M., & Duarte, M. (2000). Rambling and trembling in quiet standing. *Motor Control, 4*, 185–200.

Zatsiorsky, V. M., & Latash, M. (2008). Multifinger prehension: An overview. *Journal of Motor Behavior, 40*, 446–475.

Zelaznik, H. N., Hawkins, B., & Kisselburgh, L. (1983). Rapid visual feedback processing in single-aiming movements. *Journal of Motor Behavior, 15*, 217–236.

Zelaznik, N. H., Schmidt, R. A., & Gielen, S. C. (1986). Kinematic properties of aimed hand movements. *Journal of Motor Behavior, 18*, 353–372.

Zelazo, P. R. (1983). The development of walking: New findings and old assumptions. *Journal of Motor Behavior, 15*(2), 99–137.

Zelazo, P. R., Zelazo, N. A., & Kolb, S. (1972). Newborn walking. *Science, 176*, 314–315.

Zheng, B., Verjee, F., Lomax, A. J., & MacKenzie, C. L. (2005). Video analysis of an endoscopic cutting task performed by one vs two operators. *Surgical Endoscopy, 19*, 1388–1395.

Zillner, E. (2008). *Principles of neuropsychology*. Thomson/Wadsworth.

Zimbardo, P. G., Marshall, G., & Maslach, C. (1971). Liberating behavior from time-bound control: Expanding the present through hypnosis. *Journal of Applied Social Psychology, 4*, 305–323.

Zingale, C. M., & Kowler, E. (1987). Planning sequences of saccades. *Vision Research, 27*, 1327–1341.

Zuber, B. L., & Stark, L. (1965). Microsaccades and the velocity-amplitude relationship for saccadic eye movements. *Science, 150*, 1459–1460.

Zuchner, S., Cuccaro, M. L., Tran-Viet, K. N., Cope, H., Krishnan, R. R., Pericak-Vance, M. A., et al. (2006). SLITRK1 mutations in trichotillomania. *Molecular Psychiatry, 11*, 887.

Zwaan, R. A., & Taylor, L. J. (2006). Seeing, acting, understanding: Motor resonance in language comprehension. *Journal of Experimental Psychology: General, 135*, 1–11.

Author Index

A

Abbs, J. H., 339, 340, 341, 354
Abend, W., 236, 242
Abrams, R. A., 183, 184, 222, 229, 232, 233, 237, 250, 390, 391, 407
Accot, J., 230
Acuna, C., 80, 194
Adam, J. J., 230
Adams, J. A., 95, 96, 97, 101, 102, 132
Adams, N., 321
Adelman, P. K., 375
Adolph, K. E., 160, 161
Adolph, R., 378
Aebischer, P., 89
Aflalo, T. N., 74
Agid, Y., 230
Aglioti, S., 221, 222
Akmajian, A., 333, 334
Albus, J. S., 65
Alexander, R. M., 6, 136, 137, 138, 139
Alimi, A. M., 230
Allan, L., 134
Allard, T., 38
Allopenna, P. D., 224
Allport, A., 347
Allum, J. H., 148
Alpern, M., 187, 194, 195, 201
Alston, W., 222
Altenbuller, E., 40
Amato, I., 55
Amazeen, E. L., 17, 380
Amazeen, P. G., 17, 380
Andalman, A. S., 357
Anderson, C. M., 90
Anderson, J. R., 107, 363
Andrew, R. J., 370, 372
André-Thomas, A., 135, 154
Angel, R. W., 222
Angier, N., 220, 399
Annett, J., 214, 230
Annett, M., 214
Ansari, D., 317
Ansfield, M., 129
Anson, J. G., 134, 280

Arbib, M. A., 212
Aronov, D., 357
Aronson, E., 161, 163
Arshavsky, Y. I., 140
Arutyunyan, G. H., 113
Asanuma, H., 71, 74
Asatryan, D. G., 234, 236
Aschersleben, G., 24, 91, 129, 130, 134, 285, 293
Ashe, J., 321
Ashmead, D. H., 170, 215, 216
Aslin, R. N., 205
Athenes, S., 212, 216
Atkeson, C. G., 242, 243, 387
Augustyn, J. S., 230
Autgarden, T., 135, 154
Averbeck, B. B., 258, 321
Averill, J., 363, 371
Avraamides, M. N., 386

B

Baber, C., 250
Bachman, J. C., 396
Baddeley, A. D., 116
Bahill, A. T., 183, 188, 380
Bai, D. L., 128
Bakdash, J. Z., 31
Bakker, F. C., 380
Balash, J., 167, 388
Balasubramaniam, R., 380
Baldissera, F., 57, 58
Ballard, C., 223, 224
Balota, D. A., 390, 391
Bampton, S., 140
Bandura, A., 175
Banks, M., 363
Banks, M. S., 205
Barabási, A.-L., 423
Baraduc, P., 423
Barber, P. J., 25
Bardy, B. G., 389
Bargh, J. A., 423
Barker, A. T., 91
Barlow, H., 187

Barnes, H. J., 19, 20, 209
Bartlett, C. J., 397
Bartlett, F. C., 103
Bashore, T. R., 391
Basmajian, J. V., 49
Bastian, A. J., 170
Baylis, G. C., 249
Beamish, D., 230
Beatty, J., 177
Becker, M., 181, 182, 209
Becker, W., 189, 190
Beek, P., 238
Beek, P. J., 134, 295, 297, 380
Beek, W. J., 114, 380
Beetty, J., 177, 178
Beilock, S. L., 128, 227, 321
Bekkering, H., 131, 285
Belen'kii, V., 151
Bellugi, U., 211
Ben-Sira, D., 102
Bengtsson, S. L., 317
Bennett, S., 275
Benson, J. B., 463
Berardelli, A., 91
Berger, S. M., 175
Berkenblit, M. B., 60, 235
Berko, J., 96
Berkowitz, A. L., 317
Berman, A. J., 26, 146
Bernal, G., 175
Berndt, H., 167, 388
Bernstein, N., 15, 18, 113, 243, 381
Bertelson, P., 280
Bertenthal, B. I., 128
Berthier, N. E., 237
Berthoz, A., 205, 214
Bertram, C. P., 150, 385, 386, 387
Bhalla, M., 29
Bhatti, S. A., 230
Bierbaumer, N., 91
Biguer, B., 222
Binder, M. D., 53
Bird, G., 321
Birnholz, J., 205
Biryukova, E. V., 380
Bizzi, E., 18, 89, 198, 199, 200, 233, 234, 236, 237, 242
Bjork, R. A., 108, 115
Blake, R., 140
Blakemore, S. J., 27, 77
Blakeslee, S., 40, 41, 416, 417
Blandin, Y., 247
Bliss, J. C., 115

Bloedel, J., 65
Bloedel, J. R., 62
Boisson, D., 194
Boly, M., 79, 80
Bonnet, C. T., 389
Bonnet, M., 61, 75
Bootsma, R. J., 238, 250, 381, 382
Boschker, M. S., 380
Botvinick, M., 76, 91
Bower, B., 332, 368
Bower, G. H., 100, 165, 166
Bower, T. G. R., 215, 217
Bowman, R. W., 108, 109
Bradshaw, G., 157
Braine, M. D. S., 346
Bramble, D. M., 156
Brass, M., 91, 285
Braun, A. R., 317
Brebner, J., 283, 286, 294
Brechet, Y., 423
Breitmeyer, B., 189
Brenner, E., 212, 222, 240, 408
Bridgeman, B., 192, 204, 209
Bril, B., 380
Brindley, G. S., 203
Brinkman, C., 77
Brodsky, L., 378, 423
Brody, J. E., 66
Brooks, V. B., 48, 50, 68, 89
Brouchon, M., 121
Broughton, J. M., 215
Brown, E. L., 198
Brown, H. O., 337
Brown, L. E., 83
Brown, S., 107
Bruce, V., 364
Bruderlin, A., 393, 394
Brunia, C. H. M., 61
Bryan, W. L., 106, 107, 109
Buchanan, J. J., 114, 238
Buchthal, F., 49
Bullemer, P., 293
Bullock, D., 258, 321, 423
Buneo, C. A., 209
Bunz, H., 245, 246, 400, 401, 402
Buonomano, D. V., 36
Burdet, E., 90, 237, 423
Burgess, P. R., 54
Burkamp, C., 423
Burns, B., 297
Bushnell, E. W., 216
Butsch, R. L. C., 305
Buxbaum, L. J., 91

C

Cabel, D. W., 90
Cairney, P., 283, 286, 294
Caldwell, G. C., 47
Calvo-Merino, B., 32, 33
Cameron, L. L., 395
Campbell, F. W., 191
Campbell, J. A., 283
Cannon, W. B., 371
Caramazza, A., 265
Caramia, M. D., 91
Carello, C., 250, 380, 390, 391, 404
Carew, T. J., 146
Carlson, R. A., 108, 115, 386, 408, 423
Carlton, L. G., 228, 230, 232
Carnahan, H., 150
Carpenter, D., 50
Carpenter, R. H. S., 184, 185, 188, 194, 195
Carpenter, W. B., 129
Carr, T. H., 128, 227
Carrier, D. R., 156
Carroll, D. W., 356
Carson, L. M., 105
Carter, O., 177
Carter, S., 52
Caruso, G., 91
Cary, M., 386
Casaer, P., 17, 215
Chaffin, D. B., 230, 231
Chaffin, R., 321
Challis, J. H., 247
Chan, V., 90
Chase, R. A., 338
Chasteen, A. L., 250
Chau, T., 230
Chen, M., 423
Chen, T., 358, 362
Cheney, P. D., 75
Chevreul, M. E., 129
Chew, C.-M., 423
Chin, G., 357
Chistovich, L., 325, 338
Choi, J. T., 170
Chomsky, N., 326, 332, 334, 346, 356, 414
Christina, R. W., 134
Chua, R., 25, 230, 250
Church, R. M., 134
Churchland, P. S., 65
Ciuffreda, K. J., 184, 205
Clark, F. J., 54
Clark, M., 100
Clarkson, J. K., 326
Claxton, L. J., 216

Clayton, T. M., 163, 381
Clements, G. N., 334
Clifton, R. K., 216
Cobley, S., 34
Cock, J., 167, 388
Cockburn, J., 167, 388
Cockell, D. L., 150
Cohen, A. H., 143
Cohen, D., 363, 375, 376
Cohen, D. J., 275, 414
Cohen, I. S., 203, 204
Cohen, J., 76
Cohen, L., 230, 400
Cohen, R., 412
Cohen, R. G., 22, 24, 91, 95, 123, 128, 186, 209, 212, 270, 345, 399
Colby, C. L., 82, 83
Cole, J., 134
Cole, K. J., 339, 340, 341
Coleman, M. R., 79, 80
Coles, M. G. H., 391
Collard, R., 291, 293, 315
Collard, R. R., 216
Collewijn, H., 176, 195, 205, 209, 223
Collier, G. L., 296
Collins, R., 423
Collins, S., 18, 19
Conolly, K. J., 423
Conover, D. W., 194
Conrad, R., 116
Conway, E., 23, 308, 309
Cooke, D. F., 76
Cooke, J. D., 236
Coombes, S. A., 394
Cooper, F. S., 327, 336
Cooper, L., 90
Cooper, W. E., 304, 305, 306
Coover, J. E., 308
Cope, H., 414
Coquery, J. M., 27
Corbetta, D., 213
Corcos, D. M., 299
Coren, S., 205
Costello, J. M., 326
Cousins, N., 374
Cowan, N., 346
Cowan, W. B., 189
Cowey, A., 91
Cracco, R. Q., 91
Craft, J. L., 283
Craighero, L., 32, 128
Crane, P. K., 115
Craske, B., 244

Craske, J. D., 244
Cromer, R. F., 255
Crompton, R. H., 385
Crossman, E. R. F. W., 107, 230, 234
Crowder, R. G., 115, 293
Cruse, H., 153, 423
Crutcher, M. D., 66, 67
Csikszentmihalyi, M., 317
Cuccaro, M. L., 414
Cutting, J. E., 140, 163
Cynder, M. S., 37
Côté, L., 66, 67

D

Dalery, J., 85
Daniloff, R., 325
Daniloff, R. G., 344
Dannemiller, J. L., 205
Daprati, E., 85
Darainy, M., 90
Daroff, R. B., 198
Darwin, C. J., 115, 293
Darwin, C. R., 372, 392
David, P., 305
Davids, K., 381
Davidson, A. G., 90
Davis, M. H., 79, 80
Dawson, A. M., 247, 412
Deakin, J. M., 34
Dean, J., 153, 423
Debu, B., 159
Decety, J., 61, 170, 230
DeClerk, J., 327, 339
DeClerk, J. L., 337
Deecke, L., 71
Deffenbacher, K., 198
deGroot, A. D., 100
DeGuzman, G. C., 114
Dehaene, S., 285
Deininger, R. L., 283
Delcomyn, F., 143
Dell, B. L., 26
Dell, G. S., 21, 327, 349, 352
Dell'Osso, L. F., 198
Demaire, C., 27
Demers, R. A., 333, 334
Demonet, J.-F., 83
Demyer, W., 366
Denier van der Gon, J. J., 268
DeRenzi, E., 81
Derr, M. A., 291, 292, 293, 315
Desimone, R., 191
Desmedt, J. E., 89
Desmurget, M., 423

DeSouza, J. F., 221, 222
Deutsch, J. A., 326
Dickinson, M. H., 153
Diedrichsen, J., 247, 298, 299
Diener, H. C., 64
Dienes, Z., 380
Diestel, J. D., 140
Ding, M., 114
Ditchburn, R. W., 184, 187, 188
Divac, I., 67
Dixon, P., 249
Dizio, P., 214
Dodge, R., 27
Doidge, N., 41
Donchin, E., 391
Donelan, J. M., 419
Drachman, D. B., 46
Drews, F. A., 127
Duarte, M., 150, 380
Dubois, B., 230
Duff, S., 273
Duffy, J. R., 362
Dugas, C., 212, 216, 250
Duhamel, J.-R., 82, 83, 230
Duley, A. R., 394
Dunkeld, J., 217

E

Easton, D. E., 129
Easton, T. A., 155
Eberhard, K., 224
Ebner, T., 65
Eccles, J., 62, 63
Echallier, J. F., 222
Edelman, S., 258, 268
Eder, J. R., 249
Ehrsson, H. H., 91
Einhauser, W., 177
Ekman, P., 128, 364, 365, 368, 370, 371
Elbert, T., 38
Elble, R. J., 91
Eldridge, M. A., 269
Eliassen, J., 246
Elliott, D., 25, 230, 249, 250
Elliott, J. M., 423
Ellis, A., 263
Ellis, R., 90
Emmorey, K., 211
Engbert, R., 128, 186
Engelbrecht, S. E., 407, 408, 410
Enksen, C. W., 391
Enocka, R. M., 50
Epelboim, J., 209, 223
Epstein, W., 31

Erickson, R. P., 73
Ericsson, K. A., 34, 35, 395
Erkelens, C. J., 209, 223
Erlhagen, W., 423
Essock, E. A., 216
Estes, W. K., 98, 126, 313
Evanoff, J. N., 194
Evarts, E., 75
Evarts, E. V., 71
Everling, S., 222
Eykman-Berland, A., 220, 417

F

Fackelmann, K. A., 66
Fagan, J. W., 157
Fajen, B. R., 161
Fantz, R., 363
Farley, C. T., 153
Farné, A., 194
Farrell, J. M., 321
Fearnley, S., 288
Fee, M. S., 357
Feinstein, M. H., 283, 348
Feldman, A., 237
Feldman, A. G., 60, 234, 235, 236
Feldman, R. S., 374
Feldstein, S., 374
Feltz, D., 109
Fendrick, P., 305, 308
Fenn, W. O., 244
Ferrand, T., 250
Ferraro, M., 90, 220, 417
Fetter, M., 180, 181
Fetz, E. E., 75, 416, 417
Field, J., 215
Field, T., 363, 375, 376
Finkbeiner, M., 249
Finley, F. R., 140
Fischer, B., 189
Fischer, M. H., 230
Fischman, J., 253
Fischman, M. G., 134, 212
Fisher, D. M., 157
Fitch, H. L., 125
Fitts, P. M., 110, 111, 127, 133, 229, 231, 248, 283
Flach, J. M., 40, 214
Flanagan, J. R., 28, 40, 223, 249
Flanagan, R., 212
Flanders, M., 209
Flash, T., 19, 209, 237, 253, 258, 262, 268, 406
Fleckenstein, R., 249
Fleishman, E. A., 118, 119, 396, 397
Fletcher, S., 340
Fodor, J. A., 8

Foorman, B. R., 116
Ford, K., 222
Ford, S., 297
Fordham, C., 167, 388
Forssberg, H., 68, 147, 212
Foulke, J. A., 230, 231
Fowler, C. A., 114, 340, 358, 362
Fowler, H., 97
Fox, R., 140
Franck, N., 85
Frank, J. S., 231
Franklin, D. W., 90, 237, 423
Franz, E., 246
Franz, E. A., 17, 246, 249
Franz, V., 222
Franz, V. H., 212
Fraser, C., 240
Freed, C. R., 148
Freedman, D. G., 370
Freeman, R. N., 81
Frey, W. H., 374
Fridlund, A. J., 374
Friesen, W. V., 364, 365, 368, 371
Frith, C. D., 27, 77
Fromkin, V. A., 21, 327
Fuchs, A., 188, 194
Fuchs, A. F., 97, 189
Fucson, O. I., 60, 235
Fujii, N., 91
Full, R. J., 153
Fuller, D. C., 305

G

Gabrieli, J. D., 67
Galanter, E., 40
Galantucci, B., 358, 362
Galgano, M., 220, 417
Galin, D., 272
Gallistel, C. R., 28, 40, 283, 423
Galton, F., 34
Gardner, H., 353
Garing, A. E., 170
Garland, H., 222
Garrett, M. F., 21, 327, 352
Gauthier, G. M., 222, 223
Gawande, A., 40
Gazzaniga, M., 246
Gazzaniga, M. S., 89
Gelfan, S., 52
Gemba, H., 65
Gentile, A. M., 242
Gentner, D. R., 23, 267, 270, 303, 305, 308, 309, 311, 313, 314
Georgi, B., 357

Georgieff, N., 85
Georgopoulos, A. P., 71, 72, 80, 149, 150, 194, 385
Gergely, G., 131
Geschwin, N., 84
Geyer, S., 91
Ghez, C., 72, 85, 214, 225, 226, 409
Ghilardi, M.-F., 214
Ghosh, S. S., 362
Gibbon, J., 134
Gibson, J. J., 30, 158, 161, 163, 205, 219
Gielen, C. C. A. M., 209
Giladi, N., 167, 388
Gilbert, A. N., 374
Gilbert, D., 40
Gilbert, P. F. C., 65
Gilden, D. L., 423
Gill, E. B., 382
Gillespie, R. B., 409
Gilman, S., 62
Gilmore, R. O., 108, 115, 386, 408, 423
Giszter, S., 89, 237
Glaser, D. E., 32, 33
Glass, A. L., 134
Gleason, C. A., 86, 129
Gleick, J., 423
Glenberg, A. M., 358, 423
Glencross, D. J., 103, 396
Glover, S., 249
Glover, S. R., 222
Golby, C. W., 230
Goldberg, M. E., 82, 83, 193, 203, 204
Goldfield, E. C., 159, 160
Goldin-Meadow, S., 211
Goldman-Eisler, F., 325
Goltz, H. C., 209
Gomi, H., 237
Gonzalez, D., 383
Goodale, M. A., 29, 83, 221, 222
Goodenough, F. L., 370
Goodeve, P. J., 230, 234
Goodman, D., 244
Goodman, L. S., 337
Goodnow, J., 254
Goodnow, J. J., 254, 255
Goodwin, G. M., 52
Gopher, D., 288, 289
Gordon, A. M., 104, 212, 283, 348
Gordon, F. R., 215
Gordon, J., 72, 225, 226
Gordon, P. C., 283, 347
Gormley, J., 113
Goslow, G. E., 140
Gossweiler, R., 29
Gouras, P., 177, 180, 182, 188, 195, 201

Gracco, V. L., 339, 340, 341, 354
Grafton, S. T., 67
Graham, J., 249
Graham, K. M., 90
Gratton, G., 391
Gray, R., 227, 380
Graybiel, A. M., 91
Graziano, M., 74
Graziano, M. S., 73, 76, 383
Graziano, M. S. A., 76
Green, D. W., 269, 270
Greenberg, N., 250, 380, 423
Greenberg, R., 363, 375, 376
Greenwald, A. G., 129, 130, 283
Greer, K. L., 269, 270
Gregor, R. J., 140
Gregory, R. L., 199, 202
Grezes, J., 32, 33
Gribble, P. L., 90, 222
Grigg, P., 54
Grillner, S., 135, 143, 146, 147, 148, 149, 150, 385
Grondin, S., 321
Grosjean, M., 130, 230
Gross, C. G., 76, 383
Grossberg, S., 258, 423
Grudin, J., 23, 308, 309, 311
Grudin, J. G., 307
Guenther, F. H., 327, 339, 362
Guiard, Y., 238, 239
Guiard, Y., 250
Guic-Robles, E., 38
Guigon, E., 423
Gunilla, R., 67
Guo, H. R., 395
Gur, R. C., 364, 368
Gurfinkel, V. S., 113, 151

H

Haddad, G. M., 184, 203
Haesler, S., 357
Hager, J. C., 368
Haggard, P., 32, 33, 84, 91, 134, 167, 212, 388
Haith, M. M., 463
Haken, H., 245, 246, 400, 401, 402
Haken, H., 403
Hale, B. D., 110
Halle, M., 334, 346
Halle, M. G., 334, 346
Hallet, P. E., 190
Hallett, M., 63, 64
Halperin, W. E., 395
Halverson, A. H., 150
Hambuch, R., 297
Hammond, P. H., 75

Hampson, M., 327, 339
Handelman, G. H., 177
Hansen, R. M., 192
Hansen, S., 250
Hanson, R., 338
Hardyck, C., 12
Harnish, R. W., 333, 334
Harris, C., 293
Harris, C. M., 407
Harris, C. S., 219
Harter, N., 106, 107, 109
Hartmann, E. E., 205
Harvey, N., 328, 329, 354
Hasan, Z., 59, 60, 61
Hasegawa, A., 340
Hausdorff, J. M., 167, 171, 388, 405
Hawkins, B., 228, 231
Hay, L., 217
Hayhoe, M., 223, 224
Hazelett, W. M., 122, 123, 270, 347
Hazeltine, E., 67, 247
Hazeltine, R. E., 300
He, J., 417
Heathcote, A., 107
Heijink, H., 380
Heilman, K. M., 82
Hel-Or, H., 378, 423
Held, R., 200, 215, 218, 222
Helsen, W. F., 25, 230, 250
Henig, R. M., 364
Henis, E. A., 237
Henneman, E., 50, 53
Henry, F. M., 125, 126, 134, 189
Herman, R., 140, 222
Herrmann, U., 209
Herron, J., 272
Hess, E., 178
Heuer, H., 17
Hewitt, D. V., 115
Heyes, C. M., 321
Heyman, K., 170
Hick, W. E., 281
Hidler, J. M., 90
Hill, M. D., 299
Hinde, R. A., 354, 355
Hindorff, V., 122, 123, 270, 347
Hirose, H., 330
Hirst, W., 111
Ho, L., 102
Hockett, C. F., 337
Hoff, E., 362
Hoffer, J. A., 419
Hoffman, C., 374
Hoffman, D. S., 71

Hoffman, J. H., 205
Hofsten, C., 215
Hofsten, C.von, 216
Hogan, N., 19, 90, 238, 253, 262, 406
Holden, J. G., 423
Holder, R. L., 385
Holding, D. H., 101
Hollerbach, J. M., 243, 262, 268
Holmes, G., 63
Holmes, N. P., 91
Holst, E.von, 17, 27, 28, 202, 244
Holt, D. G., 121, 236
Holt, K. G., 121, 236
Holt, L., 321
Holub, S., 321
Hommel, B., 129, 130, 285, 293
Homskaya, E. D., 368
Honig, K., 97
Honoré, J., 27
Hooker, D., 214
Hopkins, D. A., 240
Hoss, M., 128
Houde, J. F., 362
Houk, J., 53
Hove, P., 389
Howard, L., 249
Hu, S. J., 417
Hudson, P. T., 214
Hughes, A. E., 253
Hughes, C. M., 249
Hughes, O., 340
Hulse, 97
Hulse, S. H., 97
Hultborn, H., 57, 58
Humphrey, D. R., 148
Humphreys, G. W., 364
Huttenlocher, J., 171
Huxley, A. F., 47
Hyde, J. E., 188
Hyman, R., 281

I

Iansek, R., 68
Iberall, T., 212
II, DeSota-Johnson, D., 374
Illert, M., 57, 58
Imamizu, H., 65
Imreh, G., 321
Ingvar, D. H., 374
Inhoff, A. W., 104, 189, 283
Irwin, D. E., 233, 279
Ishikura, T., 383
Ito, M., 62, 65
Ivry, R., 246, 299, 396

Ivry, R. B., 64, 67, 134, 247, 298, 299, 300
Ivry, R. I., 184, 299, 396
Izard, C. E., 371

J

Jackson, S., 249
Jacobson, E., 110
Jagacinski, R. J., 40, 214, 250, 297, 299, 380, 423
James, W., 25, 61, 94, 129
Janelle, C. M., 394
Janke, I., 40
Jankowska, E., 59
Jansen, C., 240, 407, 411
Jax, S., 249, 412
Jax, S. A., 95, 122, 123, 230, 249, 270, 345, 407
Jeannerod, M., 61, 89, 170, 212, 216, 222, 230, 240, 241
Jeka, J. J., 170
Jenkins, W. M., 38
Jessell, T. M., 89
Johansson, R. S., 55, 212, 223
Johnels, B., 68
Johnson, A., 170
Johnson, D., 327, 339
Johnson, M. H., 423
Johnson, N. F., 349
Johnson, P., 105, 111
Johnson, R., 102
Johnson-Frey, S. H., 217
Johnston, H. M., 321
Johnstone, J., 272
Jones, L. A., 250
Jones, M. R., 100, 291, 297, 299, 321
Jordan, M. I., 22, 250, 327, 343, 345, 362, 381, 406
Jordan, S., 194
Jorgensen, M. J., 122, 209
Joseph, R., 122
Juang, B. H., 362
Jungers, M. K., 321
Jurgens, R., 189, 190
Juricevic, I., 275

K

Kaas, J. H., 36
Kagan, J., 157
Kahneman, D., 177, 178, 419
Kaiser, J., 91
Kakei, S., 71
Kalaska, J. F., 72
Kalat, J. W., 146, 148
Kamara, M., 378, 423
Kaminski, T., 242
Kamm, K., 213
Kamon, E., 113

Kandel, E. R., 89, 201
Kanwisher, N., 378
Karis, D., 288, 289
Kaschak, M. P., 358, 423
Kato, A. C., 89
Katsumata, H., 380
Katzir, G., 378, 423
Kaufman, L., 174, 218
Kawato, M., 90, 237, 405
Kay, B. A., 159, 160
Kay, H., 230
Keele, S. W., 64, 124, 125, 146, 184, 228, 229, 230, 256, 279, 281, 291, 295, 299, 301, 396
Keen, R., 216
Keetch, K. M., 35, 102
Kegel, S., 383
Keller, E., 354
Keller, P., 91, 134
Keller, P. E., 91, 134, 317
Kelso, J. A. S., 114, 121, 122, 124, 136, 244, 245, 246, 262, 340, 391, 400, 401, 402
Kenneally, C., 423
Kennedy, J. M., 275
Kennerley, S., 247
Kennett, S., 84
Kenny, S., 291, 292, 293, 315
Keohl, M. A., 153
Keren, D., 378, 423
Kerr, B. A., 230
Kerr, R., 230
Kerzel, D., 246, 247
Kettner, R. E., 71
Khan, M. A., 250
Khurana, B., 275
Kim, H. H., 409
Kindermann, T., 153, 423
Kiraly, I., 131
Kirch, M., 192
Kisselburgh, L., 228
Klapp, S. T., 125, 126, 297, 299
Klatt, D. H., 339, 340
Klatzky, R., 91
Klatzky, R. L., 212
Klein, R., 219
Kleiner, K. A., 363
Kleinholdermann, U., 212
Klemmer, E. T., 279
Kliegl, R., 128, 186
Klima, E. S., 211
Kluger, J., 67
Knoblich, G., 130, 230, 246, 247, 321, 391, 392
Knoll, R. L., 126, 189, 309, 310, 311, 349
Koch, C., 177
Koch, I., 91, 134, 407

Koenig, W., 288, 289
Kolers, P. A., 107
Koller, W. C., 91
Konner, M., 372
Koretz, J. F., 177
Kornblum, S., 183, 184, 222, 229, 232, 233, 237, 287, 407
Kornhuber, H. H., 71
Kornmuller, A. E., 203
Koshland, G. F., 61
Kosslyn, S. M., 134
Koster, W. G., 267, 268, 269
Kotchoubey, B., 91
Kots, Y. M., 15, 16, 140, 243
Kowler, E., 189, 195, 196, 205, 209, 223
Kozhevnikov, V. A., 325, 338
Krakauer, J. W., 214
Kram, R., 153
Krampe, R. T., 34, 35, 395
Krebs, H. I., 90, 220, 417
Krebs, M. J., 279
Krishnan, R. R., 414
Kristofferson, A. B., 294, 295, 296, 319
Kroin, J. S., 53
Kroliczak, G., 83
Kroll, J. F., 116, 293
Krones, R., 338
Kubler, A., 91
Kunde, W., 247
Kuo, A. D., 419
Kuypers, H. G., 240
Kvalseth, T. O., 230

L

Laabs, G. J., 120
Lackner, J. R., 170, 194, 214
Lacquaniti, F., 59, 214, 243, 257, 258, 259, 261, 262, 266, 341
Ladefoged, P., 126, 327, 329, 339
Lakoff, G., 129
Lamarche, F., 268
Landers, D. M., 109
Landy, M. S., 419
Lang, P. J., 371
Langolf, G. D., 230, 231
LaRitz, T., 380
Larochelle, S., 308, 311
Larsen, B., 78, 110
Lashley, K. S., 21, 26, 94, 95, 96, 164, 278
Lassen, N. A., 78, 110
Latash, M. L., 40, 89, 115, 151, 237, 243, 321
Latour, P. L., 191
Laubrock, J., 186
Laurent, M., 128

Laureys, S., 79, 80
Lawrence, D. G., 240
Leavitt, L. A., 346
Lechtenberg, R., 62
Leckman, J. F., 414
Lecours, A., 159
Lederman, S. J., 212, 250
Lee, B. S., 326
Lee, C. Y., 338
Lee, D. N., 161, 163, 164, 166, 380, 381
Lee, T. D., 25, 35, 101, 102, 105, 247, 383
Legge, D., 25, 267
Lehman, D. M., 212
Lehman, R. S., 187
Lehman, S., 153
Lehmkuhl, G., 81
Leiman, A. L., 27
Leonard, J. A., 107, 282
Lesgold, A., 100
Lessenberry, D. D., 307
Levelt, W., 327, 352
Levenson, R. W., 371
Levine, R., 254, 255
Levy, J., 187, 270, 271, 272
Lewbel, A., 380
Li, L., 194
Li, Q., 419
Liao, M. J., 250, 380, 423
Liaw, G., 90
Liberman, A. M., 327, 336
Libet, B., 86, 129, 134
Licznerski, P., 357
Lidsky, T. I., 69
Lieberman, K., 116
Lieberman, P., 332
Lightstone, A. D., 190
Limb, C. J., 317
Lindau, M., 327, 339
Lindblom, B., 325, 326, 338, 340
Lindstrom, S., 59
Linkenauger, S. A., 31
Lisberger, S. G., 200
Lishman, J. R., 161, 163, 166
Liu, Y., 423
Llinas, R., 62, 65
Lockman, J. J., 215, 216
Loeb, G. E., 49
Loftus, E. R., 118
Loftus, G. R., 118
Logan, G. D., 126, 189, 306
Logemann, J. A., 354
Lomax, A. J., 249
Long, J., 306
Lortie, C., 249

Lotter, W. S., 397
Lotto, R. B., 158
Lough, S., 163, 381
Loukopoulos, L. D., 258, 408, 410
Low, K. A., 321
Luce, R. D., 279
Luis, M., 380
Luria, A. R., 368
Lurito, J. T., 71
Lynch, D., 90, 220, 417
Lynch, J. C., 80, 194
Lynn, D. R., 368
Lynn, J. G., 368
Lyons, D., 212
Làdavas, E., 378
Lévesque, L., 103

M

MacDonald, J., 362
MacKay, D., 347
MacKay, D. G., 108, 109, 110, 134
MacKay, D. M., 191
MacKenzie, C., 249
MacKenzie, C. L., 212, 216, 249, 250
Mackenzie, I. S., 230
MacLeod, C., 287
Macmillan, D. L., 140
MacNeilage, P. F., 96, 327, 329, 330, 337, 338, 339
Magill, R. A., 101
Magnuson, J. S., 224
Maioli, C., 59, 214
Maloney, L. T., 419
Manetto, C., 69
Mannes, C., 258, 423
Mansfield, P. K., 115
Marchak, F., 19, 20
Marchetti, E., 222, 223
Margaria, R., 139
Margolin, D. I., 264, 265, 295
Mark, L. S., 363
Marlsen-Wilson, W., 327
Marr, D., 4, 65
Marsden, C. D., 26, 59, 64, 67, 75
Marshall, G., 267
Marshall, J., 192
Marshburn, E., 297
Marteniuk, R. G., 103, 150, 212, 216, 250, 385, 386, 387
Martin, B., 409
Martin, B. J., 409
Martin, Z. E., 299
Martins, A. J., 205
Maslach, C., 267
Mason, A. H., 250

Massaro, D. W., 358, 362
Massey, J. T., 71, 72
Massion, J., 148
Mather, G., 37, 187
Matin, L., 192, 204
Matsumoto, D., 428
Mattar, A., 222
Matthews, P. B. C., 51, 52, 53, 62
Maulucci, R., 222
Mayer, E. J., 140
Mays, L. E., 190, 191
McAuley, J. D., 321
McBride, E., 110
McCarty, M. E., 215, 216
McClelland, J. L., 312, 344
McCloskey, D. J., 52
McCollum, G., 147, 148
McCormick, D. A., 65, 175
McCoy, A. M., 128
McCrary, J. M., 264, 337
McCutcheon, M., 340
McDaniel, C., 140
McDonald, P. V., 214
McFadyen, B. J., 150
McGraw, M. B., 159
McGurk, H., 362
McIntyre, J., 214
McLaughlin, C., 381
McLeod, P., 380, 381, 382
McLin, D., 123
McMahon, T. A., 18, 46, 47, 51, 58, 59, 140, 152
Mechsner, F., 119, 120, 246, 247
Meck, W. H., 134
Medendorp, W. P., 209
Meeter, M., 189
Meijer, O. G., 124
Melton, A. W., 97
Melvill Jones, G., 205
Merton, P. A., 55, 64, 75, 203
Merzenich, M. M., 36, 37, 38
Meulenbroek, R. G., 209, 212, 240, 256, 275, 380, 407, 411
Meulenbroek, R. G. J., 240, 256, 258, 407, 412
Meulenbroek, R. G. M., 408, 410
Mewhort, D. J. K., 107
Meyer, D. E., 183, 184, 222, 229, 230, 232, 233, 237, 279, 283, 347, 407
Meyers, J., 118
Miall, R. C., 170
Miceli, G., 265
Michaels, C. F., 380
Midgett, K., 29
Miller, G., 357, 366
Miller, G. A., 40, 100, 282, 332
Miller, J., 321

Miller, N., 81, 82
Miller, N. S., 321
Miller, S., 140
Milner, A. D., 29
Milner, B., 116
Milner, T. E., 90, 237, 423
Minas, S. C., 110
Mirskii, M. L., 113
Mishkin, M., 29
Misslisch, H., 180, 181
Mitchel, A. D., 249
Mitra, S., 209
Mittelstaedt, H., 27, 28, 202
Miyauchi, S., 65
Mizuno, N., 65
Moar, I., 165, 166
Mol, R., 230
Moll, K., 325
Moll, K. L., 344
Monno, A., 128
Monsell, S., 126, 189, 309, 310, 311, 349, 407
Moore, G. P., 53
Moore, M. K., 215
Moore, R. K., 175, 176
Moore, S. P., 243
Moore, T., 73
Morasso, P., 236, 242, 253, 385, 423
Morgan, R. L., 105, 106
Moritz, C. T., 416, 417
Morton, H. B., 64, 75
Moscovitch, M., 271, 272, 368
Motley, M. T., 21, 349
Mottet, D., 238, 250
Motti, F., 81
Mountcastle, V. B., 80, 194
Mowatt, M., 159
Mulder, T., 167, 388
Munhall, K. G., 307
Munte, T. F., 40
Murphy, S. T., 375
Murray, R. A. III., 308
Mussa Ivaldi, F., 222, 223
Mussa-Ivaldi, F. A., 18, 89, 90, 237
Musseler, J., 129, 130, 285, 293
Muybridge, E., 136, 415

N

Nadel, L., 170
Naing, V., 419
Naito, E., 91
Nakayama, K., 249
Nashner, L. M., 63, 147, 148
Navon, D., 321
Needham, D. M., 46
Neisser, U., 111, 115

Nelson, R. J., 37
Neves, D. M., 107
Nevo, E., 378, 423
Newcombe, N. S., 171
Newell, A. M., 107
Newell, K. M., 105, 114, 214, 232
Newhall, B., 415
Newman, R. C., 107
Newton, N., 90
Nichelli, P., 81
Niedenthal, P., 371, 378
Niedenthal, P. M., 375
Nienhuis, B., 167, 388
Nimmo-Smith, I., 262, 269, 381
Nissen, M. J., 219, 293
Nooteboom, S. G., 338, 339
Norman, D. A., 22, 98, 165, 278, 302, 305, 312, 313, 314, 320
Norton, B. J., 73
Nottebohm, F., 356
Néda, Z., 423

O

Oberg, E., 67
Obeso, J. A., 59
Ochs, M. T., 38
Ogden, R. T., 296
Ohala, J. J., 325
Ohlsson, S., 107
Oldfield, R. C., 273
Olds, J., 368
Oliveira, F., 247
Olsen, R. A., 308
Olson, B. P., 417
Olton, D. S., 165
Orlosky, G. N., 148, 149
Orlovskii, G. N., 140
Ornstein, R. E., 272
Osman, A. M., 233, 279
Osman, M., 321
Osten, P., 357
Oster, H., 365, 371
Ostry, D. J., 90, 307, 309
Osu, R., 90, 237, 423
Owen, A. M., 79, 80
O'Dell, R., 90
O'Keefe, J., 170
O'Sullivan, M., 128, 365

P

Pacherie, E., 85
Page, M. P. A., 258, 321
Pagulayan, R. J., 389
Paillard, J., 24, 121
Palazzolo, J. J., 90

Palmer, C., 321
Pal'tsev, Y. I., 151
Pantev, C., 38
Papçun, G., 126, 327, 339
Park, J.-H., 238
Park, W., 409
Parker, J. F., 396
Parker, R. F. Jr., 118, 119
Parkinson, J., 275
Pashler, H., 181, 182, 209
Passingham, R. E., 32, 33, 91
Passmore, S., 383
Patashnik, O., 300
Paterson, H. M., 393, 394
Patla, A. E., 170
Pauwels, J., 167, 388
Pavese, A., 91
Pearl, D. K., 86, 129
Pearson, K. R., 140, 141, 142, 144, 145, 149
Peleg, G., 378, 423
Peleg, O., 378, 423
Pellecchia, G. L., 128, 150, 389, 405
Pendleton, L. R., 121
Penfield, W., 69, 70, 73, 118, 354
Peper, C. E., 297
Perfetti, C. A., 116
Pericak-Vance, M. A., 414
Perkell, J. S., 339, 340
Perlmutter, S. I., 416, 417
Peschel, E. R., 330, 331
Peschel, R. E., 330, 331
Pesetsky, D., 116
Peters, M., 299
Peterson, J. R., 229
Petrides, M., 71
Petrinovich, L. F., 12
Pew, R. W., 111
Pfaltz, C. R., 148
Pfordresher, P. Q., 321
Phillips, C. G., 71
Pick, H. L., 170
Pickard, J. D., 79, 80
Picoult, E., 204
Pilloff, D., 129
Pillon, B., 230
Pinker, S., 414
Pisella, L., 194
Pittenger, J. B., 363
Pizlo, Z., 209, 223
Pizzoferrato, F., 378
Plamondon, R., 230, 268
Poeck, K., 81, 368
Poizner, H., 211

Pokorny, R. A., 299
Polanyi, M., 3, 118
Poldrak, R. A., 67
Polit, A., 233, 234, 236
Pollack, G. H., 47
Pollatsek, A., 188
Pollick, F. E., 393, 394
Popescu, F., 90
Porter, R., 68, 71
Porter, S., 378
Posner, M. I., 108, 116, 119, 188, 192, 193, 219, 228, 281
Potter, J. M., 20, 21
Potter, M. C., 116, 293
Povel, D.-J., 291, 293, 315
Powers, W. T., 40
Prabakharan, V., 67
Prablanc, C., 222
Pratt, J., 230, 249, 250
Pribram, K. H., 40
Prinz, W., 24, 91, 128, 129, 130, 134, 246, 247, 285, 293, 347, 391
Pritchard, R. M., 186
Prochazka, A., 61
Proctor, R. W., 289, 321
Proffitt, D. R., 29, 31, 140
Proteau, L., 103, 247
Proust, J., 85
Pulvermüller, F., 362
Purves, D., 158
Putnam, C. A., 244
Putz, B., 65

Q

Quinn, J. T. Jr., 231

R

Rabbitt, P. M. A., 288, 289, 306
Rabiner, L. R., 362
Raibert, M. H., 151, 152, 252
Ramachandran, V. S., 40, 41, 181, 182, 209, 220
Rashbass, C., 189, 201
Rasmssen, T., 69, 70, 73
Ravasz, E., 423
Rayner, K., 116, 188
Redding, G. M., 249
Reddish, P. E., 163, 381
Redish, A. D., 170
Reeve, T. G., 289
Reid, M. L., 270, 271, 272
Reina, G. A., 222
Reinking, R. M., 140
Repp, B., 316, 321
Repp, B. H., 316, 321

Requin, J., 61, 75
Restle, F., 100, 290
Rhodes, B. J., 258, 321
Richards, W., 191
Richardson, A., 109
Rieser, J. J., 170
Riggio, L., 128
Riggs, L. A., 27, 175, 176
Riley, M., 389
Ringel, R. L., 338
Rinkenauer, G., 321
Rinn, W. E., 365, 366, 367, 368
Risberg, J., 374
Rizzolatti, G., 32, 128
Roberts, L., 118, 354
Robinson, D. A., 183, 194
Robinson, D. L., 193
Rochefort, C., 357
Rock, I., 158, 219
Rockstroh, B., 38
Rode, G., 194
Rodionov, I. M., 140
Roeltgin, D., 264, 265, 300
Roffwarg, H. P., 205
Rogers, D. E., 125, 126, 134, 189
Rogers, D. M., 395
Rogers-Ramachandran, D., 220
Roland, P. E., 78, 110
Ron, S., 194
Rootes, T. P., 338
Rosenbaum, D., 91, 134
Rosenbaum, D. A., 19, 20, 22, 24, 47, 72, 91,
    95, 97, 98, 104, 105, 108, 115, 122, 123, 126,
    128, 134, 150, 167, 186, 189, 209, 212, 226,
    230, 240, 247, 249, 256, 258, 270, 275, 283,
    287, 291, 292, 293, 297, 300, 315, 345, 347,
    348, 349, 381, 386, 399, 407, 408, 410, 411,
    412, 423
Rosenbloom, P. S., 107
Rosenthal, R., 374
Rosenzweig, M. R., 27
Rossetti, Y., 194
Rossignol, S., 143, 147
Rossini, P. M., 91
Roth, K., 124
Roth, L. J., 82
Rothstein, A., 110
Rothwell, J. C., 26, 47, 48, 52, 53, 54, 55, 59, 89
Rovee, C. K., 157
Ruina, A., 18, 19
Rumelhart, D. E., 22, 98, 278, 302, 312, 313, 314, 320, 344
Rushworth, G., 62
Russell, D. M., 296

Ryan, E. D., 118
Rymer, W. Z., 90
Rönnqvist, L., 216

S

Sabban, Y., 308
Sabes, P. N., 250
Sackeim, H. A., 364, 368
Saggerson, A., 321
Sahrmann, S. A., 73
Sainburg, R., 273
Sainburg, R. L., 272, 273
Sakata, H., 80, 194
Salinas, E., 91
Saltzman, E., 15, 262
Sanders, M. D., 192
Sanford, A. J., 393, 394
Sanguineti, V., 423
Sarno, J. E., 395
Sasaki, K., 65
Sasaki, Y., 65
Saslow, M. G., 189
Saucy, M. C., 368
Saunders, F., 358, 362
Sawashima, M., 330
Schaal, S., 380
Schack, T., 119, 120
Scharff, C., 357
Scheerer, E., 347
Scheid, P., 71
Scheidt, R. A., 409
Schick, A. M., 27
Schieber, M. H., 90
Schlosberg, H., 279
Schmahmann, J. D., 62, 90
Schmalbruch, M., 49
Schmidt, R. A., 35, 40, 101, 102, 104, 105, 108, 115, 118,
    231, 256, 397
Schmidt, R. C., 390, 391, 404
Schmitz, J., 153, 423
Schmitz, M., 153, 423
Scholz, J. P., 114, 115
Schomaker, L. R., 256, 275
Schumm, M., 153, 423
Schutter, D. J., 90
Schwartz, A., 65
Schwartz, A. B., 71, 90, 222
Schwartz, G. E., 365
Schwartz, J. H., 89
Schwartz, M. F., 91
Schöner, G., 114, 115, 238, 391, 423
Scott, C. M., 338
Scott, S. H., 90
Scoville, W. B., 116

Seashore, C. E., 316
Sebanz, N., 391, 392
Sedivy, J., 224
Seger, C., 67
Selkirk, E. O., 348
Serino, A., 378
Severin, F. V., 148, 149
Shadmehr, R., 214, 250
Shaffer, L. H., 111, 297, 305, 306, 308, 315
Shahani, B. T., 63, 64
Shankweiler, D. P., 327, 336
Shannon, C. E., 282
Shapiro, D. C., 140
Sharp, R. H., 382
Shattuck-Hufnagle, S., 327, 352
Shatz, M., 362
Shaw, R. E., 363
Shea, C. H., 238
Shea, J. B., 105, 106
Shea, J. G., 102
Sheliga, B. M., 128
Shepard, R. N., 90
Shephard, M., 283, 286, 294
Sherrington, C. S., 61, 85, 142
Shiffrar, M., 130, 140, 230
Shik, M. L., 140
Shin, J. C., 321, 423
Shirley, M. M., 154
Shockley, K., 128, 405
Shoppmann, A., 37
Shor, R. E., 129
Shumway-Cook, A., 148, 171
Siegman, A. W., 374
Silveri, C., 265
Silverstein, R., 126
Simon, H. A., 100
Simon, J. R., 283, 286
Singh, D., 409
Siqueland, E. R., 216
Sirigu, A., 91, 230
Skavenski, A. A., 184, 192, 203, 204
Skinhoj, E., 78, 110
Skoglund, S., 54
Slater-Hammel, A. T., 126
Sloboda, J. A., 314
Slotta, J., 19, 20
Smeets, J. B., 212, 222, 240, 408
Smeets, J. B. J., 408
Smith, E. E., 134
Smith, J. E. K., 229, 230, 232, 233, 237, 407
Smith, K. U., 264, 337
Smith, L. B., 123
Smith, L. C., 271, 272
Smith, S. M., 337

Smith, T. S., 338
Smith, W. M., 264, 337
Smyth, M. M., 120, 121, 231
Smyth, T. R., 396
Soechting, J. F., 209, 243, 341
Sohn, M. A., 423
Sokolov, A. N., 336
Somjen, G., 50
Sommer, M. A., 204
Song, J. H., 249
Southard, D. L., 244
Sparks, D. L., 190, 191
Spelke, E., 111
Spence, C., 91
Spencer, J. P., 123, 213
Spencer, R. M. C., 298, 299
Sperling, A., 192
Sperling, G. A., 115, 293
Sperry, R. W., 28, 202
Spivey, M., 249, 359
Spivey-Knowlton, M., 224
Squire, L. R., 116, 117
Stark, L., 40, 183, 186, 188
Steg, G., 68
Stein, R. B., 407
Steinbach, M. J., 222
Steinberg, H., 267
Steinkühler, U., 423
Steinman, R., 176
Steinman, R. M., 184, 191, 195, 196, 203, 204, 205, 209, 223
Stelmach, G. E., 121, 265, 266
Stemwedel, M. E., 321
Stephens, B. R., 205
Stephenson, J. M., 382
Sternad, D., 238, 296, 380
Sternberg, S., 126, 189, 309, 310, 311, 349
Stetson, R. H., 329
Stevens, J. A., 170
Stevens, J. K., 204
Stewart, E., 209
Stillings, N. A., 283, 348
Stodden, D. F., 212
Stoffregen, T. A., 389
Storm, C., 363, 371
Storm, T., 363, 371
Stout, J., 177
Strasberg, S., 386
Strayer, D. L., 127
Strelow, E. R., 170
Strick, P. L., 71
Stroop, J. R., 286
Stryker, M. P., 37
Stuart, D. G., 50, 53, 140

Studdert-Kennedy, M. G., 327, 336
Summerfield, A., 267
Summers, J., 297
Summers, J. J., 301
Summers, R. J., 291, 301
Sundberg, J., 330, 338, 340, 354
Sutherland, I. E., 151, 152
Suzuki, R., 405
Swinnen, S., 17, 246
Swinnen, S. P., 17, 383
Syrovegnin, A. V., 15, 16, 243

T

Takino, R., 65
Tamada, T., 65
Tanaka, S., 395
Tanenhaus, M. K., 224
Tanji, J., 75
Tannen, B., 184
Tastevin, J., 26, 146, 170, 219
Taub, E., 38
Taylor, C. S. R., 73
Taylor, L. J., 359
Taylor-Clarke, M., 84
Tedrake, R., 18, 19
Tee, K. P., 423
Teichner, W. H., 279
Teitelman, R., 140
Temprado, J. J., 128
Ten Brinke, L., 378
Teramitsu, I., 415
Terzuolo, C., 257, 258, 259, 261, 262, 266, 267, 268, 303
Terzuolo, C. A., 301, 303, 308
Tesch-Romer, C., 34, 35, 395
Teulings, H.-L., 262, 265, 266, 269
Thach, W. T., 65
Theeuwes, J., 189
Their, P., 91
Thelen, E., 123, 156, 157, 158, 160, 213, 380
Thomassen, A. J., 256, 262, 265, 269, 275
Thomassen, A. J. W. M., 256, 258
Thompson, R. F., 65, 175
Thomson, J., 166
Thomson, J. A., 163, 164, 381
Thorndike, E. L., 101, 129
Thornton, I. M., 130
Thorpe, S. K., 385
Thuring, J. Ph., 268
Tipper, S., 249
Tipper, S. P., 249
Titzer, R., 123
Todd, J. T., 363, 381
Todorov, E., 406

Tolman, C. E., 164, 294, 385
Toman, J. E. P., 337
Tourville, J. A., 362
Touwen, B. C., 214
Towhidkhah, F., 90
Townsend, J. T., 115
Tracy, J. L., 428
Tran-Viet, K. N., 414
Treiman, R., 346
Tremblay, L., 380
Tresilian, J. R., 249
Trivedi, B. P., 357, 415
Trommershäuser, J., 419
Tsin, Y., 423
Tuller, B., 125, 340
Tuma, G., 147
Turner, A., 214, 240
Turvey, M. T., 17, 114, 115, 125, 128, 209, 243, 250, 293, 339, 358, 362, 380, 389, 390, 391, 404, 405, 423
Tversky, A., 419
Tweed, D., 180, 181
Twitchell, T. E., 214
Tyldesley, D. A., 381
Tyler, J. G., 299
Tyler, L. K., 327

U

Ullen, F., 317
Ulrich, B. D., 380
Ulrich, R., 321
Ungerleider, L. G., 29
Uswatt, G., 170

V

Vaillancourt, D. E., 114
Vallbo, A. B., 56, 57
Van der Meeche, F. G., 140
van der Steen, J., 176
van der Stigchel, S., 189
van der Wel, R., 95, 123, 270, 345, 249
van der Wel, R. P., 122, 150, 249
van Emerick, R. E. A., 114
van Emmerik, R. E., 214
van Galen, G. P., 265, 269
van Heugten, C., 47
van Honk, J., 90
van Mourik, A., 238
Van Orden, G. C., 423
Van Sommers, P., 257
van Wieringen, P. C., 381, 382
van Wieringen, P. C. W., 297
Van Zandt, T., 321
Vatikiotis-Bateson, E., 340

Vaughan, J., 19, 20, 188, 209, 212, 230, 240, 258, 407, 408, 410, 411, 412
Vercher, J.-L., 222, 223
Vereijken, B., 114, 380
Verjee, F., 249
Verwey, W. B., 258, 321
Veston, J., 357
Vickers, J. N., 170, 209
Vicsek, T., 423
Vilis, T., 209
Vince, M. A., 226
Viviani, P., 257, 258, 259, 261, 262, 266, 267, 268, 301, 303, 308
Vogel, S., 175
Vogt, S., 240
Volkmann, F. C., 27, 175, 176
Volpe, B. T., 90, 220, 417
von Holst, E., 27, 28, 202
Vorberg, D., 297
Vredenbregt, J., 209, 267, 268, 269
Vyas, S. M., 288, 289

W

Wade, D., 167, 388
Wagner, H., 381
Wagner, S. M., 211
Wallace, B., 249
Wallace, R. J., 283, 286, 294
Walsh, M. W., 249
Walsh, V., 91
Walter, C., 17, 246
Wang, J., 273
Wang, X., 203, 204
Wann, J., 262
Ward, J. A., 157
Wareham, G., 362
Warren, R. M., 327
Warren, R. P., 327
Warren, W. H., 159, 160, 161
Warren, W. H. Jr., 170, 423
Warrington, E. K., 192
Wascher, E., 91, 134
Waszak, F., 91, 134
Waynbaum, I., 373
Weaver, W., 282
Webb, W. B., 188
Weber, D. J., 419
Weber, R. J., 122, 123, 270, 347
Wegner, D. M., 86, 129
Weigelt, M., 247
Weimer, W. B., 386
Weinbruch, C., 38
Weinrich, M., 75
Weiskrantz, L., 192
Weiss, D. J., 95, 123, 270, 345

Welford, A. T., 226, 279
Wells, L. A., 321
Welsh, T. N., 249
Wentworth, N., 463
West, L. J., 308
Westheimer, G. H., 189, 194, 195, 223
Westling, G., 55, 212
White, B. L., 215
White, S., 415
Whiting, H. T. A., 114, 115, 380, 381, 382
Wickelgren, W. A., 96
Wickens, D., 283
Wicks, G. G., 102
Wiegand, R. L., 105
Wiesendanger, M., 75, 76, 78
Williams, A. M., 381
Williams, H. G., 396
Williams, J. G., 381
Willingham, D. B., 321
Willingham, D. T., 134, 321
Wilson, M., 358
Wing, A., 262, 266, 295
Wing, A. M., 134, 212, 240, 249, 264, 269, 294, 295, 296, 319
Winold, H., 380
Winstein, C. J., 102
Winzenz, D., 100
Wirta, R., 140
Wise, S., 75
Wise, S. P., 191, 214, 250
Wishart, J. G., 217
Wisse, M., 18, 19
Witt, J. K., 31, 321
Wolf, M., 340
Wolpaw, J. R., 91
Wolpert, D. M., 27, 28, 40, 77, 407
Woods, T., 383
Woodson, R., 363, 375, 376
Woodworth, R. S., 25, 227, 228, 230, 279, 280
Woollacott, M., 147, 148, 171
Woollacott, M. H., 159, 396
Wright, C. E., 126, 189, 229, 230, 232, 233, 237, 309, 310, 311, 349, 407
Wright, D., 362
Wright, E. W., 86, 129
Wu, J., 230
Wulf, G., 2, 128
Wunderlin, A., 403
Wurtz, R. H., 191, 193
Wyman, D., 184

Y

Yakolev, P., 159
Yamada, H., 288
Yamamoto, B. K., 148

Yaminishi, J., 405
Yantis, S., 233, 279
Yarbus, A. L., 187
Yonas, A., 215
Young, D. E., 35, 102
Young, D. S., 163, 381
Young, R. R., 63, 64
Young, S., 230
Yu, H., 296

Z

Zago, M., 214
Zahariev, M., 249
Zajonc, R. B., 373, 374, 375
Zanone, P. G., 128
Zatsiorsky, V. M., 150, 321

Zbrodoff, J., 189
Zelaznik, H. N., 17, 228, 231, 246, 298, 299
Zelazo, P. R., 156, 157, 158
Zernicke, R. F., 140
Zhai, S., 230
Zhang, M., 203, 204
Zheng, B., 249
Zillner, E., 91, 275
Zimbardo, P. G., 267
Zingale, C. M., 189
Zook, J. M., 37
Zuber, B. L., 186
Zuchner, S., 414
Zurif, E., 353
Zwaan, R. A., 359

Subject Index

A

Abducens nerve, extra-ocular muscles, 182
Absolute position, speech articulators, 339–340
Absolute timing, writing, 267–268
Accommodation, definition and characteristics, 177
Acoustic targets, speech control, 339–341
Actin, muscle performance, 47
Action compatibility effect, speech motor
    resonance, 358
Action slips
   categorization, 312
   definition, 22
Active movement, visual guidance studies, 219
Active tension, muscle performance, 47
Adults
   Babinski reflex, 156
   behavioral exploration, 159
   bicycle riding, 3
   bird song, 355, 357
   developmental changes, 158
   discrete vs. continuous movements, 237
   drawing, 256
   drawing strokes, 256
   facial expressions, 370, 376
   grasping, 216–217
   pharynx, 332
   reach-and-grasp, 411
   skill acquisition, 111
   skull shape, 332
   sleep postures, 159
   target tracking, 205
   visual guidance, 163
   walking, 135, 139, 154, 413
Afferent feedback, equilibrium point
    hypothesis, 237
Aiming tasks
   Fitts' task, 406–407
   hypermetria, 63
   manual, 150, 380
   phases, 25
   reaching and grasping
     back-and-forth, 238–239
     basic concept, 213
    direction, 225–226
    error correction, 227–228
    Fitts' law, 229–230
    impulse variability model, 231–232
    iterative corrections model, 230–231
    optimized initial impulse model, 232–233
    speed profiles, 225–226
   repetitive performance, 103
   short-term memory, 122
   S-R compatibility, 283
Air-hockey-playing robot, 4
Akinesia, Parkinson's disease, 66
Alcohol, and timing, 64
Algorithmic analysis level, motor control, 5–6
Allocentric frame of reference, frame of
    reference, 383–384
Allographs
   writing reaction time, 265–266
   writing stages, 263–265
Allophones, definition, 324
Alpha motor neuron, servo theory, 55–56
American English, consonants, 334
Amputees, visual therapies, 220
Amyotrophic lateral sclerosis, face control, 368
Analysis levels, motor control, 4–6
Anarchic hand, supplementary motor area, 77
Anencephalic babies, facial control, 367
Angle-angle diagram, runner knee/thigh, 142
Angular oris, facial expressions, 365
Angular velocity, two-thirds power law, 258–260
Anticipatory postural adjustments (APAs),
    locomotion, 150–151
Anti-phase patterns, finger coupling, 245–246
APAs, *see* Anticipatory postural adjustments
    (APAs)
Apes, pharynx, 332
Apple-eating posture, monkey, 74
Apraxia
   parietal cortex, 81–82
   speech production, 354
Arc length, two-thirds power law, 260–261
Arcuate fasciculus, brain disconnections, 84
Arm-hand steadiness, individual differences, 397

Arm movement
    discrete vs. continuous, 237–238
    eye-hand coordination, 222
    impulse variability model, 231–232
    joint-interpolated, 242, 387
    mental practice, 110
    motor programs, 234
    skill acquisition changes, 112
    transport and grasp phases, 240
    two-hand movement, 244
    workspace effect, 243
Articulatory mechanisms
    acoustic targets, 339–340
    consonants, 334
    speaking and singing, 331–332
Associative phase, skill acquisition stages, 111
Attention
    and saccades, 192–194
    states of mind, 127–128
Auditory feedback
    chewing sounds, 27
    voice loudness, 326
Autokinetic illusion, miniature eye
        movements, 187
Automatic stage, skill acquisition, 111–112
Autonomic activity, and facial expression, 371
Autonomous stage, skill acquisition, 111–112

B

Babies, *see also* Infants
    behavioral exploration, 159
    crawling reflex, 156
    dynamic dominance hypothesis, 272
    eye-hand coordination, 223
    facial expressions, 367, 370
    ideo-motor theory, 131
    imitation, 375
    jolly jumping, 160
    motor development, 159–161
    optimization, 407
    reach-and-grasp, 213–216, 240
    reflexes, 155–156
    stepping, 157–158
    visual guidance, 217
    walking development, 154
Babinski reflex, neonatal walking
        development, 156
Back-and-forth aiming, hand kinematics,
    238–239
Back pain, prevention and treatment, 395
Back propagation, coarticulation, 345
Backward speech
    vs. speech errors, 349
    as word game, 346–347

Balance, cognition studies, 388–389
Ballistic phase, feedback, 25
Basal ganglia
    definition, 65
    function theories, 67–69
    Huntington's disease, 66
    Parkinson's disease, 66–67
Basketball shooting, practice specificity, 35–36
Behavioral control, genetics studies, 414
Behavioral exploration, neural maturation, 159
Behavioral science, in motor control, 7
Behavioral tasks, dynamical systems theory,
    400–405
Between-hand timing, typewriting, 310
Biceps
    elbow flexion, 64
    reciprocal inhibition, 58–59
    vibration, 52
Bicycle riding, method, 3
Bilabial coordination, speech control, 341–343
Binary decisions, 282
Biomechanical efficiency, vocal control,
    325–326
Bird song
    acquisition, 356
    brain mechanisms, 356–357
    canaries, 356–357
    chaffinch studies, 354–356
    and human language, 356
    neurons, 357
    zebra finch, 357
Bits, Hick-Hyman law, 281–282
Blinking
    conditioning, 175
    optic fiber, 175–176
    purpose, 174–175
    rates, 175
    synergies, 18
    visual sensitivity, 176
Blood flow
    cerebral, finger movement sequence, 78
    and emotions, 373–374
Bouncing backpack, energy harvesting, 419
Brain, *see* also specific regions
    and bird song, 356–357
    disconnections, 84–85
    emotions and blood flow, 373–374
    human, side view, 46
    movement signals, 44
    plasticity in learning, 36–38
    and saccades, 193
    signaling studies, 416–417
    speech mechanisms, 353–354
    walking control, 147–150

Breathing, respiratory system, 329
British English, consonants, 334
Broca's aphasia, telegraphic speech, 353
Broca's area, brain disconnections, 84
Brodman's area 3a, eye movement/space
        constancy, 204
Button pressing
    R-R compatibility, 287
    S-R compatibility, 283

C

Cameras
    clinical diagnosis decentralization, 418
    early motor studies, 415
Canaries, bird song, 356–357
Castrati, 331
Cat
    decerebrate rigidity, 62
    hind limb locomotion, 142
    leg swings, 140–141
    walking sensory feedback, 146–147
Central nervous system, myelination, 158–159
Cerebellum
    coordination, 63
    event timing, 299
    function, 61–62
    and learning, 65
    muscle tone regulation, 62
    timing, 63–65
Cerebral palsy, eye-hand coordination, 223
Cerebrum, finger movement sequence, 78
Chaffinch, bird song studies, 354–356
Chess players, hierarchical models, 100
Children
    Babinski reflex, 156
    behavioral exploration, 159
    clumsy, 396
    drawing smoothly, 262
    drawing strokes, 254–256
    eye-hand coordination, 223
    language acquisition, 356
    obstacle avoidance, 412
    optokinetic nystagmus, 195
    remote coaching, 418
    response chaining, 96
    skill acquisition, 105
    timing control, 396–397
    visual acuity, 205
    visual guidance, 163–164
Choice reaction time
    chords, 288–289
    factors, 280–282
    ideo-motor theory, 285
    Simon effect, 286

Chopin etude, piano playing, 315–316
Chords, pianists, 288–289
Chorea, Huntington's disease, 66
Cigar rolling task, hierarchical learning, 107–108
Circular stomach rubs, synergy, 17
Circulatory system, head and neck, 373
Clasp knife response, definition, 53–54
Clinical diagnosis, decentralization
        technology, 418
Clock delays, keypress rhythm and
        timing, 294–295
Closed-loop control
    feedback, 26
    skill acquisition, 101–103
Clumsy children, timing control, 396–397
α-γ Coactivation, spinal cord, 57
Coarticulation
    parallel distributed processing system, 343–346
    as sequencing problem, 22–23
    speech control, 325
    typewriting, 309
Cockroach
    extensor motor neuron, 144–145
    flexor burst generator, 144–145
    gait patterns, 144
    leg swings, 140–141
    locomotion neural circuits, 143–144
    multi-leg coordination, 145
    walking machine, 153–154
Co-contraction, reciprocal inhibition, 59
Codes, see Memory codes
Coefficient of variation, keypresses, 298
Cognition
    balance, 388–389
    enactive, 386, 388
    handheld pendulum studies, 389–390
    lexical decision task, 390–391
    smooth pursuit movements, 195
    stimulus-response translation, 390
    walking, 167, 388
Cognitive entrainment, and rhythmic
        entrainment, 391
Cognitive phase, skill acquisition stages, 110
Cognitive science, in motor control, 7
Cognitive sequencing, stepping, 157
Communication, speaking and singing,
        323–324
Comparator, feedback, 25
Computational analysis level, motor
        control, 4–5
Computer animation, optimization theory, 408–409
Computer programs
    keystroke sequences, 290–291
    motor program concept, 124–125

Computers, in rehabilitation therapy, 417–418

Conditioning
  eyeblink, 175
  S-R compatibility, 283

Congruent articulation task, 243

Conjugate eye movements, characteristics, 184

Connectionist model
  coarticulation, 344–345
  typewriting, 312

Consistent practice, generalized learning programs, 105–106

Consonants
  articulation, 334
  categories, 333
  English, 333–334
  phonetic features, 335

Constriction, pupils, 177–178

Context effects, writing, 268–270

Continuous movements
  circle drawing, 298
  reaching and grasping, 213, 237–238

Contraction
  α-γ coactivation, 57
  muscle, 46–47
  reciprocal inhibition, 58–59

Control precision, individual differences, 397

Control theory, engineering, 6

Convergence, eye movements, 201

Coordinate systems
  handpaths, 385–387
  and saccades, 191

Coordination
  and cerebellum, 63
  intersegmental, 238, 240–247
  reaching and grasping, 213
  skill acquisition changes, 113
  and tonic neck reflex, 155
  vestibular ocular reflex, 198–199
  visual guidance studies, 218

Corpus callosum, apraxia, 81–82

Correction, reaching and grasping, 212

Corrective phase, feedback, 25

Corrugator, facial expressions, 365

Cortical centers, neural development, 159

Cortico-spinal tract, walking control, 149–150

Counting, enactive cognition, 386

Crank-gear-flag study, bimanual actions, 246–247

Crawling reflex, babies, 156

Critical fluctuation, dynamical systems, 402

Cross-modal integration
  parietal cortex, 82–84
  premotor cortex, 76

Current control, aiming tasks, 227

Curvature, two-thirds power law, 260

Cutaneous receptors, proprioception, 54–55

Cycling, power requirements, 139

D

Dancers, mirror neuron studies, 32–33

DBS, *see* Deep brain stimulation (DBS)

Deaf children, drawing strokes, 255–256

Decerebrate rigidity, characteristics, 62

Decision making, binariness, 282

Declarative knowledge, vs. procedural, 116–118

Deep brain stimulation (DBS), Parkinson's disease, 66–67

Degrees of freedom problem
  basics, 12–13
  efficiency, 18–19
  as everyday issue, 13–14
  hitting oncoming balls, 381
  meaning, 14
  mechanics, 18
  synergies, 14–18

Delays, response chaining thory, 95

Dementia, Huntington's disease, 66

Depressor angular oris, facial expressions, 365

Depressor anuli oris, facial expressions, 365

Depressor supercilii, facial expressions, 365

Diaphragm, respiratory system, 328

Digraph frequency, typewriting, 311

Dilation, pupils, 177–178

Direction control
  hand aiming, 225–226
  infant reach, 215
  locomotion, 148–149
  motor cortex, 71–73

Disconnections, brain, 84–85

Discrete movements, reaching and grasping, 213, 237–238

Disjunctive eye movements, characteristics, 184

Distance control, infant reach, 215

Distance reproduction, short-term memory, 120–121

Divergence, eye movements, 201

Dizziness, vestibular ocular reflex, 198

Dog
  leg swings, 140
  motor cortex, 69

Doing, in learning, 33

Donders' law, definition, 180–181

Dopamine, Parkinson's disease, 66

Doubling operator, typing models, 314

Drawing
  dynamic dominance hypothesis, 272–273
  graphic outputs, 253
  hierarchical control, 252–253
  initiation stages, 251–252
  isogeny principle, 257–258
  smoothly, 262
  stroke planning, 254–256
  two-thirds power law, 258–262
Drift, as eye movement, 184
Drinking movements, motion-emotion
    relationship, 393
Dutch, vocal control, 325
Dvorak keyboard, history, 304–305
Dynamical systems theory
  definition, 400
  finger oscillation task, 400–405
  practical applications, 405
  underlying equation, 405
Dynamic dominance hypothesis, writing and
    drawing, 272–273
Dysarthria
  and cerebellum, 63
  speech production, 354
Dysgraphia, characteristics, 263–265

E

Echoic memory, information processing, 115
Editing, speech errors, 349–350
Efficiency, degrees of freedom problem, 18–19
Egocentric frame of reference, golf putting, 383
Einstein, Albert, 4, 6
Elbow flex
  and cerebellum, 63–64
  synergy, 15–16
Electrical signals, brain studies, 416–417
Electromyographic (EMG) signals
  anticipatory postural adjustments, 151
  cerebellum, 64
  mental practice, 110
  motor cortex, 75
  speech perception, 336–337
Element-to-position associations, timing,
    97–98
EMG, see Electromyographic (EMG) signals
Emotion
  and face, 366–367
  facial expression association, 371–374
  facial expression connection, 370–371
  innateness and universality, 369–370
Emotion-motion relationship
  drinking/knocking movements, 393
  emotion activation, 393–394
  history, 392–393

  motor performance, 394–395
  point-light displays, 393
Enactive cognition, basic concept, 386, 388
Endpoint distributions, hand aiming, 225
End-state comfort effect, 20
Energy harvesting, technological innovations, 419
Engineering, in motor control, 6
English
  coarticulation, 344
  consonants, 333–334
  word components, 324
Epilepsy, and motor cortex, 69
Equifinity, definition, 235
Equilibrium point hypothesis, reaching and
    grasping
  basic concept, 213
  mass-spring model, 234–235
  monkey studies, 233–234
Erasistratus, 46
Error analysis, writing, 263
Error correction, aiming, 227–228
Errors, typewriting, 307
Event timing, keystrokes, 297–298
Exafference, definition, 28
Execution, speech production, 354
Exhalation, respiratory system, 329
Extensor activity, cat hind limb, 142
Extensor motor neuron, cockroach,
    144–145
External intercostals, respiratory
    system, 328–329
Extrafusal fibers
  definition, 51
  servo theory, 55–57
Extra-ocular muscles
  activation, 182–184
  example, 180
Eye
  cross section, 174
  saccades and attention, 192–193
  scanpath, 187–188
  visual kinesthesis, 163
Eyeblink, see Blinking
Eye-hand coordination
  cerebral palsy, 223
  eye-hand independence, 223
  eye tracks hand, 222–223
  naturalistic performance, 223
  scanpaths, 223
  speech perception, 223–224
  targeting, 222
Eye-hand span, typing, 305
Eye-head coordination, vestibular ocular
    reflex, 198–199

Eye movements
  conjugate and disjunctive, 184
  extra-ocular muscles, 182–184
  miniature, 184–187
  oculo-motor control, 205
  physical dynamics, 180–181
  purpose, 179–180
  saccades, 187–188
  saccades and attention, 192–194
  saccadic suppression, 191–192
  smooth pursuit, 194–201
  and space constancy, 201–205
  typing, 305
Eye-tracking system, example, 224

F

Face
  left-right differences, 368–369
  movement vs. structure, 363–364
  muscle, 364–365
  physical description, 364
  recognition, 363
  upper/lower control, 366
  volitional/emotional control, 366–367
Facial expression
  emotion association, 371–374
  emotion connection, 370–371
  examples, 364–365
  innateness and universality, 369–370
  married couple imitation, 375, 377
  newborn imitation, 375–376
  and social interaction, 374–377
Facial feedback, and emotions, 371
Facial nerves, control, 366–369
Factor analysis, motor control differences, 397
Falls, walking as, 139
Feedback
  afferent, 237
  auditory, 27, 326
  facial, 371
  negative loop, 25
  oral, 338
  peripheral, 124, 176, 342
  positive loop, 26
  proprioceptive, 121, 219, 234, 326
  sensory, *see* Sensory feedback
  visual, *see* Visual feedback
Feedback correction
  bat swings, 382
  keyboarding rhythm, 294–295
Feedforward, perceptual-motor integration
    problem, 26–28
Fictive locomotion, spinal cord, 143

Figure eight drawing, isogeny principle,
    257
Figure skaters, practice habits, 34
Fingering patterns, pianists, 317
Finger movements
  cerebral blood flow, 78
  coarticulation, 22–23
  coupling, 245
  cutaneous receptors, 55
  degrees of freedom problem, 12, 14
  dexterity differences, 397
  dynamical systems theory, 400–405
  and emotion, 392
  equilibrium point hypothesis, 236–237
  feedforward, 26
  finger coupling, 244–246
  grasp phase, 240
  intersegmental coordination, 240
  motor cortex, 70–71
  motor development models, 159
  motor equivalence, 341
  moving with others, 392
  muscle spindles, 52, 56
  and object size, 216
  plasticity in learning, 37–38
  R-R compatibility, 287
  short-term memory, 121
  smart spinal cord, 60
  stimulus-response compatibility,
    283, 285
  supplementary motor area, 77–78
  two-hand movement, 244–245
  vision and touch, 219–220
Finger presses
  early typewriters, 305
  keyboard sequence learning, 294
  keystroke timing, 308
  response-response compatibility, 287
  sequences, 289–290
  serial order and timing, 301
  simple reaction time, 279–280
  simultaneous strokes, 288
  typewriting models, 312–314
  typing errors, 307
Finger taps
  eye-hand coordination, 223
  individual differences, 397
  rhythm and timing, 295
  sequences, 291
  short-term memory, 121–122
  skill acquisition, 104–105
  timing amodality, 299–300
  timing problem, 23–24, 64
Fish fin, synergies, 17

Fitts' law
  aiming movements, 229–230
  and impulse variability model, 231–232
  and iterative corrections model, 230
Fixation point, saccades, 190
Flexor activity, cat hind limb, 142
Flexor burst generator, cockroach, 144–145
Fly behavior, feedforward information, 27–28
fMRI, *see* Functional magnetic resonance
    imagery (fMRI)
Force
  extra-ocular muscles, 184
  motor cortex, 71–73
  piano playing keystrokes, 315
  and timing, 299
Forward associations, response chaining, 96
Forward dynamics, basic problem, 241
Four-legged walking machine, construction, 152
Frame of reference, golf putting, 383–385
French, coarticulation, 344
Freudian slip, speech errors, 349
Frontalis, facial expressions, 365
Functional magnetic resonance imagery (fMRI)
  mirror neuron studies, 32
  supplementary motor area, 79–80

G

Gait patterns
  brain control, 148
  cockroach, 144
  genetics studies, 413
  regularities, 139–140
  speed differences, 136–137, 139
Gamma-amino-butyric acid (GABA), Huntington's
    disease, 66
Gamma motor neuron
  servo theory, 55–57
  speech production, 337–338
Gaze directions, eyeball positions, 180–181
Generalized learning programs
  advantages, 103
  definition, 103
  parameter setting, 104–105
  practice, 105–106
Genetics
  "hand walkers", 413
  Huntington's disease, 66
  Nature vs. Nurture, 412–413
  tölting, 413
  tongue trilling, 414
Genetics studies
  behavioral control, 414
  movement sequencing, 415
  psychiatric disorders, 414

speech control, 414–415
Genetic therapy, Parkinson's disease, 67
Global rate scaling, writing size, 267, 270
Goal posture, optimization theory, 409–410
Golf putting
  frame of reference, 383–385
  head displacements, 384
Golgi tendon organs, proprioception, 53–54
Grammar, Broca's aphasia, 353
Graphemes
  writing reaction time, 265
  writing stages, 263–265
Graphology, writing and drawing, 253
Graphs, writing stages, 263
Grasp reflex, *see also* Reach-and-grasp movement
  development, 214
  neonatal walking development, 155
  optimization theory, 408
Group Ia afferent, function, 51
Group II afferent, function, 52
Group IIb afferents, Golgi tendon organs, 53

H

Handedness, and writing, 270–272
Hand-eye coordination, and tonic neck reflex,
    155
Hand movements
  aiming, 225, 242
  back-and-forth aiming, 238–239
  and cerebellum, 63
  coordination, 63
  error correction, 227–228
  eye-hand coordination, 222–223
  feedforward, 27
  force and direction, 71–72
  left-right decisions, 105
  phase transitions, 245, 401
  rapid aimed, 236
  and speech motor resonance, 358
  strength, flexibility, precision, 211
  trajectories, 387
  two-hand, *see* Two-hand movements
  vision dependence, 213
  visual guidance, 218
  writing and drawing, 272
Hand orientation, infant reach, 215–216
Handpaths, coordinates, 385–387
Hand position, writing and drawing, 272
Hand-space planning, intersegmental coordination,
    241–243
"Hand walkers," genetics studies, 413
Haptic tracking, bimanual coupling, 247
Head, circulatory system, 373
Head displacements, golf putting, 384

Head movements, vestibular-oculo-motor reflex, 197–198
Hearing, speaking and singing, 326
Heart rate, and facial expression, 371
Hebrew, vocal control, 325
Hick-Hyman law
  definition, 281–282
  and stimulus-response compatibility, 282–283
Hierarchical models
  basic concept, 99–100
  context effects, 270
  dysgraphia, 264
  high-level memory, 108–109
  keypress timing, 296–297
  keystroke sequences, 291
  Morse code learning, 106–107
  skill acquisition changes, 114–115
  syllables, 347–349
  task practice, 107–108
  time keepers, 297
  writing and drawing, 252–253
High-level memory, hierarchical learning, 108–109
Hill steepness, perception, 29–31
Hindi, word components, 324
Hitch-hiking posture, monkey, 74
Hitting oncoming balls
  ball direction, 381
  basic problem, 380
  degrees of freedom problem, 381
  feedback, 382
  stroke preprogramming, 381–382
  tau principle, 380–381
Hoffman reflex (H-reflex), tuning, 61
Homologous finger substitutions, typing, 290, 307
Hookers, writing and handedness, 271
Hooke's law
  muscle performance, 47
  muscles as springs, 235
Horowitz, Vladimir, 36
Horse, walking patterns, 137
H-reflex, see Hoffman reflex (H-reflex)
Human body, general
  developmental changes, 158
  major muscles, 45
  mass-spring models, 236
Human factors, in motor control, 7
Hunt-and-peck typing, 305
Huntington's disease, and basal ganglia, 66
Hypermetria, and cerebellum, 63
Hypnosis, and writing size, 267
Hypothesis vs. model, 399
Hypothetico-deductive method, definition, 399

Hypotonia, and cerebellum, 62
Hysteresis, dynamical systems, 402

I

Iconic memory, information processing, 115
ID, see Index of difficulty (ID)
Ideational apraxia, parietal cortex, 81
Ideo-motor activity, reaction times, 284–285
Ideomotor apraxia, parietal cortex, 81
Ideo-motor theory, states of mind, 129–131
Image displacement
  eye movement/space constancy, 201
  vestibular ocular reflex, 200
Imagery, skill acquisition, 109–110
Imaging studies
  mirror neuron studies, 32
  supplementary motor area, 77–80
Imitation
  ideo-motor theory, 130–131
  married couples, 375, 377
  newborn facial expression, 375–376
Implementation analysis level, motor control, 5
Implicit knowledge, definition, 3
Impulse variability model, aiming tasks, 231–232
Incongruent articulation task, 243
Index of difficulty (ID)
  Fitts' law, 229
  movement types, 238
  two-hand movements, 244
Individual differences
  factors, 397
  motor control dimensions, 395–396
  timing control, 396
Infants, see also Babies
  grasp and object size, 216
  grasp reflex, 214
  grasp tuning, 216–217
  pharynx, 332
  reach direction, 215
  reach distance, 215
  skull shape, 332
Inflow model, eye movement/space constancy, 202–203
Information-processing system
  characteristics, 115
  codes, 115–116
  long-term memory, 118–119
Information theory
  definition, 282
  and stimulus-response compatibility, 282–283
Inhalation, respiratory system, 328–329
Initial impulse, aiming tasks, 227
Inner ear, diagram, 198
In-phase patterns, finger coupling, 245–246

Intention, states of mind, 128–129
Intention tremor, and cerebellum, 63
Inter-element inhibition, sequencing, 98–99
Interest, and pupil size, 178
Interframes, computer animation, 408–409
Inter-limb coordination, skill acquisition changes, 113–114
Intermittent circle drawing, coefficient of variation, 298
Internal intercostals, respiratory system, 329
Inter-personal coordination, studies, 391–392
Inter-response times
    keyboard sequences, 301–303
    keypresses, 294–295
    keystroke sequences, 291–292
Intersegmental coordination, reaching and grasping
    basic concept, 238, 240
    hand-space planning, 241–243
    joint-space planning, 241–243
    transport and grasp phases, 240
    two-hand movements, 244–247
Intonation, speaking, 324
Intrafusal fibers
    definition, 51
    servo theory, 55–56
Inverse dynamics, basic problem, 241
Inverted handwriting, 270
ISI, *see* Median interstroke interval (ISI)
Isogeny principle, drawing, 257–258
Isometric movements, impulse variability model, 232
Iterative corrections model, hand aiming, 230–231

J

James-Lange theory of emotion
    basic concept, 371
    chronic back pain, 395
    facial experimental, 374
Joint receptors, proprioception, 54
Joints
    muscle performance, 47
    reciprocal inhibition, 59–60
    rotation optimization, 410–411
    skill acquisition changes, 114
Joint-space planning, intersegmental coordination, 241–243
Jolly jumpers, motor developments, 159–160

K

Kafkaesque condition, supplementary motor area, 79
Keyboarding, *see also* Typewriting
    choice reaction time, 280–282
    example, 277
    ideo-motor activity, 284–285
        pianists, 278
        piano keyboard patterns, 317
        Qwerty vs. Dvorak, 304–305
        response-response compatibility, 287
        sequence learning, 293–294
        sequence rates, 301–303
        Simon effect, 286
        simple reaction time, 279–280
        SNARC effect, 285–286
        stimulus-response compatibility, 282–283
        Stroop effect, 286–287
Keyframes, computer animation, 408–409
Keystrokes
    computer program sequences, 290–291
    event timing, 297–298
    hierarchical sequences, 291
    hierarchical timing, 296–297
    inter-response times, 291–292
    piano playing, 314–317
    rhythm and timing, 294–296
    rule-based sequences, 291
    Rumelhart and Norman's model, 313
    serial choice reaction time, 289–290
    simultaneous, 288–289
    timing amodality, 299–300
    timing and serial order, 300–301
    tree-traversal process, 292–293
    typewriting timing, 307–311
    typing control units, 306–307
Kinematics
    back-and-forth aiming, 238–239
    degrees of freedom problem, 14
    motor output buffer, 126
    stepping, 157
Kinesthetic illusion, basic concept, 129
Kinetics, degrees of freedom problem, 14
Knee, angle-angle diagram, 142
Knee joint receptors, responses, 54
Knocking movements, motion-emotion relationship, 393
Knowledge, procedural vs. declarative, 116–118
Knowledge of results (KR), skill acquisition, 101–102
KR, *see* Knowledge of results (KR)

L

Languages
    acquisition, bird song studies, 356
    brain disconnections, 84
    speech components, 324–325
    speech motor resonance, 358
Larynx
    functions, 329–330
    vocal cords, 330–331
Lax vowels, 333

L-dopa
    gait pattern effects, 148
    Parkinson's disease, 66
Leaps, running as, 139
Learning
    and cerebellum, 65
    deliberate practice, 34–35
    doing, 33
    generalized, 103–106
    neural plasticity, 36–38
    specific practice, 35–36
    vestibular ocular reflex, 200
Leg movements, stepping, 157
Leg swings
    cognition studies, 390
    socially cooperative activity, 391
    walking, 140
Length-tension relation, muscle, 47–48
Lenthening, muscle, 46
Letter lists, hierarchical models, 100
Letter-production programs, *see* Graphemes
Letter strings, writing reaction times, 266
Lexical decision task
    cognition studies, 390–391
    typing speeds, 308
Limb movement
    coordination, 17, 145
    direction and force, 44
    equilibrium point hypothesis, 235–237
    impulse variability model, 231–232
    individual differences, 396
    inter-limb coordination, 113, 247
    joint angles, 19
    and learning, 65
    moving with others, 391
    multi-limb coordination, 397
    muscle spindles, 51
    population coding, 72
    proprioception, 50
    reaching and grasping, 213
    reciprocal inhibition, 59
    sensory feedback, 146
    servo theory, 56
    synergies, 15–18
    vision and touch, 220
    visual rehabilitation therapy, 220
    walking, 135–136
Limb segments
    coordination, 238–239
    reach-and-grasp, 213
Limit-cycle attractor, dynamical systems theory, 400
Linguistic hemisphere, and writing, 270
Lips
    acoustic targets, 339–341
    articulatory mechanisms, 332
    Brodman's area 3a, 204
    coarticulation, 22–23, 343–344
    consonant production, 333–335
    face control, 365
    golf putting studies, 384
    laryngeal mechanisms, 331
    motor cortex, 70
    parallel articulation, 325
    relative positioning, 341–342
    speech production, 338–340
    target hypothesis, 338
Listing's plane, definition, 181
Lobster, leg swings, 140
Location reproduction, short-term memory, 120–121
Locomotion
    anticipatory postural adjustments, 150–151
    brain control, 147–150
    forms, 135–136
    neural circuits, 143–146
    neural control
        overview, 141–143
        sensory feedback, 146–147
    and prehension, 385
Logical problems, response chaining, 95
Long jumpers, memory and feedback, 166–167
Long-loop reflexes
    motor cortex, 74–75
    tuning, 61
Long-term learning, vestibular ocular reflex, 200
Long-term memory
    function, 118–119
    information processing, 115
Looking
    accomodation, 177
    basic concept, 173–174
    blinking, 174–176
    eye movements, 179–187
    oculo-motor control, 205
    pupils, 177–178
    saccades, 187–194
    smooth pursuit movements, 194–201
    space constancy, 201–205
    vergence movements, 201
Loudness, speaking and singing, 326
Loudness profile, piano playing, 315–316
Lower face, neural control, 366
Lungs, respiratory system, 328

M

Mandarin Chinese, word components, 324
Maps, memory, 164–166
Marr, David, 4–5
Married couples, facial expression imitation, 375, 377

Masked face, Parkinson's disease, 367
Mass-spring model, equilibrium point hypothesis,
    234–235
Mechanical control, extra-ocular muscles, 184
Mechanical perturbations, anticipatory postural
    adjustments, 150–151
Mechanics, degrees of freedom problem, 18
Mechanoreceptors, definition, 55
Median interstroke interval (ISI), typing, 306
Medicine, in motor control, 7
Memory
    and feedback, 166–167
    keystroke sequences, 291
    route maps, 164–166
    survey maps, 164–166
    typewriting from, 309
Memory codes
    history effects, 122–123
    information processing, 115–116
    motor output buffer, 125–126
    motor programs, 124–125
Memory drum, definition, 126
Memory stores
    long-term, 118–119
    procedural vs. declarative knowledge, 116–118
    short-term, 119–122
Mental activity, and walking, 388
Mentalis, facial expressions, 365
Mental practice, skill acquisition, 109–110
Mesthenia gravis, muscle contraction, 46
Microsaccades, as eye movements, 185–187
Miniature eye movements
    autokinetic illusion, 187
    detection, 185
    drift, 184
    microsaccades, 185–187
    tremor, 184
    types, 185
Mini-motions, walking adjustments, 150
Minimum jerk principle
    drawing smoothly, 262
    and efficiency, 19
    motion-emotion relationship, 392
    optimization theory, 406–408
    writing and drawing, 253
Mirror neurons, and perception, 31–32
Mirror tracing task, procedural vs. declarative
    knowledge, 117
Model vs. hypothesis, 399
Monkey studies
    brain plasticity in learning, 37–38
    brain signaling studies, 416–417
    parietal cortex, 82–83
    pointing responses, 233–234

premotor cortex, 76
saccade studies, 190–191
vestibular ocular reflex, 198–199
walking sensory feedback, 146
whole-body movement, 73–74
Moro reflex, neonatal walking development, 155
Morphological level, speech errors, 352–353
Morse code, hierarchical learning, 106–107
Motion-emotion relationship
    drinking/knocking movements, 393
    emotion activation, 393–394
    history, 392–393
    motor performance, 394–395
    point-light displays, 393
Motor control basics
    analysis levels, 4–6
    contributing research, 6–7
    understanding, 2–4
Motor control theories
    dynamical systems theory, 400–405
    optimization theory, 405–412
    theorist profiles, 398–399
    theory vs. hypothesis, 399
Motor cortex
    direction control, 71–73
    force, 71–73
    function, 69–71
    long-loop reflexes, 74–75
    motor map, 70
    population coding, 72–73
    whole-body movement, 73–74
Motor delays, keypress rhythm and timing,
    294–295
Motor development
    jolly jumpers, 159–160
    models, 158–161
    neural development, 158–159
    slopes, handling, 160–161
Motor intelligence, Turing test, 3
Motor level, speech errors, 352
Motor map, example, 70
Motor memory codes, vs. spatial, 121
Motor neurons
    reciprocal inhibition, 59
    and Renshaw cells, 57
    speech production, 337–338
Motor output buffer, basic concept, 125–126
Motor potential, motor cortex, 71
Motor programs, basic concept, 124–125
Motor resonance, speech perception, 357–359
Motor skills, long-term memory, 118
Motor system
    definition, 2
    synergy types, 15

Motor theory, speech perception, 336–337, 357–359
Motor units, muscle fiber, 49–50
Mouse, movement sequencing problems, 415
Movement, general
  and emotion, 394–395
  long-term memory, 118
  and perception, 28–31
  plans, and basal ganglia, 67–68
  reaching and grasping, 213
  short-term memory, 119–122
  signals, 43–44
  whole-body, 73–74
Movement time (MT), Fitts' law, 229
MT, *see* Movement time (MT)
Multi-leg coordination, cockroach, 145
Multi-limb coordination, individual differences, 397
Muscle commands, basic concept, 125
Muscle fiber, motor units, 49–50
Muscles
  brain signal studies, 416–417
  contraction, 46–47
  eye movement/space constancy, 203
  face, 364–365
  human body, 45
  length-tension relation, 47–48
  motor units, 49–50
  proprioceptor circuitry, 51
  respiratory system, 328
  skill acquisition changes, 112
  smooth pursuit movements, 194
  as springs, 234–237
  tone regulation, 62
Muscle spindles
  proprioception, 51–53
  servo theory, 56
Myelination, CNS nerve fibers, 158–159
Myosin, muscle performance, 47

N

Nadirs, two-hand movements, 246
Nasalization, coarticulation, 22, 344
Naturalistic performance, eye-hand coordination, 223
Nature
  vs. Nurture, 412–413
  vs. walking machines, 153
Navigation
  S-R compatibility, 283
  visual guidance, 163–164
  visual kinesthesis, 161–163
Neanderthal, skull shape, 332
Neck, circulatory system, 373
Necker cube, example, 178

Negative feedback loop, 25
Negative lag-1 auto-correlations, keypresses, 294–295
Neonatal reflexes, walking development, 155–156
Nerve fibers, CNS, myelination, 158–159
Nervous system, movement signals, 44
Neural circuits, locomotion, 143–146
Neural control
  left-right face differences, 368–369
  locomotion, 141–143, 146–147
  timing, 298
  upper/lower face, 366
  volitional/emotional, face, 366–367
Neural development
  behavioral exploration, 159
  CNS myelination, 158–159
  cortical-subcortical centers, 159
  maturation direction, 159
Neural noise, timing amodality, 299
Neural plasticity, in learning, 36–38
Neurons, general
  motor cortex, 71
  movement signals, 44
  premotor cortex, 75–76
Neuroscience, in motor control, 7
Newborns, facial expression imitation, 375–376
Nodes, typing models, 312–313
Nurture vs. Nature, 412–413

O

Object manipulation
  coarticulation, 22–24
  patient "D.F.", 29–30
Object size, infant grasping, 216
Obstacle-avoidance
  Fitts' law, 230
  reach-and-grasp movement, 411–412
Ockham's razor, definition, 407
Oculo-motor activities
  blinking, 174–176
  development and plasticity, 205
  eye movement/space constancy, 201–202
Oculo-motor nerve, extra-ocular muscles, 182–183
OKN, *see* Optokinetic nystagmus (OKN)
One-person task, task sharing, 391–392
Open-loop control
  feedback, 26
  feedforward, 26
Optic fiber, and blinking, 175–176
Optimization theory
  computer animation, 408–409
  criterion, 406–407
  definition, 405–406
  goal posture, 409–410

joint rotation, 410–411
   reach-and-grasp movement, 408, 411–412
   variables, 407
Optimized initial impulse model, aiming tasks, 232–233
Optokinetic nystagmus (OKN), smooth pursuit movements, 195, 197
Optomotor reflex, feedforward, 27
Oral feedback, speech production, 338
Orbital coordinates, saccades, 191
Orientation, infant reach, 215–216
Oscillation
   finger coupling, 244–246
   finger tasks, 402
Oscillatory model, drawing smoothly, 262
Ouija game, and intention, 128
Outflow model, eye movement/space constancy, 201–204

P

Parallel distributed processing system, coarticulation, 343–346
Paralysis, treatment technologies, 415–416
Parameter remapping effect, motor memory, 122–124
Parameter-setting models, generalized programs, 104–105
Parietal cortex
   apraxia, 81–82
   cross-modal integration, 82–84
   function, 80
Parietal lobe, dysgraphia, 264–265
Parkinson's disease
   and basal ganglia, 66–67
   dynamical systems theories, 405
   face control, 367
   motor and clock delays, 295
Passive dynamics walkers, 18
Passive movement, visual guidance studies, 219
Passive tension, muscle performance, 47
Pen-direction reversal times, 269
Pendulums
   cognition studies, 389–390
   two-hand swinging, 406
Perception
   bimanual coupling, 247
   gait patterns, 139–140
   mirror neurons, 31–32
   and movement, 28–31
   speech motor theory, 336–337
   and tapping, 299
   timing amodality, 300
   vision for action, 221
   and walking control, 167

Perceptual changes, feedforward, 27
Perceptual deficits, dysgraphia, 264–265
Perceptual-motor coordination, visual guidance studies, 218
Perceptual-motor integration problem
   and attention, 127
   basal ganglia, 69
   choices, 419–420
   feedback, 25–26
   feedforward, 26–28
   mirror neurons, 31–32
   movement and perception, 28–31
Perceptual trace, definition, 101
Performance
   attention role, 127–128
   and emotion, 394–395
   eye-hand coordination, 223
   motor memory, 122
Performance speed
   and skill acquisition, 107
   typing, 311
Peripheral feedback
   blinking, 176
   motor programs, 124
   speech, 342
PET, see Positron emission tomography (PET)
Phantom limb, visual therapies, 220
Pharynx, speech evolution, 332
Phonemes
   backward talking, 346–347
   definition, 324
   speaking issues, 324
   speech rates, 325
Phonemic restoration, definition, 327
Phones, definition, 324
Phonetic features
   consonants, 335
   definition, 324
   speech errors, 352
Phonology
   speech errors, 352–353
   standard theory, 334–335
Photodiodes, extra-ocular muscle studies, 183
Photoreceptors, and eye movement, 186
Physical changes, skill acquisition, 112–115
Physical control, face, 364–365
Physical mechanics, degrees of freedom problem, 18
Physical response, swinging room studies, 163
Physics, in motor control, 6
Physiological constraints, coarticulation, 22
Physiology, in motor control, 7
Pianists
   chords, 288–289
   keyboarding, 278

Piano playing
    Chopin etude, 315–316
    keyboard patterns, 317
    rubato control, 316–317
    scores and notes, 314–315
    vs. typing, 314
Pig Latin, as word game, 346
Pitch
    gaze direction, 181
    speaking, 324
    vocal cords, 330
Planning
    drawing strokes, 254–256
    hand- and joint-space, 241–243
    reaching and grasping, 212
    speech production, 353–354
Plant, feedback, 25
Plasticity
    in learning, 36–38
    oculo-motor control, 205
Point attractor, dynamical systems theory, 400
Point-light displays, motion-emotion relationship, 393
Population coding, motor cortex, 72–73
Portable eye-tracking system, example, 224
Positions, speech articulators, 339–340
Positive feedback loop, 26
Positron emission tomography (PET), supplementary motor area, 77–78
Posterior parietal cortex, and saccades, 193–194
Posture
    degrees of freedom problem, 19
    walking, 147, 150–151
Posture neurons, monkey, 74
Potential landscape, dynamical systems, 404
Power requirements, walking, running, cycling, 139
Practice
    deliberate, 34–35
    generalized learning programs, 105–106
    hierarchical learning, 107–108
    specificity, 35–36
Precision, grasp tuning, 216–217
Preflex, Nature vs. walking machines, 153
Prehension, and locomotion, 385
Premotor cortex, function, 75–76
Procedural analysis level, motor control, 5–6
Procedural knowledge, vs. declarative, 116–118
Procerus, facial expressions, 365
Programming, speech production, 354
Pronunciation rules
    response chaining, 96
    rule-governed behavior, 97
Proportionality constant, two-thirds power law, 260–261

Proprioception
    cutaneous receptors, 54–55
    definition, 50–51
    eye movement/space constancy, 203–204
    Golgi tendon organs, 53–54
    joint receptors, 54
    muscle spindles, 51–53
Proprioceptive feedback
    equilibrium point hypothesis, 234
    short-term memory, 121
    speech production, 326
    visual guidance, 219
Pseudobulbar palsy, facial control, 367
Psychiatric disorders, genetics studies, 414
Psychogenic motor disorders, prevention and treatment, 395
Psychological constraints, coarticulation, 22
Pupil responses, constriction/dilation, 177–178

Q

Qwerty keyboard, history, 304–305

R

Random jitter, *see* Tremor
Rapid eye movement (REM) sleep
    saccades, 188
    smooth pursuit movements, 194
Rapid movements, impulse variability model, 231–232
Rate scaling, writing size, 266–267
Reach-and-grasp movement
    aiming, 213
        direction, 225–226
        error correction, 227–228
        Fitts' law, 229–230
        impulse variability model, 231–232
        iterative corrections model, 230–231
        optimized initial impulse model, 232–233
        speed profiles, 225–226
    basic concept, 212
    development, 213, 214–217
    direction, 215
    distance, 215
    equilibrium point hypothesis, 213
        mass-spring model, 234–235
        monkey studies, 233–237
    grasp tuning, 216–217
    intersegmental coordination
        basic concept, 238, 240
        hand-space planning, 241–243
        joint-space planning, 241–243
        transport and grasp phases, 240
        two-hand movements, 244–247

limb coordination, 213
movement types, 213, 237–238
object size, 216
optimization theory, 411–412
orientation, 215–216
visual guidance, 213
  basic concept, 217–218
  early studies, 218–219
  eye-hand coordination, 222–224
  vision for action, 221–222
  vision and touch, 219–220
Reaching
  aiming, 213
  basic concept, 212
  development, 213
  equilibrium point hypothesis, 213
  limb coordination, 213
  movement types, 213
  optimization theory, 408
  visual guidance, 213
  and walking, 385–386
Reaction time (RT)
  allograph selection, 265–266
  choice, 280–282
  chords, 288–289
  grapheme selection, 265
  ideo-motor activity, 284–285
  individual differences, 397
  keyboard sequence learning, 293
  keystroke sequences, 289–290
  response-response compatibility, 287
  Simon effect, 286
  simple, 279–280
  stimulus-response compatibility, 282–283
  Stroop effect, 286–287
Reafference
  definition, 28
  S-R compatibility, 285
Reciprocal inhibition, spinal cord, 58–60
Recitation speed, hierarchical learning, 109–110
Recurrent inhibition, spinal cord, 57–58
Reference signal, feedback, 25
Reflex
  brain control, 148
  Nature vs. walking machines, 153
  neonatal walking development, 155–156
  optomotor, 27
  wiping, spinal frogs, 60–61
Reflex tuning, spinal, 61
Regime, dynamical systems, 400–405
Rehabilitation therapy
  technological innovations, 417–418
  vision and touch, 220

Relative phase, dynamical systems, 402
Relative positioning
  mechanism, 341–342
  speech articulators, 339–341
Relative timing, writing, 267–268
REM, *see* Rapid eye movement (REM) sleep
Renshaw cells, recurrent inhibition, 57–58
Repetitive aiming task, and knowledge of
  results, 103
Respiratory system, components, 328–329
Response chaining
  basic theory, 94–95
  feedback, 96
  forward associations, 96
  logical problem, 95
  pronunciation rules, 96
  timing problem, 95
Response competition, Stroop effect, 286
Response-response (R-R) compatibility
  characteristics, 287
  keystroke sequences, 290
Response speed, skill acquisition, 112
Resting length, muscles as springs, 237
Resting tremor, Parkinson's disease, 66
Restricted pathway movement, Fitts' law, 230
Retina
  eye movement/space constancy, 201–202
  saccades, 190
Retinal stabilization, characteristics, 186–187
Rhythm
  keypresses, 294–296
  piano playing, 315–316
  timing amodality, 299–300
Rhythmic entrainment, and cognitive
  entrainment, 391
Right frontal lobe, dysgraphia, 264–265
Righting reflex, neonatal walking
  development, 155
Rigidity, Parkinson's disease, 66
Robots, *see also* Walking machines
  humanoid, development, 3–4
  limb movement therapy, 220
  passive dynamics walkers, 18
  in rehabilitation therapy, 417–418
Roll, gaze direction, 181
Route maps, memory, 164–166
R-R, *see* Response-response (R-R) compatibility
RT, *see* Reaction time (RT)
Rubato control, piano playing, 316–317
Rubber hand illusion, premotor cortex, 76
Rule-governed behavior
  keystroke sequences, 291
  pronunciation rules, 97

Running
  knee/thigh angle-angle diagram, 142
  power requirements, 139
  speed, 97
  stages, 138
  vs. walking, 139

S

Saccades
  and attention, 192–194
  and brain areas, 193
  coordinate systems, 191
  definition, 187
  extra-ocular muscles, 183
  fixation point, 190
  initiation, 188–189
  latencies, 189
  monkey studies, 190–191
  and optokinetic nystagmus, 195
  REM sleep, 188
  retinal location, 190
  scanpath timing, 187–188
  and smooth pursuit movements, 194–195
  stopping, 189
Saccadic suppression
  causes, 191–192
  feedforward, 27
Scanpath
  eye-hand coordination, 223
  eyes, 187–188
Schemas
  advantages, 103
  definition, 103
Schizophrenia, brain disconnections, 84–85
Semantic level, speech errors, 352
Sensory feedback
  equilibrium point hypothesis, 234, 236
  leg movement sequencing, 145–146
  locomotion control, 143, 150
  long-loop reflexex, 74
  monkey studies, 26
  motor programs, 124
  response chaining, 96
  speech production, 338
  visual guidance, 218
  in walking, 146–147
Sensory nerve fibers
  Ia afferent, 51
  II afferent, 52
Sentences
  speech errors, 352
  speech perception, 358–359
Sequences of actions
  keyboard learning, 293–294

keyboard rates, 301–303
keystrokes, 289–293
long-term memory, 118–119
Sequencing problem
  coarticulation, 22–23
  inter-element inhibition, 98–99
  leg movements, 145–146
  speech errors, 20–22
Serial choice reaction time
  keyboard sequence learning, 293
  keystroke sequences, 289–290
Serial order problem
  definition, 94
  element-to-position associations, 97
  hierarchies, 99–100
  response chaining, 94–97
  speech output, 345
  and timing, 300–301
  typing, 313
Servomechanism, feedback, 25
Servo theory
  smooth pursuit movements, 195
  spinal cord, 55–57
Shadowing, definition, 327
Short-latency reflexes, tuning, 61
Short-term memory
  history effects, 122–123
  information processing, 115
  movements, 119–122
Simon effect, characteristics, 286
Simple reaction time, factors, 279–280
Simultaneous keystrokes, chords, 288–289
Singing
  articulatory mechanisms, 331–332
  bird song, 354–357
  communication, 323–324
  and hearing, 326
  laryngeal mechanisms, 329–331
  loudness control, 326
  properties, 323
  and respiratory system, 328–329
Sinusoidal oscillation, finger tasks, 402
Six-legged walking machine, construction, 152–153
Size principle, muscles, 50
Skill acquisition
  closed-loop theory, 101–103
  generalized programs, 103–106
  hierarchical learning, 106–109
  imagery, 109–110
  mental practice, 109–110
  physical changes, 112–115
  stage theory, 110–112
Ski simulator, skill acquisition changes, 114
Skulls, Neanderthal vs. human, 332

Slips of the pen, writing errors, 263
Slopes, motor development behavior, 160–161
SMA, *see* Supplementary motor area (SMA)
Smart spinal cord, spinal frog studies, 60–61
Smiling
    and blood flow, 374
    characteristics, 363–364
    emotional expression, 369–374
    face neural control, 366–369
    face physical control, 364–365
    social interaction, 374–377
Smooth pursuit movements
    anticipatory, 196
    cognitive states, 195
    control, 194–195
    definition, 194
    initiation, 194
    muscles, 194
    optokinetic nystagmus, 195, 197
    velocity, 194
    vestibular-oculo-motor reflex,
        197–201
SNARC effect, S-R compatibility,
    285–286
Social interaction, and facial expression,
    374–377
Socially cooperative activity, leg swinging,
    391
Somesthetic feedback, speech production, 338
Song learning, zebra finches, 415
Space constancy, and eye movements, 201–205
Spatial attention, and saccades, 192–193
Spatial coordinates, saccades, 191
Spatial memory codes, vs. motor, 121
Spatial neglect, definition, 194
Spatial targets, speech control, 339
Speaking, *see also* Speech control
    articulatory mechanisms, 331–332
    communication, 323–324
    and hearing, 326
    laryngeal mechanisms, 329–331
    loudness control, 326
    properties, 323
    and respiratory system, 328–329
    S-R compatibility, 283
    variations, 324
    vocal apparatus, 326
    word components, 324
Specificity of practice, definition, 35–36
Speech control, *see also* Speaking
    acoustic targets, 339–341
    brain mechanisms, 353–354
    coarticulation, 343–346
    consonants, 333–335

genetics studies, 414–415
    high-level, 346–353
    motor theory, 336–337
    pharynx, 332
    relative positions, 339–342
    speed studies, 347–349
    target hypothesis, 337–338
    timing, 325
    variability, 335
    vocal cords, 330–331
    vowels, 332–333
    word games, 346–347
Speech errors
    and cerebellum, 63
    definition, 349
    editing, 349–350
    Freudian slip, 349
    processing, 352–353
    sentence representation, 352
    as sequencing problem, 20–22
    types, 350–352
Speech perception
    eye-hand coordination, 223–224
    motor resonance, 357–359
Speed control
    degrees of freedom problem, 12
    digraph typing, 311
    element-to-position associations, 98
    enactive cognition, 386
    gait patterns, 136–139, 144
    hammering, 227
    hierarchical time keepers, 297
    keyboarding, 278–279
    keypress sequences, 291
    keystroke timing, 307–308
    locomotion, 146, 148–149
    reaching distance, 215
    reaction time, 279
    response chaining, 95
    singers' breathing, 329
    speaking, 347–349
    and time, 15
    transport and grasp phases, 240
    two-hand movements, 245–246
    typing, 302–303, 305–306
    typing coarticulation, 23
    vocal output, 325
    walking, 135–136
    walking and mental activity, 388
    whole-body movement, 74
Speed profiles
    equilibrium point hypothesis, 236
    hand aiming, 226–227
    positioning movements, 407

Spinal cord
    α-γ coactivation, 57
    fictive locomotion, 143
    monkey pointing responses, 234
    reciprocal inhibition, 58–60
    recurrent inhibition, 57–58
    reflex tuning, 61
    servo theory, 55–57
    smart, 60–61
    spinal reflexes, 55
    in walking, 147
Spinal frogs, spinal cord studies, 60–61
Spinal pathways, movement signals, 44
Spirals, drawing, 261
Spooner, William Archibald, 20–21
Spoonerisms, 20–21
Spring system, muscles as, 234–236
Squeezing task, short-term memory, 121–122
S-R, see Stimulus-response (S-R) compatibility
Stage theory, skill acquisition, 110–112
Stance phase, walking, 140–141
Startle reflex, neonatal walking development, 155
States of mind
    attention, 127–128
    ideo-motor theory, 129–131
    intention, 128–129
Stationarity, motor and clock delays, 296
Statistics, in motor control, 7
Stepping reflex
    disappearance/reappearance, 156–158
    neonatal walking development, 155–156
Stiffness, muscles as springs, 236–237
Stimulus-response (S-R) compatibility
    arrangements, 284
    ideo-motor accounts, 284–285
    keyboard sequence learning, 294
    reaction time (RT), 282–283
    Simon effect, 286
    SNARC effect, 285–286
Stimulus-response translation
    choice reaction time, 280–281
    chord performance, 289
    cognition studies, 390
Strabismus, definition, 181
Stress, speaking, 324
Stretch (muscle)
    clasp knife response, 53–54
    decerebrate rigidity, 62
    muscle, 46
    proprioception, 52
Stroboscopic photography, touch typing, 308
Stroke patients, limb movement therapy, 220
Stroke planning, drawing, 254–256
Stroop effect, characteristics, 286–287

Sub-cortical centers, neural development, 159
Superior colliculus, and saccades, 193
Supplementary motor area (SMA)
    action sequence extension, 79–80
    anarchic hand, 77
    finger movement sequence, 78
    Kafkaesque condition, 79
    location, 76–77
Suppression effects, feedforward, 27
Survey maps, memory, 164–166
Swimming reflex, neonatal walking
        development, 156
Swinging room, navigation studies, 161–163
Swing phase, walking, 140–141
Syllables, hierarchical organization, 347–349
Synchronization, feedback-based, 24–25
Synergies
    blinking, 18
    concept, 14–15
    fish fins, 17
    between limbs, 17
    within limb, 15–16, 18
    types, 15
Syntactic level, speech errors, 352

T

Tabes dorsalis, characteristics, 146
Tacit knowledge, definition, 3
Tapping
    coefficient of variation, 298
    and perception, 299
Target hypothesis, speech control, 337–338
Task sharing, one- vs. two-person, 391–392
Tau principle, hitting oncoming balls, 380–381
Technological innovations
    brain signal studies, 416–417
    diagnosis decentralization, 418
    early cameras, 415
    energy harvesting, 419
    paralysis treatment, 415–416
    in rehabilitation therapy, 417–418
Telegraphic speech, Broca's aphasia, 353
Tense vowels, 333
Testosterone, in bird song, 357
Theory space, optimization theory, 408
Thigh, angle-angle diagram, 142
3D tracking skills, long-term memory, 119
Tics, prevention and treatment, 395
Timing
    amodality, 299–300
    basic problem, 23–25
    and cerebellum, 63–65
    degrees of freedom problem, 14
    element-to-position associations, 97–98

extra-ocular muscles, 184
and force, 299
hierarchical, 296–297
individual differences, 396
intersegmental coordination, 240
isogeny principle, 258
keypresses, 294–296
keypress events, 297–298
neural control, 298
respiratory system, 329
response chaining, 94–97
Rumelhart and Norman's typing model, 313
and serial order, 300–301
skill acquisition changes, 113
speech control, 325
typewriting keystrokes, 307–311
writing, 267–268
Toddlers
obstacle avoidance, 412
visual guidance, 163–164
Token nodes, typing models, 314
Tölting, genetics studies, 413
Tone, speaking, 324
Tongue trilling, genetics studies, 414
Tonic neck reflex, neonatal walking
development, 155–156
Topographic representations, motor
cortex, 69
Touch, vision correlation, 219–220
Touching nose task, degrees of freedom
problem, 12–13
Touch typing, stroboscopic photograph, 308
Transition, dynamical systems, 400
Transport phase, intersegmental coordination,
240
Tree-traversal process, keystroke sequences,
292–293
Tremor, as eye movement, 184
Triceps
elbow flexion, 64
reciprocal inhibition, 58–59
Trichotillomania, genetics studies, 414
Trochlear nerve, extra-ocular muscles, 182
Tuning
infant grasping, 216–217
skill acquisition changes, 113
spinal reflexes, 61
Turing, Alan, 3
Turing test, basics, 3
Twitch (muscle)
motor cortex, 70–71
responses to, 53
Two-hand movements
arm interactions, 244

conditions, 246
crank-gear-flag study, 246–247
finger coupling, 244–246
mechanism, 244
and perception, 247
Two-person task, task sharing, 392
Two-thirds power law
angular velocity, 258–260
drawing smoothly, 262
mechanisms, 262
spiral drawings, 261
terms, 260–261
Typewriting
coarticulation, 22–23, 309
digraph frequency, 311
errors, 307
historical issues, 304–306
keystroke timing, 307–311
from memory, 309
vs. piano playing, 314
Rumelhart and Norman's model, 312–314
units of control, 306–307
word frequency, 310–311

U

Uncontrolled manifold, skill acquisition
changes, 114
Upper face, neural control, 366
Utterances, speaking speed, 347–348

V

Variable practice, generalized learning
programs, 105–106
Velocity, aiming tasks, 227–228
Verbal labels, drawing strokes, 256
Vergence movements, types, 201
Vestibular ocular reflex (VOR)
adaptation components, 200–201
damage adaptation, 199–200
development and plasticity, 205
head movements, 197–198
image displacement, 200
inner ear, 198
and learning, 65
long-term learning, 200
Vibration, muscle spindles, 52
Violinists, practice habits, 34
Virtual-reality (VR) technology
perception studies, 31
in rehabilitation therapy, 418
Vision, touch correlation, 219–220
Visual attention, and brain areas, 193
Visual cortex, and saccades, 193
Visual dominance, vs. touch, 219–220

Visual feedback
  aiming tasks, 227, 228
  cutaneous receptors, 55
  dysgraphia, 264
  and memory, 166–167
  monkey studies, 416
  premotor cortex, 76–77
  reaching-and-grasping, 215, 217, 234
  short-term memory, 119–120
  skill acquisition, 103
Visual guidance
  developments, 163–164
  reaching and grasping
    basic concept, 213, 217–218
    early studies, 218–219
    eye-hand coordination, 222–224
    vision for action, 221–222
    vision and touch, 219–220
  walking control, 149–150
Visual kinethesis
  basic concept, 161
  swinging room studies, 161–163
Visual rearrangement, adaptation studies, 218
Visual sensitivity, eyeblink, 176
Visual stimulus, and learning, 65
Vocal control
  consonant production, 333–335
  speaking and singing, 325–326
Vocal cords
  pitch and voicing, 330
  speech production, 330–331
Vocal system, schematic diagram, 328
Vocal tract
  articulatory mechanisms, 331–332
  cross section, 328
  laryngeal mechanisms, 329–331
  pharynx, 332
  respiratory system, 328–329
  vowel production, 332–333
Voicing
  larynx function, 329–330
  vocal cords, 330
Volitional control, face, 366–367
VOR, *see* Vestibular ocular reflex (VOR)
Vowels, and speech, 332–333

W

Walking
  anticipatory postural adjustments, 150–151
  body structure changes, 158
  brain's role, 147–150
  camera-based studies, 416
  cognition studies, 388

degrees of freedom problem, 18–19
energy harvesting, 419
gait pattern regularities, 139–140
gait pattern speed, 136–137, 139
locomotion control, 141–143
locomotion forms, 135–136
locomotion neural circuits, 143–146
memory and feedback, 166–167
memory maps, 164–166
motor development models, 158–161
navigation, 161–164
neonatal reflexes, 155–156
Parkinson's disease, 68
power requirements, 139
and reaching, 385–386
vs. running, 139
sensory feedback role, 146–147
simplified model, 138
stages, 138
stepping, 156–158
visual guidance, 163–164
visual kinesthesis, 161–163
Walking machines
  construction, 151–152
  early designs, 152–153
  requirements, 151
Wernicke's area, brain disconnections, 84
Whole-body movement, motor cortex,
      73–74
Wiping reflex, spinal frogs, 60–61
Within-hand timing, typewriting, 310
Woods, Tiger, 383
Word games, speech control, 346–347
Words
  language components, 324
  speech errors, 352
  typing timing, 310–311
  typing transcription, 305
  writing stages, 263–265
Working memory
  history effects, 123
  information processing, 115
Wrist flex, synergy, 15–16
Writing
  allograph selection, 265–266
  context effects, 268–270
  dynamic dominance hypothesis,
      272–273
  dysgraphia, 263–265
  error analysis, 263
  grapheme selection, 265
  graphic outputs, 253
  and handedness, 270–272

hierarchical control, 252–253
initiation stages, 251–252
size control, 266–268
S-R compatibility, 283
style preservation, 252
timing distinctions, 267–268
Writing machine, characteristics, 267–269

Y

Yaw, gaze direction, 181

Z

Zebra finch
  bird song, 357
  song learning, 415
Zenith, two-hand movements, 246
Zygomatic major, facial expressions, 365
Zygomatic muscles
  facial expressions, 365
  and smiling, 374